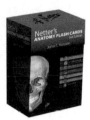

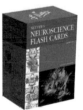
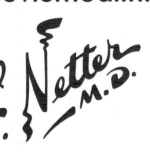

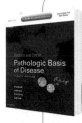
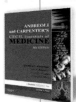
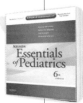
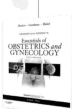
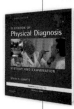
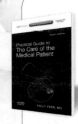

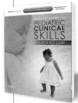
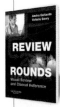
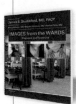

Atlas of
Human Anatomy

Fifth Edition

Frank H. Netter, MD

SAUNDERS
ELSEVIER

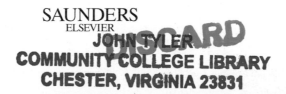

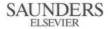

1600 John F. Kennedy Blvd.
Ste 1800
Philadelphia, PA 19103-2899

(handwritten) Ref QM 25 .N46 2011

ATLAS OF HUMAN ANATOMY
Fifth Edition

Standard Edition:	978-1-4160-5951-6
International Edition:	978-0-8089-2423-4
Enhanced International Edition:	978-0-8089-2422-7
Professional Edition:	978-1-4377-0970-4

Notice

Neither the Publisher nor the Editors assume any responsibility for any loss or injury and/or damage to persons or property arising out of or related to any use of the material contained in this book. It is the responsibility of the treating practitioner, relying on independent expertise and knowledge of the patient, to determine the best treatment and method of application for the patient.

The Publisher

Previous editions copyrighted 2006, 2003, 1997, 1989.

Library of Congress Cataloging-in-Publication Data
Netter, Frank H. (Frank Henry), 1906-1991.
 Atlas of human anatomy / Frank H. Netter.—5th ed.
  p. ; cm.
 Includes index.
 ISBN 978–1–4160–5951–6
 1. Human anatomy—Atlases. I. Title.
 [DNLM: 1. Anatomy—Atlases. QS 17 N474a 2010]
 QM25.N46 2010
 611.0022'2—dc22   2009034216

Director of Netter Products: Anne Lenehan
Online Editor: Elyse O'Grady
Developmental Editor: Marybeth Thiel
Publishing Services Manager: Linda Van Pelt
Design Direction: Lou Forgione
Illustrations Manager: Karen Giacomucci
Marketing Manager: Jason Oberacker

Printed in United States of America.

Last digit is the print number: 9 8 7 6 5 4 3 2 1

Consulting Editors

John T. Hansen, PhD
Lead Editor
Professor of Neurobiology and Anatomy
Associate Dean for Admissions
University of Rochester School of Medicine and Dentistry
Rochester, New York

Brion Benninger, MD, MS
Department of Surgery
Department of Oral & Maxillofacial Surgery
Department of Integrated Biosciences
Course Director
Oregon Health Sciences University
Portland, Oregon

Jennifer K. Brueckner, PhD
Assistant Dean for Student Affairs
University of Kentucky College of Medicine
Office of the Dean, Student Affairs
Lexington, Kentucky

Stephen W. Carmichael, PhD, DSc
International Consultant
Professor Emeritus of Anatomy
Professor Emeritus of Orthopedic Surgery
Mayo Clinic
Rochester, Minnesota

Noelle A. Granger, PhD
Professor Emeritus
Department of Cell and Developmental Biology
University of North Carolina at Chapel Hill
Chapel Hill, North Carolina

R. Shane Tubbs, MS, PA-C, PhD
Pediatric Neurosurgery
Children's Hospital
Birmingham, Alabama

Acknowledgments

Brion Benninger, MD, MS

I would like to thank my wife Alison for her support and for our son Jack, who keeps it all worthwhile. I want to thank Elsevier, especially Anne Lenehan, Marybeth Thiel, and Linda Van Pelt, for their insight and direction, enabling my fellow coeditors and Carlos Machado to work in such a rich environment. I particularly want to thank my first clinical anatomy mentors, Gerald Tressidor and Harold Ellis (Guy's Hospital); my clinical mentors, Peter Bell, Chris Colton, and David deBono; all my past and future patients and students; and OHSU clinical colleagues who bring anatomy to life (DT, LL). Thanks to my colleagues in the Department of Radiology at OHSU. Lastly, I thank my mother for her love of education and my father for his inquisitive mind.

Jennifer K. Brueckner, PhD

I am eternally grateful to my fiancé Kurt and to my parents, John and Rheba, for their patience, support, encouragement, and inspiration. Many thanks to John Hansen for the kind invitation and opportunity to contribute to this premier atlas! I would also like to thank the University of Kentucky College of Medicine Class of 2012 for their excellent input and suggestions for this edition; I am so lucky to have the privilege of working with such wonderful medical students! I am indebted to Carlos Machado for making the anatomical visions in my imagination come alive on paper with his magical artwork. Last but not least, I am so thankful for the Elsevier staff for their patience and support, including Marybeth Thiel, Anne Lenehan, and Linda Van Pelt.

Stephen W. Carmichael, PhD, DSc

I would like to thank Anne Lenehan and Elyse O'Grady for their administrative support during the preparation of this edition.

Noelle A. Granger, PhD

I am deeply grateful to my husband, Gene, for his support of my efforts during the work on this new edition. I also want to acknowledge two of my colleagues from the University of North Carolina School of Medicine: James Scatliff, MD, former Chair of the Department of Radiology, and O.W. Henson, PhD, Professor Emeritus of Anatomy, who showed me the beauty and complexity of anatomy. Special recognition goes to the supremely talented Carlos Machado and the artists at Elsevier, who did such exceptional work on this edition. Lastly, thanks go to the wonderful staff at Elsevier, in particular Marybeth Thiel and Anne Lenehan, for their leadership and patience with us academics.

John T. Hansen, PhD

I would like to thank Marybeth Thiel, Developmental Editor; Anne Lenehan, Acquisitions Editor; and Linda Van Pelt, Publishing Services Manager, for their meticulous shepherding of this fifth edition of the *Atlas of Human Anatomy* through each step of the publishing process. They, along with the entire Editorial, Production, Design, Illustration, and Marketing team at Elsevier, have been the epitome of professionalism. Also, I wish to express my thanks to my teaching colleagues at Rochester, and all my past and present students who have enriched my career and taught me much more than I have taught them. Finally, I am indebted to my entire family for their continued support, and especially to my wife Paula, whose love and encouragement has been the constant in my life and is the source of all the joy I know.

R. Shane Tubbs, MS, PA-C, PhD

I am indebted to the fantastic staff at Elsevier, including Anne Lenehan, Marybeth Thiel, and Elyse O'Grady. Dr. Carlos Machado's artwork has been a most welcomed contribution. I thank my wonderful wife Susan and son Isaiah for their patience during this endeavor. Colleagues and friends that supported me during the production of this edition include Drs. W. Jerry Oakes, E. George Salter, Marios Loukas, Arthur McAdams, Mohammadali Shoja, and Aaron Cohen-Gadol, and I thank each of them. Finally, without God and His wonderful design of the human body, we, as anatomists, would be left with nothing to describe or name!

Foreword

The fifth edition of *Atlas of Human Anatomy* by Frank H. Netter, MD, has been updated by the Consulting Editor team, led by John T. Hansen, of Brion Benninger, Jennifer K. Brueckner, Stephen W. Carmichael, Noelle A. Granger, and R. Shane Tubbs. We have each reviewed, modified, and updated a section of the *Atlas*. In this new edition, the editorial team has updated the radiologic images in the print book and in the online ancillaries, bringing clinical imaging into context with anatomy. As anatomy does require new material, Carlos A.G. Machado, MD, has added outstanding new images and anatomic views to this edition. The Consulting Editor team has relied heavily on *Terminologica Anatomica* as the basis for updates to nomenclature and terminology. The genius of Dr. Netter's paintings is that the anatomy is portrayed clearly, realistically, and in a clinically relatable fashion while maintaining the balance between complexity and oversimplification. This fifth edition owes much to the consulting editors of the earlier editions, Drs. Sharon Colacino (Oberg) (first edition), Arthur F. Dalley II (second edition), and John T. Hansen (third edition), who shepherded their editions with great skill and uncompromising professionalism, making our task significantly easier. The fourth edition was the first published under Elsevier and included the contributions of Anil Walji and Thomas Gest, as well as many members of the current consulting editor team.

Overall global changes to all sections of the *Atlas* include re-organization of plate order to more accurately reflect the current practice of teaching anatomy; reduction of labeling of some images; and removal of dated clinical plates. The flow of images in each section is now oriented from superficial to deep layers. In the upper and lower limb sections, the images have been changed to reflect the orientation common for imaging anatomy. In addition, many plates throughout the book have been updated to improve the artwork for a more contemporary view of anatomic aspects. We hope you enjoy this new edition of the *Atlas of Human Anatomy* and that you find it useful for learning and for your career.

About the Online versions:

For the standard edition and enhanced international edition of the *Atlas*, we have included access to the website *www.studentconsult.com*. From student and faculty feedback, we learned that the inclusion of Netter: *Atlas of Human Anatomy* in Student Consult would further enrich this excellent site. Many of the tools that were available on *www.Netteranatomy.com* are now available on Student Consult, and there are extra features as well. In addition to the 80+ images from the print *Atlas*, there are over 250 clinical images that the Consulting Editors have added to the site, including many Netter clinical images. These images are clinical and radiologic images showing both normal anatomy and pathologic conditions. The Integration Links from Netter on Student Consult are expanded and enable the user to link to the major brands and products on this site that students and faculty love. Also on Student Consult are videos created from Interact Elsevier, *Netter's 3D Interactive Anatomy* product, and the Interactive Dissection Modules from the University of North Carolina, Chapel Hill. Additional online resources such as radiologic images, videos from UNC Dissection Modules, and many other resources are indicated by the symbol . The symbol indicates videos from *Netter's 3D Interactive Anatomy*.

For the Professional edition of the Atlas, the online resource is through *www.netterreference.com*, the site for clinical Netter products. The *Atlas* online will have 80+ Netter images and the clinical images, as well as videos from *Netter's 3D Interactive Anatomy*. This site will be the jumping-off point for the new version of the Netter Presenter, which allows users to create custom Netter images.

Brion Benninger, MD, MS
Jennifer K. Brueckner, PhD
Stephen W. Carmichael, PhD, DSc
Noelle A. Granger, PhD
John T. Hansen, PhD
R. Shane Tubbs, MS, PA-C, PhD

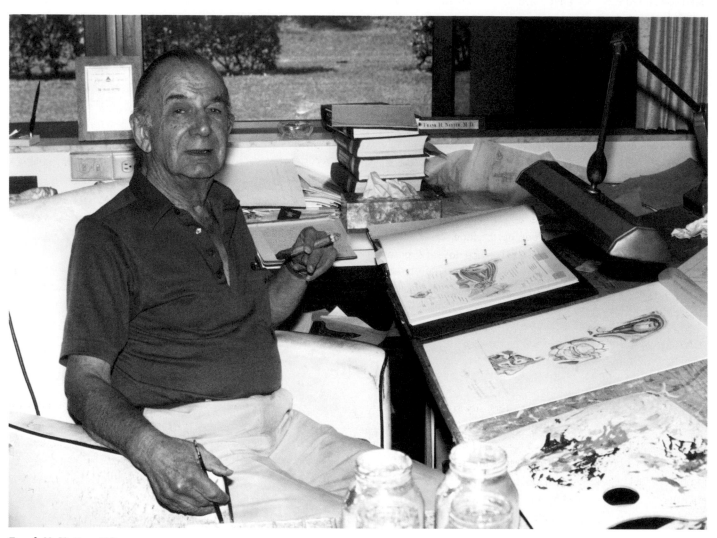

Frank H. Netter, MD
Photograph by James L. Clayton

To my dear wife, Vera

Preface to the First Edition

I have often said that my career as a medical artist for almost 50 years has been a sort of "command performance" in the sense that it has grown in response to the desires and requests of the medical profession. Over these many years, I have produced almost 4,000 illustrations, mostly for *The CIBA (now Netter) Collection of Medical Illustrations* but also for *Clinical Symposia*. These pictures have been concerned with the varied subdivisions of medical knowledge such as gross anatomy, histology, embryology, physiology, pathology, diagnostic modalities, surgical and therapeutic techniques, and clinical manifestations of a multitude of diseases. As the years went by, however, there were more and more requests from physicians and students for me to produce an atlas purely of gross anatomy. Thus, this atlas has come about, not through any inspiration on my part but rather, like most of my previous works, as a fulfillment of the desires of the medical profession.

It involved going back over all the illustrations I had made over so many years, selecting those pertinent to gross anatomy, classifying them and organizing them by system and region, adapting them to page size and space, and arranging them in logical sequence. Anatomy of course does not change, but our understanding of anatomy and its clinical significance does change, as do anatomical terminology and nomenclature. This therefore required much updating of many of the older pictures and even revision of a number of them in order to make them more pertinent to today's ever-expanding scope of medical and surgical practice. In addition, I found that there were gaps in the portrayal of medical knowledge as pictorialized in the illustrations I had previously done, and this necessitated my making a number of new pictures that are included in this volume.

In creating an atlas such as this, it is important to achieve a happy medium between complexity and simplification. If the pictures are too complex, they may be difficult and confusing to read; if oversimplified, they may not be adequately definitive or may even be misleading. I have therefore striven for a middle course of realism without the clutter of confusing minutiae. I hope that the students and members of the medical and allied professions will find the illustrations readily understandable, yet instructive and useful.

At one point, the publisher and I thought it might be nice to include a foreword by a truly outstanding and renowned anatomist, but there are so many in that category that we could not make a choice. We did think of men like Vesalius, Leonardo da Vinci, William Hunter, and Henry Gray, who of course are unfortunately unavailable, but I do wonder what their comments might have been about this atlas.

Frank H. Netter, MD
(1906–1991)

Frank H. Netter, MD

Frank H. Netter was born in New York City in 1906. He studied art at the Art Students League and the National Academy of Design before entering medical school at New York University, where he received his Doctor of Medicine degree in 1931. During his student years, Dr. Netter's notebook sketches attracted the attention of the medical faculty and other physicians, allowing him to augment his income by illustrating articles and textbooks. He continued illustrating as a sideline after establishing a surgical practice in 1933, but he ultimately opted to give up his practice in favor of a full-time commitment to art. After service in the United States Army during World War II, Dr. Netter began his long collaboration with the CIBA Pharmaceutical Company (now Novartis Pharmaceuticals). This 45-year partnership resulted in the production of the extraordinary collection of medical art so familiar to physicians and other medical professionals worldwide.

Icon Learning Systems acquired the Netter Collection in July 2000 and continued to update Dr. Netter's original paintings and to add newly commissioned paintings by artists trained in the style of Dr. Netter. In 2005, Elsevier Inc. purchased the Netter Collection and all publications from Icon Learning Systems. There are now over 50 publications featuring the art of Dr. Netter available through Elsevier Inc.

Dr. Netter's works are among the finest examples of the use of illustration in the teaching of medical concepts. The 13-book *Netter Collection of Medical Illustrations*, which includes the greater part of the more than 20,000 paintings created by Dr. Netter, became and remains one of the most famous medical works ever published. *The Netter Atlas of Human Anatomy*, first published in 1989, presents the anatomic paintings from the Netter Collection. Now translated into 16 languages, it is the anatomy atlas of choice among medical and health professions students the world over.

The Netter illustrations are appreciated not only for their aesthetic qualities, but also, more important, for their intellectual content. As Dr. Netter wrote in 1949, "Clarification of a subject is the aim and goal of illustration. No matter how beautifully painted, how delicately and subtly rendered a subject may be, it is of little value as a *medical illustration* if it does not serve to make clear some medical point." Dr. Netter's planning, conception, point of view, and approach are what inform his paintings and what make them so intellectually valuable.

Frank H. Netter, MD, physician and artist, died in 1991.

Contents

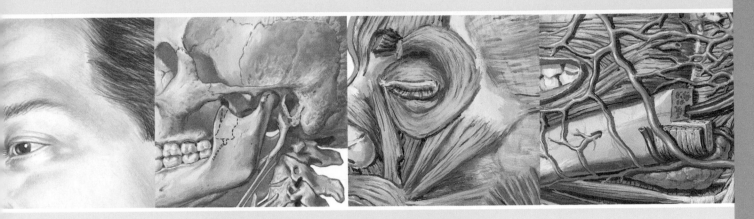

Section 1 HEAD AND NECK

1 HEAD AND NECK

Atlas of Human Anatomy

Orbit and Contents
Plates 81-91

Ear
Plates 92-98

Meninges and Brain
Plates 99-114

Cranial and Cervical Nerves
Plates 115-134

Cerebral Vasculature
Plates 135-146

Regional Scans

Plates 147-148

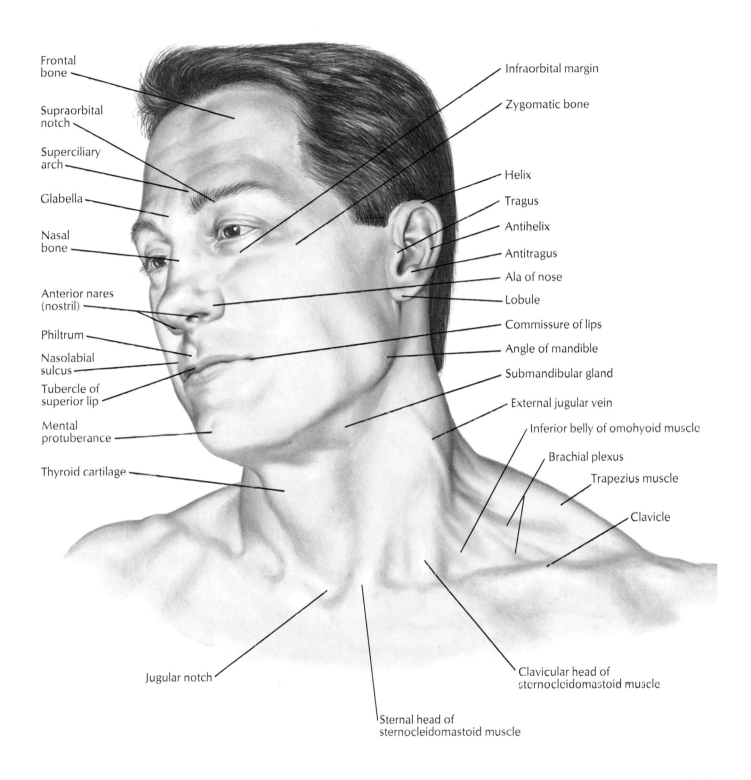

Frontal bone

Supraorbital notch

Superciliary arch

Glabella

Nasal bone

Anterior nares (nostril)

Philtrum

Nasolabial sulcus

Tubercle of superior lip

Mental protuberance

Thyroid cartilage

Jugular notch

Sternal head of sternocleidomastoid muscle

Infraorbital margin

Zygomatic bone

Helix

Tragus

Antihelix

Antitragus

Ala of nose

Lobule

Commissure of lips

Angle of mandible

Submandibular gland

External jugular vein

Inferior belly of omohyoid muscle

Brachial plexus

Trapezius muscle

Clavicle

Clavicular head of sternocleidomastoid muscle

C. Machado
_M.D.

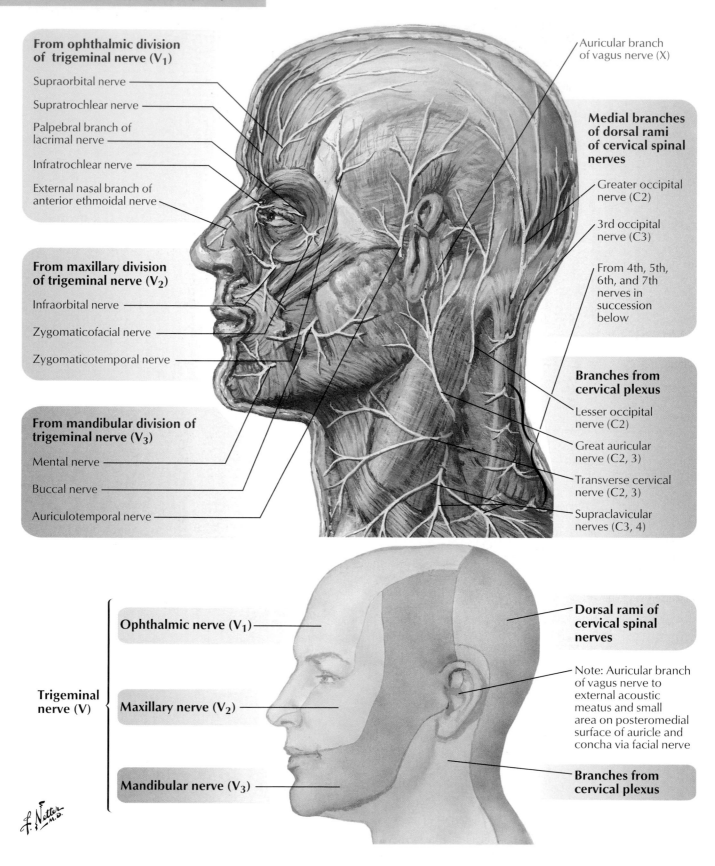

From ophthalmic division of trigeminal nerve (V₁)

Supraorbital nerve

Supratrochlear nerve

Palpebral branch of lacrimal nerve

Infratrochlear nerve

External nasal branch of anterior ethmoidal nerve

From maxillary division of trigeminal nerve (V₂)

Infraorbital nerve

Zygomaticofacial nerve

Zygomaticotemporal nerve

From mandibular division of trigeminal nerve (V₃)

Mental nerve

Buccal nerve

Auriculotemporal nerve

Auricular branch of vagus nerve (X)

Medial branches of dorsal rami of cervical spinal nerves

Greater occipital nerve (C2)

3rd occipital nerve (C3)

From 4th, 5th, 6th, and 7th nerves in succession below

Branches from cervical plexus

Lesser occipital nerve (C2)

Great auricular nerve (C2, 3)

Transverse cervical nerve (C2, 3)

Supraclavicular nerves (C3, 4)

Trigeminal nerve (V)

Ophthalmic nerve (V₁)

Maxillary nerve (V₂)

Mandibular nerve (V₃)

Dorsal rami of cervical spinal nerves

Note: Auricular branch of vagus nerve to external acoustic meatus and small area on posteromedial surface of auricle and concha via facial nerve

Branches from cervical plexus

Plate 2

Superficial Head and Neck

Scalp {
Skin and subcutaneous tissue
Epicranial aponeurosis (galea aponeurotica) (*cut to reveal skull*)

Middle temporal artery and vein

Zygomaticoorbital artery

Transverse facial artery and vein

Supraorbital artery and vein

Supratrochlear artery and vein

Nasofrontal vein

Dorsal nasal artery and vein

Zygomaticotemporal artery and vein

Angular artery and vein

Zygomatico-facial artery and vein

Infraorbital artery and vein

Deep facial vein (from pterygoid plexus)

Facial artery and vein

Parietal emissary vein

Frontal }
Parietal }
Branches of superficial temporal artery and vein

Anterior auricular arteries

Mastoid emissary vein and meningeal branch of occipital artery (posterior meningeal artery)

Occipital artery and vein (*cut*)

Posterior auricular artery and vein

External jugular vein (*cut*)

Retromandibular vein

Common facial vein

Internal jugular vein

Internal carotid artery

External carotid artery

Common carotid artery

Lingual artery and vein

Sources of arterial supply of face

Black: from internal carotid artery (via ophthalmic artery)

Red: from external carotid artery

f. Netter M.D.

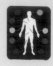

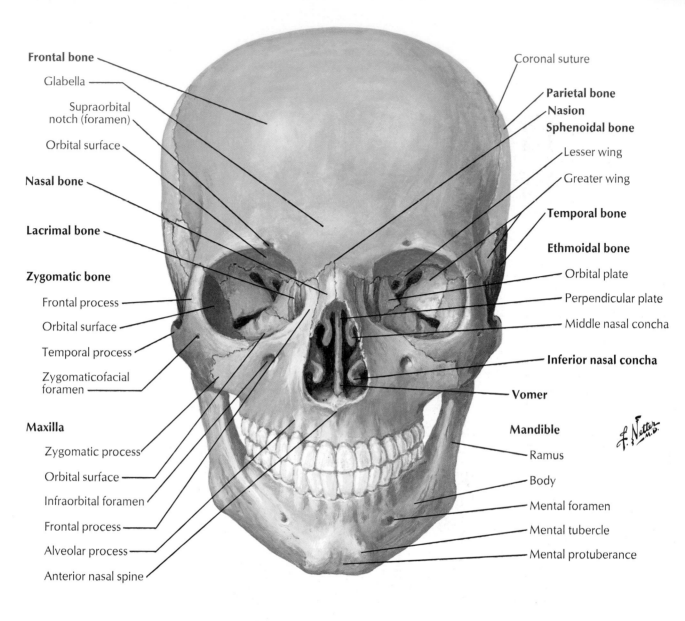

Frontal bone

Glabella

Supraorbital
notch (foramen)

Orbital surface

Nasal bone

Lacrimal bone

Zygomatic bone

Frontal process

Orbital surface

Temporal process

Zygomaticofacial
foramen

Maxilla

Zygomatic process

Orbital surface

Infraorbital foramen

Frontal process

Alveolar process

Anterior nasal spine

Coronal suture

Parietal bone
Nasion
Sphenoidal bone

Lesser wing

Greater wing

Temporal bone

Ethmoidal bone

Orbital plate

Perpendicular plate

Middle nasal concha

Inferior nasal concha

Vomer

Mandible

Ramus

Body

Mental foramen

Mental tubercle

Mental protuberance

Right orbit: frontal and slightly lateral view

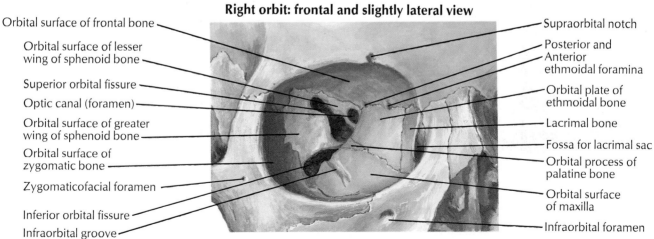

Orbital surface of frontal bone

Orbital surface of lesser
wing of sphenoid bone

Superior orbital fissure

Optic canal (foramen)

Orbital surface of greater
wing of sphenoid bone

Orbital surface of
zygomatic bone

Zygomaticofacial foramen

Inferior orbital fissure

Infraorbital groove

Supraorbital notch

Posterior and
Anterior
ethmoidal foramina

Orbital plate of
ethmoidal bone

Lacrimal bone

Fossa for lacrimal sac

Orbital process of
palatine bone

Orbital surface
of maxilla

Infraorbital foramen

Plate 4 | **Bones and Ligaments**

See also **Plate 4**

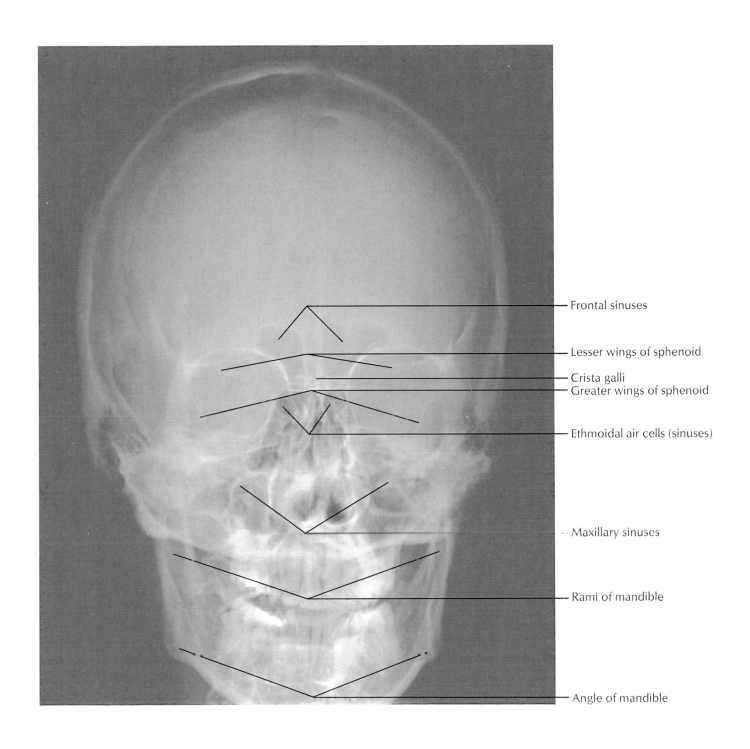

Frontal sinuses

Lesser wings of sphenoid

Crista galli

Greater wings of sphenoid

Ethmoidal air cells (sinuses)

Maxillary sinuses

Rami of mandible

Angle of mandible

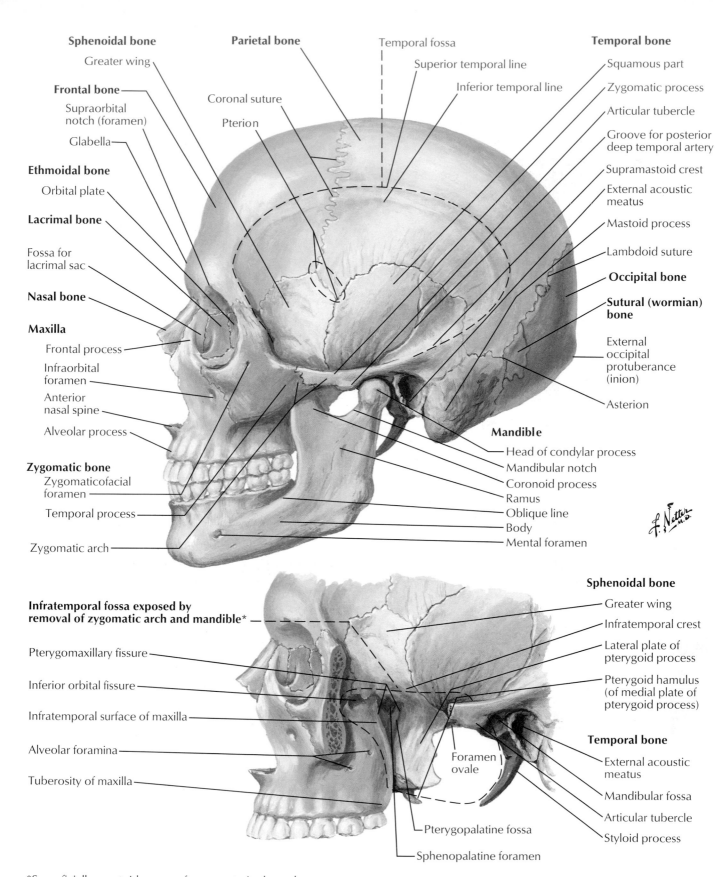

Sphenoidal bone
Greater wing

Frontal bone
Supraorbital notch (foramen)
Glabella

Ethmoidal bone
Orbital plate

Lacrimal bone
Fossa for lacrimal sac

Nasal bone

Maxilla
Frontal process
Infraorbital foramen
Anterior nasal spine
Alveolar process

Zygomatic bone
Zygomaticofacial foramen
Temporal process
Zygomatic arch

Parietal bone
Coronal suture
Pterion

Temporal fossa
Superior temporal line
Inferior temporal line

Temporal bone
Squamous part
Zygomatic process
Articular tubercle
Groove for posterior deep temporal artery
Supramastoid crest
External acoustic meatus
Mastoid process
Lambdoid suture

Occipital bone

Sutural (wormian) bone

External occipital protuberance (inion)

Asterion

Mandible
Head of condylar process
Mandibular notch
Coronoid process
Ramus
Oblique line
Body
Mental foramen

Infratemporal fossa exposed by removal of zygomatic arch and mandible*

Pterygomaxillary fissure

Inferior orbital fissure

Infratemporal surface of maxilla

Alveolar foramina

Tuberosity of maxilla

Foramen ovale

Sphenoidal bone
Greater wing
Infratemporal crest
Lateral plate of pterygoid process
Pterygoid hamulus (of medial plate of pterygoid process)

Temporal bone
External acoustic meatus
Mandibular fossa
Articular tubercle
Styloid process

Pterygopalatine fossa

Sphenopalatine foramen

*Superficially, mastoid process forms posterior boundary.

Plate 6

Bones and Ligaments

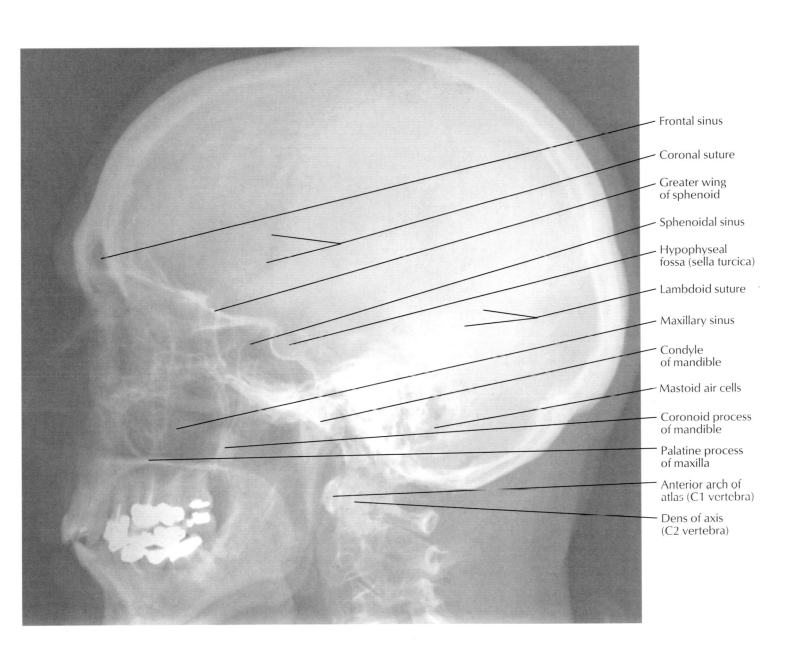

Frontal sinus

Coronal suture

Greater wing
of sphenoid

Sphenoidal sinus

Hypophyseal
fossa (sella turcica)

Lambdoid suture

Maxillary sinus

Condyle
of mandible

Mastoid air cells

Coronoid process
of mandible

Palatine process
of maxilla

Anterior arch of
atlas (C1 vertebra)

Dens of axis
(C2 vertebra)

Skull: Midsagittal Section

See also **Plates 36, 37**

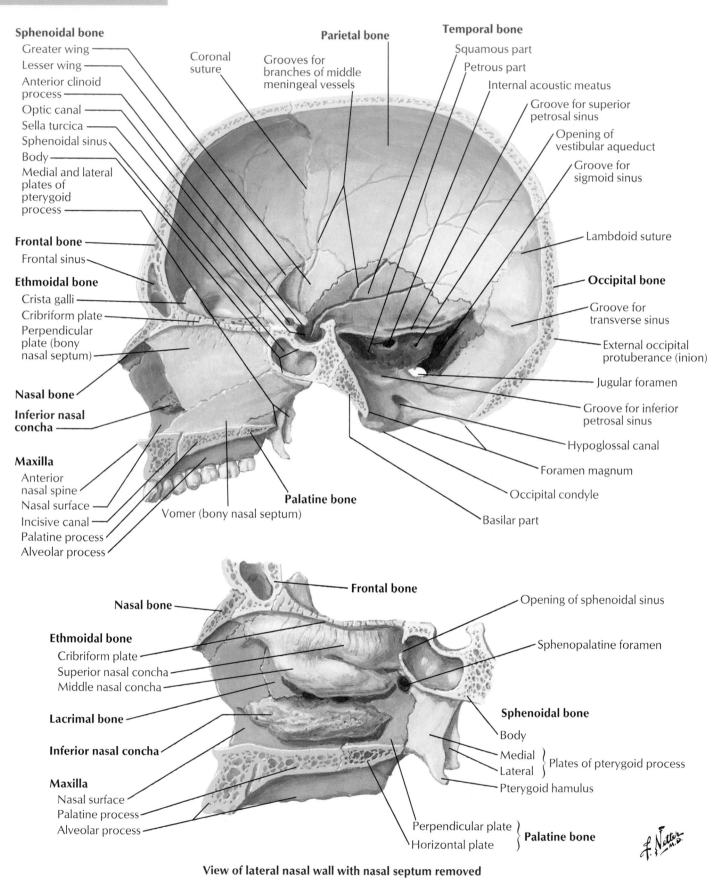

Sphenoidal bone
Greater wing
Lesser wing
Anterior clinoid process
Optic canal
Sella turcica
Sphenoidal sinus
Body
Medial and lateral plates of pterygoid process

Frontal bone
Frontal sinus

Ethmoidal bone
Crista galli
Cribriform plate
Perpendicular plate (bony nasal septum)

Nasal bone

Inferior nasal concha

Maxilla
Anterior nasal spine
Nasal surface
Incisive canal
Palatine process
Alveolar process

Coronal suture

Parietal bone

Grooves for branches of middle meningeal vessels

Temporal bone
Squamous part
Petrous part
Internal acoustic meatus
Groove for superior petrosal sinus
Opening of vestibular aqueduct
Groove for sigmoid sinus

Lambdoid suture

Occipital bone
Groove for transverse sinus
External occipital protuberance (inion)
Jugular foramen
Groove for inferior petrosal sinus
Hypoglossal canal
Foramen magnum
Occipital condyle
Basilar part

Palatine bone
Vomer (bony nasal septum)

Nasal bone

Ethmoidal bone
Cribriform plate
Superior nasal concha
Middle nasal concha

Lacrimal bone

Inferior nasal concha

Maxilla
Nasal surface
Palatine process
Alveolar process

Frontal bone

Opening of sphenoidal sinus

Sphenopalatine foramen

Sphenoidal bone
Body
Medial }
Lateral } Plates of pterygoid process
Pterygoid hamulus

Perpendicular plate }
Horizontal plate } **Palatine bone**

View of lateral nasal wall with nasal septum removed

F. Netter M.D.

Plate 8

Bones and Ligaments

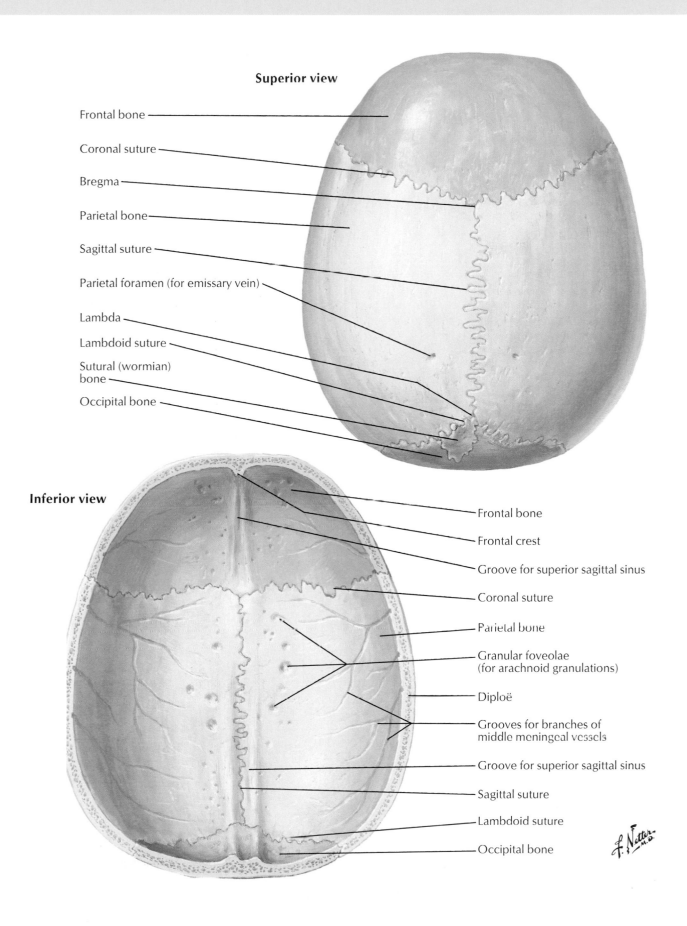

Superior view

Frontal bone

Coronal suture

Bregma

Parietal bone

Sagittal suture

Parietal foramen (for emissary vein)

Lambda

Lambdoid suture

Sutural (wormian) bone

Occipital bone

Inferior view

Frontal bone

Frontal crest

Groove for superior sagittal sinus

Coronal suture

Parietal bone

Granular foveolae (for arachnoid granulations)

Diploë

Grooves for branches of middle meningeal vessels

Groove for superior sagittal sinus

Sagittal suture

Lambdoid suture

Occipital bone

Maxilla
Incisive fossa
Palatine process
Intermaxillary suture
Zygomatic process

Zygomatic bone

Frontal bone

Sphenoidal bone
Pterygoid process
Hamulus
Medial plate
Pterygoid fossa
Lateral plate
Scaphoid fossa
Greater wing
Foramen ovale
Foramen spinosum
Spine

Temporal bone
Zygomatic process
Articular tubercle
Mandibular fossa
Styloid process
Petrotympanic fissure
Carotid canal (external opening)
Tympanic canaliculus
External acoustic meatus
Mastoid canaliculus
Mastoid process
Stylomastoid foramen
Petrous part
Mastoid notch (for
      digastric muscle)
Occipital groove
      (for occipital artery)
Jugular fossa
      (jugular foramen in its depth)
Mastoid foramen

Parietal bone

Occipital bone
Hypoglossal canal
Occipital condyle
Condylar canal and fossa
Basilar part
Pharyngeal tubercle
Foramen magnum
Inferior nuchal line
External occipital crest
Superior nuchal line
External occipital protuberance

Palatomaxillary suture

Palatine bone
Horizontal plate
Greater palatine foramen
Pyramidal process
Lesser palatine foramina
Posterior nasal spine

Choanae

Vomer

Ala

Groove for auditory
(pharyngotympanic,
eustachian) tube

Foramen lacerum

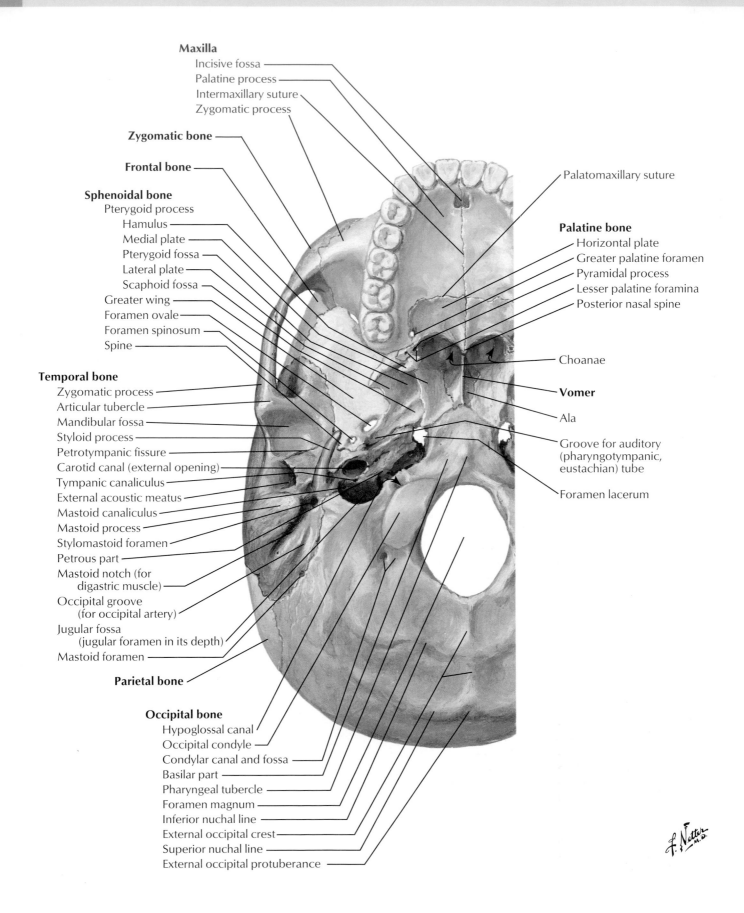

Plate 10

Bones and Ligaments

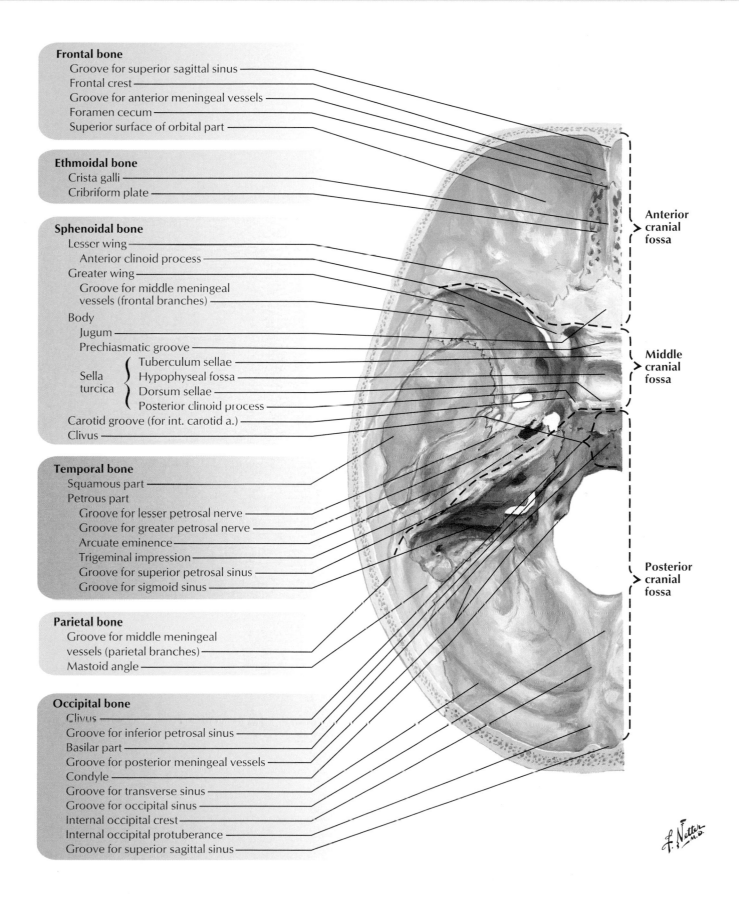

Frontal bone
Groove for superior sagittal sinus
Frontal crest
Groove for anterior meningeal vessels
Foramen cecum
Superior surface of orbital part

Ethmoidal bone
Crista galli
Cribriform plate

Sphenoidal bone
Lesser wing
Anterior clinoid process
Greater wing
Groove for middle meningeal vessels (frontal branches)
Body
Jugum
Prechiasmatic groove
Sella turcica { Tuberculum sellae
Hypophyseal fossa
Dorsum sellae
Posterior clinoid process
Carotid groove (for int. carotid a.)
Clivus

Temporal bone
Squamous part
Petrous part
Groove for lesser petrosal nerve
Groove for greater petrosal nerve
Arcuate eminence
Trigeminal impression
Groove for superior petrosal sinus
Groove for sigmoid sinus

Parietal bone
Groove for middle meningeal vessels (parietal branches)
Mastoid angle

Occipital bone
Clivus
Groove for inferior petrosal sinus
Basilar part
Groove for posterior meningeal vessels
Condyle
Groove for transverse sinus
Groove for occipital sinus
Internal occipital crest
Internal occipital protuberance
Groove for superior sagittal sinus

Anterior cranial fossa

Middle cranial fossa

Posterior cranial fossa

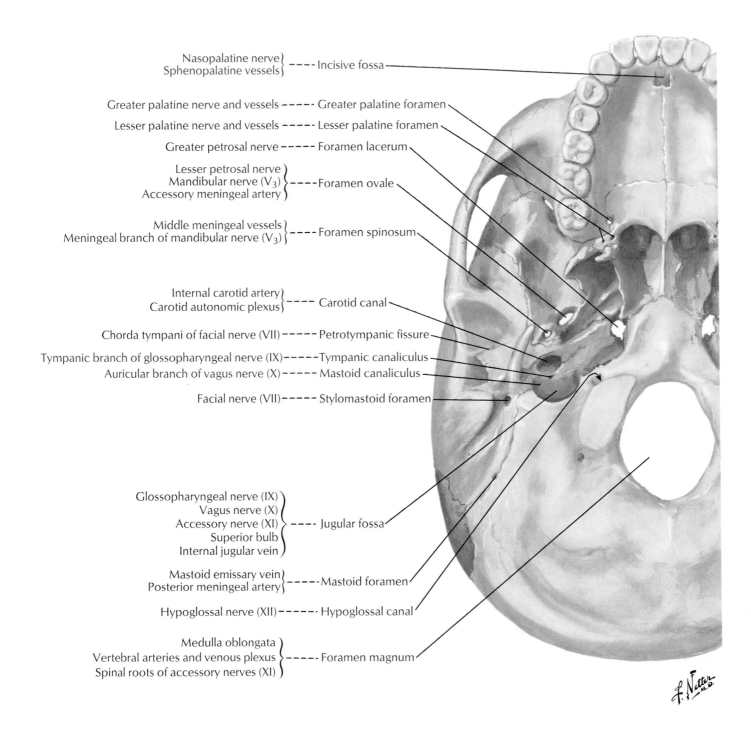

Nasopalatine nerve⎫
Sphenopalatine vessels⎭ ---- Incisive fossa

Greater palatine nerve and vessels ---- Greater palatine foramen

Lesser palatine nerve and vessels ---- Lesser palatine foramen

Greater petrosal nerve ---- Foramen lacerum

Lesser petrosal nerve⎫
Mandibular nerve (V₃)⎬ ---- Foramen ovale
Accessory meningeal artery⎭

Middle meningeal vessels⎫
Meningeal branch of mandibular nerve (V₃)⎭ ---- Foramen spinosum

Internal carotid artery⎫
Carotid autonomic plexus⎭ ---- Carotid canal

Chorda tympani of facial nerve (VII) ---- Petrotympanic fissure

Tympanic branch of glossopharyngeal nerve (IX) ---- Tympanic canaliculus

Auricular branch of vagus nerve (X) ---- Mastoid canaliculus

Facial nerve (VII) ---- Stylomastoid foramen

Glossopharyngeal nerve (IX)⎫
Vagus nerve (X)⎪
Accessory nerve (XI)⎬ ---- Jugular fossa
Superior bulb⎪
Internal jugular vein⎭

Mastoid emissary vein⎫
Posterior meningeal artery⎭ ---- Mastoid foramen

Hypoglossal nerve (XII) ---- Hypoglossal canal

Medulla oblongata⎫
Vertebral arteries and venous plexus⎬ ---- Foramen magnum
Spinal roots of accessory nerves (XI)⎭

Plate 12

Bones and Ligaments

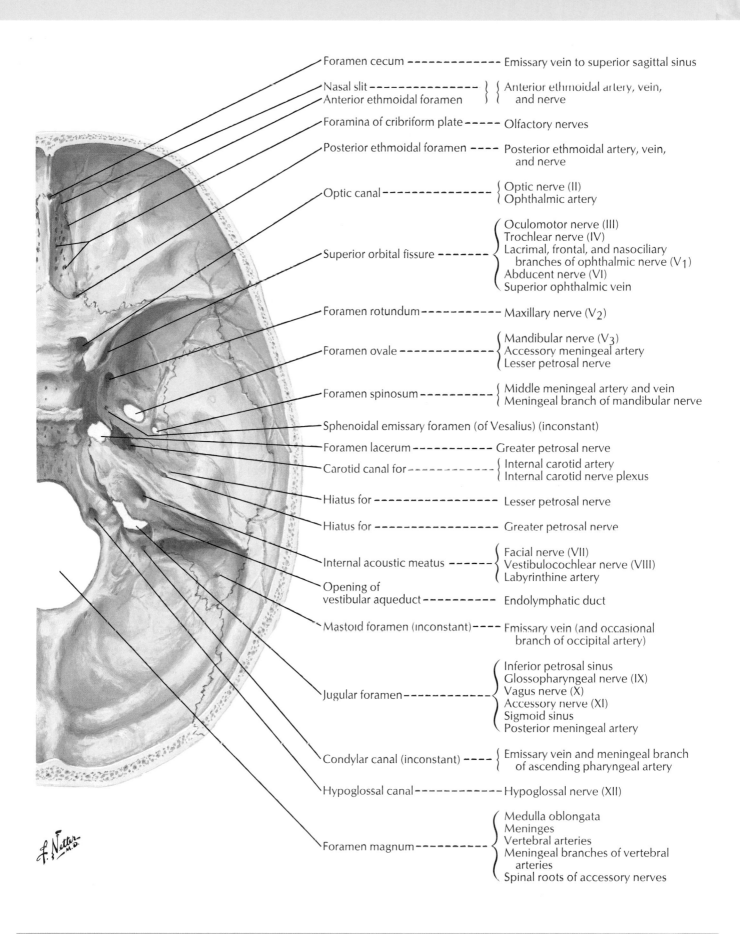

Foramen cecum ------------ Emissary vein to superior sagittal sinus

Nasal slit --------------- ⎫ ⎧ Anterior ethmoidal artery, vein,
Anterior ethmoidal foramen ⎭ ⎩ and nerve

Foramina of cribriform plate ----- Olfactory nerves

Posterior ethmoidal foramen ---- Posterior ethmoidal artery, vein, and nerve

Optic canal --------------- ⎧ Optic nerve (II)
⎩ Ophthalmic artery

Superior orbital fissure ------- ⎧ Oculomotor nerve (III)
⎪ Trochlear nerve (IV)
⎨ Lacrimal, frontal, and nasociliary
⎪   branches of ophthalmic nerve (V₁)
⎪ Abducent nerve (VI)
⎩ Superior ophthalmic vein

Foramen rotundum ---------- Maxillary nerve (V₂)

Foramen ovale ------------ ⎧ Mandibular nerve (V₃)
⎨ Accessory meningeal artery
⎩ Lesser petrosal nerve

Foramen spinosum ---------- ⎧ Middle meningeal artery and vein
⎩ Meningeal branch of mandibular nerve

Sphenoidal emissary foramen (of Vesalius) (inconstant)

Foramen lacerum ----------- Greater petrosal nerve

Carotid canal for ---------- ⎧ Internal carotid artery
⎩ Internal carotid nerve plexus

Hiatus for --------------- Lesser petrosal nerve

Hiatus for --------------- Greater petrosal nerve

Internal acoustic meatus ------ ⎧ Facial nerve (VII)
⎨ Vestibulocochlear nerve (VIII)
⎩ Labyrinthine artery

Opening of
vestibular aqueduct --------- Endolymphatic duct

Mastoid foramen (inconstant) ---- Emissary vein (and occasional
branch of occipital artery)

Jugular foramen ----------- ⎧ Inferior petrosal sinus
⎪ Glossopharyngeal nerve (IX)
⎨ Vagus nerve (X)
⎪ Accessory nerve (XI)
⎪ Sigmoid sinus
⎩ Posterior meningeal artery

Condylar canal (inconstant) ---- ⎧ Emissary vein and meningeal branch
⎩ of ascending pharyngeal artery

Hypoglossal canal ---------- Hypoglossal nerve (XII)

Foramen magnum ---------- ⎧ Medulla oblongata
⎪ Meninges
⎪ Vertebral arteries
⎨ Meningeal branches of vertebral
⎪   arteries
⎩ Spinal roots of accessory nerves

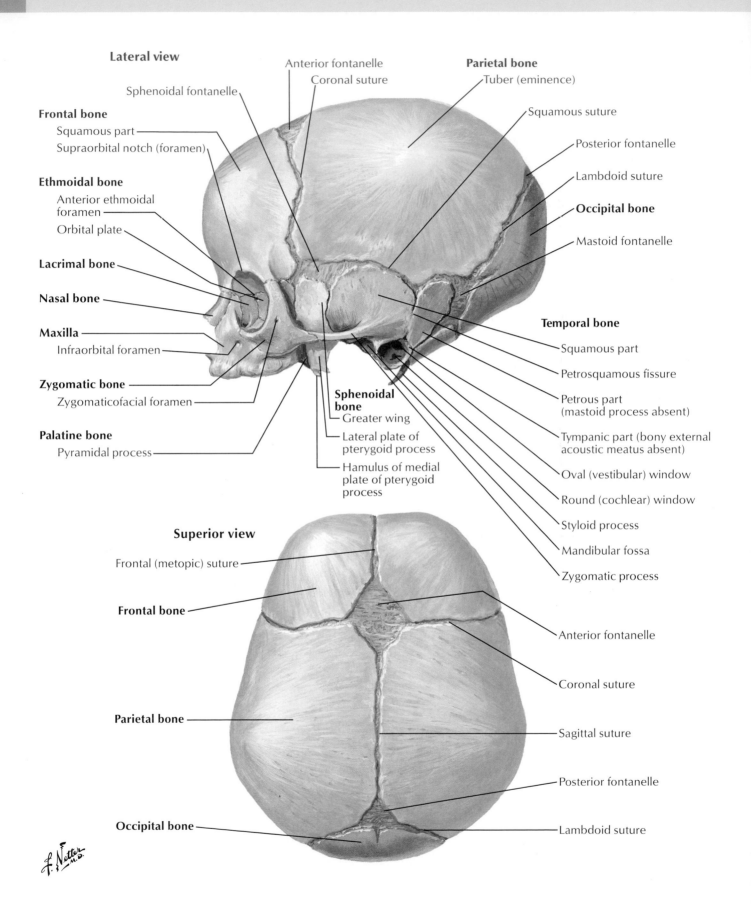

Lateral view

Frontal bone
- Squamous part
- Supraorbital notch (foramen)

Ethmoidal bone
- Anterior ethmoidal foramen
- Orbital plate

Lacrimal bone

Nasal bone

Maxilla
- Infraorbital foramen

Zygomatic bone
- Zygomaticofacial foramen

Palatine bone
- Pyramidal process

Sphenoidal fontanelle

Anterior fontanelle
Coronal suture

Sphenoidal bone
- Greater wing
- Lateral plate of pterygoid process
- Hamulus of medial plate of pterygoid process

Parietal bone
- Tuber (eminence)
- Squamous suture
- Posterior fontanelle
- Lambdoid suture

Occipital bone
- Mastoid fontanelle

Temporal bone
- Squamous part
- Petrosquamous fissure
- Petrous part (mastoid process absent)
- Tympanic part (bony external acoustic meatus absent)
- Oval (vestibular) window
- Round (cochlear) window
- Styloid process
- Mandibular fossa
- Zygomatic process

Superior view

Frontal (metopic) suture

Frontal bone

Parietal bone

Occipital bone

Anterior fontanelle

Coronal suture

Sagittal suture

Posterior fontanelle

Lambdoid suture

Plate 14

Bones and Ligaments

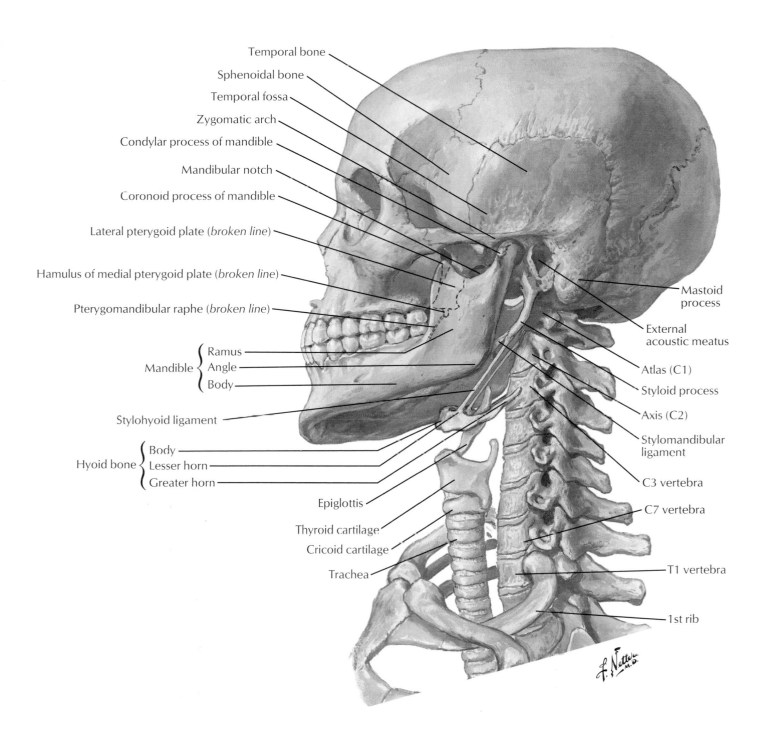

Temporal bone

Sphenoidal bone

Temporal fossa

Zygomatic arch

Condylar process of mandible

Mandibular notch

Coronoid process of mandible

Lateral pterygoid plate (*broken line*)

Hamulus of medial pterygoid plate (*broken line*)

Pterygomandibular raphe (*broken line*)

Mandible
{
Ramus
Angle
Body
}

Stylohyoid ligament

Hyoid bone
{
Body
Lesser horn
Greater horn
}

Epiglottis

Thyroid cartilage

Cricoid cartilage

Trachea

Mastoid process

External acoustic meatus

Atlas (C1)

Styloid process

Axis (C2)

Stylomandibular ligament

C3 vertebra

C7 vertebra

T1 vertebra

1st rib

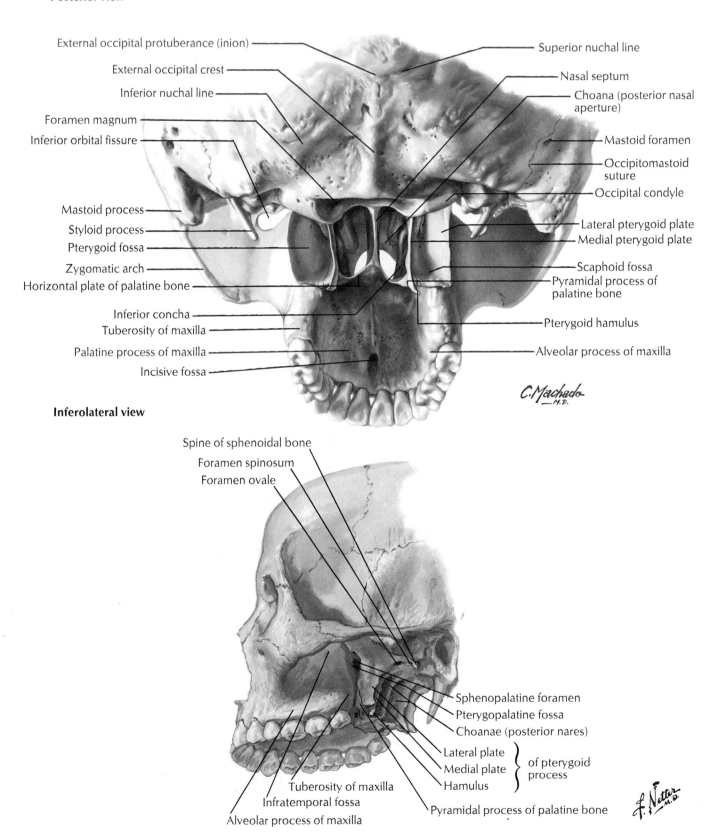

Posterior view

External occipital protuberance (inion) — Superior nuchal line

External occipital crest — Nasal septum

Inferior nuchal line — Choana (posterior nasal aperture)

Foramen magnum — Mastoid foramen

Inferior orbital fissure — Occipitomastoid suture

— Occipital condyle

Mastoid process — Lateral pterygoid plate

Styloid process — Medial pterygoid plate

Pterygoid fossa — Scaphoid fossa

Zygomatic arch — Pyramidal process of palatine bone

Horizontal plate of palatine bone

Inferior concha — Pterygoid hamulus

Tuberosity of maxilla

Palatine process of maxilla — Alveolar process of maxilla

Incisive fossa

C. Machado M.D.

Inferolateral view

Spine of sphenoidal bone

Foramen spinosum

Foramen ovale

Sphenopalatine foramen

Pterygopalatine fossa

Choanae (posterior nares)

Lateral plate ⎫
Medial plate ⎬ of pterygoid process
Hamulus ⎭

Tuberosity of maxilla

Infratemporal fossa

Alveolar process of maxilla

Pyramidal process of palatine bone

F. Netter M.D.

Plate 16   **Bones and Ligaments**

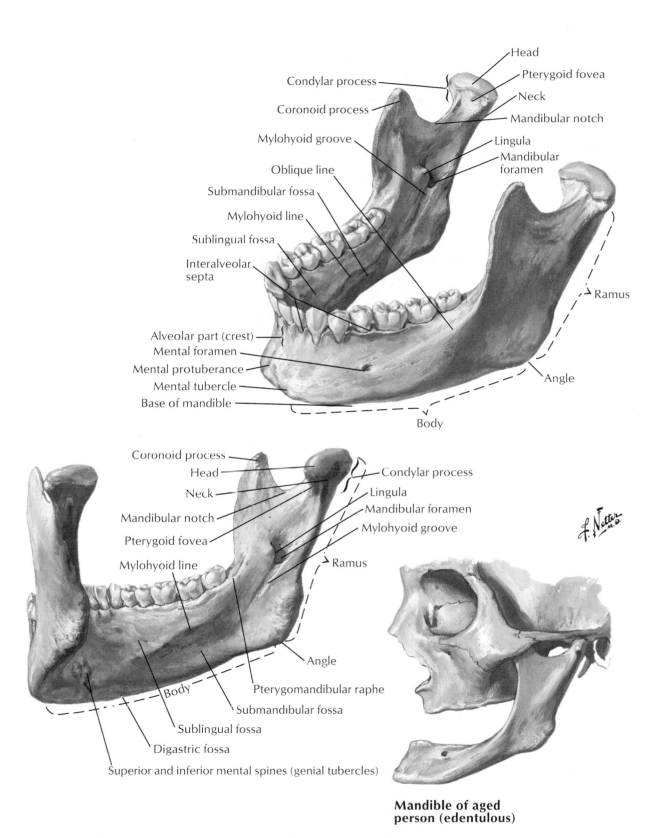

Head
Pterygoid fovea
Neck
Mandibular notch
Lingula
Mandibular foramen

Condylar process
Coronoid process
Mylohyoid groove
Oblique line
Submandibular fossa
Mylohyoid line
Sublingual fossa
Interalveolar septa

Ramus

Alveolar part (crest)
Mental foramen
Mental protuberance
Mental tubercle
Base of mandible

Angle

Body

Coronoid process
Head
Neck
Mandibular notch
Pterygoid fovea
Mylohyoid line

Condylar process
Lingula
Mandibular foramen
Mylohyoid groove

Ramus

Angle

Body
Pterygomandibular raphe
Submandibular fossa
Sublingual fossa
Digastric fossa
Superior and inferior mental spines (genial tubercles)

Mandible of aged person (edentulous)

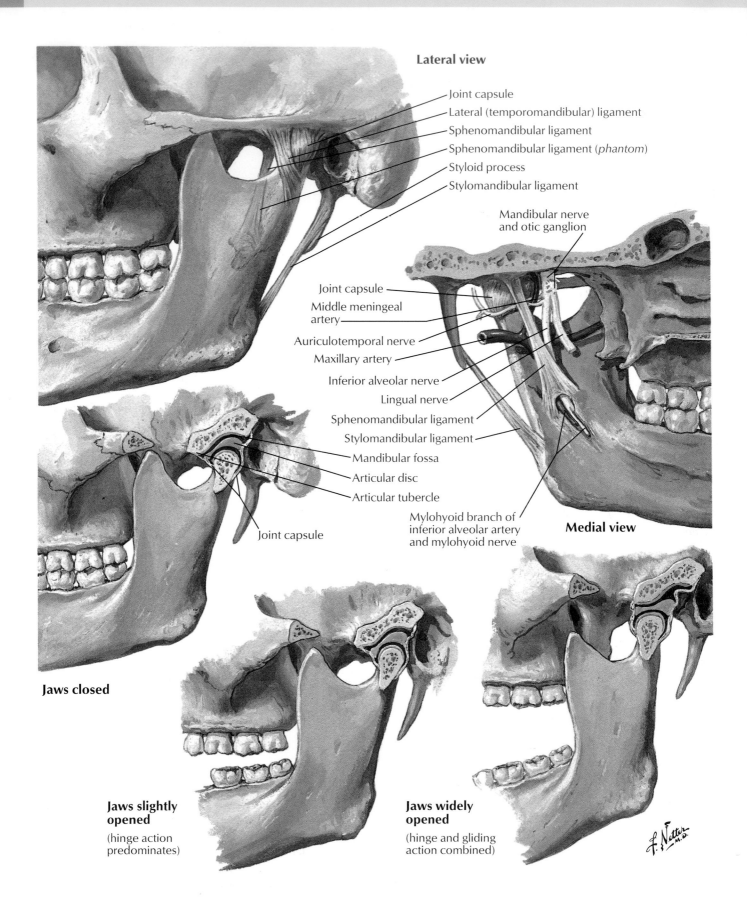

Lateral view

Joint capsule

Lateral (temporomandibular) ligament

Sphenomandibular ligament

Sphenomandibular ligament (*phantom*)

Styloid process

Stylomandibular ligament

Mandibular nerve and otic ganglion

Joint capsule

Middle meningeal artery

Auriculotemporal nerve

Maxillary artery

Inferior alveolar nerve

Lingual nerve

Sphenomandibular ligament

Stylomandibular ligament

Mandibular fossa

Articular disc

Articular tubercle

Joint capsule

Mylohyoid branch of inferior alveolar artery and mylohyoid nerve

Medial view

Jaws closed

Jaws slightly opened

(hinge action predominates)

Jaws widely opened

(hinge and gliding action combined)

Plate 18

Bones and Ligaments

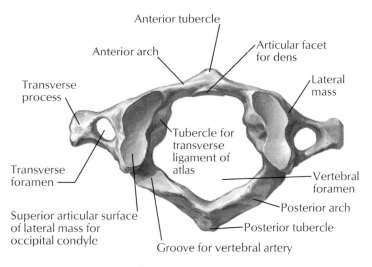

Anterior tubercle

Anterior arch

Articular facet for dens

Transverse process

Lateral mass

Transverse foramen

Tubercle for transverse ligament of atlas

Vertebral foramen

Superior articular surface of lateral mass for occipital condyle

Posterior arch

Posterior tubercle

Groove for vertebral artery

Atlas (C1): superior view

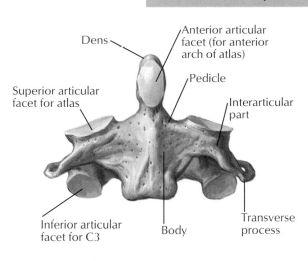

Dens

Anterior articular facet (for anterior arch of atlas)

Superior articular facet for atlas

Pedicle

Interarticular part

Inferior articular facet for C3

Body

Transverse process

Axis (C2): anterior view

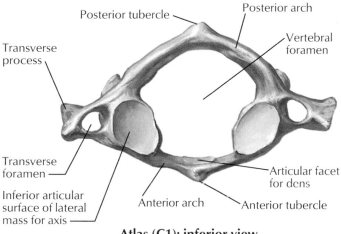

Posterior tubercle

Posterior arch

Transverse process

Vertebral foramen

Transverse foramen

Articular facet for dens

Inferior articular surface of lateral mass for axis

Anterior arch

Anterior tubercle

Atlas (C1): inferior view

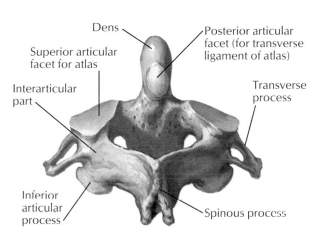

Dens

Posterior articular facet (for transverse ligament of atlas)

Superior articular facet for atlas

Interarticular part

Transverse process

Inferior articular process

Spinous process

Axis (C2): posterosuperior view

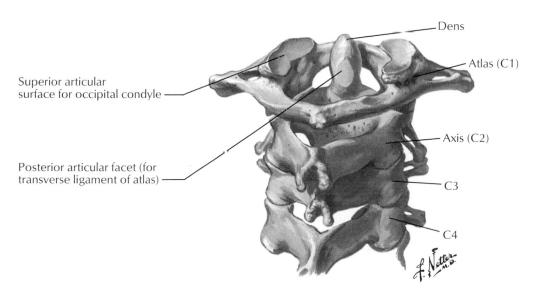

Dens

Atlas (C1)

Superior articular surface for occipital condyle

Axis (C2)

C3

Posterior articular facet (for transverse ligament of atlas)

C4

Upper cervical vertebrae, assembled: posterosuperior view

Cervical Vertebrae (continued)

See also **Plates 15, 150**

Inferior aspect of C3 and superior aspect of C4 showing the sites of the facet and uncovertebral articulations

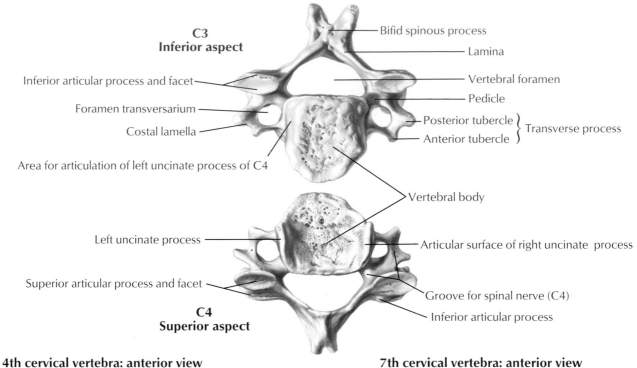

C3
Inferior aspect

- Bifid spinous process
- Lamina
- Inferior articular process and facet
- Vertebral foramen
- Foramen transversarium
- Pedicle
- Costal lamella
- Posterior tubercle } Transverse process
- Anterior tubercle }
- Area for articulation of left uncinate process of C4
- Vertebral body
- Left uncinate process
- Articular surface of right uncinate process
- Superior articular process and facet
- Groove for spinal nerve (C4)
- Inferior articular process

C4
Superior aspect

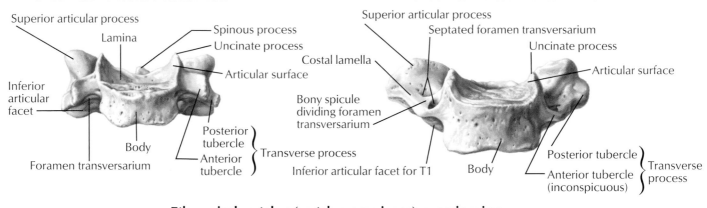

4th cervical vertebra: anterior view

- Superior articular process
- Lamina
- Spinous process
- Uncinate process
- Articular surface
- Inferior articular facet
- Posterior tubercle }
- Body
- Anterior tubercle } Transverse process
- Foramen transversarium

7th cervical vertebra: anterior view

- Superior articular process
- Septated foramen transversarium
- Uncinate process
- Costal lamella
- Articular surface
- Bony spicule dividing foramen transversarium
- Posterior tubercle }
- Inferior articular facet for T1
- Body
- Anterior tubercle (inconspicuous) } Transverse process

7th cervical vertebra (vertebra prominens): superior view

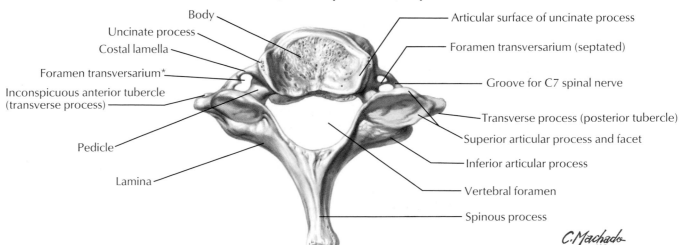

- Body
- Uncinate process
- Costal lamella
- Foramen transversarium*
- Inconspicuous anterior tubercle (transverse process)
- Pedicle
- Lamina
- Articular surface of uncinate process
- Foramen transversarium (septated)
- Groove for C7 spinal nerve
- Transverse process (posterior tubercle)
- Superior articular process and facet
- Inferior articular process
- Vertebral foramen
- Spinous process

C.Machado M.D.

*The foramina transversaria of C7 transmit vertebral veins, but usually not the vertebral artery, and are asymmetrical in this specimen.

Plate 20   **Bones and Ligaments**

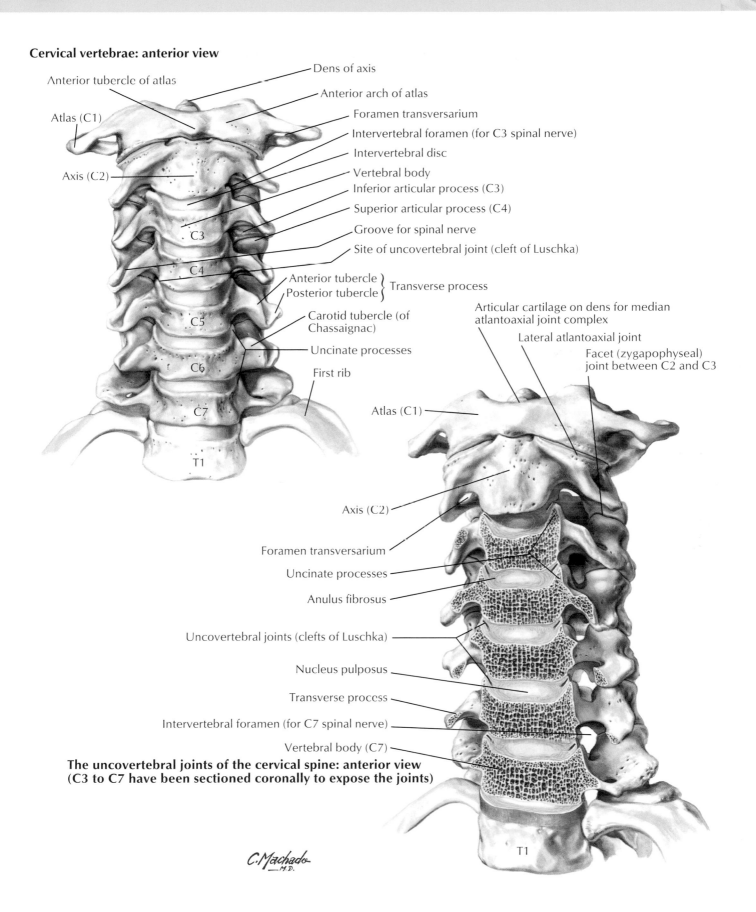

Cervical vertebrae: anterior view

Anterior tubercle of atlas

Dens of axis

Anterior arch of atlas

Atlas (C1)

Foramen transversarium

Intervertebral foramen (for C3 spinal nerve)

Intervertebral disc

Axis (C2)

Vertebral body

Inferior articular process (C3)

Superior articular process (C4)

C3

Groove for spinal nerve

Site of uncovertebral joint (cleft of Luschka)

C4

Anterior tubercle ⎫
Posterior tubercle ⎭ Transverse process

C5

Carotid tubercle (of Chassaignac)

Articular cartilage on dens for median atlantoaxial joint complex

Lateral atlantoaxial joint

Facet (zygapophyseal) joint between C2 and C3

Uncinate processes

C6

First rib

Atlas (C1)

C7

T1

Axis (C2)

Foramen transversarium

Uncinate processes

Anulus fibrosus

Uncovertebral joints (clefts of Luschka)

Nucleus pulposus

Transverse process

Intervertebral foramen (for C7 spinal nerve)

Vertebral body (C7)

The uncovertebral joints of the cervical spine: anterior view (C3 to C7 have been sectioned coronally to expose the joints)

T1

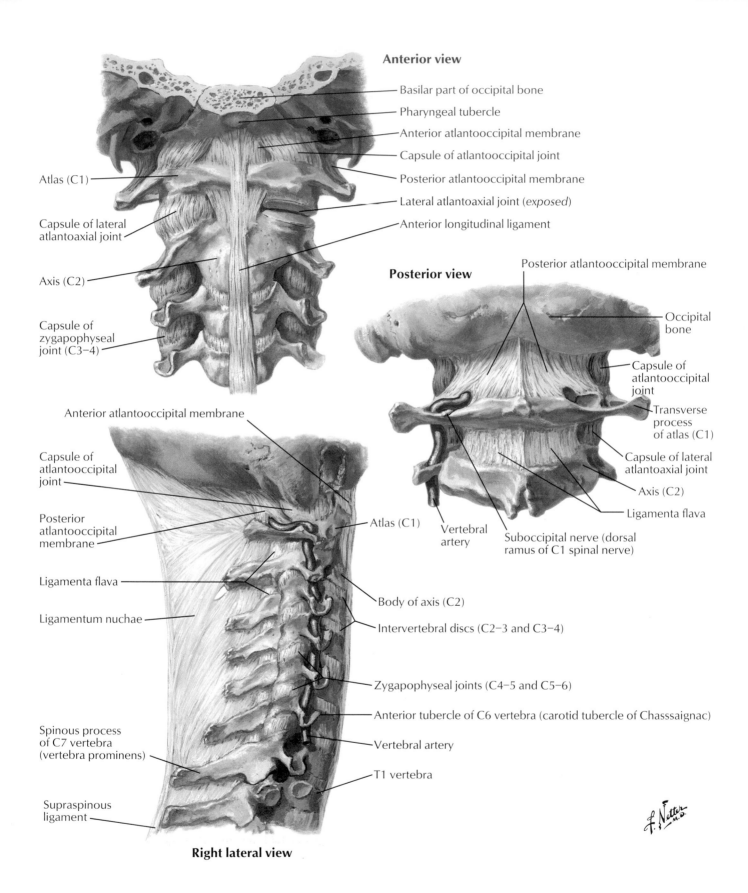

Anterior view

Basilar part of occipital bone

Pharyngeal tubercle

Anterior atlantooccipital membrane

Capsule of atlantooccipital joint

Posterior atlantooccipital membrane

Lateral atlantoaxial joint (*exposed*)

Anterior longitudinal ligament

Atlas (C1)

Capsule of lateral atlantoaxial joint

Axis (C2)

Capsule of zygapophyseal joint (C3–4)

Posterior view

Posterior atlantooccipital membrane

Occipital bone

Capsule of atlantooccipital joint

Transverse process of atlas (C1)

Capsule of lateral atlantoaxial joint

Axis (C2)

Ligamenta flava

Vertebral artery

Suboccipital nerve (dorsal ramus of C1 spinal nerve)

Anterior atlantooccipital membrane

Capsule of atlantooccipital joint

Posterior atlantooccipital membrane

Ligamenta flava

Ligamentum nuchae

Atlas (C1)

Body of axis (C2)

Intervertebral discs (C2–3 and C3–4)

Zygapophyseal joints (C4–5 and C5–6)

Anterior tubercle of C6 vertebra (carotid tubercle of Chasssaignac)

Vertebral artery

T1 vertebra

Spinous process of C7 vertebra (vertebra prominens)

Supraspinous ligament

Right lateral view

Plate 22

Bones and Ligaments

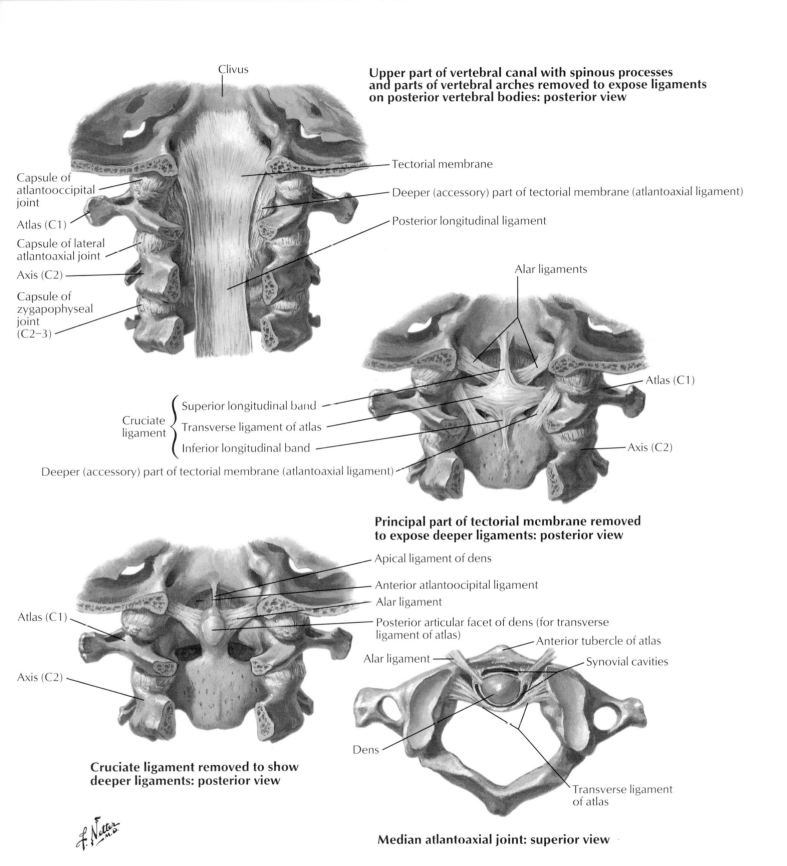

Clivus

Upper part of vertebral canal with spinous processes and parts of vertebral arches removed to expose ligaments on posterior vertebral bodies: posterior view

Tectorial membrane

Deeper (accessory) part of tectorial membrane (atlantoaxial ligament)

Posterior longitudinal ligament

Capsule of atlantooccipital joint

Atlas (C1)

Capsule of lateral atlantoaxial joint

Axis (C2)

Capsule of zygapophyseal joint (C2–3)

Alar ligaments

Atlas (C1)

Axis (C2)

Cruciate ligament
- Superior longitudinal band
- Transverse ligament of atlas
- Inferior longitudinal band

Deeper (accessory) part of tectorial membrane (atlantoaxial ligament)

Principal part of tectorial membrane removed to expose deeper ligaments: posterior view

Apical ligament of dens

Anterior atlantooccipital ligament

Alar ligament

Posterior articular facet of dens (for transverse ligament of atlas)

Atlas (C1)

Axis (C2)

Anterior tubercle of atlas

Alar ligament

Synovial cavities

Dens

Transverse ligament of atlas

Cruciate ligament removed to show deeper ligaments: posterior view

Median atlantoaxial joint: superior view

Facial Nerve Branches and Parotid Gland

See also **Plates 61, 71, 122**

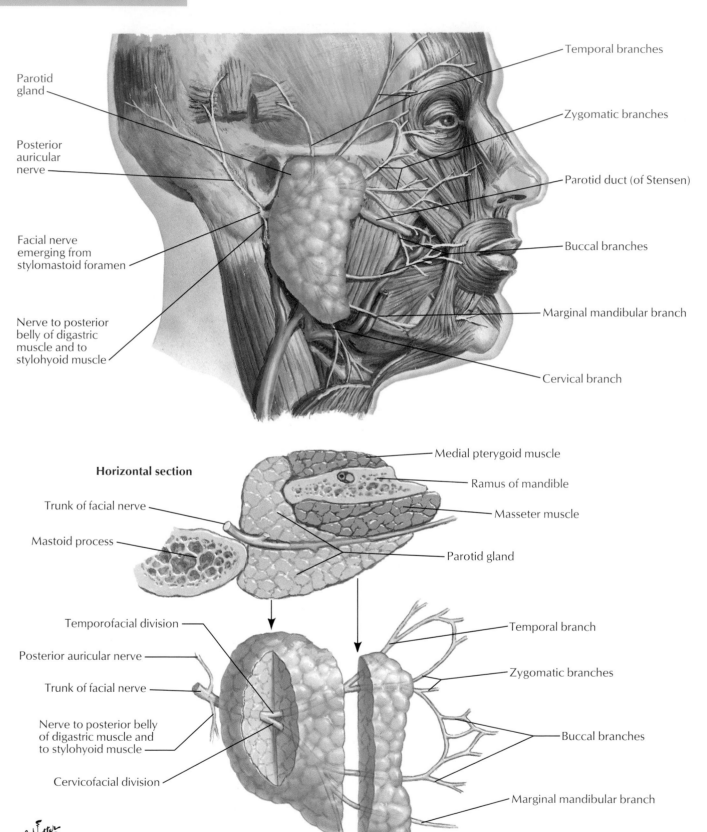

Parotid gland

Posterior auricular nerve

Facial nerve emerging from stylomastoid foramen

Nerve to posterior belly of digastric muscle and to stylohyoid muscle

Temporal branches

Zygomatic branches

Parotid duct (of Stensen)

Buccal branches

Marginal mandibular branch

Cervical branch

Horizontal section

Trunk of facial nerve

Mastoid process

Medial pterygoid muscle

Ramus of mandible

Masseter muscle

Parotid gland

Temporofacial division

Posterior auricular nerve

Trunk of facial nerve

Nerve to posterior belly of digastric muscle and to stylohyoid muscle

Cervicofacial division

Temporal branch

Zygomatic branches

Buccal branches

Marginal mandibular branch

Cervical branch

Plate 24

Superficial Face

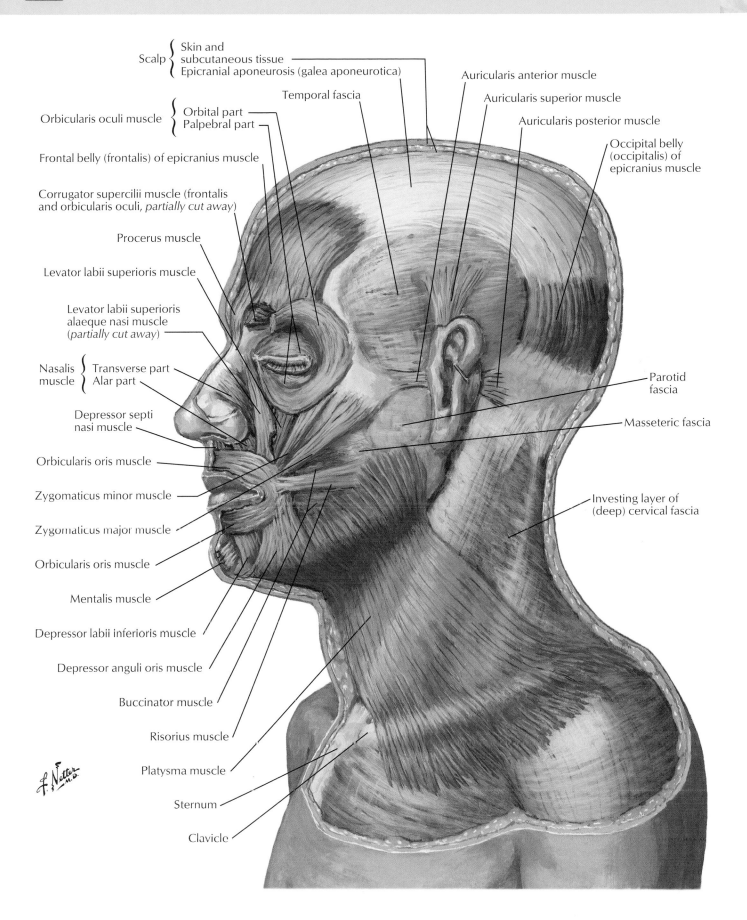

Scalp
- Skin and subcutaneous tissue
- Epicranial aponeurosis (galea aponeurotica)

Temporal fascia

Auricularis anterior muscle

Auricularis superior muscle

Auricularis posterior muscle

Occipital belly (occipitalis) of epicranius muscle

Orbicularis oculi muscle
- Orbital part
- Palpebral part

Frontal belly (frontalis) of epicranius muscle

Corrugator supercilii muscle (frontalis and orbicularis oculi, *partially cut away*)

Procerus muscle

Levator labii superioris muscle

Levator labii superioris alaeque nasi muscle (*partially cut away*)

Nasalis muscle
- Transverse part
- Alar part

Depressor septi nasi muscle

Orbicularis oris muscle

Zygomaticus minor muscle

Zygomaticus major muscle

Orbicularis oris muscle

Mentalis muscle

Depressor labii inferioris muscle

Depressor anguli oris muscle

Buccinator muscle

Risorius muscle

Platysma muscle

Sternum

Clavicle

Parotid fascia

Masseteric fascia

Investing layer of (deep) cervical fascia

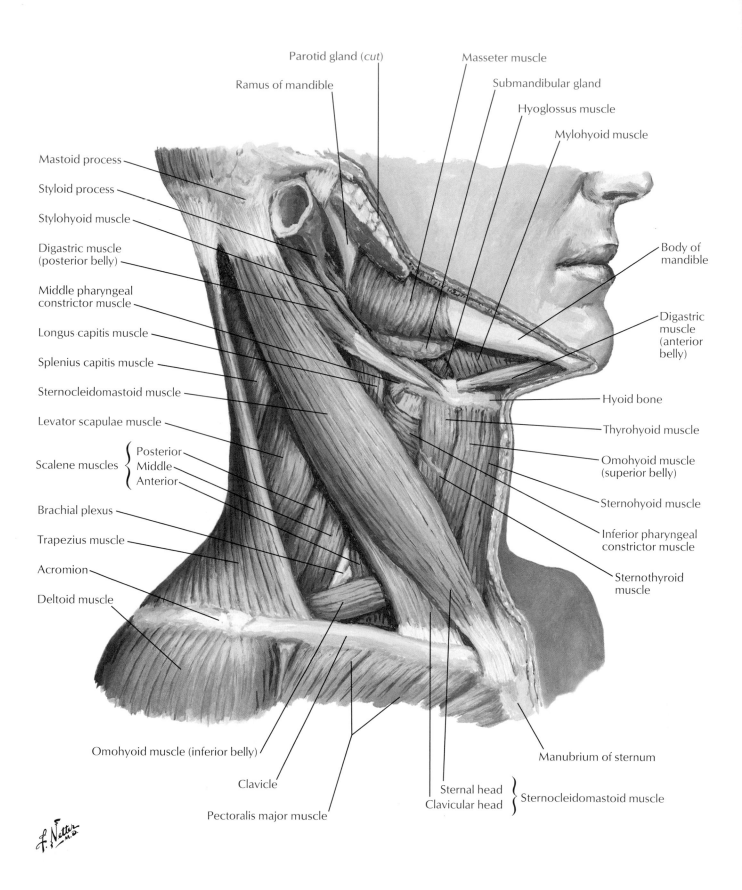

Parotid gland (cut)

Masseter muscle

Ramus of mandible

Submandibular gland

Hyoglossus muscle

Mylohyoid muscle

Mastoid process

Styloid process

Stylohyoid muscle

Digastric muscle (posterior belly)

Middle pharyngeal constrictor muscle

Longus capitis muscle

Splenius capitis muscle

Sternocleidomastoid muscle

Levator scapulae muscle

Scalene muscles { Posterior / Middle / Anterior }

Brachial plexus

Trapezius muscle

Acromion

Deltoid muscle

Body of mandible

Digastric muscle (anterior belly)

Hyoid bone

Thyrohyoid muscle

Omohyoid muscle (superior belly)

Sternohyoid muscle

Inferior pharyngeal constrictor muscle

Sternothyroid muscle

Omohyoid muscle (inferior belly)

Clavicle

Pectoralis major muscle

Sternal head / Clavicular head } Sternocleidomastoid muscle

Manubrium of sternum

Plate 26

Neck

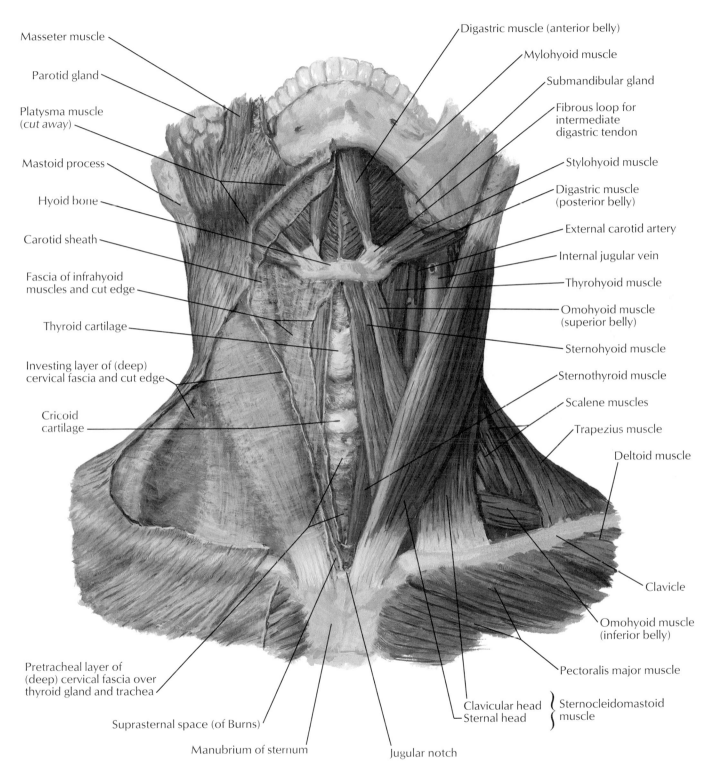

Masseter muscle

Parotid gland

Platysma muscle (*cut away*)

Mastoid process

Hyoid bone

Carotid sheath

Fascia of infrahyoid muscles and cut edge

Thyroid cartilage

Investing layer of (deep) cervical fascia and cut edge

Cricoid cartilage

Pretracheal layer of (deep) cervical fascia over thyroid gland and trachea

Suprasternal space (of Burns)

Manubrium of sternum

Digastric muscle (anterior belly)

Mylohyoid muscle

Submandibular gland

Fibrous loop for intermediate digastric tendon

Stylohyoid muscle

Digastric muscle (posterior belly)

External carotid artery

Internal jugular vein

Thyrohyoid muscle

Omohyoid muscle (superior belly)

Sternohyoid muscle

Sternothyroid muscle

Scalene muscles

Trapezius muscle

Deltoid muscle

Clavicle

Omohyoid muscle (inferior belly)

Pectoralis major muscle

Clavicular head
Sternal head } Sternocleidomastoid muscle

Jugular notch

Infrahyoid and Suprahyoid Muscles

See also **Plate 53**

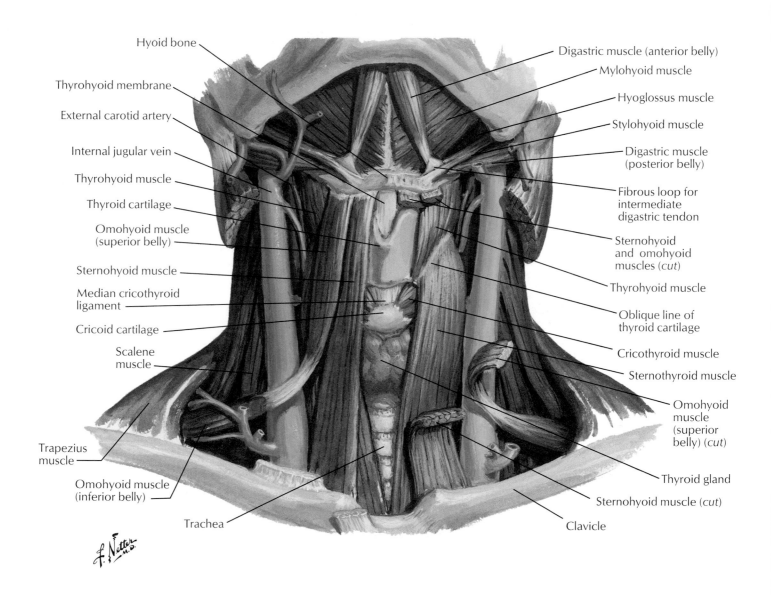

Hyoid bone

Thyrohyoid membrane

External carotid artery

Internal jugular vein

Thyrohyoid muscle

Thyroid cartilage

Omohyoid muscle (superior belly)

Sternohyoid muscle

Median cricothyroid ligament

Cricoid cartilage

Scalene muscle

Trapezius muscle

Omohyoid muscle (inferior belly)

Trachea

Digastric muscle (anterior belly)

Mylohyoid muscle

Hyoglossus muscle

Stylohyoid muscle

Digastric muscle (posterior belly)

Fibrous loop for intermediate digastric tendon

Sternohyoid and omohyoid muscles (cut)

Thyrohyoid muscle

Oblique line of thyroid cartilage

Cricothyroid muscle

Sternothyroid muscle

Omohyoid muscle (superior belly) (cut)

Thyroid gland

Sternohyoid muscle (cut)

Clavicle

Plate 28 **Neck**

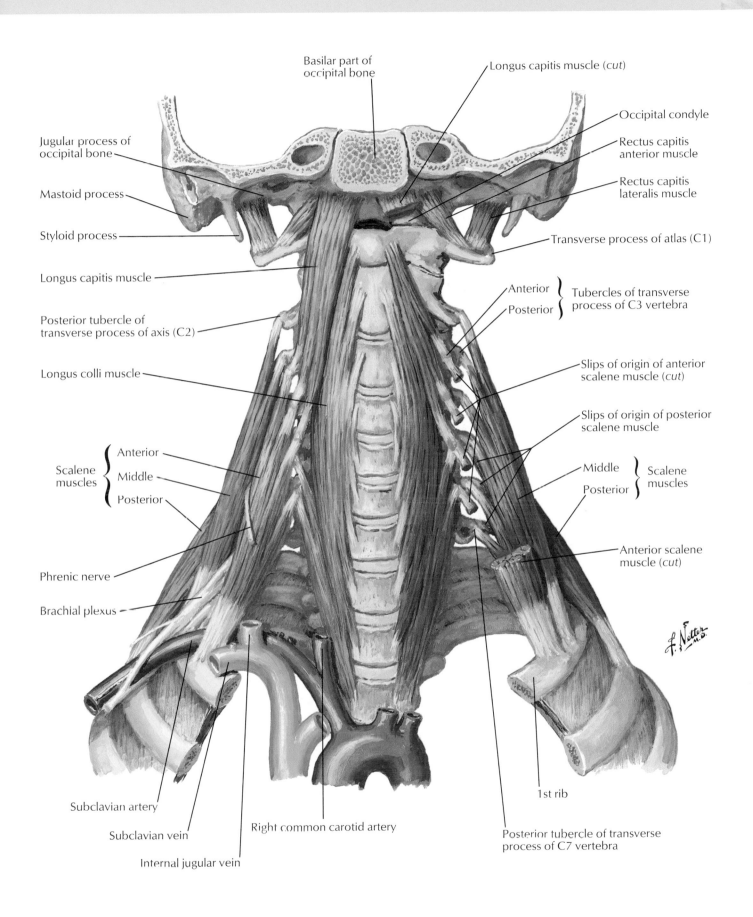

Basilar part of occipital bone

Longus capitis muscle (cut)

Occipital condyle

Jugular process of occipital bone

Rectus capitis anterior muscle

Mastoid process

Rectus capitis lateralis muscle

Styloid process

Transverse process of atlas (C1)

Longus capitis muscle

Anterior

Posterior

Tubercles of transverse process of C3 vertebra

Posterior tubercle of transverse process of axis (C2)

Slips of origin of anterior scalene muscle (cut)

Longus colli muscle

Slips of origin of posterior scalene muscle

Scalene muscles

Anterior

Middle

Posterior

Middle

Posterior

Scalene muscles

Phrenic nerve

Anterior scalene muscle (cut)

Brachial plexus

1st rib

Subclavian artery

Posterior tubercle of transverse process of C7 vertebra

Subclavian vein

Right common carotid artery

Internal jugular vein

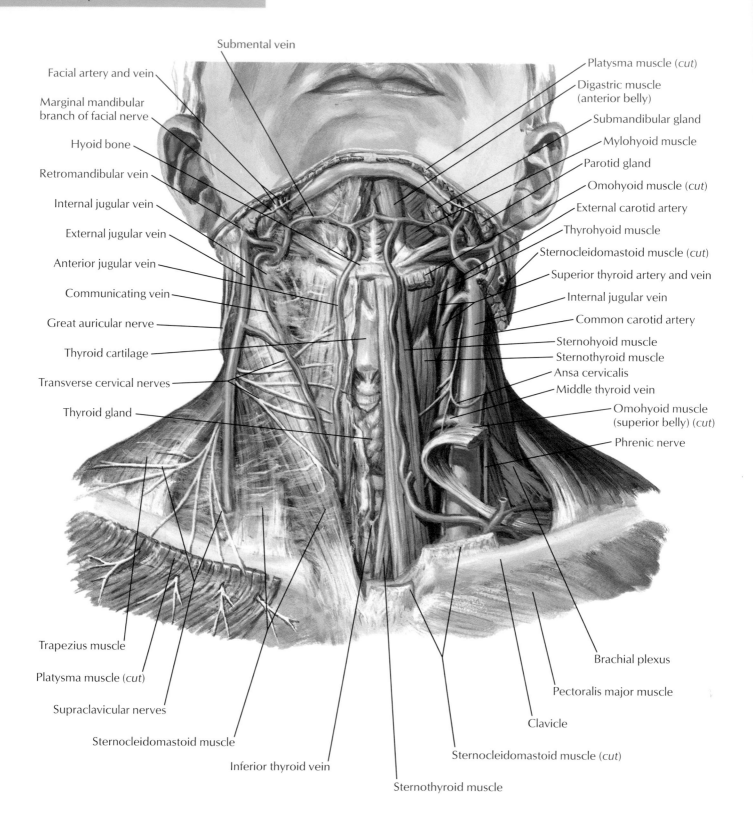

Submental vein

Facial artery and vein

Marginal mandibular branch of facial nerve

Hyoid bone

Retromandibular vein

Internal jugular vein

External jugular vein

Anterior jugular vein

Communicating vein

Great auricular nerve

Thyroid cartilage

Transverse cervical nerves

Thyroid gland

Platysma muscle (*cut*)

Digastric muscle (anterior belly)

Submandibular gland

Mylohyoid muscle

Parotid gland

Omohyoid muscle (*cut*)

External carotid artery

Thyrohyoid muscle

Sternocleidomastoid muscle (*cut*)

Superior thyroid artery and vein

Internal jugular vein

Common carotid artery

Sternohyoid muscle

Sternothyroid muscle

Ansa cervicalis

Middle thyroid vein

Omohyoid muscle (superior belly) (*cut*)

Phrenic nerve

Trapezius muscle

Platysma muscle (*cut*)

Supraclavicular nerves

Sternocleidomastoid muscle

Inferior thyroid vein

Sternothyroid muscle

Sternocleidomastoid muscle (*cut*)

Clavicle

Pectoralis major muscle

Brachial plexus

Plate 30

Neck

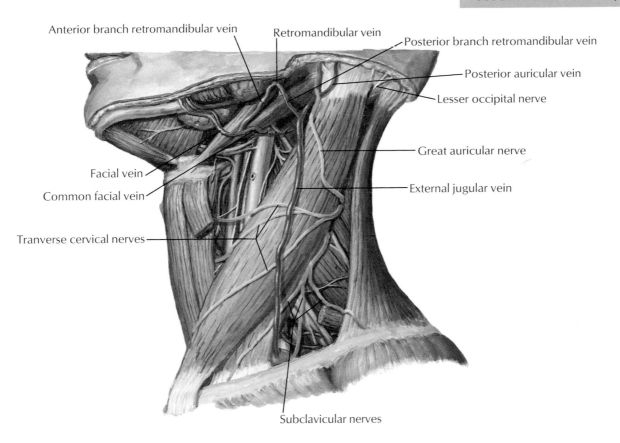

Anterior branch retromandibular vein — Retromandibular vein — Posterior branch retromandibular vein

Posterior auricular vein

Lesser occipital nerve

Great auricular nerve

Facial vein

Common facial vein

External jugular vein

Tranverse cervical nerves

Subclavicular nerves

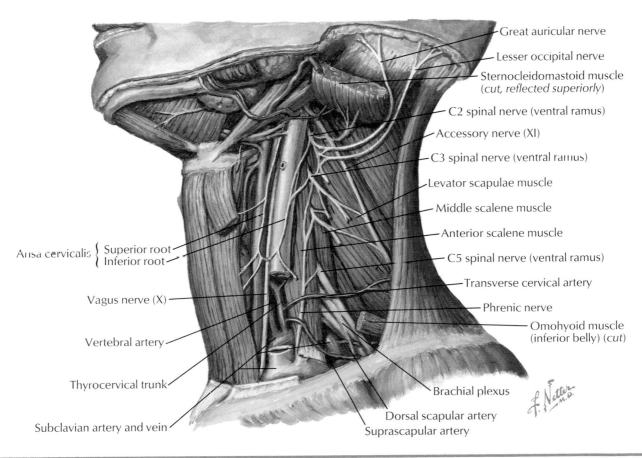

Great auricular nerve

Lesser occipital nerve

Sternocleidomastoid muscle (*cut, reflected superiorly*)

C2 spinal nerve (ventral ramus)

Accessory nerve (XI)

C3 spinal nerve (ventral ramus)

Levator scapulae muscle

Middle scalene muscle

Anterior scalene muscle

Ansa cervicalis { Superior root / Inferior root

C5 spinal nerve (ventral ramus)

Transverse cervical artery

Vagus nerve (X)

Phrenic nerve

Omohyoid muscle (inferior belly) (*cut*)

Vertebral artery

Thyrocervical trunk

Brachial plexus

Subclavian artery and vein

Dorsal scapular artery

Suprascapular artery

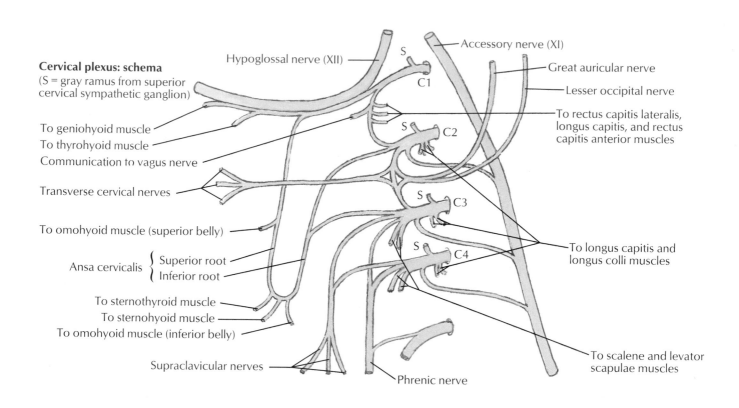

Cervical plexus: schema
(S = gray ramus from superior
cervical sympathetic ganglion)

Hypoglossal nerve (XII)

S

C1

Accessory nerve (XI)

Great auricular nerve

Lesser occipital nerve

To geniohyoid muscle
To thyrohyoid muscle
Communication to vagus nerve

S

C2

To rectus capitis lateralis,
longus capitis, and rectus
capitis anterior muscles

Transverse cervical nerves

S

C3

To omohyoid muscle (superior belly)

Ansa cervicalis { Superior root
                 Inferior root

S

C4

To longus capitis and
longus colli muscles

To sternothyroid muscle
To sternohyoid muscle
To omohyoid muscle (inferior belly)

Supraclavicular nerves

Phrenic nerve

To scalene and levator
scapulae muscles

Right anterior dissection

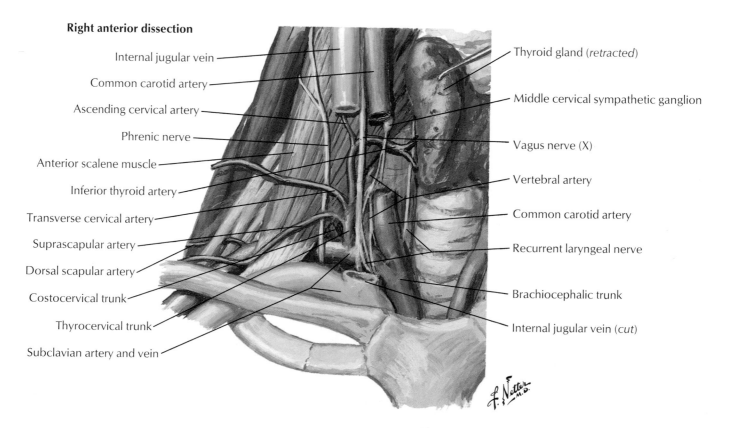

Internal jugular vein

Common carotid artery

Ascending cervical artery

Phrenic nerve

Anterior scalene muscle

Inferior thyroid artery

Transverse cervical artery

Suprascapular artery

Dorsal scapular artery

Costocervical trunk

Thyrocervical trunk

Subclavian artery and vein

Thyroid gland (retracted)

Middle cervical sympathetic ganglion

Vagus nerve (X)

Vertebral artery

Common carotid artery

Recurrent laryngeal nerve

Brachiocephalic trunk

Internal jugular vein (cut)

Plate 32

Neck

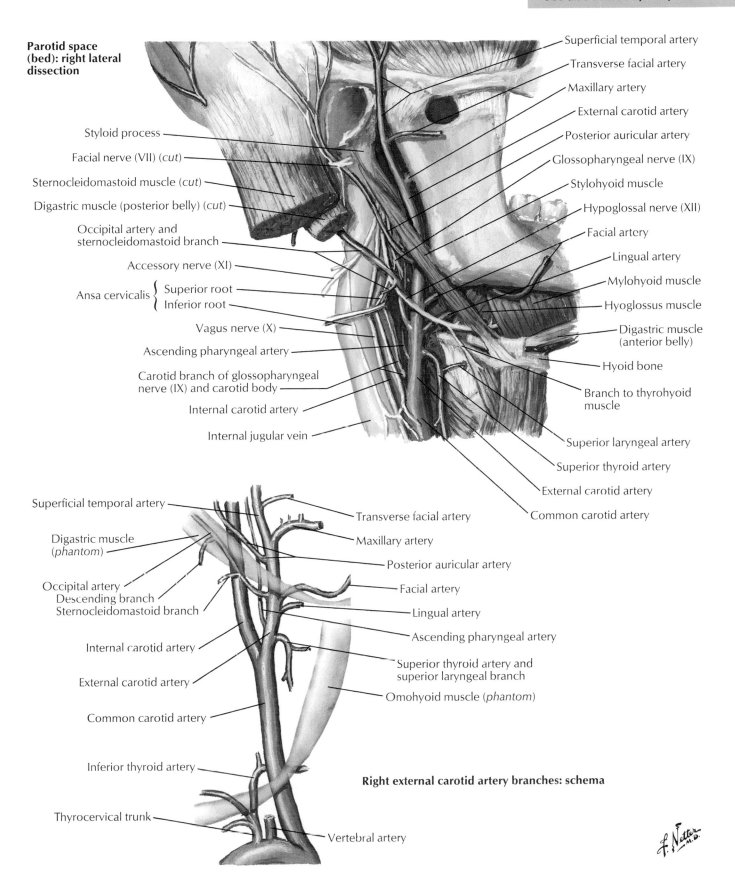

Parotid space (bed): right lateral dissection

Styloid process

Facial nerve (VII) (*cut*)

Sternocleidomastoid muscle (*cut*)

Digastric muscle (posterior belly) (*cut*)

Occipital artery and sternocleidomastoid branch

Accessory nerve (XI)

Ansa cervicalis { Superior root
Inferior root

Vagus nerve (X)

Ascending pharyngeal artery

Carotid branch of glossopharyngeal nerve (IX) and carotid body

Internal carotid artery

Internal jugular vein

Superficial temporal artery

Transverse facial artery

Maxillary artery

External carotid artery

Posterior auricular artery

Glossopharyngeal nerve (IX)

Stylohyoid muscle

Hypoglossal nerve (XII)

Facial artery

Lingual artery

Mylohyoid muscle

Hyoglossus muscle

Digastric muscle (anterior belly)

Hyoid bone

Branch to thyrohyoid muscle

Superior laryngeal artery

Superior thyroid artery

External carotid artery

Common carotid artery

Superficial temporal artery

Digastric muscle (*phantom*)

Occipital artery

Descending branch

Sternocleidomastoid branch

Internal carotid artery

External carotid artery

Common carotid artery

Inferior thyroid artery

Thyrocervical trunk

Transverse facial artery

Maxillary artery

Posterior auricular artery

Facial artery

Lingual artery

Ascending pharyngeal artery

Superior thyroid artery and superior laryngeal branch

Omohyoid muscle (*phantom*)

Right external carotid artery branches: schema

Vertebral artery

For contents of carotid sheath see **Plates 69–71**

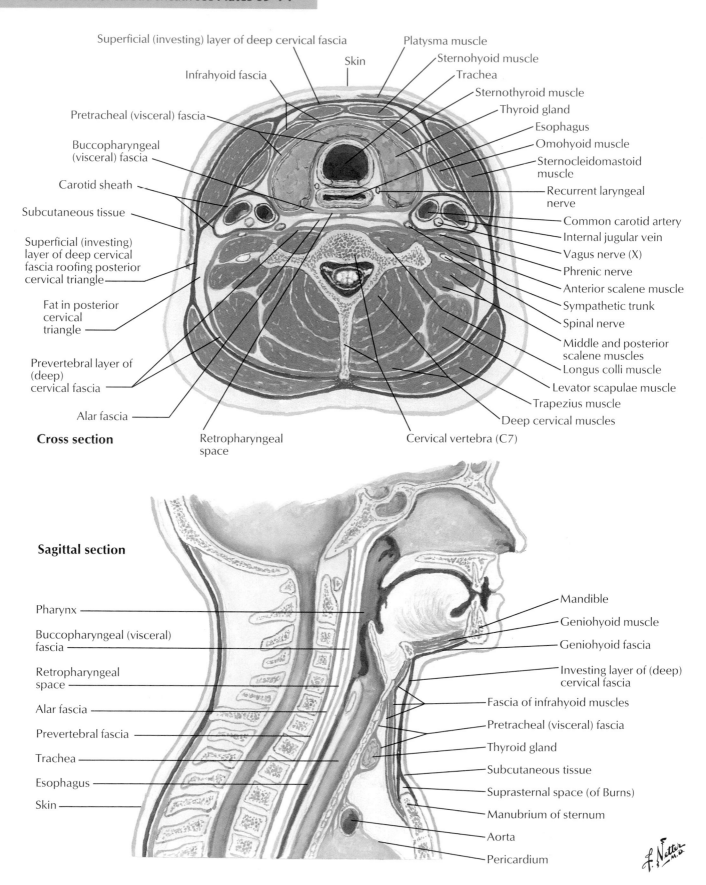

Superficial (investing) layer of deep cervical fascia

Infrahyoid fascia

Platysma muscle

Skin

Sternohyoid muscle

Trachea

Pretracheal (visceral) fascia

Sternothyroid muscle

Thyroid gland

Esophagus

Buccopharyngeal (visceral) fascia

Omohyoid muscle

Sternocleidomastoid muscle

Carotid sheath

Recurrent laryngeal nerve

Subcutaneous tissue

Common carotid artery

Internal jugular vein

Superficial (investing) layer of deep cervical fascia roofing posterior cervical triangle

Vagus nerve (X)

Phrenic nerve

Anterior scalene muscle

Fat in posterior cervical triangle

Sympathetic trunk

Spinal nerve

Middle and posterior scalene muscles

Prevertebral layer of (deep) cervical fascia

Longus colli muscle

Levator scapulae muscle

Trapezius muscle

Alar fascia

Deep cervical muscles

Cross section

Retropharyngeal space

Cervical vertebra (C7)

Sagittal section

Pharynx

Mandible

Buccopharyngeal (visceral) fascia

Geniohyoid muscle

Geniohyoid fascia

Retropharyngeal space

Investing layer of (deep) cervical fascia

Alar fascia

Fascia of infrahyoid muscles

Prevertebral fascia

Pretracheal (visceral) fascia

Trachea

Thyroid gland

Esophagus

Subcutaneous tissue

Skin

Suprasternal space (of Burns)

Manubrium of sternum

Aorta

Pericardium

Anterolateral view

Frontal bone

Nasal bones

Frontal process of maxilla

Lateral process of septal nasal cartilages

Septal cartilage

Minor alar cartilage

Accessory nasal cartilage

Major alar cartilage { Lateral crus

Medial crus

Nasal septal cartilage

Anterior nasal spine of maxilla

Alar fibrofatty tissue

Infraorbital foramen

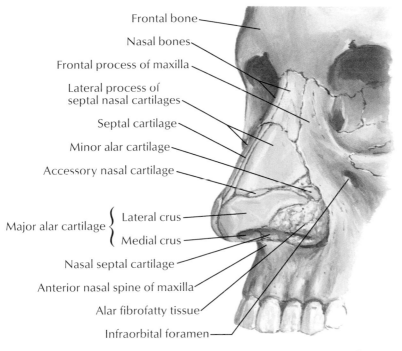

Inferior view

Major alar cartilage

Lateral crus   Medial crus

Alar fibrofatty tissue

Nasal septal cartilage

Anterior nasal spine of maxilla

Intermaxillary suture

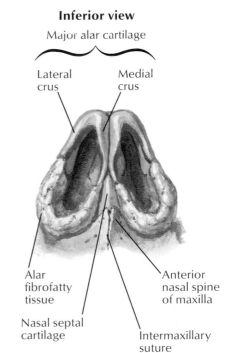

Superficial temporal artery

Frontalis muscle

Supraorbital artery and nerve

Supratrochlear artery and nerve

Procerus muscle

Corrugator supercilii muscle

Dorsal nasal artery

Infratrochlear nerve

Angular artery

External nasal artery and nerve

Nasalis muscle (transverse part)

Infraorbital artery and nerve

Lateral nasal artery

Transverse facial artery

Nasalis muscle (alar part)

Depressor septi nasi muscle

Orbicularis oris muscle

Facial artery

Superior and inferior labial arteries

Nasal Region

Plate 35

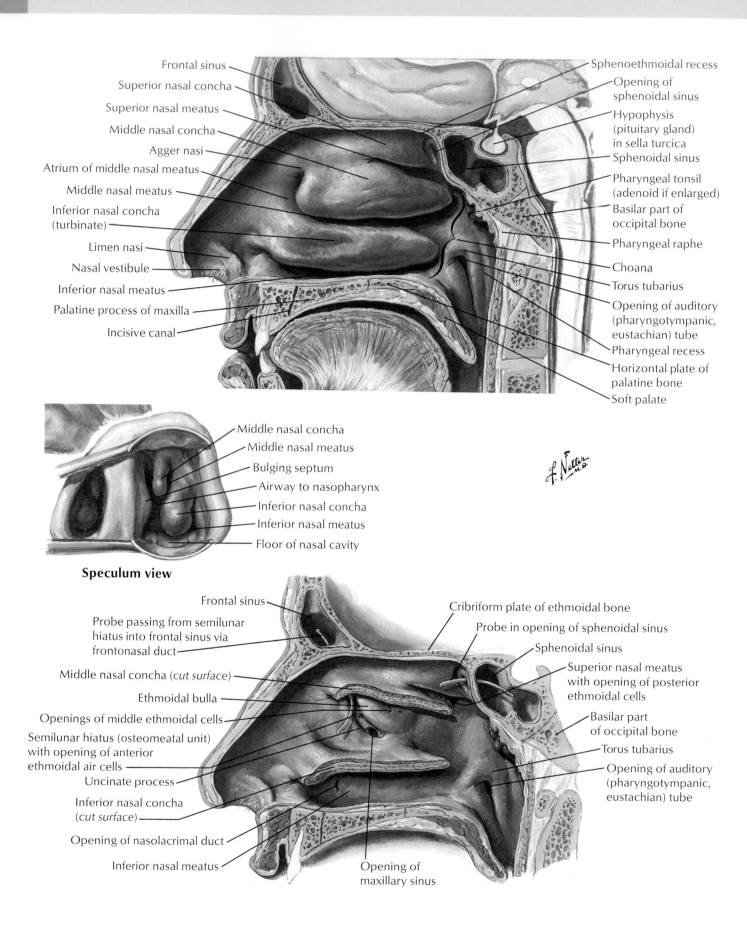

Frontal sinus

Superior nasal concha

Superior nasal meatus

Middle nasal concha

Agger nasi

Atrium of middle nasal meatus

Middle nasal meatus

Inferior nasal concha (turbinate)

Limen nasi

Nasal vestibule

Inferior nasal meatus

Palatine process of maxilla

Incisive canal

Sphenoethmoidal recess

Opening of sphenoidal sinus

Hypophysis (pituitary gland) in sella turcica

Sphenoidal sinus

Pharyngeal tonsil (adenoid if enlarged)

Basilar part of occipital bone

Pharyngeal raphe

Choana

Torus tubarius

Opening of auditory (pharyngotympanic, eustachian) tube

Pharyngeal recess

Horizontal plate of palatine bone

Soft palate

Middle nasal concha

Middle nasal meatus

Bulging septum

Airway to nasopharynx

Inferior nasal concha

Inferior nasal meatus

Floor of nasal cavity

Speculum view

Frontal sinus

Probe passing from semilunar hiatus into frontal sinus via frontonasal duct

Middle nasal concha (cut surface)

Ethmoidal bulla

Openings of middle ethmoidal cells

Semilunar hiatus (osteomeatal unit) with opening of anterior ethmoidal air cells

Uncinate process

Inferior nasal concha (cut surface)

Opening of nasolacrimal duct

Inferior nasal meatus

Cribriform plate of ethmoidal bone

Probe in opening of sphenoidal sinus

Sphenoidal sinus

Superior nasal meatus with opening of posterior ethmoidal cells

Basilar part of occipital bone

Torus tubarius

Opening of auditory (pharyngotympanic, eustachian) tube

Opening of maxillary sinus

Plate 36   **Nasal Region**

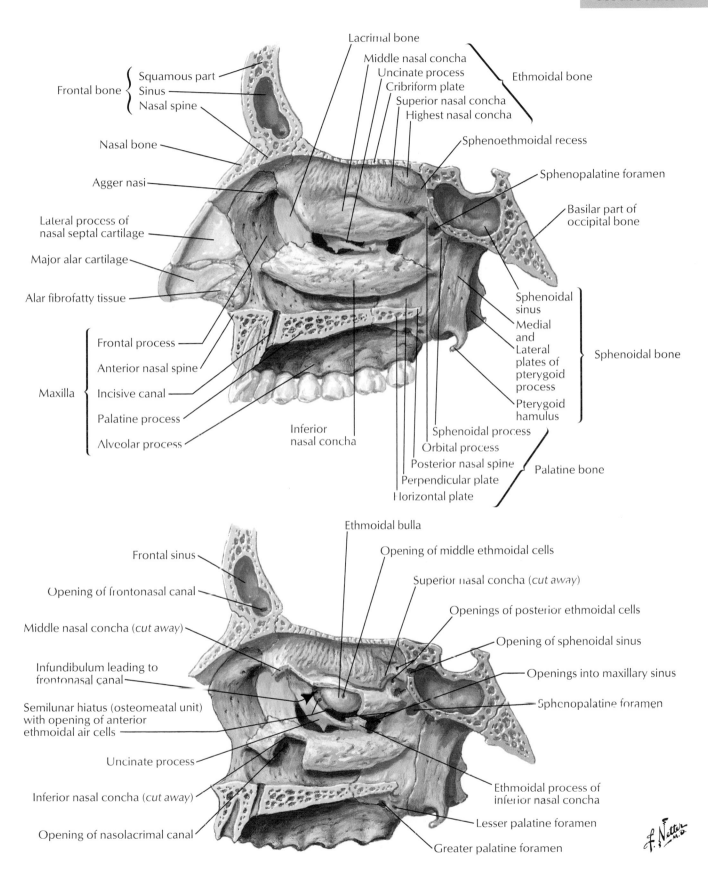

Lacrimal bone

Middle nasal concha

Uncinate process

Cribriform plate

Superior nasal concha

Highest nasal concha

Ethmoidal bone

Frontal bone — Squamous part / Sinus / Nasal spine

Nasal bone

Agger nasi

Lateral process of nasal septal cartilage

Major alar cartilage

Alar fibrofatty tissue

Sphenoethmoidal recess

Sphenopalatine foramen

Basilar part of occipital bone

Sphenoidal sinus

Medial and Lateral plates of pterygoid process

Pterygoid hamulus

Sphenoidal bone

Maxilla — Frontal process / Anterior nasal spine / Incisive canal / Palatine process / Alveolar process

Inferior nasal concha

Sphenoidal process

Orbital process

Posterior nasal spine

Perpendicular plate

Horizontal plate

Palatine bone

Ethmoidal bulla

Frontal sinus

Opening of frontonasal canal

Middle nasal concha (*cut away*)

Infundibulum leading to frontonasal canal

Semilunar hiatus (osteomeatal unit) with opening of anterior ethmoidal air cells

Uncinate process

Inferior nasal concha (*cut away*)

Opening of nasolacrimal canal

Opening of middle ethmoidal cells

Superior nasal concha (*cut away*)

Openings of posterior ethmoidal cells

Opening of sphenoidal sinus

Openings into maxillary sinus

Sphenopalatine foramen

Ethmoidal process of inferior nasal concha

Lesser palatine foramen

Greater palatine foramen

Medial Wall of Nasal Cavity (Nasal Septum)

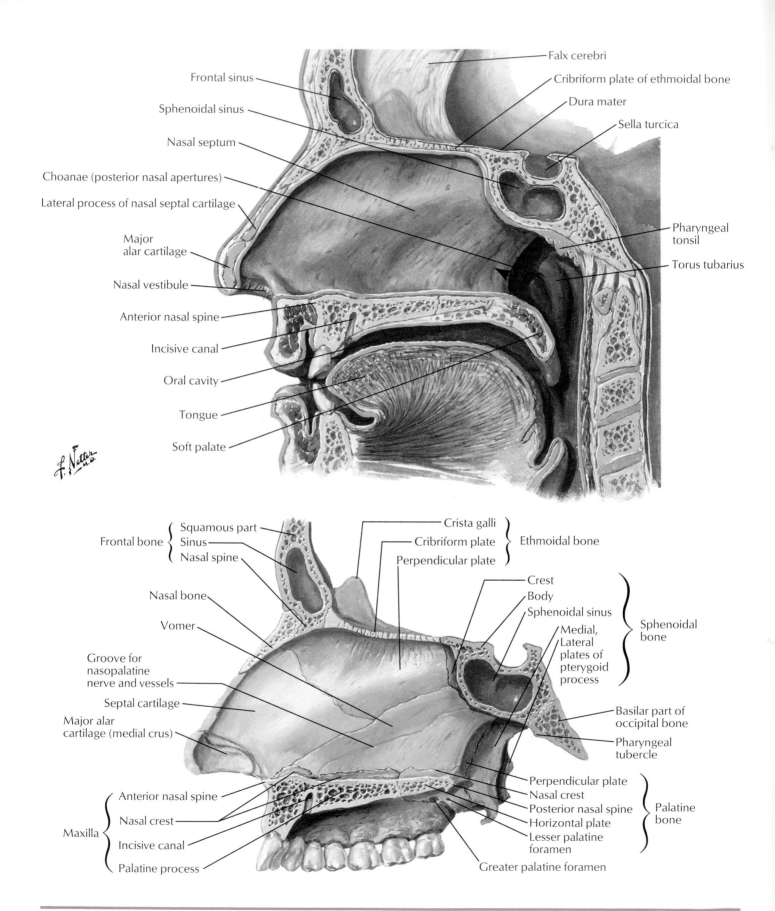

Frontal sinus

Sphenoidal sinus

Nasal septum

Choanae (posterior nasal apertures)

Lateral process of nasal septal cartilage

Major alar cartilage

Nasal vestibule

Anterior nasal spine

Incisive canal

Oral cavity

Tongue

Soft palate

Falx cerebri

Cribriform plate of ethmoidal bone

Dura mater

Sella turcica

Pharyngeal tonsil

Torus tubarius

Frontal bone
  Squamous part
  Sinus
  Nasal spine

Nasal bone

Vomer

Groove for nasopalatine nerve and vessels

Septal cartilage

Major alar cartilage (medial crus)

Maxilla
  Anterior nasal spine
  Nasal crest
  Incisive canal
  Palatine process

Crista galli
Cribriform plate
Perpendicular plate
} Ethmoidal bone

Crest
Body
Sphenoidal sinus
Medial, Lateral plates of pterygoid process
} Sphenoidal bone

Basilar part of occipital bone

Pharyngeal tubercle

Perpendicular plate
Nasal crest
Posterior nasal spine
Horizontal plate
Lesser palatine foramen
} Palatine bone

Greater palatine foramen

Plate 38   **Nasal Region**

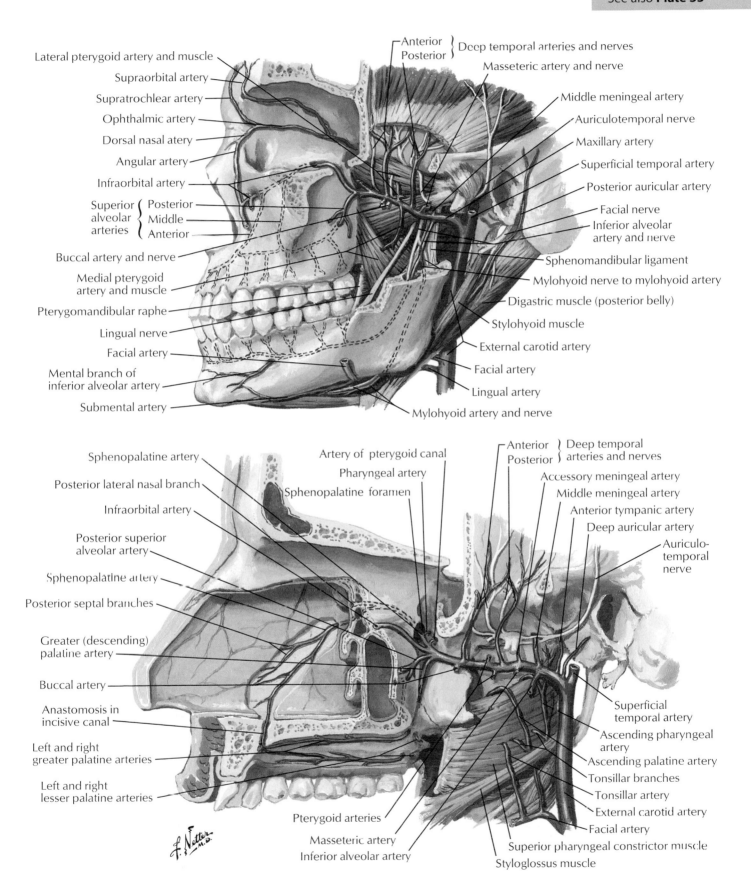

Lateral pterygoid artery and muscle
Supraorbital artery
Supratrochlear artery
Ophthalmic artery
Dorsal nasal atery
Angular artery
Infraorbital artery
Superior { Posterior / Middle / Anterior } alveolar arteries
Buccal artery and nerve
Medial pterygoid artery and muscle
Pterygomandibular raphe
Lingual nerve
Facial artery
Mental branch of inferior alveolar artery
Submental artery

Anterior } Deep temporal arteries and nerves
Posterior }
Masseteric artery and nerve
Middle meningeal artery
Auriculotemporal nerve
Maxillary artery
Superficial temporal artery
Posterior auricular artery
Facial nerve
Inferior alveolar artery and nerve
Sphenomandibular ligament
Mylohyoid nerve to mylohyoid artery
Digastric muscle (posterior belly)
Stylohyoid muscle
External carotid artery
Facial artery
Lingual artery
Mylohyoid artery and nerve

Sphenopalatine artery
Posterior lateral nasal branch
Infraorbital artery
Posterior superior alveolar artery
Sphenopalatine artery
Posterior septal branches
Greater (descending) palatine artery
Buccal artery
Anastomosis in incisive canal
Left and right greater palatine arteries
Left and right lesser palatine arteries

Artery of pterygoid canal
Pharyngeal artery
Sphenopalatine foramen

Anterior } Deep temporal
Posterior } arteries and nerves
Accessory meningeal artery
Middle meningeal artery
Anterior tympanic artery
Deep auricular artery
Auriculo-temporal nerve
Superficial temporal artery
Ascending pharyngeal artery
Ascending palatine artery
Tonsillar branches
Tonsillar artery
External carotid artery
Facial artery

Pterygoid arteries
Masseteric artery
Inferior alveolar artery
Superior pharyngeal constrictor muscle
Styloglossus muscle

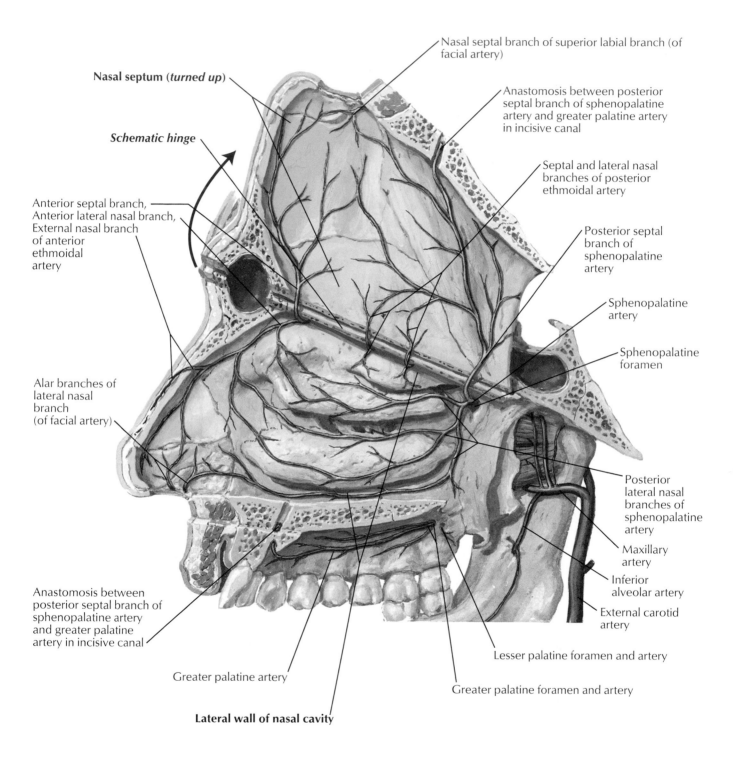

Nasal septal branch of superior labial branch (of facial artery)

Nasal septum (*turned up*)

Anastomosis between posterior septal branch of sphenopalatine artery and greater palatine artery in incisive canal

Schematic hinge

Septal and lateral nasal branches of posterior ethmoidal artery

Anterior septal branch, Anterior lateral nasal branch, External nasal branch of anterior ethmoidal artery

Posterior septal branch of sphenopalatine artery

Sphenopalatine artery

Sphenopalatine foramen

Alar branches of lateral nasal branch (of facial artery)

Posterior lateral nasal branches of sphenopalatine artery

Maxillary artery

Inferior alveolar artery

External carotid artery

Anastomosis between posterior septal branch of sphenopalatine artery and greater palatine artery in incisive canal

Lesser palatine foramen and artery

Greater palatine artery

Greater palatine foramen and artery

Lateral wall of nasal cavity

Plate 40

Nasal Region

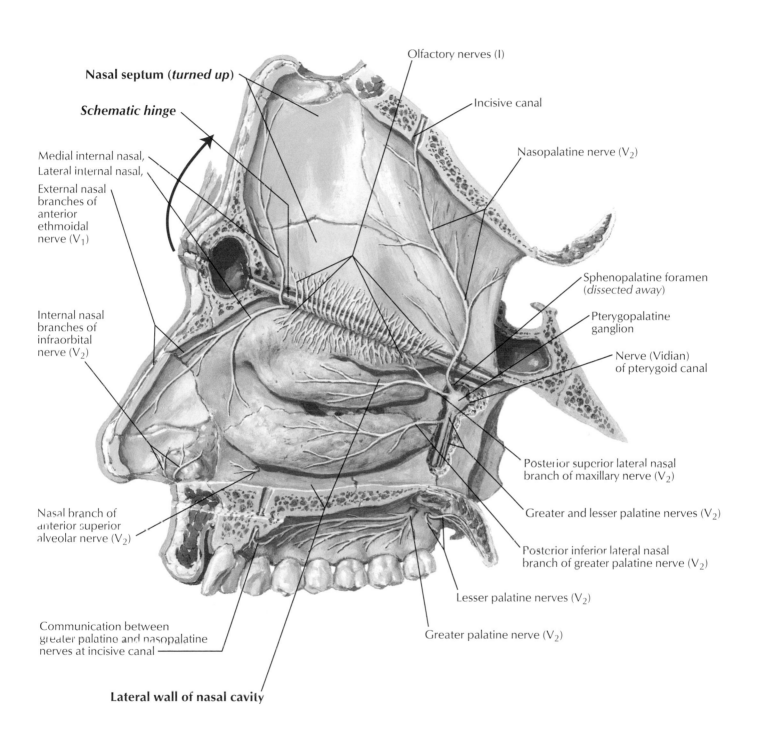

Nasal septum (*turned up*)

Schematic hinge

Medial internal nasal,
Lateral internal nasal,
External nasal
branches of
anterior
ethmoidal
nerve (V₁)

Internal nasal
branches of
infraorbital
nerve (V₂)

Nasal branch of
anterior superior
alveolar nerve (V₂)

Communication between
greater palatine and nasopalatine
nerves at incisive canal

Lateral wall of nasal cavity

Olfactory nerves (I)

Incisive canal

Nasopalatine nerve (V₂)

Sphenopalatine foramen
(*dissected away*)

Pterygopalatine
ganglion

Nerve (Vidian)
of pterygoid canal

Posterior superior lateral nasal
branch of maxillary nerve (V₂)

Greater and lesser palatine nerves (V₂)

Posterior inferior lateral nasal
branch of greater palatine nerve (V₂)

Lesser palatine nerves (V₂)

Greater palatine nerve (V₂)

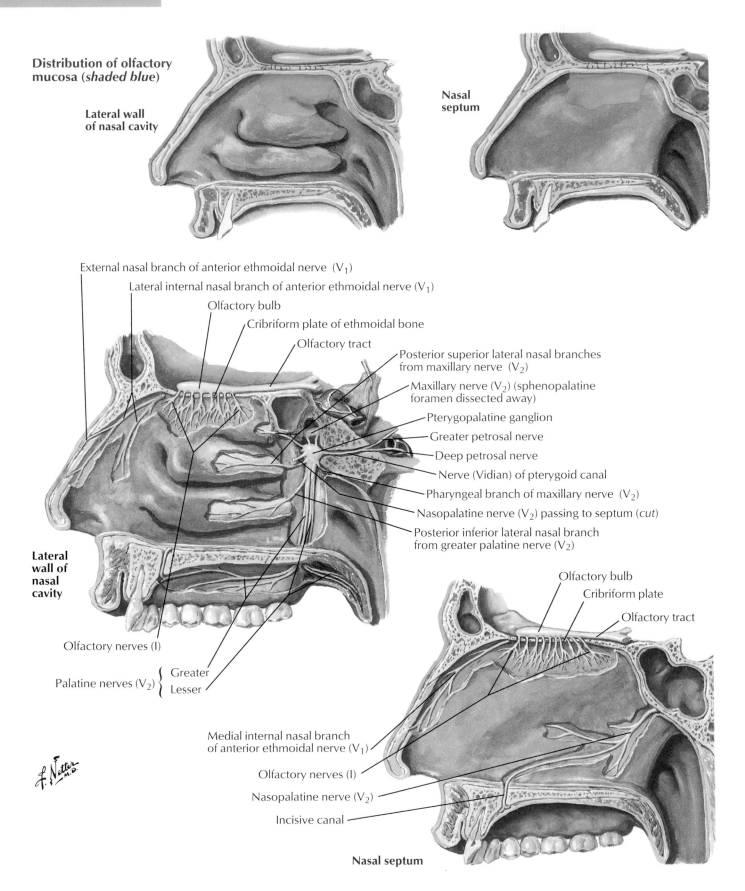

Distribution of olfactory mucosa (*shaded blue*)

Lateral wall of nasal cavity

Nasal septum

External nasal branch of anterior ethmoidal nerve (V₁)

Lateral internal nasal branch of anterior ethmoidal nerve (V₁)

Olfactory bulb

Cribriform plate of ethmoidal bone

Olfactory tract

Posterior superior lateral nasal branches from maxillary nerve (V₂)

Maxillary nerve (V₂) (sphenopalatine foramen dissected away)

Pterygopalatine ganglion

Greater petrosal nerve

Deep petrosal nerve

Nerve (Vidian) of pterygoid canal

Pharyngeal branch of maxillary nerve (V₂)

Nasopalatine nerve (V₂) passing to septum (*cut*)

Posterior inferior lateral nasal branch from greater palatine nerve (V₂)

Lateral wall of nasal cavity

Olfactory nerves (I)

Palatine nerves (V₂) { Greater / Lesser

Olfactory bulb

Cribriform plate

Olfactory tract

Medial internal nasal branch of anterior ethmoidal nerve (V₁)

Olfactory nerves (I)

Nasopalatine nerve (V₂)

Incisive canal

Nasal septum

Plate 42

Nasal Region

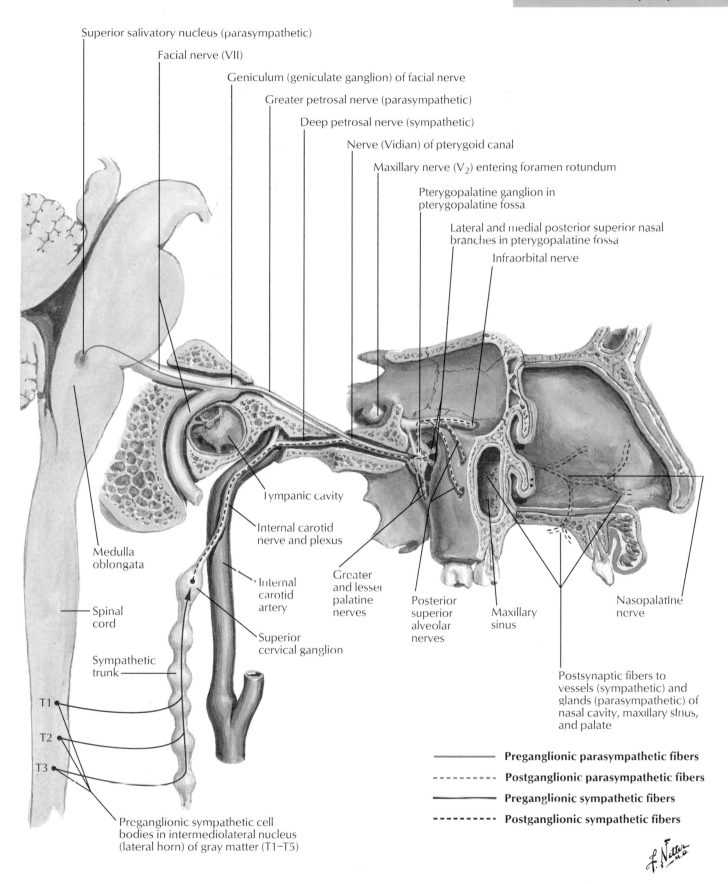

Superior salivatory nucleus (parasympathetic)

Facial nerve (VII)

Geniculum (geniculate ganglion) of facial nerve

Greater petrosal nerve (parasympathetic)

Deep petrosal nerve (sympathetic)

Nerve (Vidian) of pterygoid canal

Maxillary nerve (V$_2$) entering foramen rotundum

Pterygopalatine ganglion in pterygopalatine fossa

Lateral and medial posterior superior nasal branches in pterygopalatine fossa

Infraorbital nerve

Tympanic cavity

Internal carotid nerve and plexus

Medulla oblongata

Internal carotid artery

Greater and lesser palatine nerves

Posterior superior alveolar nerves

Maxillary sinus

Nasopalatine nerve

Spinal cord

Sympathetic trunk

Superior cervical ganglion

T1

T2

T3

Preganglionic sympathetic cell bodies in intermediolateral nucleus (lateral horn) of gray matter (T1–T5)

Postsynaptic fibers to vessels (sympathetic) and glands (parasympathetic) of nasal cavity, maxillary sinus, and palate

————————	**Preganglionic parasympathetic fibers**
- - - - - - - - -	**Postganglionic parasympathetic fibers**
————————	**Preganglionic sympathetic fibers**
- - - - - - - - -	**Postganglionic sympathetic fibers**

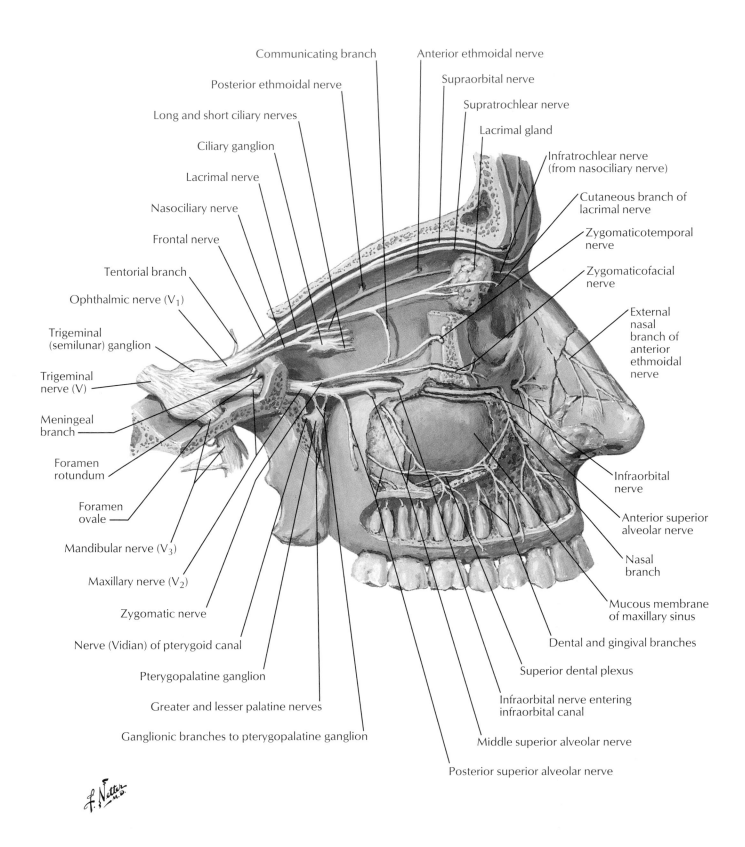

Communicating branch

Anterior ethmoidal nerve

Posterior ethmoidal nerve

Supraorbital nerve

Long and short ciliary nerves

Supratrochlear nerve

Ciliary ganglion

Lacrimal gland

Lacrimal nerve

Infratrochlear nerve
(from nasociliary nerve)

Nasociliary nerve

Cutaneous branch of
lacrimal nerve

Frontal nerve

Zygomaticotemporal
nerve

Tentorial branch

Zygomaticofacial
nerve

Ophthalmic nerve (V₁)

External
nasal
branch of
anterior
ethmoidal
nerve

Trigeminal
(semilunar) ganglion

Trigeminal
nerve (V)

Meningeal
branch

Foramen
rotundum

Infraorbital
nerve

Foramen
ovale

Anterior superior
alveolar nerve

Mandibular nerve (V₃)

Nasal
branch

Maxillary nerve (V₂)

Zygomatic nerve

Mucous membrane
of maxillary sinus

Nerve (Vidian) of pterygoid canal

Dental and gingival branches

Pterygopalatine ganglion

Superior dental plexus

Greater and lesser palatine nerves

Infraorbital nerve entering
infraorbital canal

Ganglionic branches to pterygopalatine ganglion

Middle superior alveolar nerve

Posterior superior alveolar nerve

Plate 44

Nasal Region

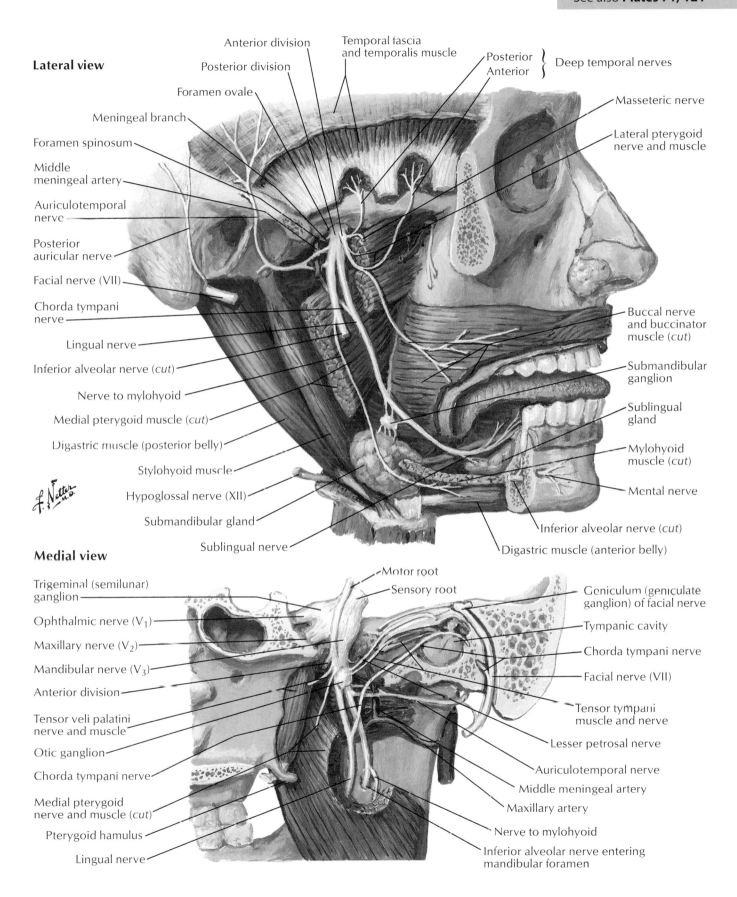

Lateral view

Anterior division
Posterior division
Foramen ovale
Meningeal branch
Foramen spinosum
Middle meningeal artery
Auriculotemporal nerve
Posterior auricular nerve
Facial nerve (VII)
Chorda tympani nerve
Lingual nerve
Inferior alveolar nerve (*cut*)
Nerve to mylohyoid
Medial pterygoid muscle (*cut*)
Digastric muscle (posterior belly)
Stylohyoid muscle
Hypoglossal nerve (XII)
Submandibular gland
Sublingual nerve

Temporal fascia and temporalis muscle
Posterior
Anterior } Deep temporal nerves
Masseteric nerve
Lateral pterygoid nerve and muscle
Buccal nerve and buccinator muscle (*cut*)
Submandibular ganglion
Sublingual gland
Mylohyoid muscle (*cut*)
Mental nerve
Inferior alveolar nerve (*cut*)
Digastric muscle (anterior belly)

Medial view

Trigeminal (semilunar) ganglion
Ophthalmic nerve (V₁)
Maxillary nerve (V₂)
Mandibular nerve (V₃)
Anterior division
Tensor veli palatini nerve and muscle
Otic ganglion
Chorda tympani nerve
Medial pterygoid nerve and muscle (*cut*)
Pterygoid hamulus
Lingual nerve

Motor root
Sensory root
Geniculum (geniculate ganglion) of facial nerve
Tympanic cavity
Chorda tympani nerve
Facial nerve (VII)
Tensor tympani muscle and nerve
Lesser petrosal nerve
Auriculotemporal nerve
Middle meningeal artery
Maxillary artery
Nerve to mylohyoid
Inferior alveolar nerve entering mandibular foramen

Nasal Region

Plate 45

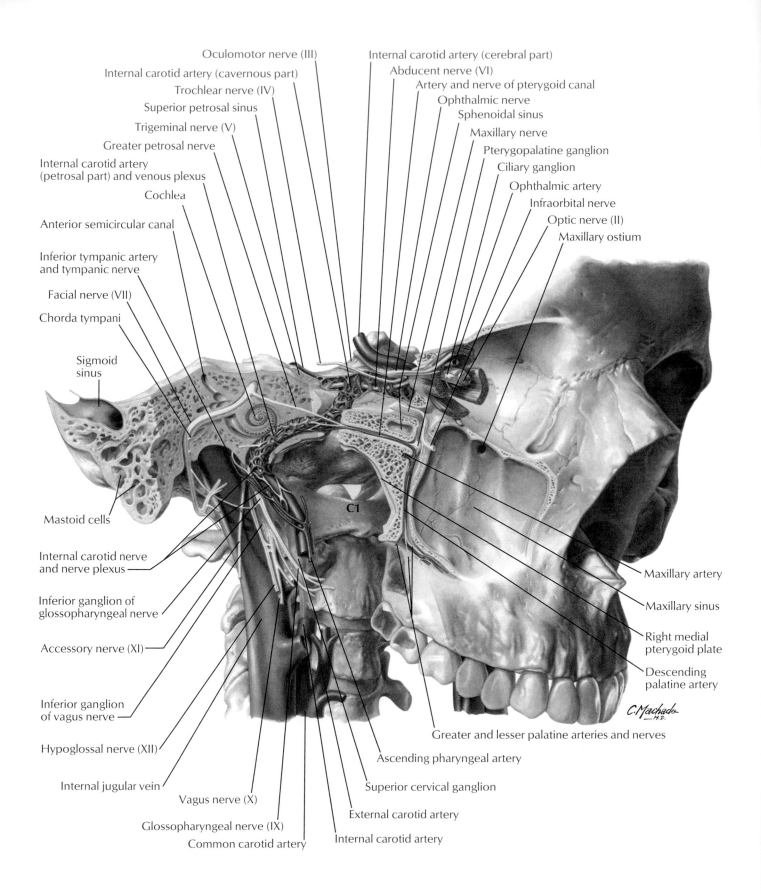

Oculomotor nerve (III)

Internal carotid artery (cavernous part)

Trochlear nerve (IV)

Superior petrosal sinus

Trigeminal nerve (V)

Greater petrosal nerve

Internal carotid artery
(petrosal part) and venous plexus

Cochlea

Anterior semicircular canal

Inferior tympanic artery
and tympanic nerve

Facial nerve (VII)

Chorda tympani

Sigmoid
sinus

Mastoid cells

Internal carotid nerve
and nerve plexus

Inferior ganglion of
glossopharyngeal nerve

Accessory nerve (XI)

Inferior ganglion
of vagus nerve

Hypoglossal nerve (XII)

Internal jugular vein

Vagus nerve (X)

Glossopharyngeal nerve (IX)

Common carotid artery

Internal carotid artery (cerebral part)

Abducent nerve (VI)

Artery and nerve of pterygoid canal

Ophthalmic nerve

Sphenoidal sinus

Maxillary nerve

Pterygopalatine ganglion

Ciliary ganglion

Ophthalmic artery

Infraorbital nerve

Optic nerve (II)

Maxillary ostium

Maxillary artery

Maxillary sinus

Right medial
pterygoid plate

Descending
palatine artery

Greater and lesser palatine arteries and nerves

Ascending pharyngeal artery

Superior cervical ganglion

External carotid artery

Internal carotid artery

C1

C.Machado
M.D.

Plate 46   **Nasal Region**

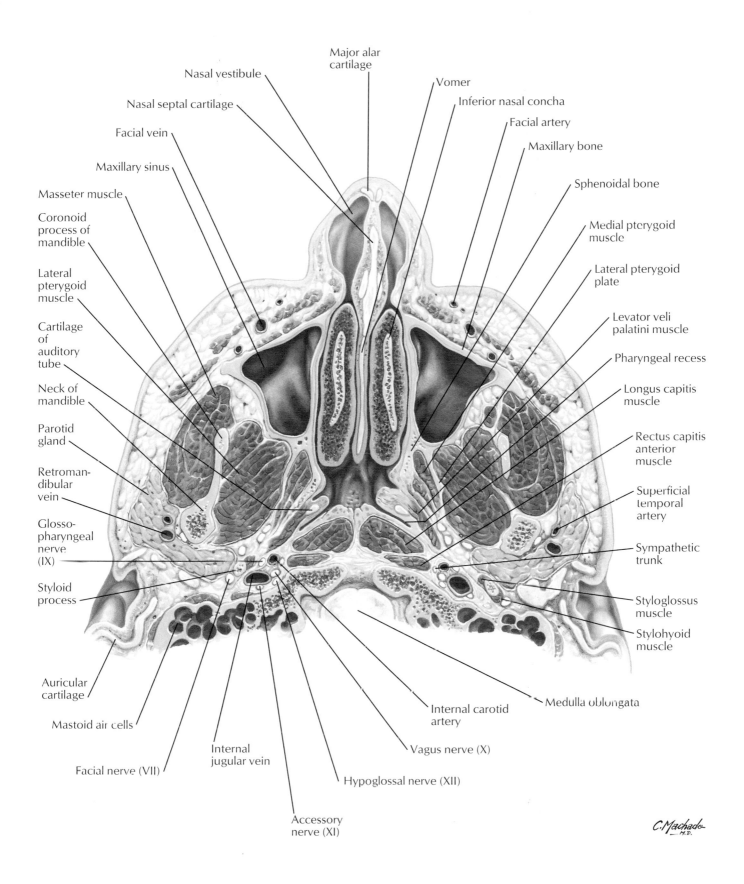

Major alar cartilage

Nasal vestibule

Nasal septal cartilage

Facial vein

Maxillary sinus

Masseter muscle

Coronoid process of mandible

Lateral pterygoid muscle

Cartilage of auditory tube

Neck of mandible

Parotid gland

Retromandibular vein

Glossopharyngeal nerve (IX)

Styloid process

Auricular cartilage

Mastoid air cells

Facial nerve (VII)

Internal jugular vein

Accessory nerve (XI)

Hypoglossal nerve (XII)

Vagus nerve (X)

Internal carotid artery

Medulla oblongata

Stylohyoid muscle

Styloglossus muscle

Sympathetic trunk

Superficial temporal artery

Rectus capitis anterior muscle

Longus capitis muscle

Pharyngeal recess

Levator veli palatini muscle

Lateral pterygoid plate

Medial pterygoid muscle

Sphenoidal bone

Maxillary bone

Facial artery

Inferior nasal concha

Vomer

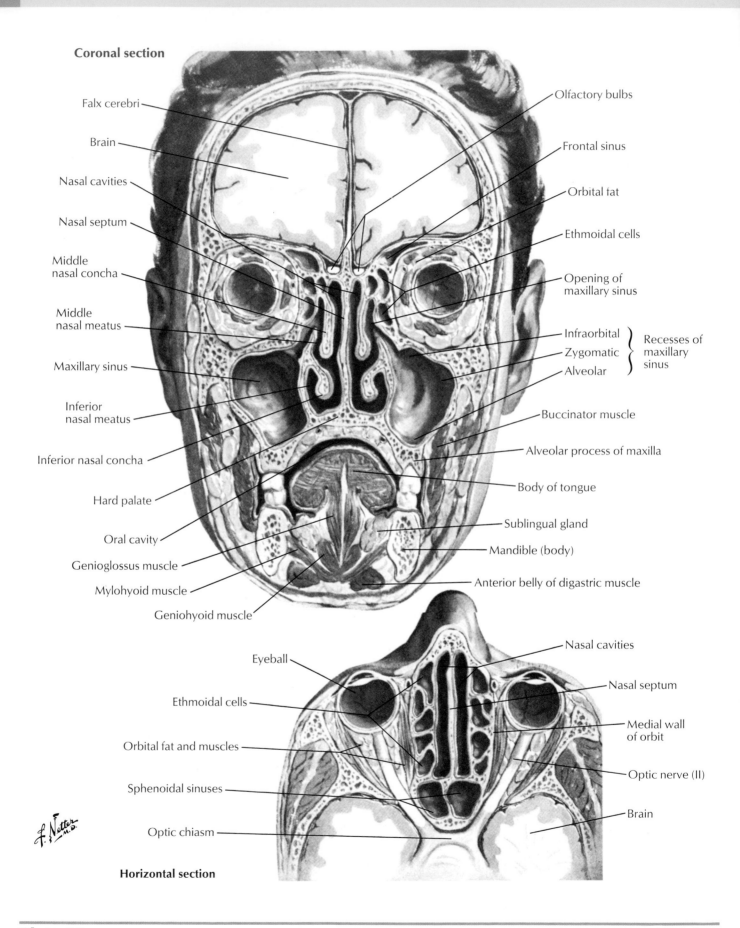

Coronal section

Falx cerebri

Brain

Nasal cavities

Nasal septum

Middle nasal concha

Middle nasal meatus

Maxillary sinus

Inferior nasal meatus

Inferior nasal concha

Hard palate

Oral cavity

Genioglossus muscle

Mylohyoid muscle

Geniohyoid muscle

Olfactory bulbs

Frontal sinus

Orbital fat

Ethmoidal cells

Opening of maxillary sinus

Infraorbital

Zygomatic — Recesses of maxillary sinus

Alveolar

Buccinator muscle

Alveolar process of maxilla

Body of tongue

Sublingual gland

Mandible (body)

Anterior belly of digastric muscle

Eyeball

Ethmoidal cells

Orbital fat and muscles

Sphenoidal sinuses

Optic chiasm

Nasal cavities

Nasal septum

Medial wall of orbit

Optic nerve (II)

Brain

Horizontal section

Plate 48   **Nasal Region**

Sagittal section

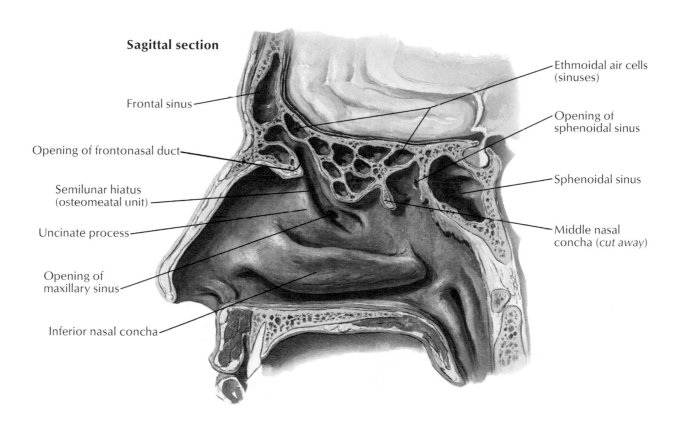

Frontal sinus

Opening of frontonasal duct

Semilunar hiatus
(osteomeatal unit)

Uncinate process

Opening of
maxillary sinus

Inferior nasal concha

Ethmoidal air cells
(sinuses)

Opening of
sphenoidal sinus

Sphenoidal sinus

Middle nasal
concha (cut away)

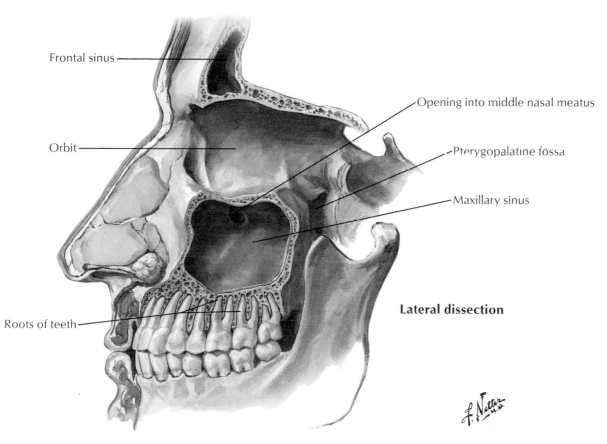

Frontal sinus

Orbit

Roots of teeth

Opening into middle nasal meatus

Pterygopalatine fossa

Maxillary sinus

Lateral dissection

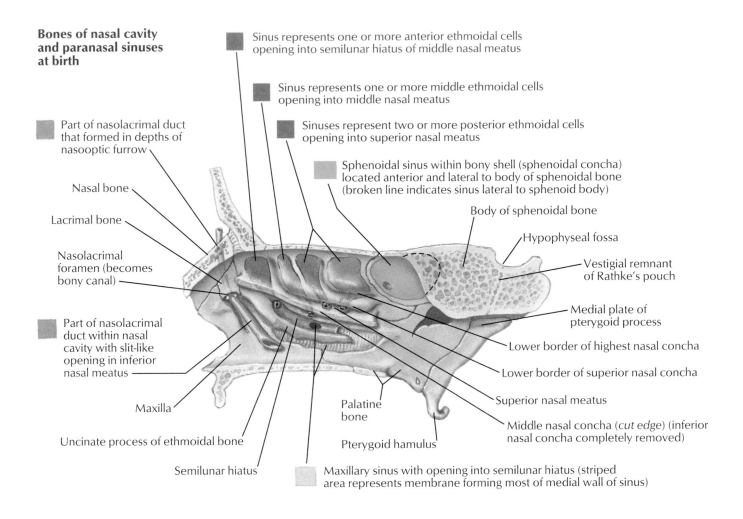

Bones of nasal cavity and paranasal sinuses at birth

Sinus represents one or more anterior ethmoidal cells opening into semilunar hiatus of middle nasal meatus

Sinus represents one or more middle ethmoidal cells opening into middle nasal meatus

Sinuses represent two or more posterior ethmoidal cells opening into superior nasal meatus

Sphenoidal sinus within bony shell (sphenoidal concha) located anterior and lateral to body of sphenoidal bone (broken line indicates sinus lateral to sphenoid body)

Part of nasolacrimal duct that formed in depths of nasooptic furrow

Nasal bone

Lacrimal bone

Nasolacrimal foramen (becomes bony canal)

Body of sphenoidal bone

Hypophyseal fossa

Vestigial remnant of Rathke's pouch

Medial plate of pterygoid process

Lower border of highest nasal concha

Part of nasolacrimal duct within nasal cavity with slit-like opening in inferior nasal meatus

Lower border of superior nasal concha

Maxilla

Superior nasal meatus

Middle nasal concha (*cut edge*) (inferior nasal concha completely removed)

Uncinate process of ethmoidal bone

Palatine bone

Pterygoid hamulus

Semilunar hiatus

Maxillary sinus with opening into semilunar hiatus (striped area represents membrane forming most of medial wall of sinus)

Growth of frontal and maxillary sinuses throughout life

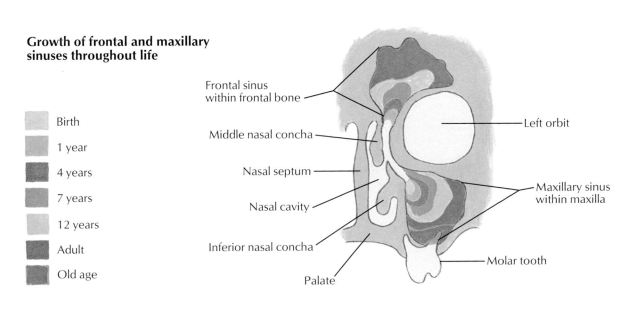

Birth

1 year

4 years

7 years

12 years

Adult

Old age

Frontal sinus within frontal bone

Left orbit

Middle nasal concha

Nasal septum

Nasal cavity

Maxillary sinus within maxilla

Inferior nasal concha

Molar tooth

Palate

Plate 50 **Nasal Region**

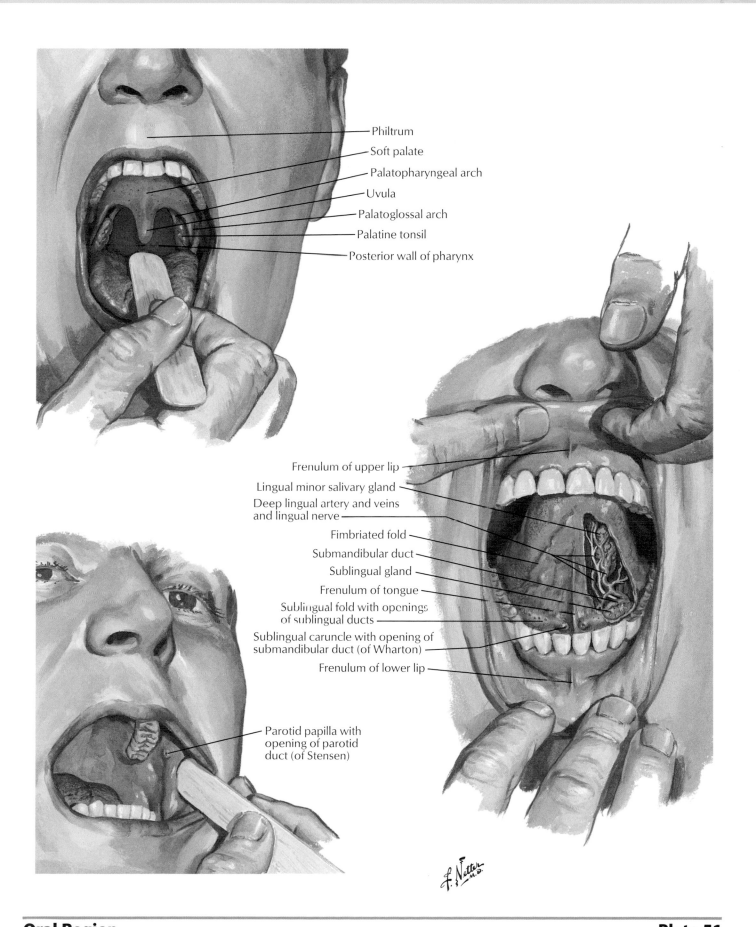

Philtrum
Soft palate
Palatopharyngeal arch
Uvula
Palatoglossal arch
Palatine tonsil
Posterior wall of pharynx

Frenulum of upper lip
Lingual minor salivary gland
Deep lingual artery and veins and lingual nerve
Fimbriated fold
Submandibular duct
Sublingual gland
Frenulum of tongue
Sublingual fold with openings of sublingual ducts
Sublingual caruncle with opening of submandibular duct (of Wharton)
Frenulum of lower lip

Parotid papilla with opening of parotid duct (of Stensen)

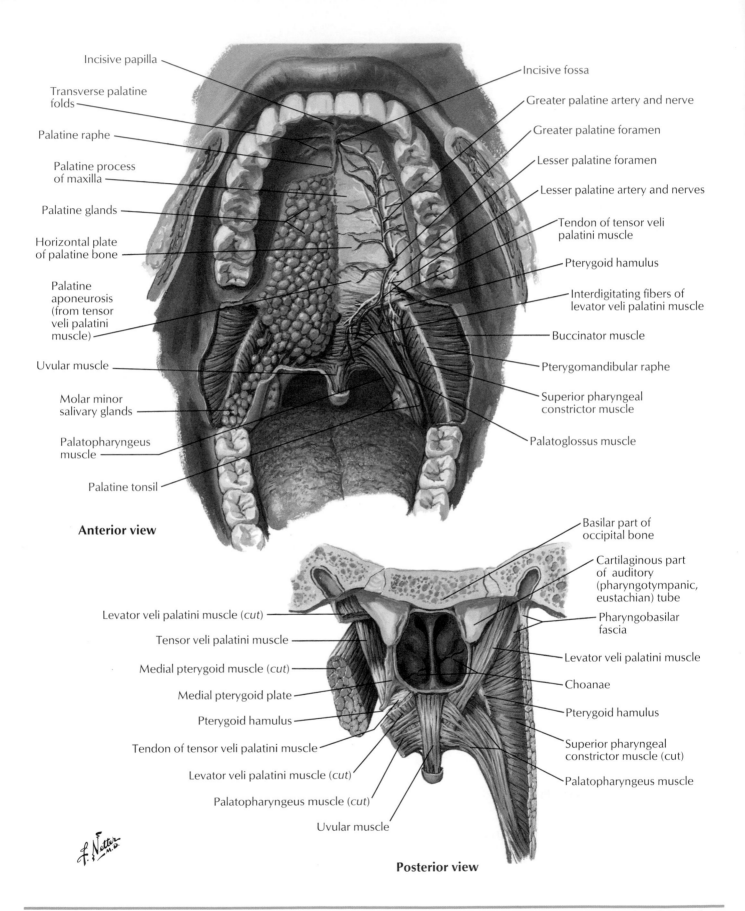

Incisive papilla

Transverse palatine folds

Palatine raphe

Palatine process of maxilla

Palatine glands

Horizontal plate of palatine bone

Palatine aponeurosis (from tensor veli palatini muscle)

Uvular muscle

Molar minor salivary glands

Palatopharyngeus muscle

Palatine tonsil

Incisive fossa

Greater palatine artery and nerve

Greater palatine foramen

Lesser palatine foramen

Lesser palatine artery and nerves

Tendon of tensor veli palatini muscle

Pterygoid hamulus

Interdigitating fibers of levator veli palatini muscle

Buccinator muscle

Pterygomandibular raphe

Superior pharyngeal constrictor muscle

Palatoglossus muscle

Anterior view

Levator veli palatini muscle (*cut*)

Tensor veli palatini muscle

Medial pterygoid muscle (*cut*)

Medial pterygoid plate

Pterygoid hamulus

Tendon of tensor veli palatini muscle

Levator veli palatini muscle (*cut*)

Palatopharyngeus muscle (*cut*)

Uvular muscle

Basilar part of occipital bone

Cartilaginous part of auditory (pharyngotympanic, eustachian) tube

Pharyngobasilar fascia

Levator veli palatini muscle

Choanae

Pterygoid hamulus

Superior pharyngeal constrictor muscle (cut)

Palatopharyngeus muscle

Posterior view

Plate 52   **Oral Region**

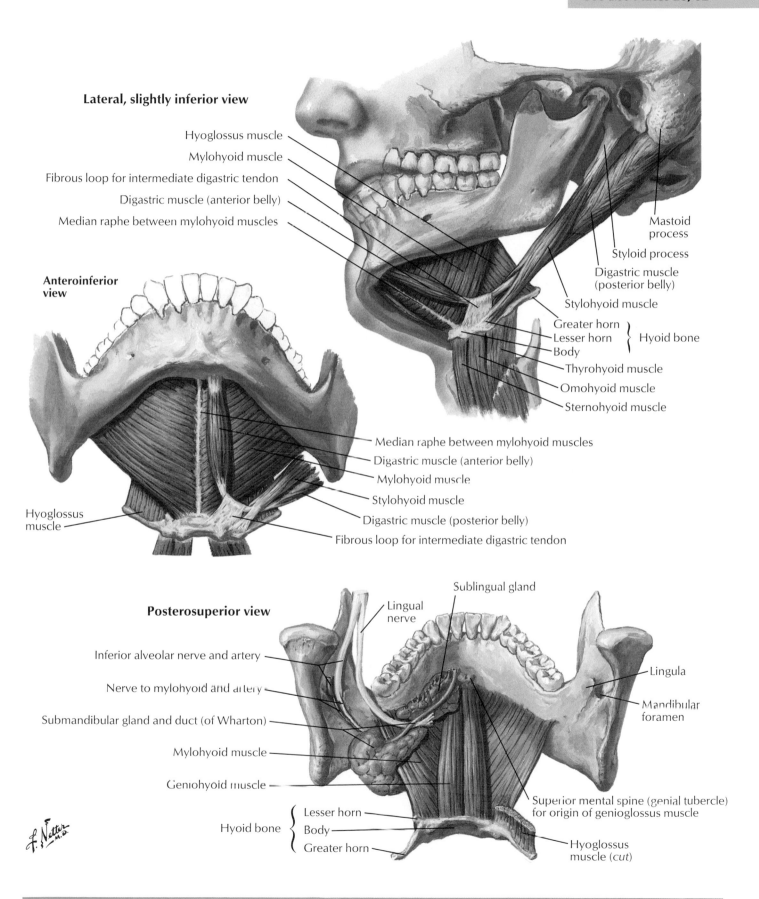

Lateral, slightly inferior view

Hyoglossus muscle

Mylohyoid muscle

Fibrous loop for intermediate digastric tendon

Digastric muscle (anterior belly)

Median raphe between mylohyoid muscles

Mastoid process

Styloid process

Digastric muscle (posterior belly)

Stylohyoid muscle

Greater horn
Lesser horn } Hyoid bone
Body

Thyrohyoid muscle

Omohyoid muscle

Sternohyoid muscle

Anteroinferior view

Hyoglossus muscle

Median raphe between mylohyoid muscles

Digastric muscle (anterior belly)

Mylohyoid muscle

Stylohyoid muscle

Digastric muscle (posterior belly)

Fibrous loop for intermediate digastric tendon

Posterosuperior view

Sublingual gland

Lingual nerve

Inferior alveolar nerve and artery

Nerve to mylohyoid and artery

Submandibular gland and duct (of Wharton)

Mylohyoid muscle

Geniohyoid muscle

Lingula

Mandibular foramen

Superior mental spine (genial tubercle) for origin of genioglossus muscle

Hyoglossus muscle (*cut*)

Hyoid bone { Lesser horn
Body
Greater horn

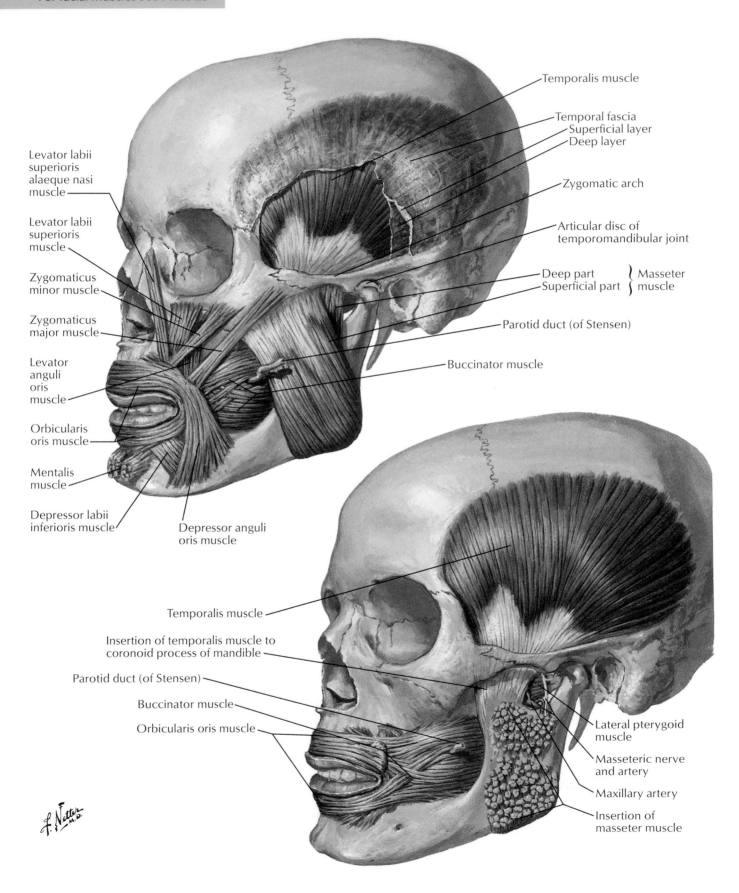

Temporalis muscle

Temporal fascia
Superficial layer
Deep layer

Zygomatic arch

Articular disc of
temporomandibular joint

Deep part } Masseter
Superficial part } muscle

Parotid duct (of Stensen)

Buccinator muscle

Levator labii
superioris
alaeque nasi
muscle

Levator labii
superioris
muscle

Zygomaticus
minor muscle

Zygomaticus
major muscle

Levator
anguli
oris
muscle

Orbicularis
oris muscle

Mentalis
muscle

Depressor labii
inferioris muscle

Depressor anguli
oris muscle

Temporalis muscle

Insertion of temporalis muscle to
coronoid process of mandible

Parotid duct (of Stensen)

Buccinator muscle

Orbicularis oris muscle

Lateral pterygoid
muscle

Masseteric nerve
and artery

Maxillary artery

Insertion of
masseter muscle

Plate 54

Oral Region

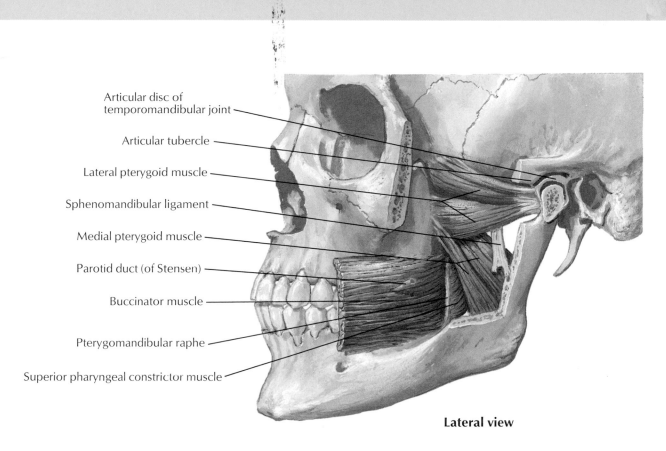

Articular disc of temporomandibular joint

Articular tubercle

Lateral pterygoid muscle

Sphenomandibular ligament

Medial pterygoid muscle

Parotid duct (of Stensen)

Buccinator muscle

Pterygomandibular raphe

Superior pharyngeal constrictor muscle

Lateral view

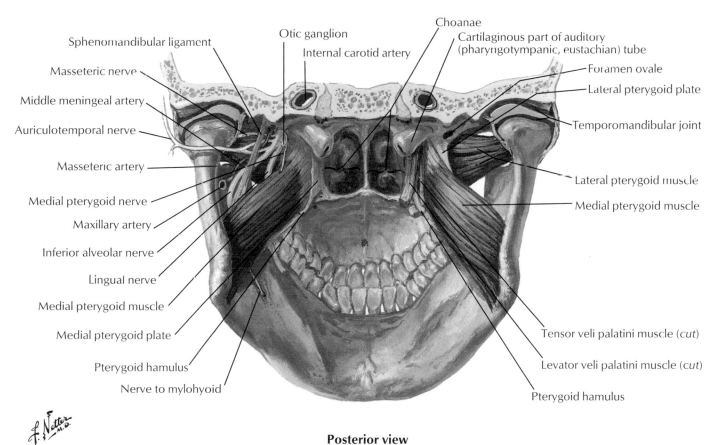

Sphenomandibular ligament

Masseteric nerve

Middle meningeal artery

Auriculotemporal nerve

Masseteric artery

Medial pterygoid nerve

Maxillary artery

Inferior alveolar nerve

Lingual nerve

Medial pterygoid muscle

Medial pterygoid plate

Pterygoid hamulus

Nerve to mylohyoid

Otic ganglion

Internal carotid artery

Choanae

Cartilaginous part of auditory (pharyngotympanic, eustachian) tube

Foramen ovale

Lateral pterygoid plate

Temporomandibular joint

Lateral pterygoid muscle

Medial pterygoid muscle

Tensor veli palatini muscle (*cut*)

Levator veli palatini muscle (*cut*)

Pterygoid hamulus

Posterior view

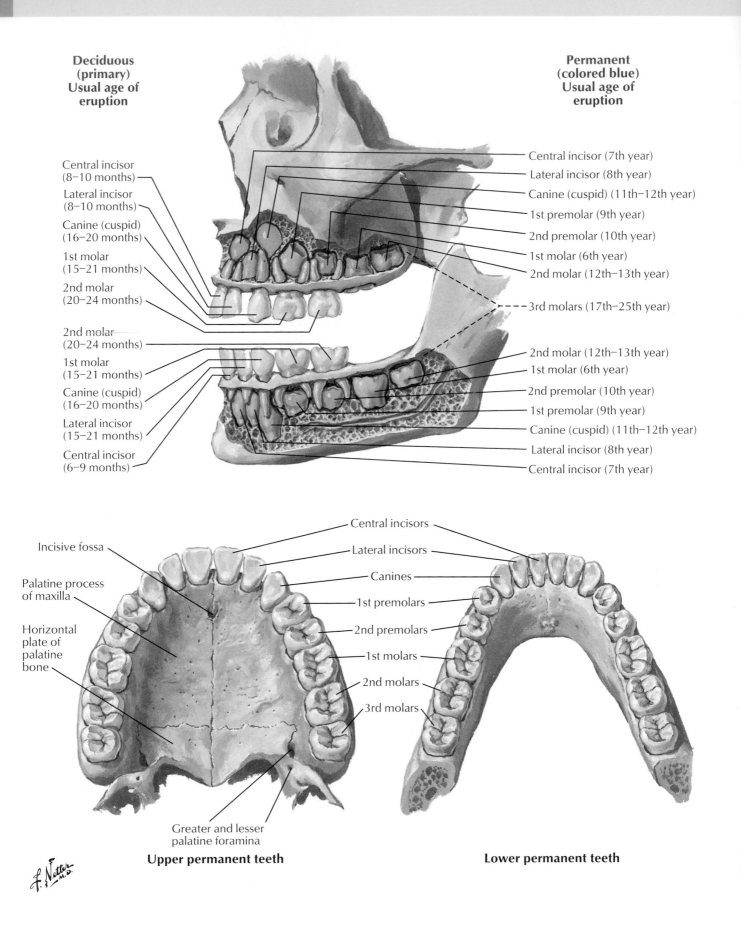

Deciduous (primary) Usual age of eruption

Central incisor (8–10 months)
Lateral incisor (8–10 months)
Canine (cuspid) (16–20 months)
1st molar (15–21 months)
2nd molar (20–24 months)

2nd molar (20–24 months)
1st molar (15–21 months)
Canine (cuspid) (16–20 months)
Lateral incisor (15–21 months)
Central incisor (6–9 months)

Permanent (colored blue) Usual age of eruption

Central incisor (7th year)
Lateral incisor (8th year)
Canine (cuspid) (11th–12th year)
1st premolar (9th year)
2nd premolar (10th year)
1st molar (6th year)
2nd molar (12th–13th year)
3rd molars (17th–25th year)
2nd molar (12th–13th year)
1st molar (6th year)
2nd premolar (10th year)
1st premolar (9th year)
Canine (cuspid) (11th–12th year)
Lateral incisor (8th year)
Central incisor (7th year)

Incisive fossa
Palatine process of maxilla
Horizontal plate of palatine bone
Greater and lesser palatine foramina

Central incisors
Lateral incisors
Canines
1st premolars
2nd premolars
1st molars
2nd molars
3rd molars

Upper permanent teeth

Lower permanent teeth

Plate 56

Oral Region

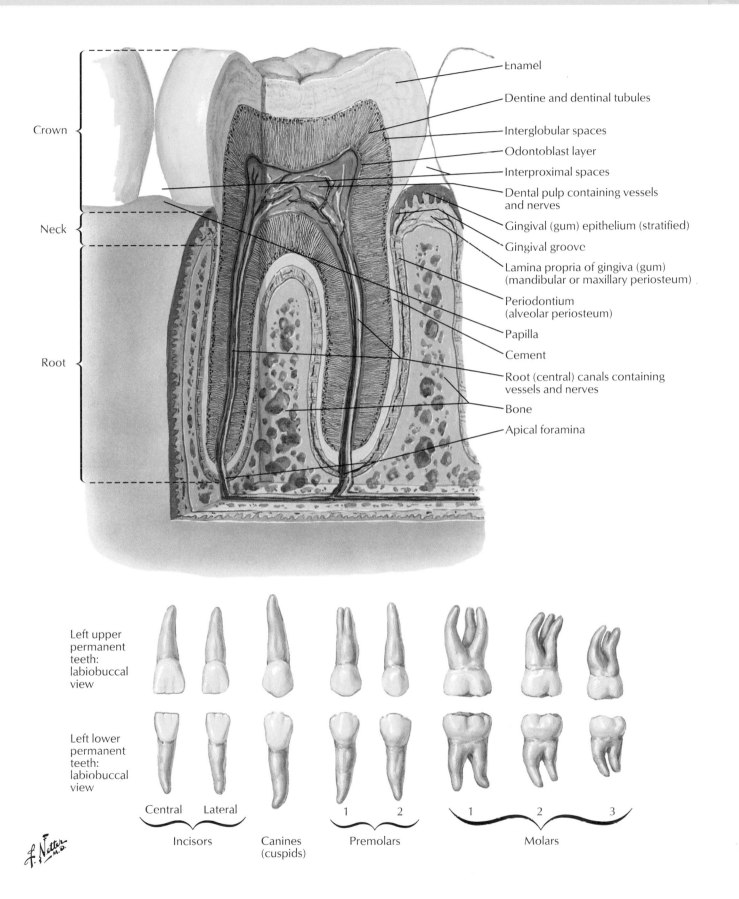

Crown

Neck

Root

Enamel

Dentine and dentinal tubules

Interglobular spaces

Odontoblast layer

Interproximal spaces

Dental pulp containing vessels and nerves

Gingival (gum) epithelium (stratified)

Gingival groove

Lamina propria of gingiva (gum) (mandibular or maxillary periosteum)

Periodontium (alveolar periosteum)

Papilla

Cement

Root (central) canals containing vessels and nerves

Bone

Apical foramina

Left upper permanent teeth: labiobuccal view

Left lower permanent teeth: labiobuccal view

Central   Lateral

Incisors

Canines (cuspids)

1   2

Premolars

1   2   3

Molars

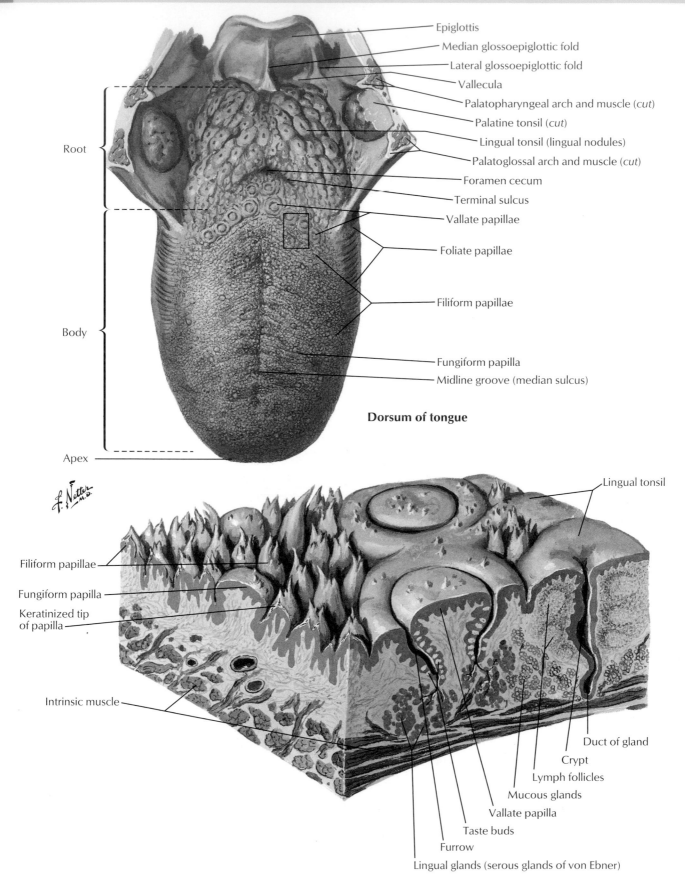

Epiglottis

Median glossoepiglottic fold

Lateral glossoepiglottic fold

Vallecula

Palatopharyngeal arch and muscle (*cut*)

Palatine tonsil (*cut*)

Lingual tonsil (lingual nodules)

Palatoglossal arch and muscle (*cut*)

Foramen cecum

Terminal sulcus

Vallate papillae

Foliate papillae

Filiform papillae

Fungiform papilla

Midline groove (median sulcus)

Root

Body

Apex

Dorsum of tongue

Lingual tonsil

Filiform papillae

Fungiform papilla

Keratinized tip of papilla

Intrinsic muscle

Duct of gland

Crypt

Lymph follicles

Mucous glands

Vallate papilla

Taste buds

Furrow

Lingual glands (serous glands of von Ebner)

Schematic stereogram: area indicated above

Plate 58

Oral Region

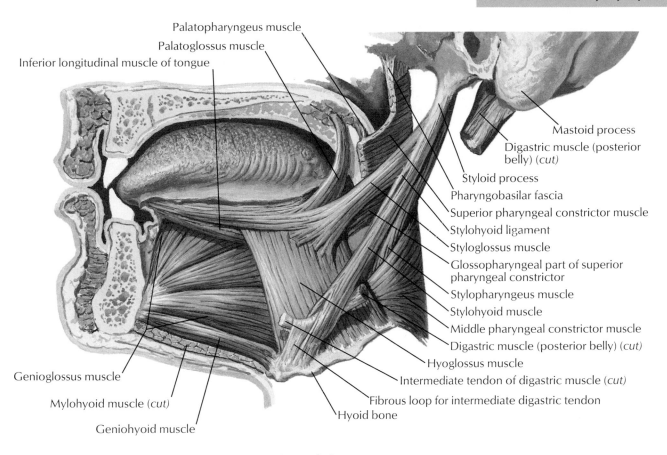

Palatopharyngeus muscle

Palatoglossus muscle

Inferior longitudinal muscle of tongue

Mastoid process

Digastric muscle (posterior belly) (*cut*)

Styloid process

Pharyngobasilar fascia

Superior pharyngeal constrictor muscle

Stylohyoid ligament

Styloglossus muscle

Glossopharyngeal part of superior pharyngeal constrictor

Stylopharyngeus muscle

Stylohyoid muscle

Middle pharyngeal constrictor muscle

Digastric muscle (posterior belly) (*cut*)

Hyoglossus muscle

Intermediate tendon of digastric muscle (*cut*)

Fibrous loop for intermediate digastric tendon

Hyoid bone

Genioglossus muscle

Mylohyoid muscle (*cut*)

Geniohyoid muscle

Lateral view

Lingual nerve

Submandibular ganglion

Deep lingual artery and venae comitantes

Artery to frenulum

Submandibular duct (of Wharton)

Genioglossus muscle

Sublingual artery and vein

Geniohyoid muscle

Hyoid bone

Hypoglossal nerve (XII)

Vena comitans of hypoglossal nerve

Dorsal lingual artery and vein

Suprahyoid artery

Superior pharyngeal constrictor muscle

Styloglossus muscle

Palatoglossus muscle (*cut*)

Stylohyoid ligament

Stylopharyngeus muscle

Hyoglossus muscle (*cut*)

Lingual artery

External carotid artery

Internal jugular vein

Retromandibular vein

Facial vein

Common trunk for facial, retromandibular, and lingual veins (common facial vein)

Lingual vein

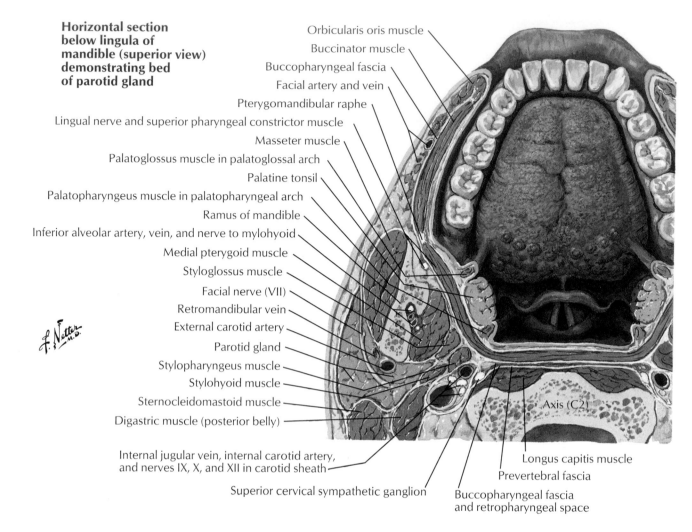

Horizontal section below lingula of mandible (superior view) demonstrating bed of parotid gland

Orbicularis oris muscle

Buccinator muscle

Buccopharyngeal fascia

Facial artery and vein

Pterygomandibular raphe

Lingual nerve and superior pharyngeal constrictor muscle

Masseter muscle

Palatoglossus muscle in palatoglossal arch

Palatine tonsil

Palatopharyngeus muscle in palatopharyngeal arch

Ramus of mandible

Inferior alveolar artery, vein, and nerve to mylohyoid

Medial pterygoid muscle

Styloglossus muscle

Facial nerve (VII)

Retromandibular vein

External carotid artery

Parotid gland

Stylopharyngeus muscle

Stylohyoid muscle

Sternocleidomastoid muscle

Digastric muscle (posterior belly)

Internal jugular vein, internal carotid artery, and nerves IX, X, and XII in carotid sheath

Superior cervical sympathetic ganglion

Axis (C2)

Longus capitis muscle

Prevertebral fascia

Buccopharyngeal fascia and retropharyngeal space

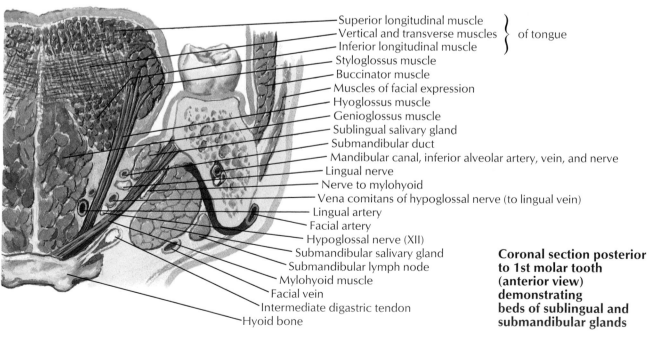

Superior longitudinal muscle

Vertical and transverse muscles } of tongue

Inferior longitudinal muscle

Styloglossus muscle

Buccinator muscle

Muscles of facial expression

Hyoglossus muscle

Genioglossus muscle

Sublingual salivary gland

Submandibular duct

Mandibular canal, inferior alveolar artery, vein, and nerve

Lingual nerve

Nerve to mylohyoid

Vena comitans of hypoglossal nerve (to lingual vein)

Lingual artery

Facial artery

Hypoglossal nerve (XII)

Submandibular salivary gland

Submandibular lymph node

Mylohyoid muscle

Facial vein

Intermediate digastric tendon

Hyoid bone

Coronal section posterior to 1st molar tooth (anterior view) demonstrating beds of sublingual and submandibular glands

Plate 60

Oral Region

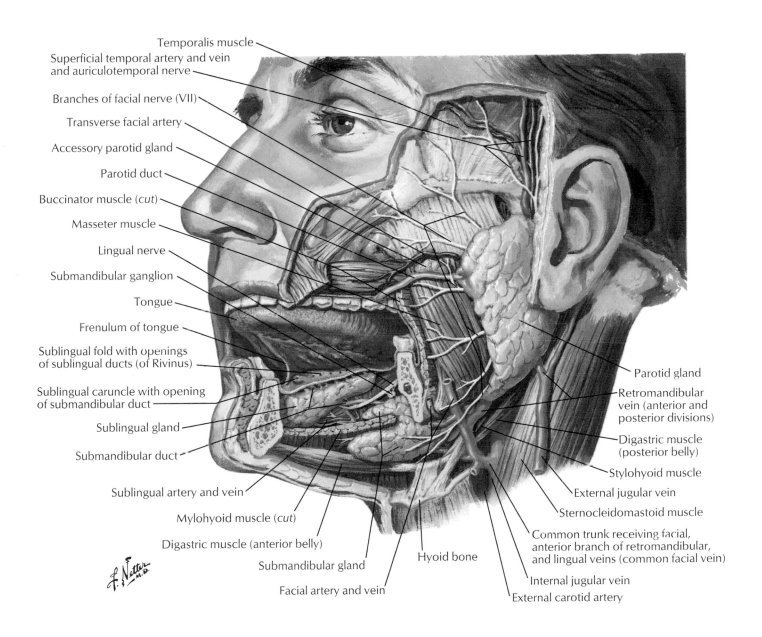

Temporalis muscle

Superficial temporal artery and vein and auriculotemporal nerve

Branches of facial nerve (VII)

Transverse facial artery

Accessory parotid gland

Parotid duct

Buccinator muscle (*cut*)

Masseter muscle

Lingual nerve

Submandibular ganglion

Tongue

Frenulum of tongue

Sublingual fold with openings of sublingual ducts (of Rivinus)

Sublingual caruncle with opening of submandibular duct

Sublingual gland

Submandibular duct

Sublingual artery and vein

Mylohyoid muscle (*cut*)

Digastric muscle (anterior belly)

Submandibular gland

Facial artery and vein

Hyoid bone

Parotid gland

Retromandibular vein (anterior and posterior divisions)

Digastric muscle (posterior belly)

Stylohyoid muscle

External jugular vein

Sternocleidomastoid muscle

Common trunk receiving facial, anterior branch of retromandibular, and lingual veins (common facial vein)

Internal jugular vein

External carotid artery

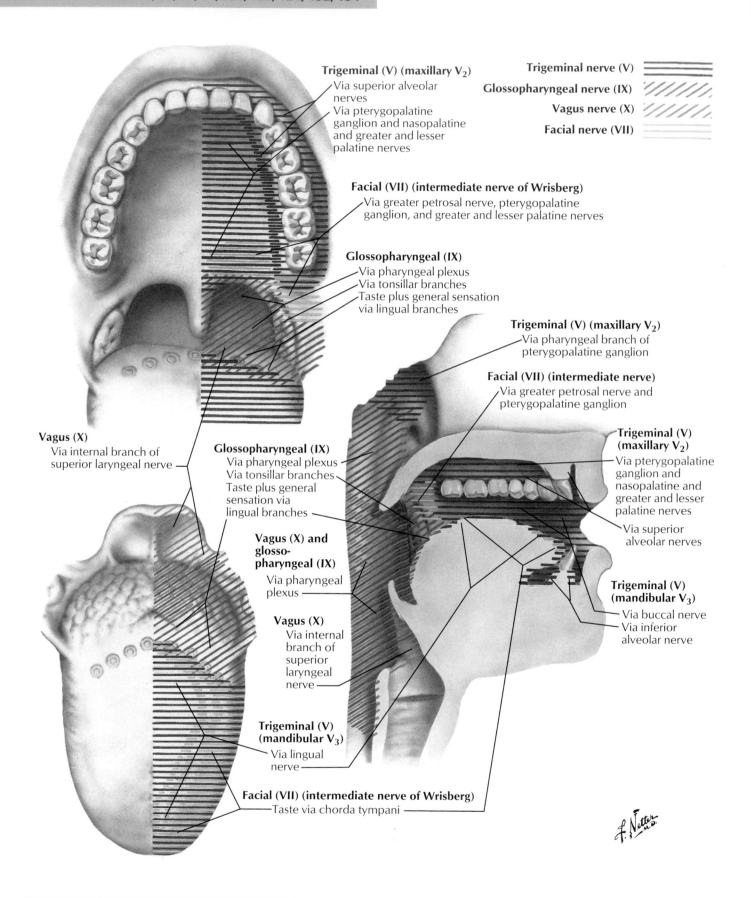

Trigeminal (V) (maxillary V₂)
Via superior alveolar nerves
Via pterygopalatine ganglion and nasopalatine and greater and lesser palatine nerves

Facial (VII) (intermediate nerve of Wrisberg)
Via greater petrosal nerve, pterygopalatine ganglion, and greater and lesser palatine nerves

Glossopharyngeal (IX)
Via pharyngeal plexus
Via tonsillar branches
Taste plus general sensation via lingual branches

Trigeminal (V) (maxillary V₂)
Via pharyngeal branch of pterygopalatine ganglion

Facial (VII) (intermediate nerve)
Via greater petrosal nerve and pterygopalatine ganglion

Trigeminal (V) (maxillary V₂)
Via pterygopalatine ganglion and nasopalatine and greater and lesser palatine nerves
Via superior alveolar nerves

Vagus (X)
Via internal branch of superior laryngeal nerve

Glossopharyngeal (IX)
Via pharyngeal plexus
Via tonsillar branches
Taste plus general sensation via lingual branches

Vagus (X) and glosso-pharyngeal (IX)
Via pharyngeal plexus

Vagus (X)
Via internal branch of superior laryngeal nerve

Trigeminal (V) (mandibular V₃)
Via buccal nerve
Via inferior alveolar nerve

Trigeminal (V) (mandibular V₃)
Via lingual nerve

Facial (VII) (intermediate nerve of Wrisberg)
Taste via chorda tympani

Trigeminal nerve (V)
Glossopharyngeal nerve (IX)
Vagus nerve (X)
Facial nerve (VII)

Plate 62

Oral Region

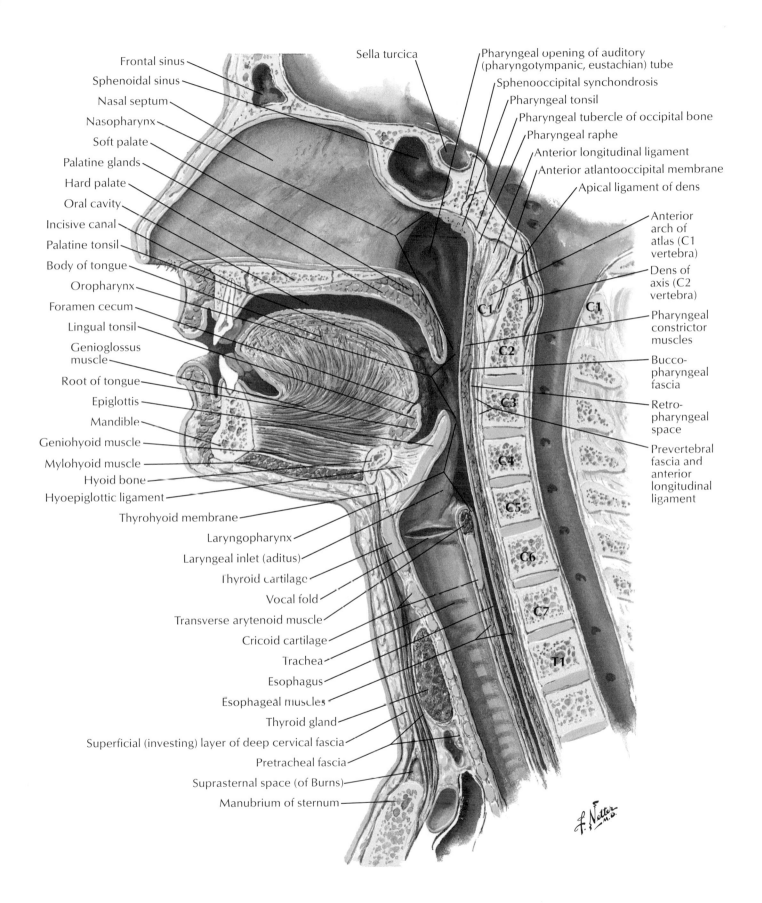

Frontal sinus

Sphenoidal sinus

Nasal septum

Nasopharynx

Soft palate

Palatine glands

Hard palate

Oral cavity

Incisive canal

Palatine tonsil

Body of tongue

Oropharynx

Foramen cecum

Lingual tonsil

Genioglossus muscle

Root of tongue

Epiglottis

Mandible

Geniohyoid muscle

Mylohyoid muscle

Hyoid bone

Hyoepiglottic ligament

Thyrohyoid membrane

Laryngopharynx

Laryngeal inlet (aditus)

Thyroid cartilage

Vocal fold

Transverse arytenoid muscle

Cricoid cartilage

Trachea

Esophagus

Esophageal muscles

Thyroid gland

Superficial (investing) layer of deep cervical fascia

Pretracheal fascia

Suprasternal space (of Burns)

Manubrium of sternum

Sella turcica

Pharyngeal opening of auditory (pharyngotympanic, eustachian) tube

Sphenooccipital synchondrosis

Pharyngeal tonsil

Pharyngeal tubercle of occipital bone

Pharyngeal raphe

Anterior longitudinal ligament

Anterior atlantooccipital membrane

Apical ligament of dens

Anterior arch of atlas (C1 vertebra)

Dens of axis (C2 vertebra)

Pharyngeal constrictor muscles

Bucco-pharyngeal fascia

Retro-pharyngeal space

Prevertebral fascia and anterior longitudinal ligament

C1

C2

C3

C4

C5

C6

C7

T1

C1

f. Netter m.d.

**Medial view
sagittal section**

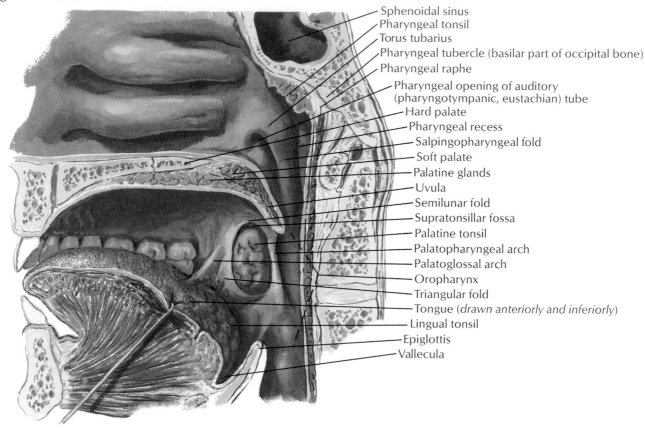

Sphenoidal sinus
Pharyngeal tonsil
Torus tubarius
Pharyngeal tubercle (basilar part of occipital bone)
Pharyngeal raphe
Pharyngeal opening of auditory
(pharyngotympanic, eustachian) tube
Hard palate
Pharyngeal recess
Salpingopharyngeal fold
Soft palate
Palatine glands
Uvula
Semilunar fold
Supratonsillar fossa
Palatine tonsil
Palatopharyngeal arch
Palatoglossal arch
Oropharynx
Triangular fold
Tongue (*drawn anteriorly and inferiorly*)
Lingual tonsil
Epiglottis
Vallecula

Pharyngeal mucosa removed

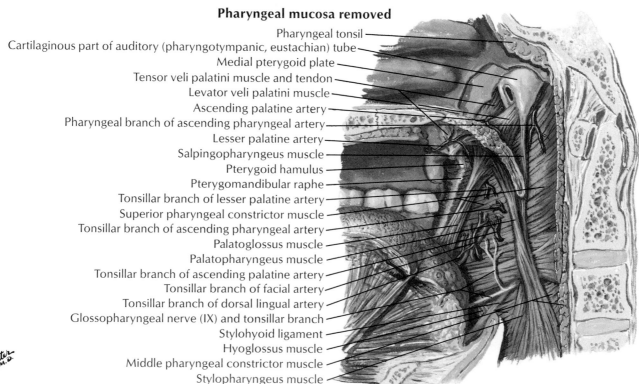

Pharyngeal tonsil
Cartilaginous part of auditory (pharyngotympanic, eustachian) tube
Medial pterygoid plate
Tensor veli palatini muscle and tendon
Levator veli palatini muscle
Ascending palatine artery
Pharyngeal branch of ascending pharyngeal artery
Lesser palatine artery
Salpingopharyngeus muscle
Pterygoid hamulus
Pterygomandibular raphe
Tonsillar branch of lesser palatine artery
Superior pharyngeal constrictor muscle
Tonsillar branch of ascending pharyngeal artery
Palatoglossus muscle
Palatopharyngeus muscle
Tonsillar branch of ascending palatine artery
Tonsillar branch of facial artery
Tonsillar branch of dorsal lingual artery
Glossopharyngeal nerve (IX) and tonsillar branch
Stylohyoid ligament
Hyoglossus muscle
Middle pharyngeal constrictor muscle
Stylopharyngeus muscle

Plate 64

Pharynx

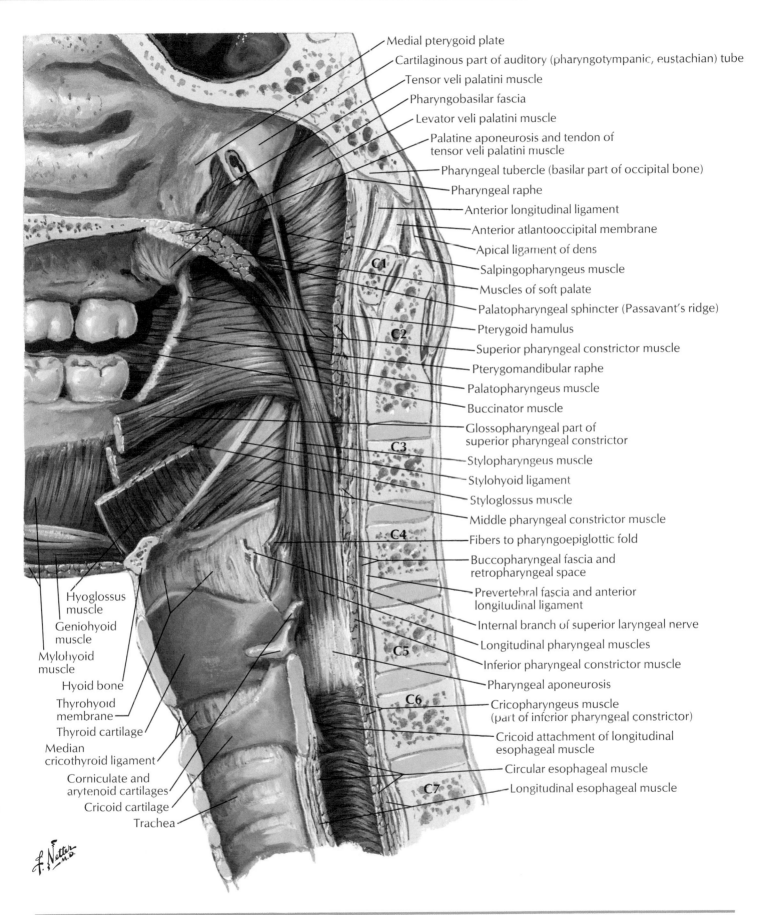

Medial pterygoid plate

Cartilaginous part of auditory (pharyngotympanic, eustachian) tube

Tensor veli palatini muscle

Pharyngobasilar fascia

Levator veli palatini muscle

Palatine aponeurosis and tendon of tensor veli palatini muscle

Pharyngeal tubercle (basilar part of occipital bone)

Pharyngeal raphe

Anterior longitudinal ligament

Anterior atlantooccipital membrane

Apical ligament of dens

Salpingopharyngeus muscle

Muscles of soft palate

Palatopharyngeal sphincter (Passavant's ridge)

Pterygoid hamulus

Superior pharyngeal constrictor muscle

Pterygomandibular raphe

Palatopharyngeus muscle

Buccinator muscle

Glossopharyngeal part of superior pharyngeal constrictor

Stylopharyngeus muscle

Stylohyoid ligament

Styloglossus muscle

Middle pharyngeal constrictor muscle

Fibers to pharyngoepiglottic fold

Buccopharyngeal fascia and retropharyngeal space

Prevertebral fascia and anterior longitudinal ligament

Internal branch of superior laryngeal nerve

Longitudinal pharyngeal muscles

Inferior pharyngeal constrictor muscle

Pharyngeal aponeurosis

Cricopharyngeus muscle (part of inferior pharyngeal constrictor)

Cricoid attachment of longitudinal esophageal muscle

Circular esophageal muscle

Longitudinal esophageal muscle

Hyoglossus muscle

Geniohyoid muscle

Mylohyoid muscle

Hyoid bone

Thyrohyoid membrane

Thyroid cartilage

Median cricothyroid ligament

Corniculate and arytenoid cartilages

Cricoid cartilage

Trachea

C1

C2

C3

C4

C5

C6

C7

Pharynx

Plate 65

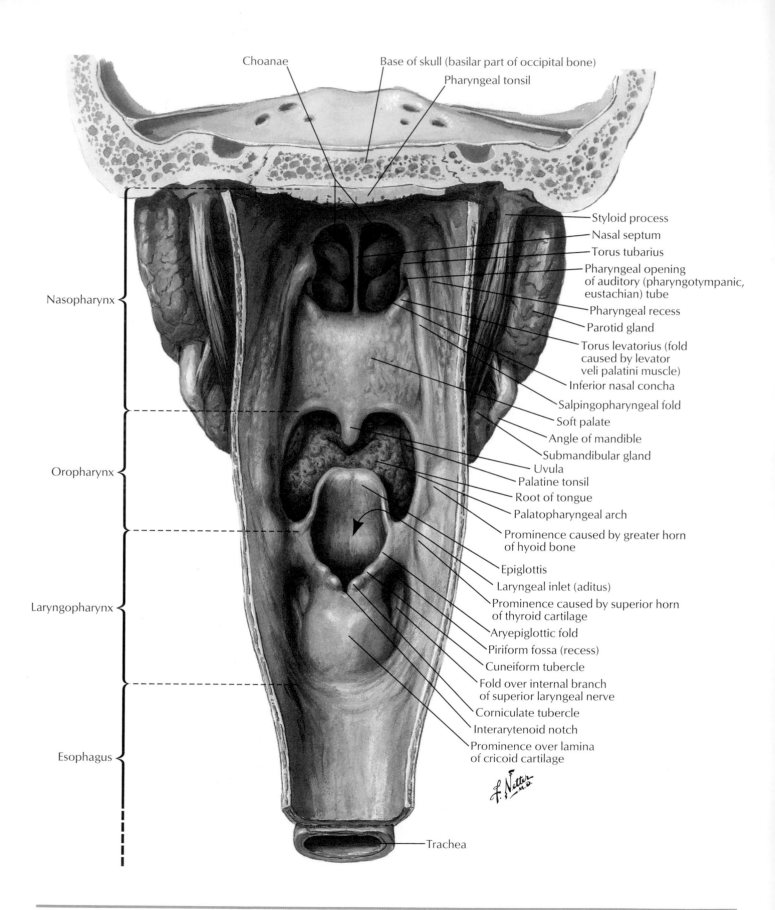

Choanae

Base of skull (basilar part of occipital bone)

Pharyngeal tonsil

Styloid process

Nasal septum

Torus tubarius

Pharyngeal opening of auditory (pharyngotympanic, eustachian) tube

Pharyngeal recess

Parotid gland

Torus levatorius (fold caused by levator veli palatini muscle)

Inferior nasal concha

Salpingopharyngeal fold

Soft palate

Angle of mandible

Submandibular gland

Uvula

Palatine tonsil

Root of tongue

Palatopharyngeal arch

Prominence caused by greater horn of hyoid bone

Epiglottis

Laryngeal inlet (aditus)

Prominence caused by superior horn of thyroid cartilage

Aryepiglottic fold

Piriform fossa (recess)

Cuneiform tubercle

Fold over internal branch of superior laryngeal nerve

Corniculate tubercle

Interarytenoid notch

Prominence over lamina of cricoid cartilage

Trachea

Nasopharynx

Oropharynx

Laryngopharynx

Esophagus

Plate 66   **Pharynx**

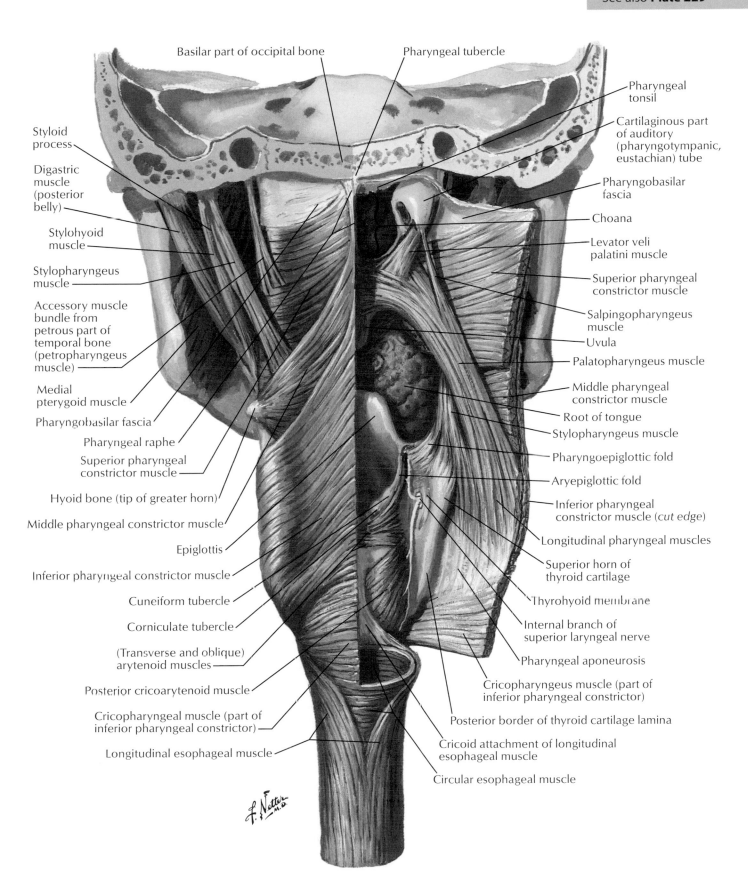

Basilar part of occipital bone

Pharyngeal tubercle

Pharyngeal tonsil

Cartilaginous part of auditory (pharyngotympanic, eustachian) tube

Styloid process

Digastric muscle (posterior belly)

Stylohyoid muscle

Stylopharyngeus muscle

Accessory muscle bundle from petrous part of temporal bone (petropharyngeus muscle)

Medial pterygoid muscle

Pharyngobasilar fascia

Pharyngeal raphe

Superior pharyngeal constrictor muscle

Hyoid bone (tip of greater horn)

Middle pharyngeal constrictor muscle

Epiglottis

Inferior pharyngeal constrictor muscle

Cuneiform tubercle

Corniculate tubercle

(Transverse and oblique) arytenoid muscles

Posterior cricoarytenoid muscle

Cricopharyngeal muscle (part of inferior pharyngeal constrictor)

Longitudinal esophageal muscle

Pharyngobasilar fascia

Choana

Levator veli palatini muscle

Superior pharyngeal constrictor muscle

Salpingopharyngeus muscle

Uvula

Palatopharyngeus muscle

Middle pharyngeal constrictor muscle

Root of tongue

Stylopharyngeus muscle

Pharyngoepiglottic fold

Aryepiglottic fold

Inferior pharyngeal constrictor muscle (*cut edge*)

Longitudinal pharyngeal muscles

Superior horn of thyroid cartilage

Thyrohyoid membrane

Internal branch of superior laryngeal nerve

Pharyngeal aponeurosis

Cricopharyngeus muscle (part of inferior pharyngeal constrictor)

Posterior border of thyroid cartilage lamina

Cricoid attachment of longitudinal esophageal muscle

Circular esophageal muscle

Muscles of Pharynx: Lateral View

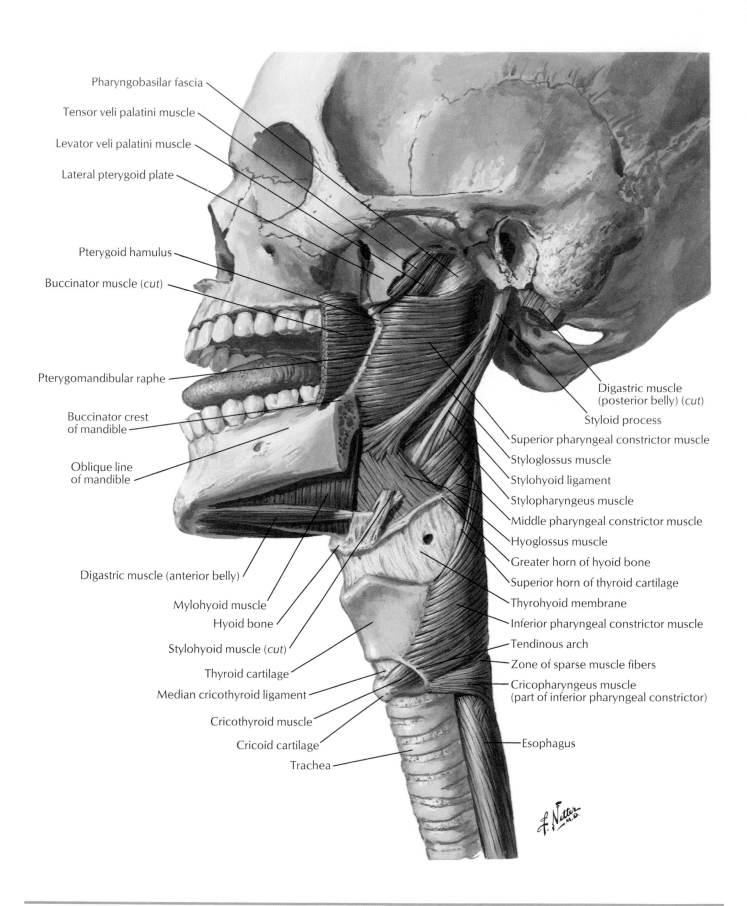

Pharyngobasilar fascia

Tensor veli palatini muscle

Levator veli palatini muscle

Lateral pterygoid plate

Pterygoid hamulus

Buccinator muscle (*cut*)

Pterygomandibular raphe

Buccinator crest
of mandible

Oblique line
of mandible

Digastric muscle (anterior belly)

Mylohyoid muscle

Hyoid bone

Stylohyoid muscle (*cut*)

Thyroid cartilage

Median cricothyroid ligament

Cricothyroid muscle

Cricoid cartilage

Trachea

Digastric muscle
(posterior belly) (*cut*)

Styloid process

Superior pharyngeal constrictor muscle

Styloglossus muscle

Stylohyoid ligament

Stylopharyngeus muscle

Middle pharyngeal constrictor muscle

Hyoglossus muscle

Greater horn of hyoid bone

Superior horn of thyroid cartilage

Thyrohyoid membrane

Inferior pharyngeal constrictor muscle

Tendinous arch

Zone of sparse muscle fibers

Cricopharyngeus muscle
(part of inferior pharyngeal constrictor)

Esophagus

Plate 68　　　　　　　　　　　　　　　　　　　　　　　　　　　**Pharynx**

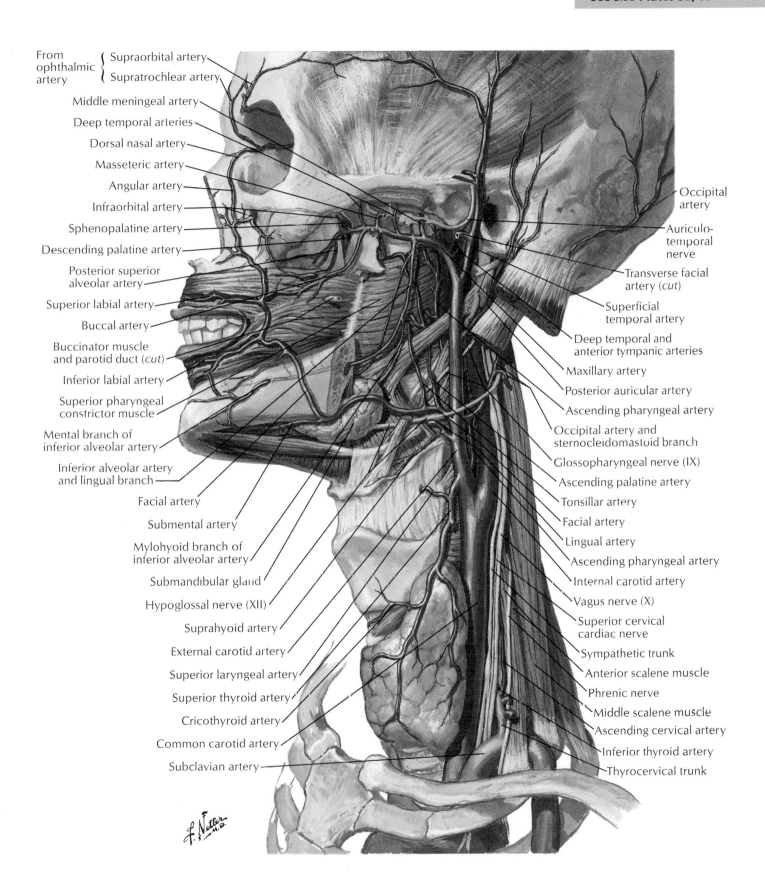

From ophthalmic artery
{ Supraorbital artery
{ Supratrochlear artery

Middle meningeal artery

Deep temporal arteries

Dorsal nasal artery

Masseteric artery

Angular artery

Infraorbital artery

Sphenopalatine artery

Descending palatine artery

Posterior superior alveolar artery

Superior labial artery

Buccal artery

Buccinator muscle and parotid duct (cut)

Inferior labial artery

Superior pharyngeal constrictor muscle

Mental branch of inferior alveolar artery

Inferior alveolar artery and lingual branch

Facial artery

Submental artery

Mylohyoid branch of inferior alveolar artery

Submandibular gland

Hypoglossal nerve (XII)

Suprahyoid artery

External carotid artery

Superior laryngeal artery

Superior thyroid artery

Cricothyroid artery

Common carotid artery

Subclavian artery

Occipital artery

Auriculo-temporal nerve

Transverse facial artery (cut)

Superficial temporal artery

Deep temporal and anterior tympanic arteries

Maxillary artery

Posterior auricular artery

Ascending pharyngeal artery

Occipital artery and sternocleidomastoid branch

Glossopharyngeal nerve (IX)

Ascending palatine artery

Tonsillar artery

Facial artery

Lingual artery

Ascending pharyngeal artery

Internal carotid artery

Vagus nerve (X)

Superior cervical cardiac nerve

Sympathetic trunk

Anterior scalene muscle

Phrenic nerve

Middle scalene muscle

Ascending cervical artery

Inferior thyroid artery

Thyrocervical trunk

Pharynx

Plate 69

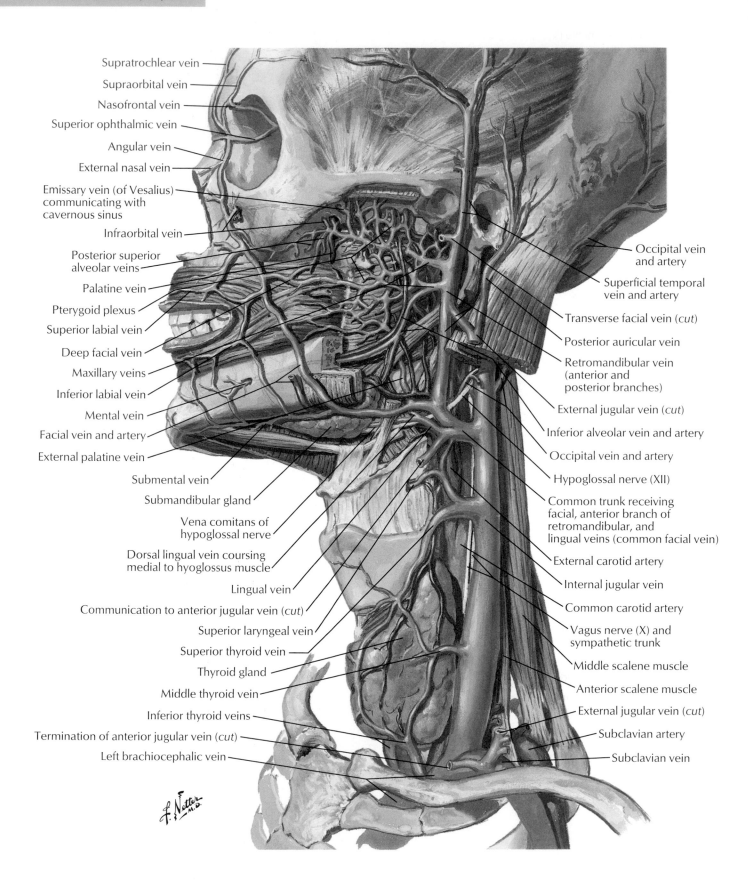

Supratrochlear vein

Supraorbital vein

Nasofrontal vein

Superior ophthalmic vein

Angular vein

External nasal vein

Emissary vein (of Vesalius) communicating with cavernous sinus

Infraorbital vein

Posterior superior alveolar veins

Palatine vein

Pterygoid plexus

Superior labial vein

Deep facial vein

Maxillary veins

Inferior labial vein

Mental vein

Facial vein and artery

External palatine vein

Submental vein

Submandibular gland

Vena comitans of hypoglossal nerve

Dorsal lingual vein coursing medial to hyoglossus muscle

Lingual vein

Communication to anterior jugular vein (cut)

Superior laryngeal vein

Superior thyroid vein

Thyroid gland

Middle thyroid vein

Inferior thyroid veins

Termination of anterior jugular vein (cut)

Left brachiocephalic vein

Occipital vein and artery

Superficial temporal vein and artery

Transverse facial vein (cut)

Posterior auricular vein

Retromandibular vein (anterior and posterior branches)

External jugular vein (cut)

Inferior alveolar vein and artery

Occipital vein and artery

Hypoglossal nerve (XII)

Common trunk receiving facial, anterior branch of retromandibular, and lingual veins (common facial vein)

External carotid artery

Internal jugular vein

Common carotid artery

Vagus nerve (X) and sympathetic trunk

Middle scalene muscle

Anterior scalene muscle

External jugular vein (cut)

Subclavian artery

Subclavian vein

Plate 70

Pharynx

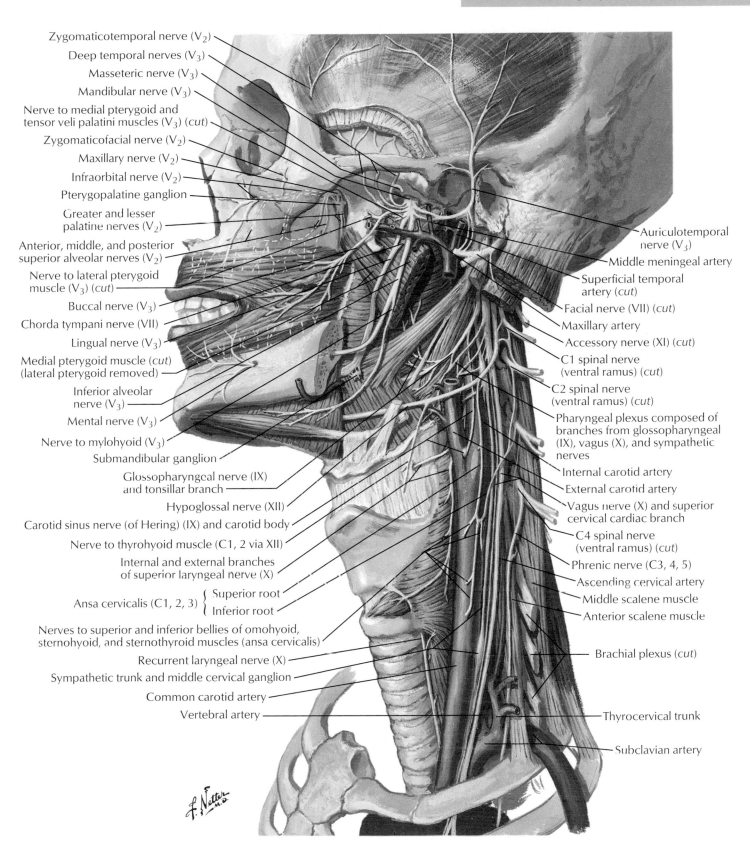

Zygomaticotemporal nerve (V₂)

Deep temporal nerves (V₃)

Masseteric nerve (V₃)

Mandibular nerve (V₃)

Nerve to medial pterygoid and tensor veli palatini muscles (V₃) (cut)

Zygomaticofacial nerve (V₂)

Maxillary nerve (V₂)

Infraorbital nerve (V₂)

Pterygopalatine ganglion

Greater and lesser palatine nerves (V₂)

Anterior, middle, and posterior superior alveolar nerves (V₂)

Nerve to lateral pterygoid muscle (V₃) (cut)

Buccal nerve (V₃)

Chorda tympani nerve (VII)

Lingual nerve (V₃)

Medial pterygoid muscle (cut) (lateral pterygoid removed)

Inferior alveolar nerve (V₃)

Mental nerve (V₃)

Nerve to mylohyoid (V₃)

Submandibular ganglion

Glossopharyngeal nerve (IX) and tonsillar branch

Hypoglossal nerve (XII)

Carotid sinus nerve (of Hering) (IX) and carotid body

Nerve to thyrohyoid muscle (C1, 2 via XII)

Internal and external branches of superior laryngeal nerve (X)

Ansa cervicalis (C1, 2, 3) { Superior root / Inferior root }

Nerves to superior and inferior bellies of omohyoid, sternohyoid, and sternothyroid muscles (ansa cervicalis)

Recurrent laryngeal nerve (X)

Sympathetic trunk and middle cervical ganglion

Common carotid artery

Vertebral artery

Auriculotemporal nerve (V₃)

Middle meningeal artery

Superficial temporal artery (cut)

Facial nerve (VII) (cut)

Maxillary artery

Accessory nerve (XI) (cut)

C1 spinal nerve (ventral ramus) (cut)

C2 spinal nerve (ventral ramus) (cut)

Pharyngeal plexus composed of branches from glossopharyngeal (IX), vagus (X), and sympathetic nerves

Internal carotid artery

External carotid artery

Vagus nerve (X) and superior cervical cardiac branch

C4 spinal nerve (ventral ramus) (cut)

Phrenic nerve (C3, 4, 5)

Ascending cervical artery

Middle scalene muscle

Anterior scalene muscle

Brachial plexus (cut)

Thyrocervical trunk

Subclavian artery

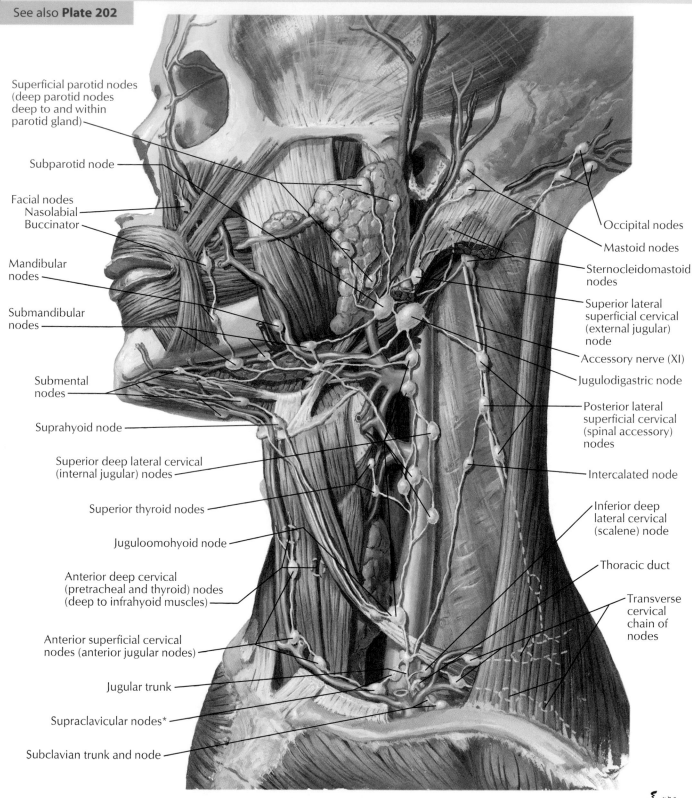

Superficial parotid nodes (deep parotid nodes deep to and within parotid gland)

Subparotid node

Facial nodes
Nasolabial
Buccinator

Mandibular nodes

Submandibular nodes

Submental nodes

Suprahyoid node

Superior deep lateral cervical (internal jugular) nodes

Superior thyroid nodes

Juguloomohyoid node

Anterior deep cervical (pretracheal and thyroid) nodes (deep to infrahyoid muscles)

Anterior superficial cervical nodes (anterior jugular nodes)

Jugular trunk

Supraclavicular nodes*

Subclavian trunk and node

Occipital nodes

Mastoid nodes

Sternocleidomastoid nodes

Superior lateral superficial cervical (external jugular) node

Accessory nerve (XI)

Jugulodigastric node

Posterior lateral superficial cervical (spinal accessory) nodes

Intercalated node

Inferior deep lateral cervical (scalene) node

Thoracic duct

Transverse cervical chain of nodes

*The supraclavicular group of nodes (also known as the lower deep cervical group), especially on the left, are also sometimes referred to as the signal or sentinel lymph nodes of Virchow or Troisier, especially when sufficiently enlarged and palpable. These nodes (or a single node) are so termed because they may be the first recognized presumptive evidence of malignant disease in the viscera.

Plate 72

Pharynx

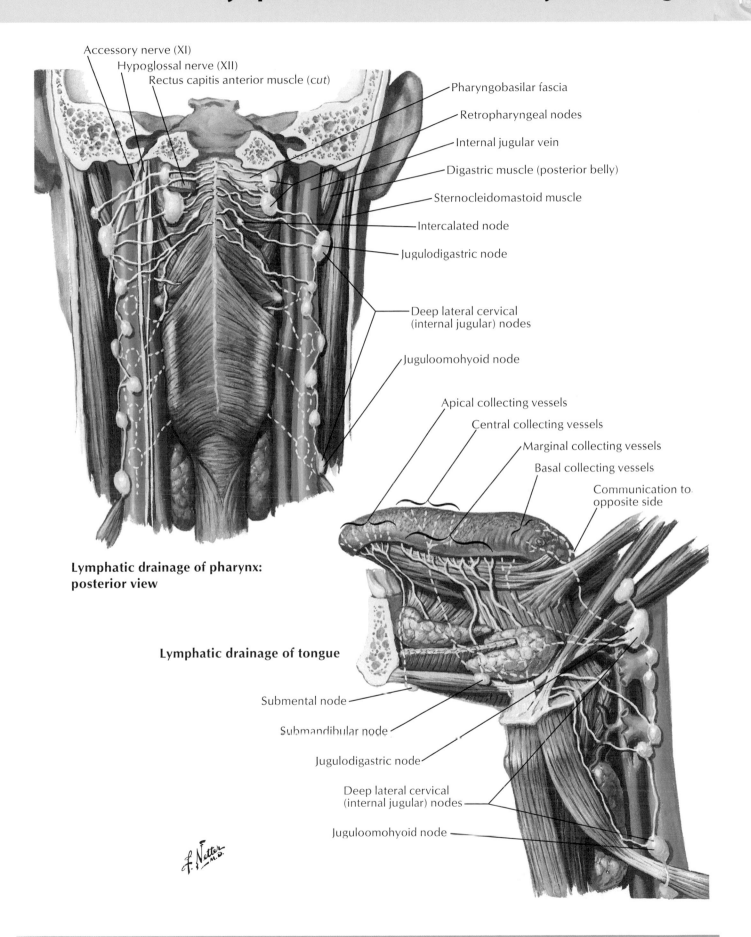

Accessory nerve (XI)

Hypoglossal nerve (XII)

Rectus capitis anterior muscle (*cut*)

Pharyngobasilar fascia

Retropharyngeal nodes

Internal jugular vein

Digastric muscle (posterior belly)

Sternocleidomastoid muscle

Intercalated node

Jugulodigastric node

Deep lateral cervical (internal jugular) nodes

Juguloomohyoid node

Lymphatic drainage of pharynx: posterior view

Apical collecting vessels

Central collecting vessels

Marginal collecting vessels

Basal collecting vessels

Communication to opposite side

Lymphatic drainage of tongue

Submental node

Submandibular node

Jugulodigastric node

Deep lateral cervical (internal jugular) nodes

Juguloomohyoid node

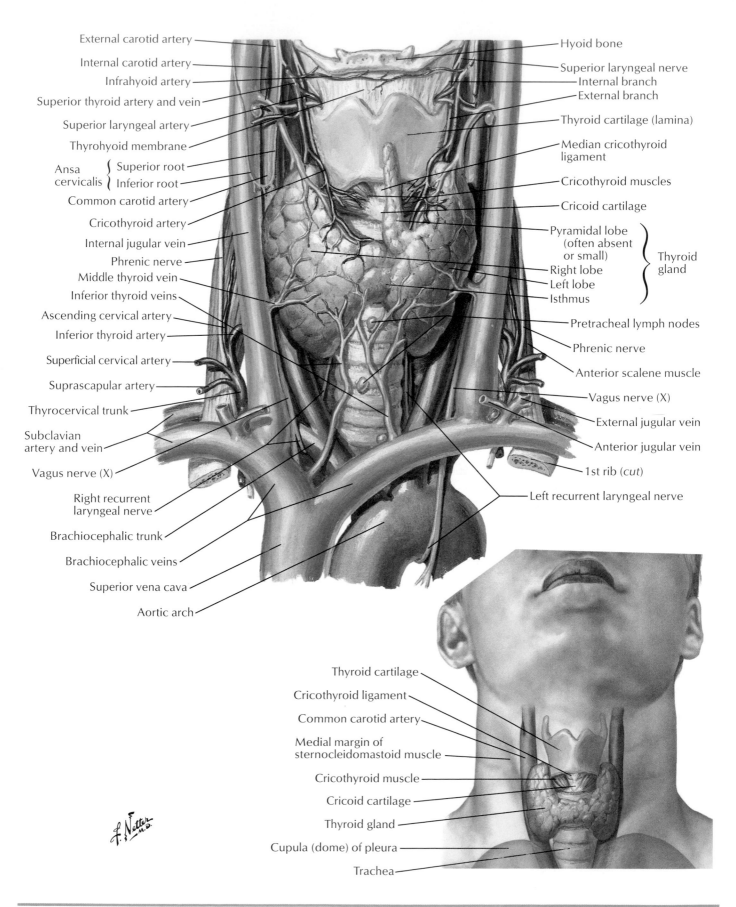

External carotid artery

Internal carotid artery

Infrahyoid artery

Superior thyroid artery and vein

Superior laryngeal artery

Thyrohyoid membrane

Ansa cervicalis { Superior root / Inferior root

Common carotid artery

Cricothyroid artery

Internal jugular vein

Phrenic nerve

Middle thyroid vein

Inferior thyroid veins

Ascending cervical artery

Inferior thyroid artery

Superficial cervical artery

Suprascapular artery

Thyrocervical trunk

Subclavian artery and vein

Vagus nerve (X)

Right recurrent laryngeal nerve

Brachiocephalic trunk

Brachiocephalic veins

Superior vena cava

Aortic arch

Hyoid bone

Superior laryngeal nerve

Internal branch

External branch

Thyroid cartilage (lamina)

Median cricothyroid ligament

Cricothyroid muscles

Cricoid cartilage

Pyramidal lobe (often absent or small)

Right lobe

Left lobe

Isthmus

Thyroid gland

Pretracheal lymph nodes

Phrenic nerve

Anterior scalene muscle

Vagus nerve (X)

External jugular vein

Anterior jugular vein

1st rib (cut)

Left recurrent laryngeal nerve

Thyroid cartilage

Cricothyroid ligament

Common carotid artery

Medial margin of sternocleidomastoid muscle

Cricothyroid muscle

Cricoid cartilage

Thyroid gland

Cupula (dome) of pleura

Trachea

Plate 74

Thyroid Gland and Larynx

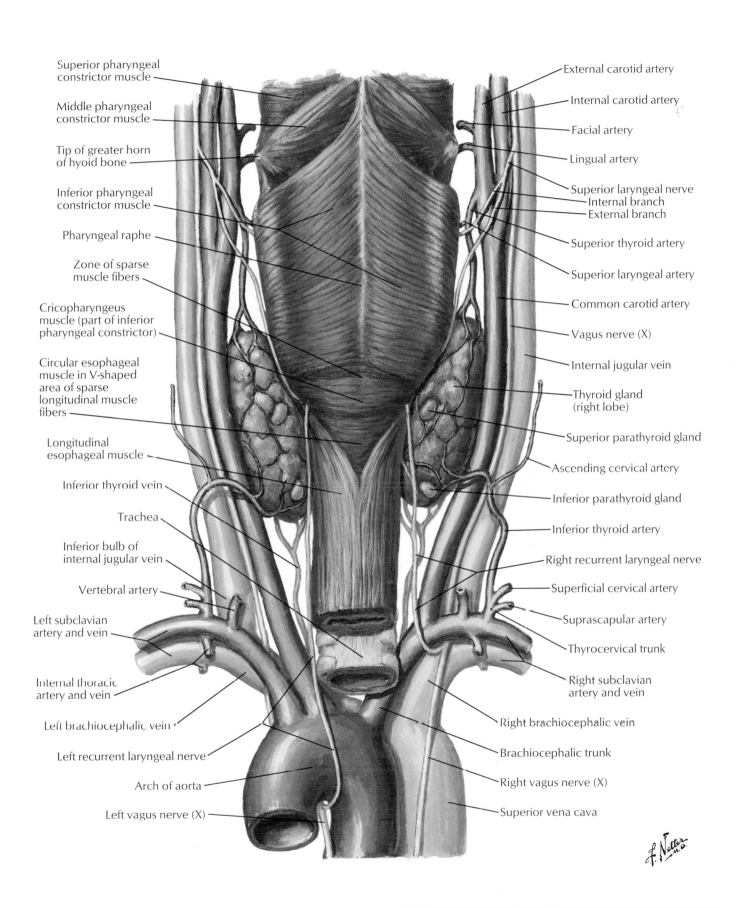

Superior pharyngeal constrictor muscle

Middle pharyngeal constrictor muscle

Tip of greater horn of hyoid bone

Inferior pharyngeal constrictor muscle

Pharyngeal raphe

Zone of sparse muscle fibers

Cricopharyngeus muscle (part of inferior pharyngeal constrictor)

Circular esophageal muscle in V-shaped area of sparse longitudinal muscle fibers

Longitudinal esophageal muscle

Inferior thyroid vein

Trachea

Inferior bulb of internal jugular vein

Vertebral artery

Left subclavian artery and vein

Internal thoracic artery and vein

Left brachiocephalic vein

Left recurrent laryngeal nerve

Arch of aorta

Left vagus nerve (X)

External carotid artery

Internal carotid artery

Facial artery

Lingual artery

Superior laryngeal nerve
Internal branch
External branch

Superior thyroid artery

Superior laryngeal artery

Common carotid artery

Vagus nerve (X)

Internal jugular vein

Thyroid gland (right lobe)

Superior parathyroid gland

Ascending cervical artery

Inferior parathyroid gland

Inferior thyroid artery

Right recurrent laryngeal nerve

Superficial cervical artery

Suprascapular artery

Thyrocervical trunk

Right subclavian artery and vein

Right brachiocephalic vein

Brachiocephalic trunk

Right vagus nerve (X)

Superior vena cava

Parathyroid Glands

See also **Plates 74, 75, 80, 227, 229**

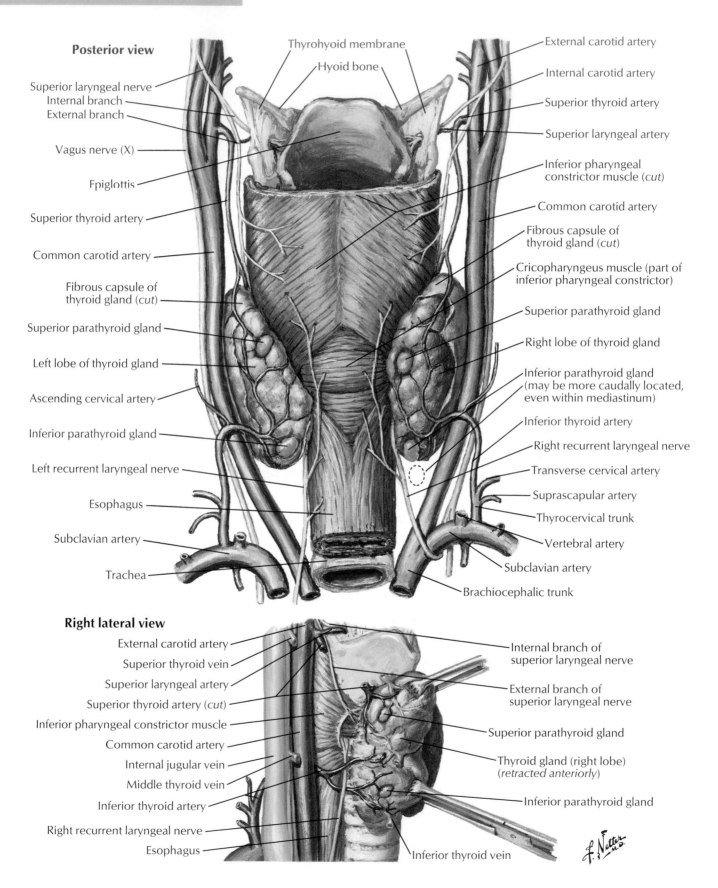

Posterior view

Superior laryngeal nerve
Internal branch
External branch

Vagus nerve (X)

Epiglottis

Superior thyroid artery

Common carotid artery

Fibrous capsule of
thyroid gland (cut)

Superior parathyroid gland

Left lobe of thyroid gland

Ascending cervical artery

Inferior parathyroid gland

Left recurrent laryngeal nerve

Esophagus

Subclavian artery

Trachea

Thyrohyoid membrane
Hyoid bone

External carotid artery

Internal carotid artery

Superior thyroid artery

Superior laryngeal artery

Inferior pharyngeal
constrictor muscle (cut)

Common carotid artery

Fibrous capsule of
thyroid gland (cut)

Cricopharyngeus muscle (part of
inferior pharyngeal constrictor)

Superior parathyroid gland

Right lobe of thyroid gland

Inferior parathyroid gland
(may be more caudally located,
even within mediastinum)

Inferior thyroid artery

Right recurrent laryngeal nerve

Transverse cervical artery

Suprascapular artery

Thyrocervical trunk

Vertebral artery

Subclavian artery

Brachiocephalic trunk

Right lateral view

External carotid artery

Superior thyroid vein

Superior laryngeal artery

Superior thyroid artery (cut)

Inferior pharyngeal constrictor muscle

Common carotid artery

Internal jugular vein

Middle thyroid vein

Inferior thyroid artery

Right recurrent laryngeal nerve

Esophagus

Internal branch of
superior laryngeal nerve

External branch of
superior laryngeal nerve

Superior parathyroid gland

Thyroid gland (right lobe)
(retracted anteriorly)

Inferior parathyroid gland

Inferior thyroid vein

Plate 76

Thyroid Gland and Larynx

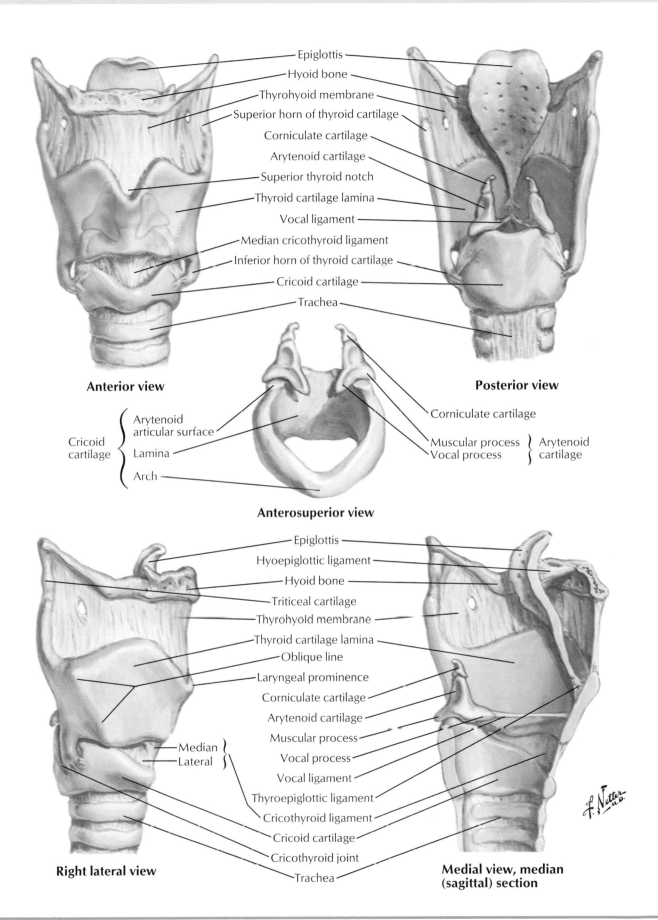

Epiglottis
Hyoid bone
Thyrohyoid membrane
Superior horn of thyroid cartilage
Corniculate cartilage
Arytenoid cartilage
Superior thyroid notch
Thyroid cartilage lamina
Vocal ligament
Median cricothyroid ligament
Inferior horn of thyroid cartilage
Cricoid cartilage
Trachea

Anterior view

Posterior view

Corniculate cartilage
Muscular process
Vocal process
Arytenoid cartilage

Cricoid cartilage {
Arytenoid articular surface
Lamina
Arch
}

Anterosuperior view

Epiglottis
Hyoepiglottic ligament
Hyoid bone
Triticeal cartilage
Thyrohyoid membrane
Thyroid cartilage lamina
Oblique line
Laryngeal prominence
Corniculate cartilage
Arytenoid cartilage
Muscular process
Vocal process
Vocal ligament
Thyroepiglottic ligament
Cricothyroid ligament
Cricoid cartilage
Cricothyroid joint
Trachea

Median }
Lateral }

Right lateral view

Medial view, median (sagittal) section

f. Netter M.D.

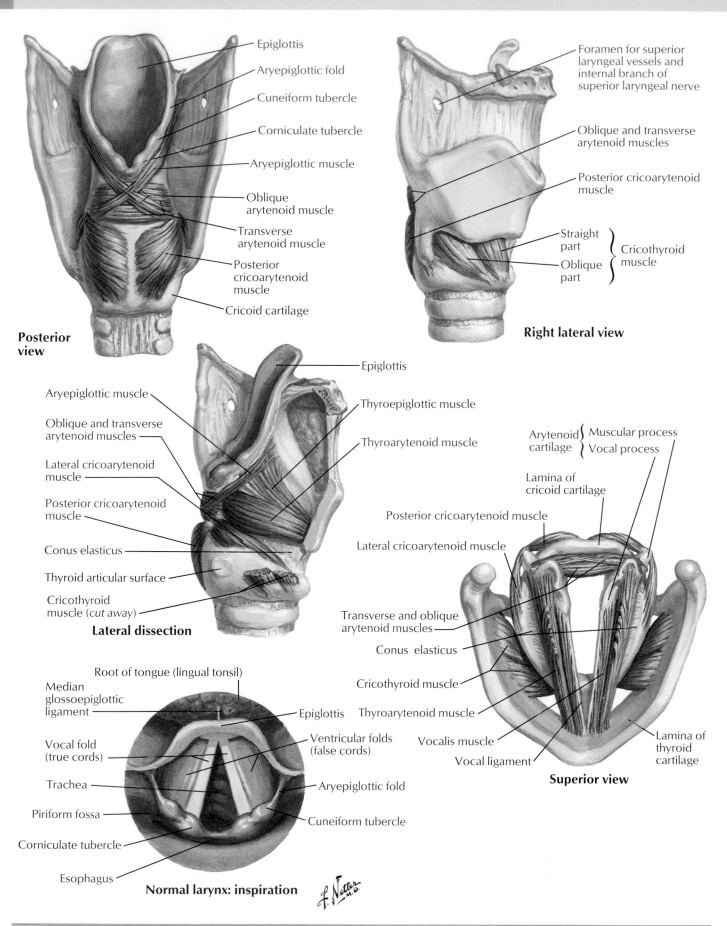

Posterior view

- Epiglottis
- Aryepiglottic fold
- Cuneiform tubercle
- Corniculate tubercle
- Aryepiglottic muscle
- Oblique arytenoid muscle
- Transverse arytenoid muscle
- Posterior cricoarytenoid muscle
- Cricoid cartilage

Right lateral view

- Foramen for superior laryngeal vessels and internal branch of superior laryngeal nerve
- Oblique and transverse arytenoid muscles
- Posterior cricoarytenoid muscle
- Straight part
- Oblique part
- Cricothyroid muscle

Lateral dissection

- Aryepiglottic muscle
- Oblique and transverse arytenoid muscles
- Lateral cricoarytenoid muscle
- Posterior cricoarytenoid muscle
- Conus elasticus
- Thyroid articular surface
- Cricothyroid muscle (*cut away*)
- Epiglottis
- Thyroepiglottic muscle
- Thyroarytenoid muscle

Superior view

- Arytenoid cartilage { Muscular process / Vocal process }
- Lamina of cricoid cartilage
- Posterior cricoarytenoid muscle
- Lateral cricoarytenoid muscle
- Transverse and oblique arytenoid muscles
- Conus elasticus
- Cricothyroid muscle
- Thyroarytenoid muscle
- Vocalis muscle
- Vocal ligament
- Lamina of thyroid cartilage

Normal larynx: inspiration

- Root of tongue (lingual tonsil)
- Median glossoepiglottic ligament
- Vocal fold (true cords)
- Trachea
- Piriform fossa
- Corniculate tubercle
- Esophagus
- Epiglottis
- Ventricular folds (false cords)
- Aryepiglottic fold
- Cuneiform tubercle

Plate 78

Thyroid Gland and Larynx

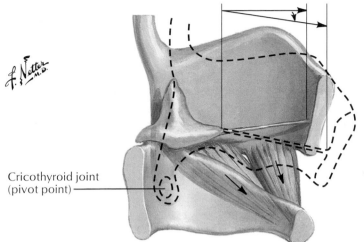

Cricothyroid joint
(pivot point)

Action of cricothyroid muscles
Lengthening (increasing tension)
of vocal ligaments

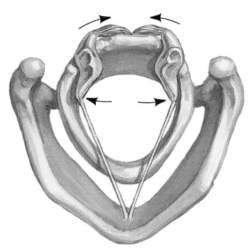

Action of posterior cricoarytenoid muscles
Abduction of vocal ligaments

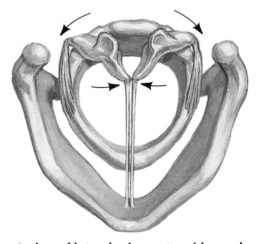

Action of lateral cricoarytenoid muscles
Adduction of vocal ligaments

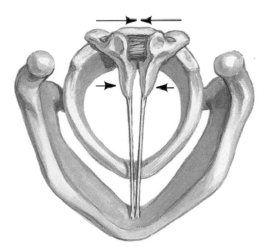

Action of transverse and oblique arytenoid muscles
Adduction of vocal ligaments

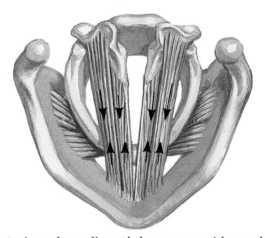

Action of vocalis and thyroarytenoid muscles
Shortening (relaxation) of vocal ligaments

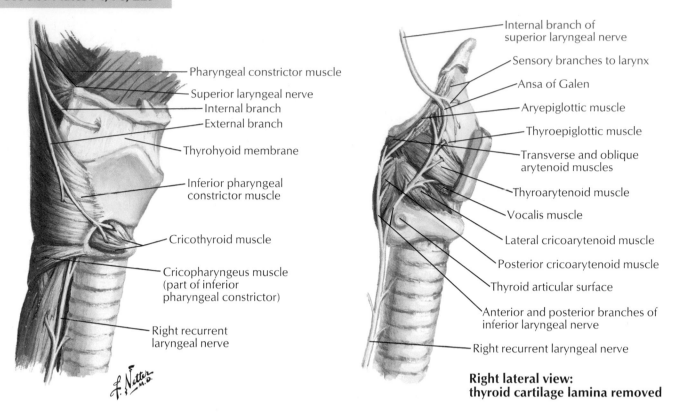

Pharyngeal constrictor muscle

Superior laryngeal nerve

Internal branch

External branch

Thyrohyoid membrane

Inferior pharyngeal constrictor muscle

Cricothyroid muscle

Cricopharyngeus muscle (part of inferior pharyngeal constrictor)

Right recurrent laryngeal nerve

Internal branch of superior laryngeal nerve

Sensory branches to larynx

Ansa of Galen

Aryepiglottic muscle

Thyroepiglottic muscle

Transverse and oblique arytenoid muscles

Thyroarytenoid muscle

Vocalis muscle

Lateral cricoarytenoid muscle

Posterior cricoarytenoid muscle

Thyroid articular surface

Anterior and posterior branches of inferior laryngeal nerve

Right recurrent laryngeal nerve

Right lateral view: thyroid cartilage lamina removed

Coronal section through larynx

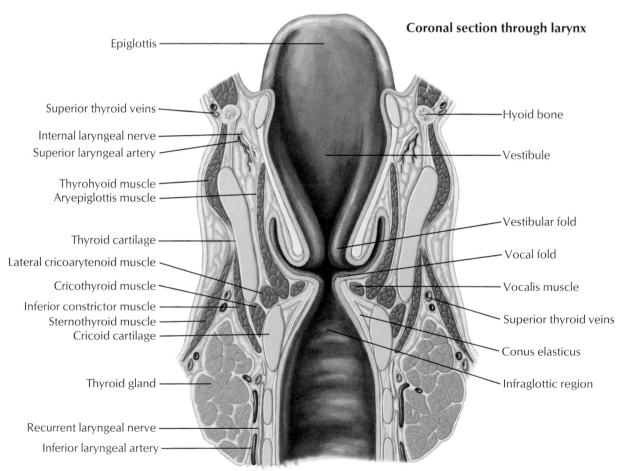

Epiglottis

Superior thyroid veins

Internal laryngeal nerve

Superior laryngeal artery

Thyrohyoid muscle

Aryepiglottis muscle

Thyroid cartilage

Lateral cricoarytenoid muscle

Cricothyroid muscle

Inferior constrictor muscle

Sternothyroid muscle

Cricoid cartilage

Thyroid gland

Recurrent laryngeal nerve

Inferior laryngeal artery

Hyoid bone

Vestibule

Vestibular fold

Vocal fold

Vocalis muscle

Superior thyroid veins

Conus elasticus

Infraglottic region

Plate 80

Thyroid Gland and Larynx

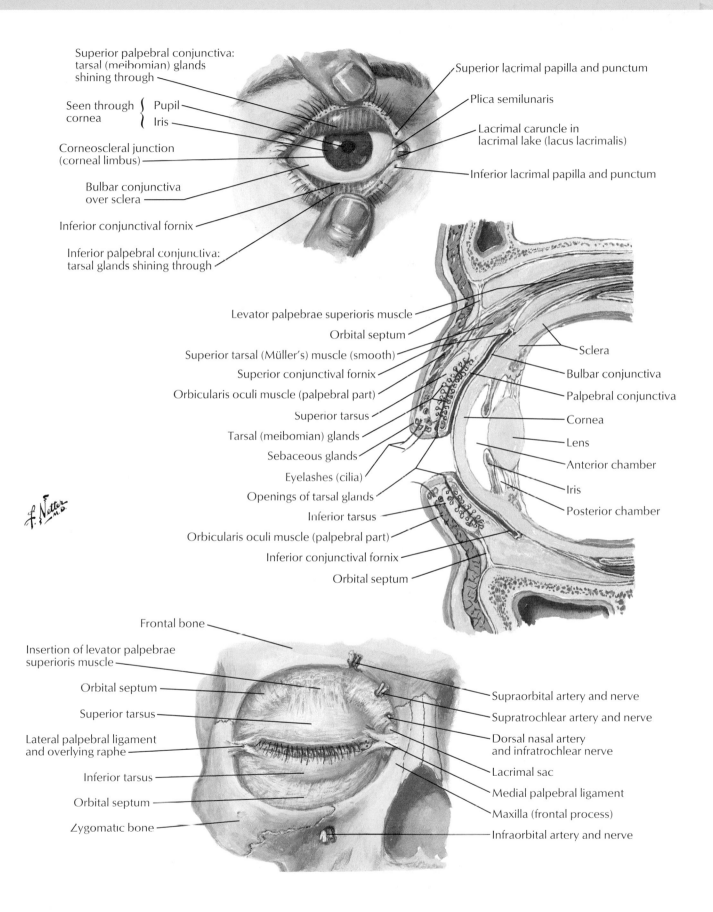

Superior palpebral conjunctiva: tarsal (meibomian) glands shining through

Seen through cornea { Pupil / Iris

Corneoscleral junction (corneal limbus)

Bulbar conjunctiva over sclera

Inferior conjunctival fornix

Inferior palpebral conjunctiva: tarsal glands shining through

Superior lacrimal papilla and punctum

Plica semilunaris

Lacrimal caruncle in lacrimal lake (lacus lacrimalis)

Inferior lacrimal papilla and punctum

Levator palpebrae superioris muscle

Orbital septum

Superior tarsal (Müller's) muscle (smooth)

Superior conjunctival fornix

Orbicularis oculi muscle (palpebral part)

Superior tarsus

Tarsal (meibomian) glands

Sebaceous glands

Eyelashes (cilia)

Openings of tarsal glands

Inferior tarsus

Orbicularis oculi muscle (palpebral part)

Inferior conjunctival fornix

Orbital septum

Sclera

Bulbar conjunctiva

Palpebral conjunctiva

Cornea

Lens

Anterior chamber

Iris

Posterior chamber

Frontal bone

Insertion of levator palpebrae superioris muscle

Orbital septum

Superior tarsus

Lateral palpebral ligament and overlying raphe

Inferior tarsus

Orbital septum

Zygomatic bone

Supraorbital artery and nerve

Supratrochlear artery and nerve

Dorsal nasal artery and infratrochlear nerve

Lacrimal sac

Medial palpebral ligament

Maxilla (frontal process)

Infraorbital artery and nerve

Lacrimal Apparatus

See also **Plates 44, 132**

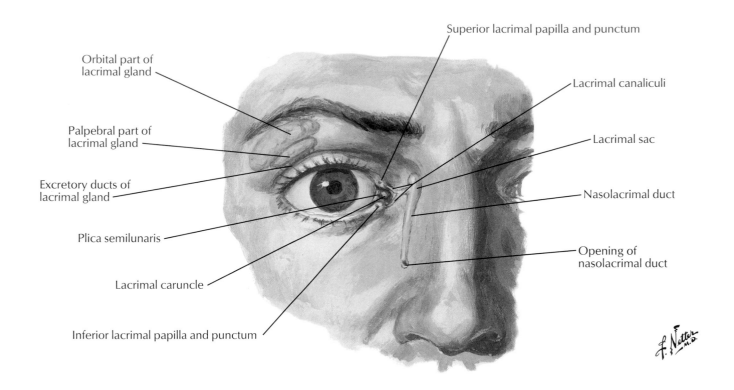

Orbital part of lacrimal gland

Palpebral part of lacrimal gland

Excretory ducts of lacrimal gland

Plica semilunaris

Lacrimal caruncle

Inferior lacrimal papilla and punctum

Superior lacrimal papilla and punctum

Lacrimal canaliculi

Lacrimal sac

Nasolacrimal duct

Opening of nasolacrimal duct

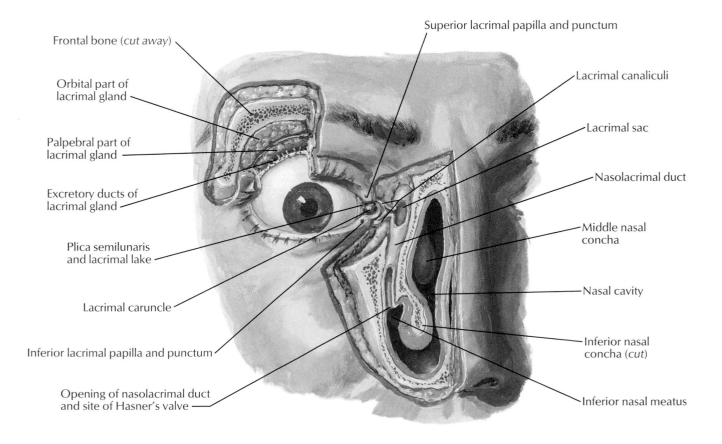

Frontal bone (cut away)

Orbital part of lacrimal gland

Palpebral part of lacrimal gland

Excretory ducts of lacrimal gland

Plica semilunaris and lacrimal lake

Lacrimal caruncle

Inferior lacrimal papilla and punctum

Opening of nasolacrimal duct and site of Hasner's valve

Superior lacrimal papilla and punctum

Lacrimal canaliculi

Lacrimal sac

Nasolacrimal duct

Middle nasal concha

Nasal cavity

Inferior nasal concha (cut)

Inferior nasal meatus

Plate 82   **Orbit and Contents**

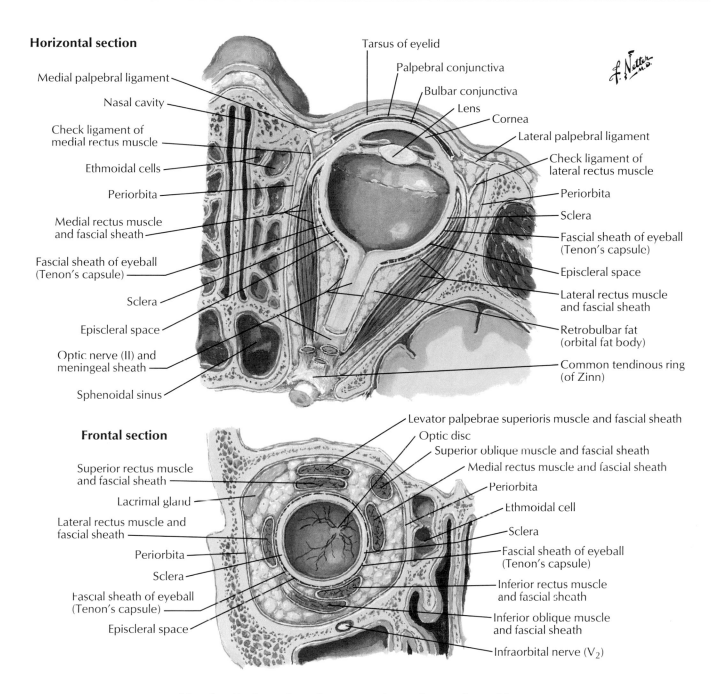

Horizontal section

- Medial palpebral ligament
- Nasal cavity
- Check ligament of medial rectus muscle
- Ethmoidal cells
- Periorbita
- Medial rectus muscle and fascial sheath
- Fascial sheath of eyeball (Tenon's capsule)
- Sclera
- Episcleral space
- Optic nerve (II) and meningeal sheath
- Sphenoidal sinus

- Tarsus of eyelid
- Palpebral conjunctiva
- Bulbar conjunctiva
- Lens
- Cornea
- Lateral palpebral ligament
- Check ligament of lateral rectus muscle
- Periorbita
- Sclera
- Fascial sheath of eyeball (Tenon's capsule)
- Episcleral space
- Lateral rectus muscle and fascial sheath
- Retrobulbar fat (orbital fat body)
- Common tendinous ring (of Zinn)

Frontal section

- Superior rectus muscle and fascial sheath
- Lacrimal gland
- Lateral rectus muscle and fascial sheath
- Periorbita
- Sclera
- Fascial sheath of eyeball (Tenon's capsule)
- Episcleral space

- Levator palpebrae superioris muscle and fascial sheath
- Optic disc
- Superior oblique muscle and fascial sheath
- Medial rectus muscle and fascial sheath
- Periorbita
- Ethmoidal cell
- Sclera
- Fascial sheath of eyeball (Tenon's capsule)
- Inferior rectus muscle and fascial sheath
- Inferior oblique muscle and fascial sheath
- Infraorbital nerve (V$_2$)

Muscle attachments and nerves and vessels entering orbit

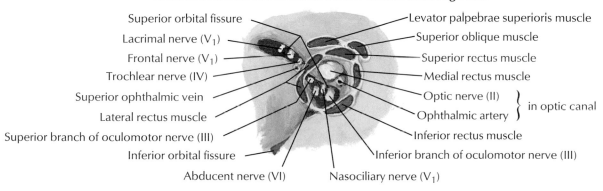

- Superior orbital fissure
- Lacrimal nerve (V$_1$)
- Frontal nerve (V$_1$)
- Trochlear nerve (IV)
- Superior ophthalmic vein
- Lateral rectus muscle
- Superior branch of oculomotor nerve (III)
- Inferior orbital fissure
- Abducent nerve (VI)
- Nasociliary nerve (V$_1$)

- Levator palpebrae superioris muscle
- Superior oblique muscle
- Superior rectus muscle
- Medial rectus muscle
- Optic nerve (II)
- Ophthalmic artery } in optic canal
- Inferior rectus muscle
- Inferior branch of oculomotor nerve (III)

Extrinsic Eye Muscles

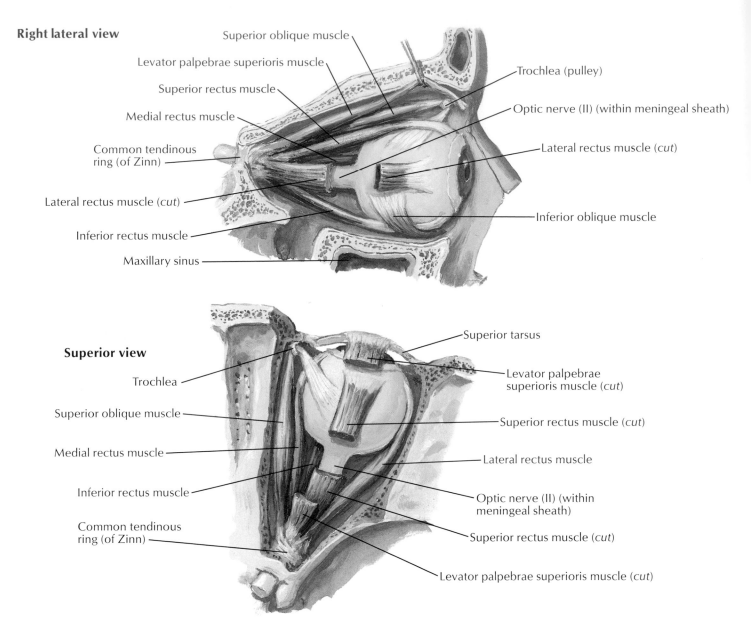

Right lateral view

Superior oblique muscle

Levator palpebrae superioris muscle

Superior rectus muscle

Medial rectus muscle

Common tendinous ring (of Zinn)

Lateral rectus muscle (*cut*)

Inferior rectus muscle

Maxillary sinus

Trochlea (pulley)

Optic nerve (II) (within meningeal sheath)

Lateral rectus muscle (*cut*)

Inferior oblique muscle

Superior view

Trochlea

Superior oblique muscle

Medial rectus muscle

Inferior rectus muscle

Common tendinous ring (of Zinn)

Superior tarsus

Levator palpebrae superioris muscle (*cut*)

Superior rectus muscle (*cut*)

Lateral rectus muscle

Optic nerve (II) (within meningeal sheath)

Superior rectus muscle (*cut*)

Levator palpebrae superioris muscle (*cut*)

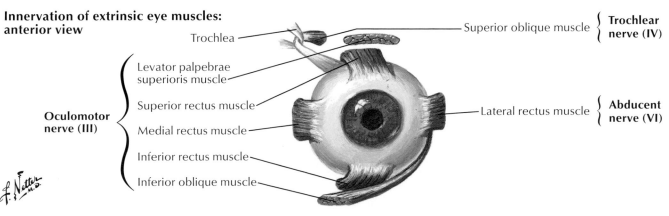

Innervation of extrinsic eye muscles: anterior view

Trochlea

Levator palpebrae superioris muscle

Superior rectus muscle

Medial rectus muscle

Inferior rectus muscle

Inferior oblique muscle

Oculomotor nerve (III)

Superior oblique muscle **Trochlear nerve (IV)**

Lateral rectus muscle **Abducent nerve (VI)**

Plate 84   **Orbit and Contents**

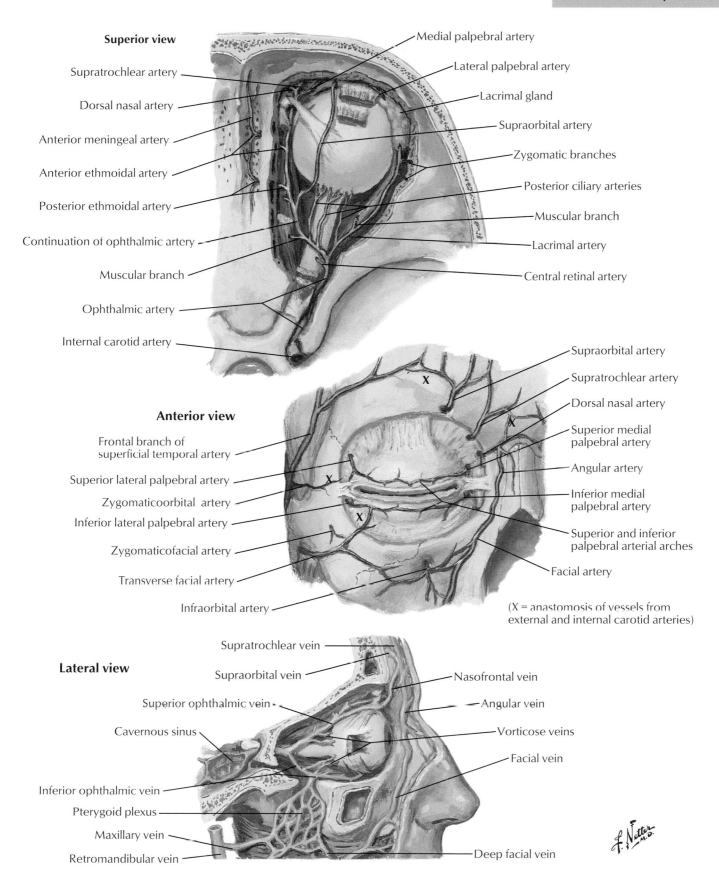

Superior view

Supratrochlear artery

Dorsal nasal artery

Anterior meningeal artery

Anterior ethmoidal artery

Posterior ethmoidal artery

Continuation of ophthalmic artery

Muscular branch

Ophthalmic artery

Internal carotid artery

Medial palpebral artery

Lateral palpebral artery

Lacrimal gland

Supraorbital artery

Zygomatic branches

Posterior ciliary arteries

Muscular branch

Lacrimal artery

Central retinal artery

Anterior view

Frontal branch of superficial temporal artery

Superior lateral palpebral artery

Zygomaticoorbital artery

Inferior lateral palpebral artery

Zygomaticofacial artery

Transverse facial artery

Infraorbital artery

Supraorbital artery

Supratrochlear artery

Dorsal nasal artery

Superior medial palpebral artery

Angular artery

Inferior medial palpebral artery

Superior and inferior palpebral arterial arches

Facial artery

(X = anastomosis of vessels from external and internal carotid arteries)

Lateral view

Supratrochlear vein

Supraorbital vein

Superior ophthalmic vein

Cavernous sinus

Inferior ophthalmic vein

Pterygoid plexus

Maxillary vein

Retromandibular vein

Nasofrontal vein

Angular vein

Vorticose veins

Facial vein

Deep facial vein

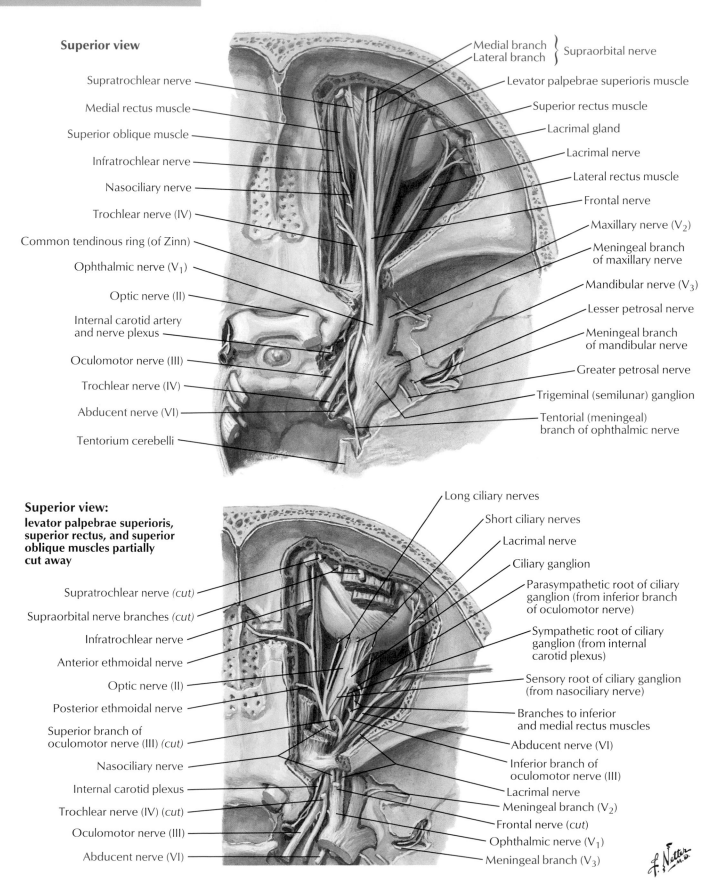

Superior view

Supratrochlear nerve

Medial rectus muscle

Superior oblique muscle

Infratrochlear nerve

Nasociliary nerve

Trochlear nerve (IV)

Common tendinous ring (of Zinn)

Ophthalmic nerve (V₁)

Optic nerve (II)

Internal carotid artery and nerve plexus

Oculomotor nerve (III)

Trochlear nerve (IV)

Abducent nerve (VI)

Tentorium cerebelli

Medial branch } Supraorbital nerve
Lateral branch

Levator palpebrae superioris muscle

Superior rectus muscle

Lacrimal gland

Lacrimal nerve

Lateral rectus muscle

Frontal nerve

Maxillary nerve (V₂)

Meningeal branch of maxillary nerve

Mandibular nerve (V₃)

Lesser petrosal nerve

Meningeal branch of mandibular nerve

Greater petrosal nerve

Trigeminal (semilunar) ganglion

Tentorial (meningeal) branch of ophthalmic nerve

Superior view:
levator palpebrae superioris,
superior rectus, and superior
oblique muscles partially
cut away

Supratrochlear nerve (cut)

Supraorbital nerve branches (cut)

Infratrochlear nerve

Anterior ethmoidal nerve

Optic nerve (II)

Posterior ethmoidal nerve

Superior branch of oculomotor nerve (III) (cut)

Nasociliary nerve

Internal carotid plexus

Trochlear nerve (IV) (cut)

Oculomotor nerve (III)

Abducent nerve (VI)

Long ciliary nerves

Short ciliary nerves

Lacrimal nerve

Ciliary ganglion

Parasympathetic root of ciliary ganglion (from inferior branch of oculomotor nerve)

Sympathetic root of ciliary ganglion (from internal carotid plexus)

Sensory root of ciliary ganglion (from nasociliary nerve)

Branches to inferior and medial rectus muscles

Abducent nerve (VI)

Inferior branch of oculomotor nerve (III)

Lacrimal nerve

Meningeal branch (V₂)

Frontal nerve (cut)

Ophthalmic nerve (V₁)

Meningeal branch (V₃)

Plate 86   **Orbit and Contents**

Horizontal section

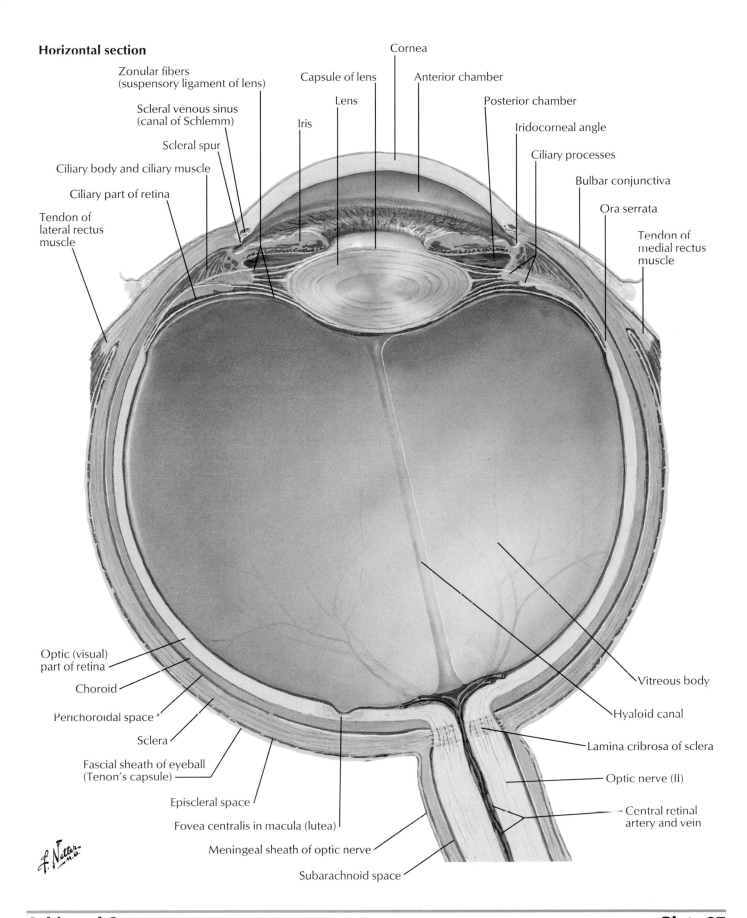

Cornea

Capsule of lens

Lens

Iris

Zonular fibers
(suspensory ligament of lens)

Scleral venous sinus
(canal of Schlemm)

Scleral spur

Ciliary body and ciliary muscle

Ciliary part of retina

Tendon of
lateral rectus
muscle

Anterior chamber

Posterior chamber

Iridocorneal angle

Ciliary processes

Bulbar conjunctiva

Ora serrata

Tendon of
medial rectus
muscle

Optic (visual)
part of retina

Choroid

Perichoroidal space

Sclera

Fascial sheath of eyeball
(Tenon's capsule)

Episcleral space

Fovea centralis in macula (lutea)

Meningeal sheath of optic nerve

Subarachnoid space

Vitreous body

Hyaloid canal

Lamina cribrosa of sclera

Optic nerve (II)

Central retinal
artery and vein

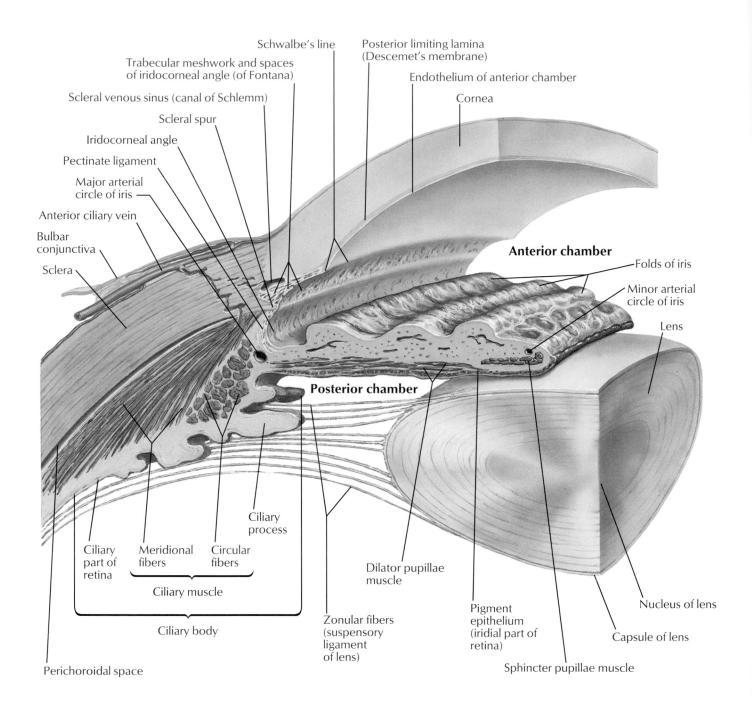

Schwalbe's line

Posterior limiting lamina (Descemet's membrane)

Trabecular meshwork and spaces of iridocorneal angle (of Fontana)

Endothelium of anterior chamber

Scleral venous sinus (canal of Schlemm)

Cornea

Scleral spur

Iridocorneal angle

Pectinate ligament

Major arterial circle of iris

Anterior ciliary vein

Bulbar conjunctiva

Sclera

Anterior chamber

Folds of iris

Minor arterial circle of iris

Lens

Posterior chamber

Ciliary process

Ciliary part of retina

Meridional fibers

Circular fibers

Dilator pupillae muscle

Pigment epithelium (iridial part of retina)

Nucleus of lens

Capsule of lens

Sphincter pupillae muscle

Ciliary muscle

Zonular fibers (suspensory ligament of lens)

Ciliary body

Perichoroidal space

Note: For clarity, only single plane of zonular fibers shown; actually, fibers surround entire circumference of lens.

Plate 88

Orbit and Contents

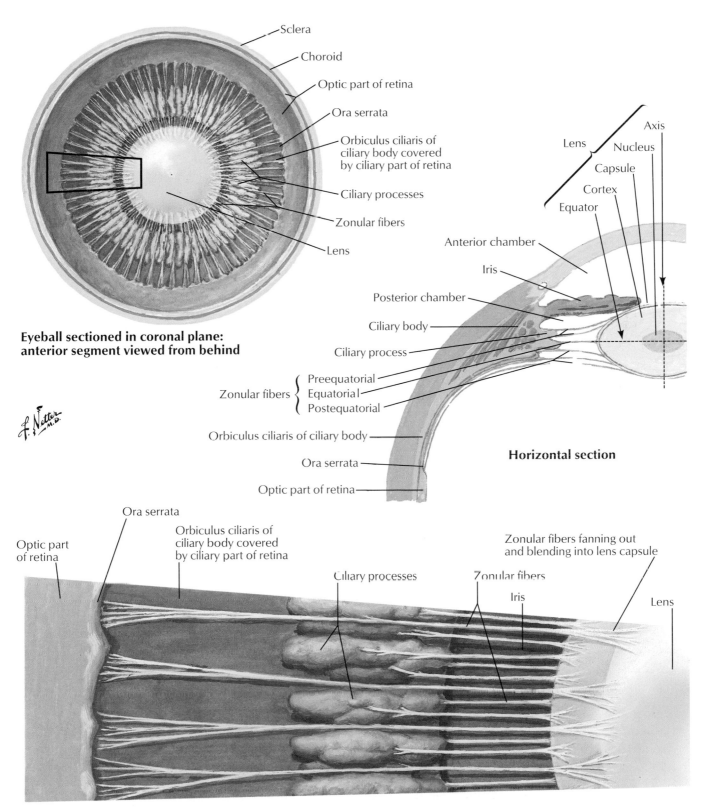

Sclera

Choroid

Optic part of retina

Ora serrata

Orbiculus ciliaris of ciliary body covered by ciliary part of retina

Ciliary processes

Zonular fibers

Lens

Eyeball sectioned in coronal plane: anterior segment viewed from behind

Axis

Lens { Nucleus, Capsule, Cortex, Equator

Anterior chamber

Iris

Posterior chamber

Ciliary body

Ciliary process

Zonular fibers {
Preequatorial
Equatorial
Postequatorial

Orbiculus ciliaris of ciliary body

Ora serrata

Optic part of retina

Horizontal section

Ora serrata

Optic part of retina

Orbiculus ciliaris of ciliary body covered by ciliary part of retina

Zonular fibers fanning out and blending into lens capsule

Ciliary processes

Zonular fibers

Iris

Lens

Enlargement of segment outlined in top illustration (semischematic)

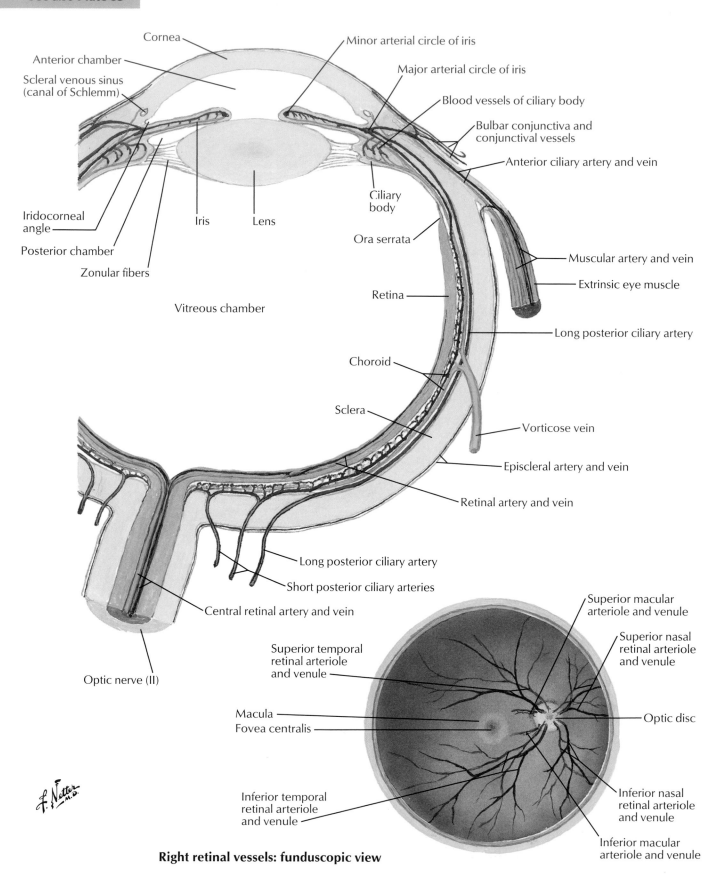

Cornea

Anterior chamber

Scleral venous sinus
(canal of Schlemm)

Minor arterial circle of iris

Major arterial circle of iris

Blood vessels of ciliary body

Bulbar conjunctiva and
conjunctival vessels

Anterior ciliary artery and vein

Iridocorneal
angle

Posterior chamber

Zonular fibers

Iris

Lens

Ciliary
body

Ora serrata

Muscular artery and vein

Extrinsic eye muscle

Vitreous chamber

Retina

Long posterior ciliary artery

Choroid

Sclera

Vorticose vein

Episcleral artery and vein

Retinal artery and vein

Long posterior ciliary artery

Short posterior ciliary arteries

Central retinal artery and vein

Optic nerve (II)

Superior temporal
retinal arteriole
and venule

Macula

Fovea centralis

Superior macular
arteriole and venule

Superior nasal
retinal arteriole
and venule

Optic disc

Inferior nasal
retinal arteriole
and venule

Inferior temporal
retinal arteriole
and venule

Inferior macular
arteriole and venule

Right retinal vessels: funduscopic view

Plate 90

Orbit and Contents

Vascular arrangements within the choroid (vascular tunic) of the eyeball

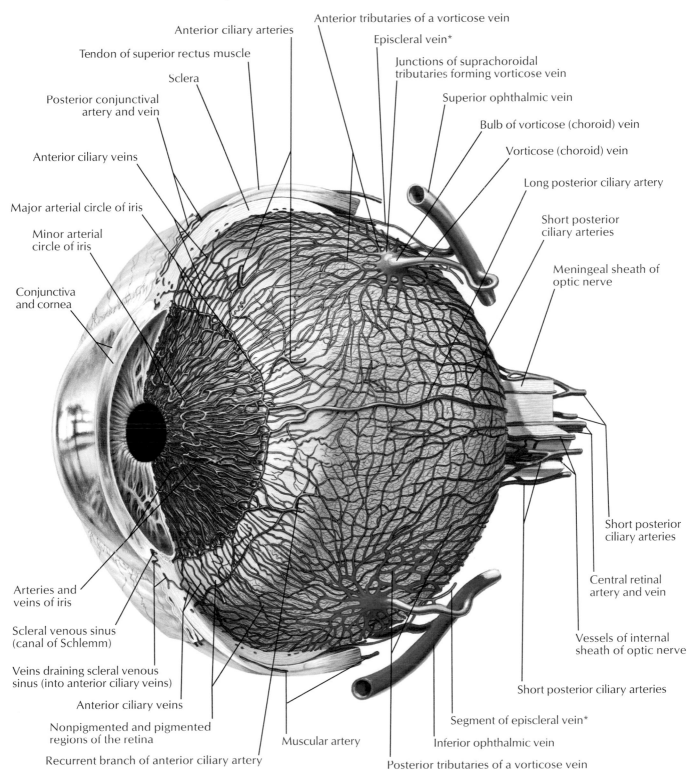

Anterior ciliary arteries

Anterior tributaries of a vorticose vein

Episcleral vein*

Tendon of superior rectus muscle

Junctions of suprachoroidal tributaries forming vorticose vein

Sclera

Superior ophthalmic vein

Posterior conjunctival artery and vein

Bulb of vorticose (choroid) vein

Vorticose (choroid) vein

Anterior ciliary veins

Long posterior ciliary artery

Major arterial circle of iris

Short posterior ciliary arteries

Minor arterial circle of iris

Meningeal sheath of optic nerve

Conjunctiva and cornea

Short posterior ciliary arteries

Central retinal artery and vein

Arteries and veins of iris

Vessels of internal sheath of optic nerve

Scleral venous sinus (canal of Schlemm)

Veins draining scleral venous sinus (into anterior ciliary veins)

Short posterior ciliary arteries

Anterior ciliary veins

Segment of episcleral vein*

Nonpigmented and pigmented regions of the retina

Inferior ophthalmic vein

Muscular artery

Recurrent branch of anterior ciliary artery

Posterior tributaries of a vorticose vein

The episcleral veins are shown here anastomosing with the vorticose veins, which they do; however, they also drain into the anterior ciliary veins.

C. Machado
M.D.

Pathway of Sound Reception

Frontal section

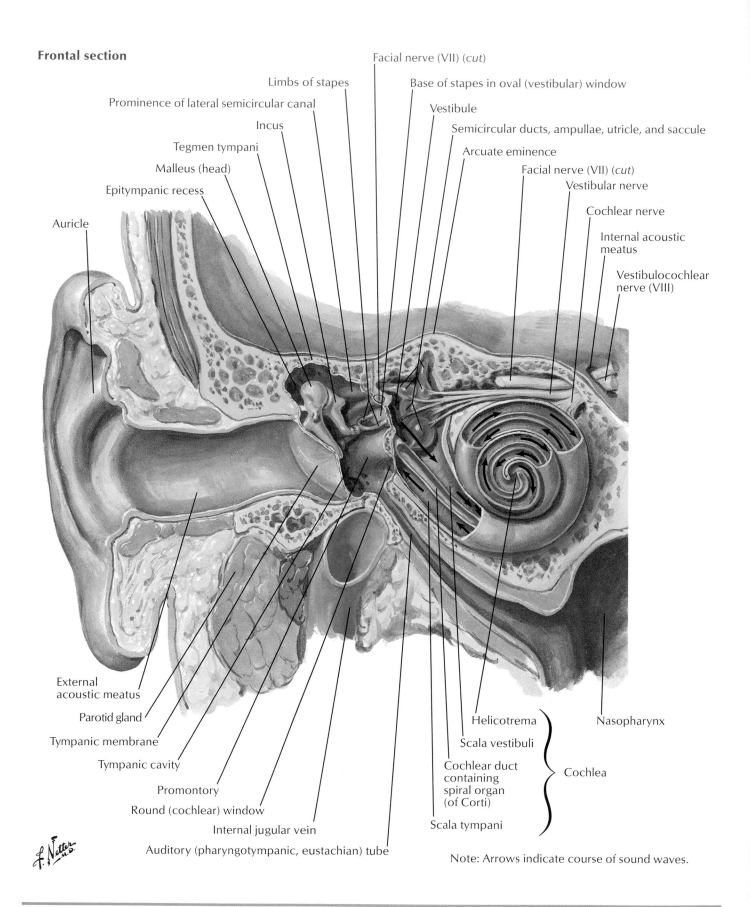

Facial nerve (VII) (*cut*)

Limbs of stapes

Base of stapes in oval (vestibular) window

Prominence of lateral semicircular canal

Vestibule

Incus

Semicircular ducts, ampullae, utricle, and saccule

Tegmen tympani

Arcuate eminence

Malleus (head)

Facial nerve (VII) (*cut*)

Epitympanic recess

Vestibular nerve

Auricle

Cochlear nerve

Internal acoustic meatus

Vestibulocochlear nerve (VIII)

External acoustic meatus

Parotid gland

Tympanic membrane

Tympanic cavity

Promontory

Helicotrema

Nasopharynx

Round (cochlear) window

Scala vestibuli

Internal jugular vein

Cochlear duct containing spiral organ (of Corti)

Cochlea

Auditory (pharyngotympanic, eustachian) tube

Scala tympani

Note: Arrows indicate course of sound waves.

Plate 92

Ear

Right auricle (pinna)

Triangular fossa
Crux of helix
Helix
External acoustic meatus
Scaphoid fossa
Crura of antihelix
Auricular tubercle (of Darwin)
Antihelix
Tragus
Concha of auricle
Intertragic notch
Lobule of auricle
Antitragus

Otoscopic view of right tympanic membrane

Pars flaccida
Lateral process of malleus
Posterior mallear fold
Anterior mallear fold
Long limb of incus
Handle of malleus
Umbo
Cone of light
Pars tensa

Coronal oblique section of external acoustic meatus and middle ear (tympanic cavity)

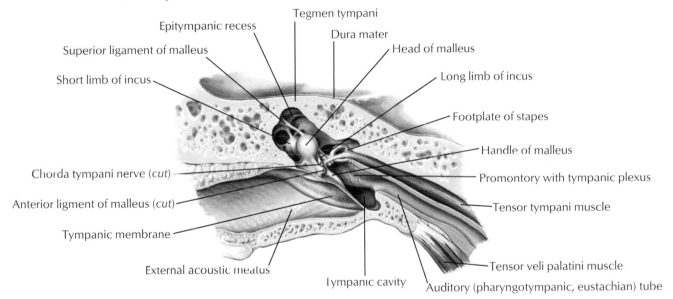

Epitympanic recess
Tegmen tympani
Dura mater
Superior ligament of malleus
Head of malleus
Short limb of incus
Long limb of incus
Footplate of stapes
Handle of malleus
Chorda tympani nerve (cut)
Promontory with tympanic plexus
Anterior ligment of malleus (cut)
Tensor tympani muscle
Tympanic membrane
External acoustic meatus
Tensor veli palatini muscle
Tympanic cavity
Auditory (pharyngotympanic, eustachian) tube

Right tympanic cavity after removal of tympanic membrane (lateral view)

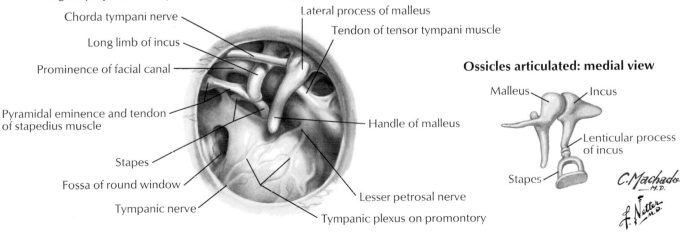

Chorda tympani nerve
Lateral process of malleus
Long limb of incus
Tendon of tensor tympani muscle
Prominence of facial canal
Pyramidal eminence and tendon of stapedius muscle
Handle of malleus
Stapes
Fossa of round window
Tympanic nerve
Lesser petrosal nerve
Tympanic plexus on promontory

Ossicles articulated: medial view

Malleus
Incus
Lenticular process of incus
Stapes

C. Machado M.D.

F. Netter M.D.

Lateral wall of tympanic cavity: medial (internal) view

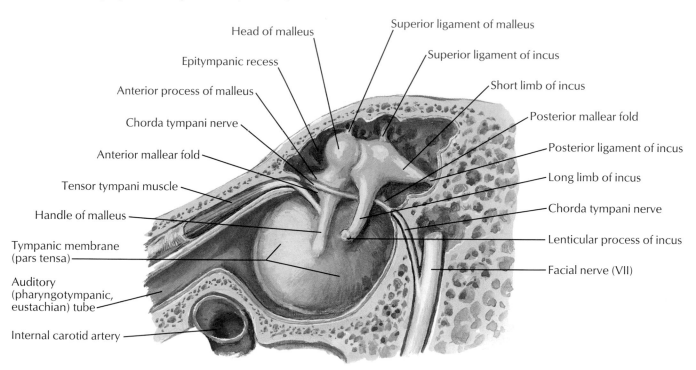

Head of malleus

Epitympanic recess

Anterior process of malleus

Chorda tympani nerve

Anterior mallear fold

Tensor tympani muscle

Handle of malleus

Tympanic membrane
(pars tensa)

Auditory
(pharyngotympanic,
eustachian) tube

Internal carotid artery

Superior ligament of malleus

Superior ligament of incus

Short limb of incus

Posterior mallear fold

Posterior ligament of incus

Long limb of incus

Chorda tympani nerve

Lenticular process of incus

Facial nerve (VII)

Medial wall of tympanic cavity: lateral view

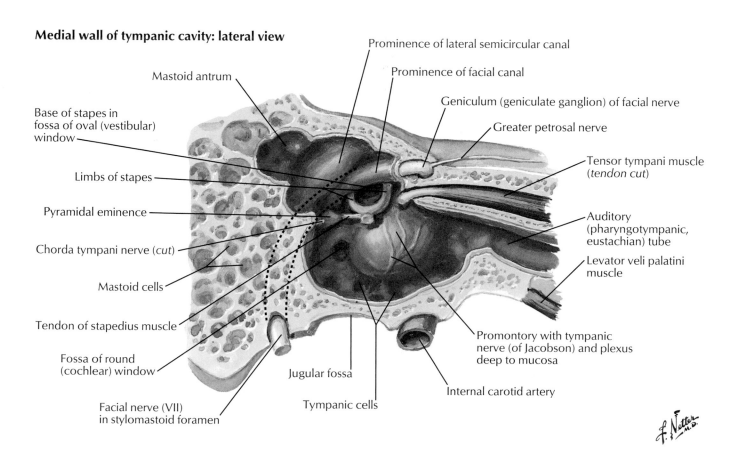

Mastoid antrum

Base of stapes in
fossa of oval (vestibular)
window

Limbs of stapes

Pyramidal eminence

Chorda tympani nerve (cut)

Mastoid cells

Tendon of stapedius muscle

Fossa of round
(cochlear) window

Facial nerve (VII)
in stylomastoid foramen

Jugular fossa

Tympanic cells

Prominence of lateral semicircular canal

Prominence of facial canal

Geniculum (geniculate ganglion) of facial nerve

Greater petrosal nerve

Tensor tympani muscle
(tendon cut)

Auditory
(pharyngotympanic,
eustachian) tube

Levator veli palatini
muscle

Promontory with tympanic
nerve (of Jacobson) and plexus
deep to mucosa

Internal carotid artery

Plate 94

Ear

Right bony labyrinth (otic capsule), anterolateral view: surrounding cancellous bone removed

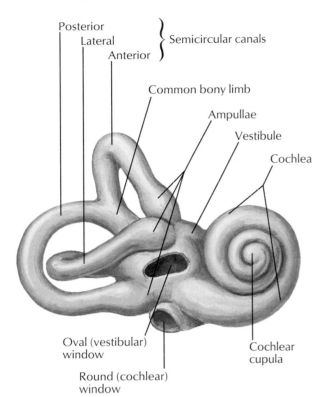

Posterior
Lateral
Anterior
} Semicircular canals

Common bony limb

Ampullae

Vestibule

Cochlea

Oval (vestibular) window

Round (cochlear) window

Cochlear cupula

Dissected right bony labyrinth (otic capsule): membranous labyrinth removed

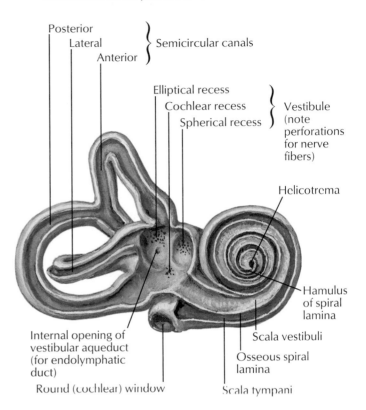

Posterior
Lateral
Anterior
} Semicircular canals

Elliptical recess
Cochlear recess
Spherical recess
} Vestibule (note perforations for nerve fibers)

Helicotrema

Internal opening of vestibular aqueduct (for endolymphatic duct)

Round (cochlear) window

Hamulus of spiral lamina

Scala vestibuli

Osseous spiral lamina

Scala tympani

Right membranous labyrinth with nerves: medial view

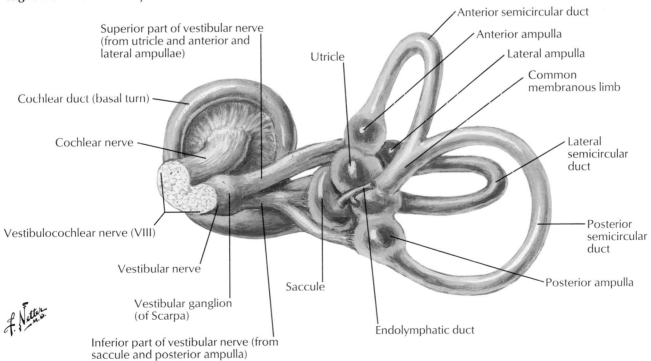

Superior part of vestibular nerve (from utricle and anterior and lateral ampullae)

Cochlear duct (basal turn)

Cochlear nerve

Vestibulocochlear nerve (VIII)

Vestibular nerve

Vestibular ganglion (of Scarpa)

Inferior part of vestibular nerve (from saccule and posterior ampulla)

Saccule

Endolymphatic duct

Utricle

Anterior semicircular duct

Anterior ampulla

Lateral ampulla

Common membranous limb

Lateral semicircular duct

Posterior semicircular duct

Posterior ampulla

Bony and membranous labyrinths: schema

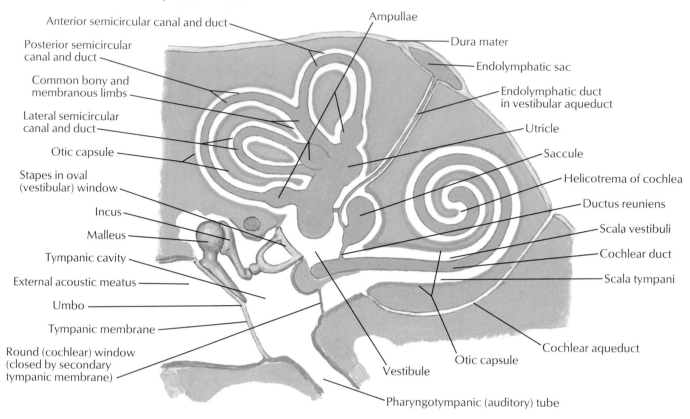

Anterior semicircular canal and duct

Posterior semicircular canal and duct

Common bony and membranous limbs

Lateral semicircular canal and duct

Otic capsule

Stapes in oval (vestibular) window

Incus

Malleus

Tympanic cavity

External acoustic meatus

Umbo

Tympanic membrane

Round (cochlear) window (closed by secondary tympanic membrane)

Ampullae

Dura mater

Endolymphatic sac

Endolymphatic duct in vestibular aqueduct

Utricle

Saccule

Helicotrema of cochlea

Ductus reuniens

Scala vestibuli

Cochlear duct

Scala tympani

Cochlear aqueduct

Otic capsule

Vestibule

Pharyngotympanic (auditory) tube

Section through turn of cochlea

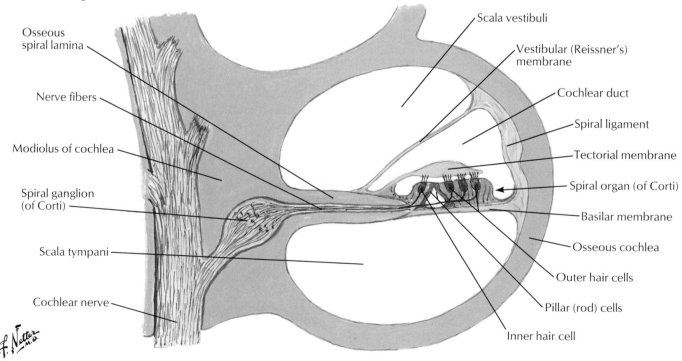

Osseous spiral lamina

Nerve fibers

Modiolus of cochlea

Spiral ganglion (of Corti)

Scala tympani

Cochlear nerve

Scala vestibuli

Vestibular (Reissner's) membrane

Cochlear duct

Spiral ligament

Tectorial membrane

Spiral organ (of Corti)

Basilar membrane

Osseous cochlea

Outer hair cells

Pillar (rod) cells

Inner hair cell

Plate 96

Ear

Superior projection of right bony labyrinth on floor of skull

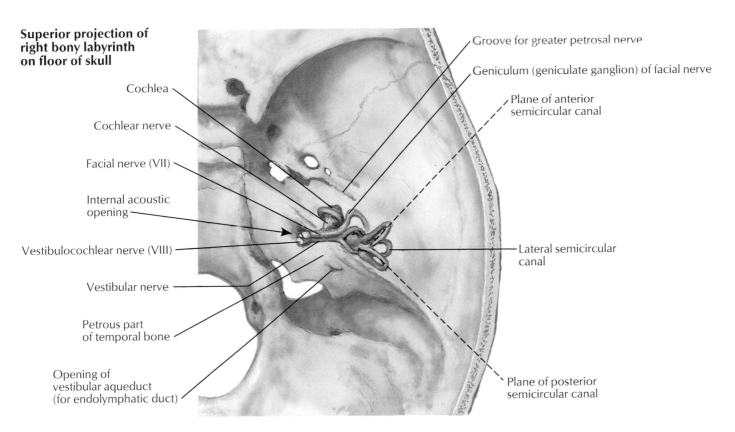

Cochlea

Cochlear nerve

Facial nerve (VII)

Internal acoustic opening

Vestibulocochlear nerve (VIII)

Vestibular nerve

Petrous part of temporal bone

Opening of vestibular aqueduct (for endolymphatic duct)

Groove for greater petrosal nerve

Geniculum (geniculate ganglion) of facial nerve

Plane of anterior semicircular canal

Lateral semicircular canal

Plane of posterior semicircular canal

Lateral projection of right membranous labyrinth

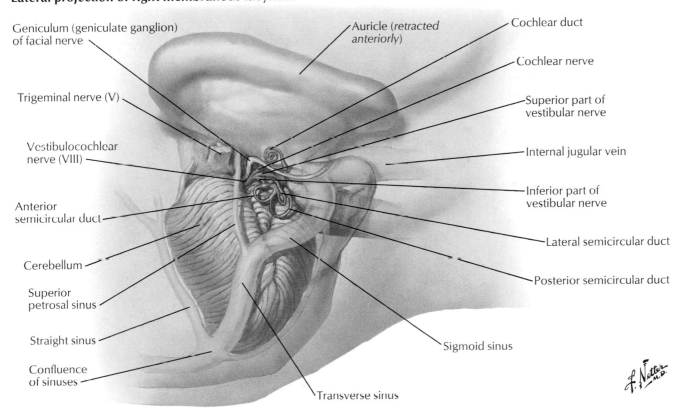

Geniculum (geniculate ganglion) of facial nerve

Trigeminal nerve (V)

Vestibulocochlear nerve (VIII)

Anterior semicircular duct

Cerebellum

Superior petrosal sinus

Straight sinus

Confluence of sinuses

Auricle (*retracted anteriorly*)

Transverse sinus

Cochlear duct

Cochlear nerve

Superior part of vestibular nerve

Internal jugular vein

Inferior part of vestibular nerve

Lateral semicircular duct

Posterior semicircular duct

Sigmoid sinus

Cartilaginous part of auditory (pharyngotympanic, eustachian) tube at base of skull: inferior view

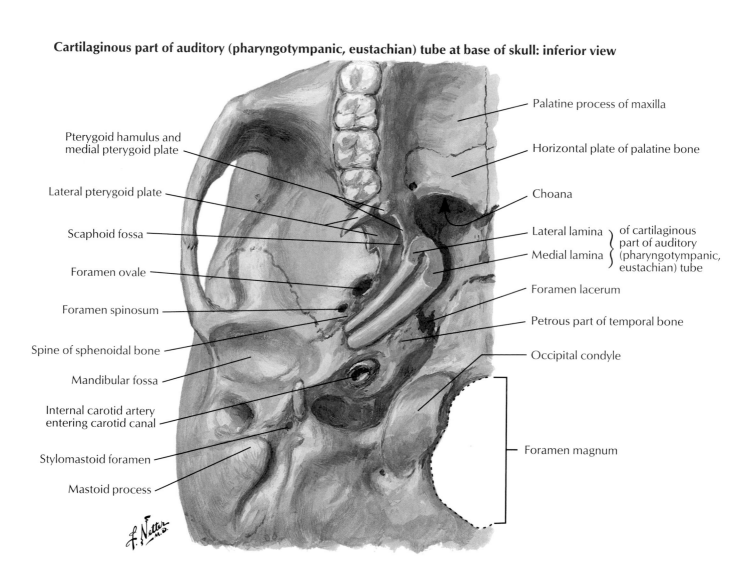

Pterygoid hamulus and medial pterygoid plate

Lateral pterygoid plate

Scaphoid fossa

Foramen ovale

Foramen spinosum

Spine of sphenoidal bone

Mandibular fossa

Internal carotid artery entering carotid canal

Stylomastoid foramen

Mastoid process

Palatine process of maxilla

Horizontal plate of palatine bone

Choana

Lateral lamina ⎫ of cartilaginous
⎬ part of auditory
Medial lamina ⎭ (pharyngotympanic, eustachian) tube

Foramen lacerum

Petrous part of temporal bone

Occipital condyle

Foramen magnum

Plate 98

Ear

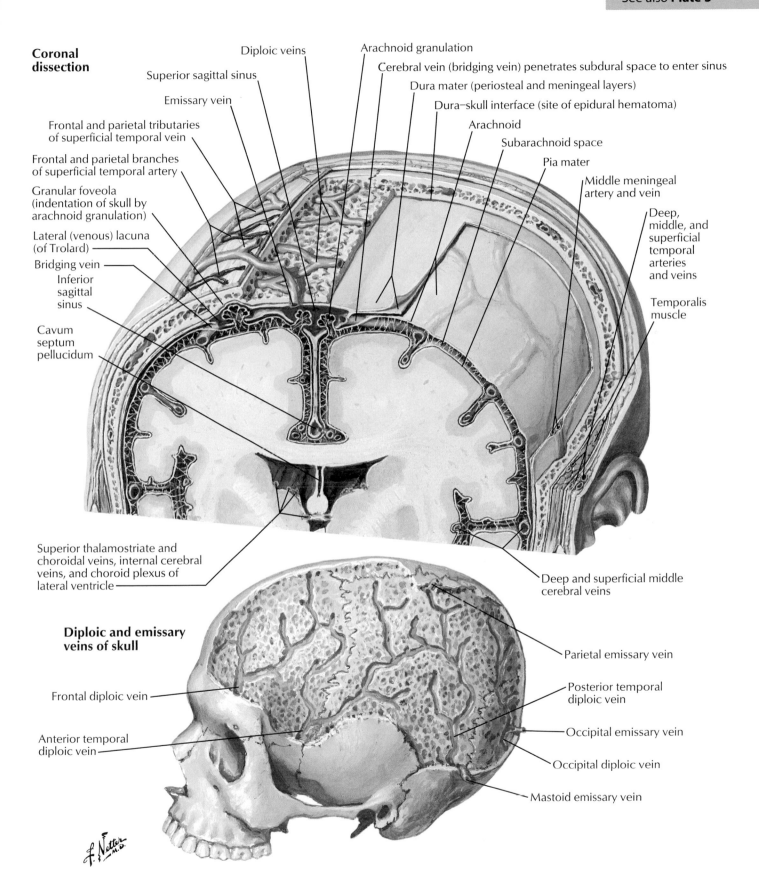

Coronal dissection

Diploic veins

Superior sagittal sinus

Emissary vein

Frontal and parietal tributaries of superficial temporal vein

Frontal and parietal branches of superficial temporal artery

Granular foveola (indentation of skull by arachnoid granulation)

Lateral (venous) lacuna (of Trolard)

Bridging vein

Inferior sagittal sinus

Cavum septum pellucidum

Arachnoid granulation

Cerebral vein (bridging vein) penetrates subdural space to enter sinus

Dura mater (periosteal and meningeal layers)

Dura–skull interface (site of epidural hematoma)

Arachnoid

Subarachnoid space

Pia mater

Middle meningeal artery and vein

Deep, middle, and superficial temporal arteries and veins

Temporalis muscle

Superior thalamostriate and choroidal veins, internal cerebral veins, and choroid plexus of lateral ventricle

Deep and superficial middle cerebral veins

Diploic and emissary veins of skull

Frontal diploic vein

Anterior temporal diploic vein

Parietal emissary vein

Posterior temporal diploic vein

Occipital emissary vein

Occipital diploic vein

Mastoid emissary vein

Meninges and Brain

Plate 99

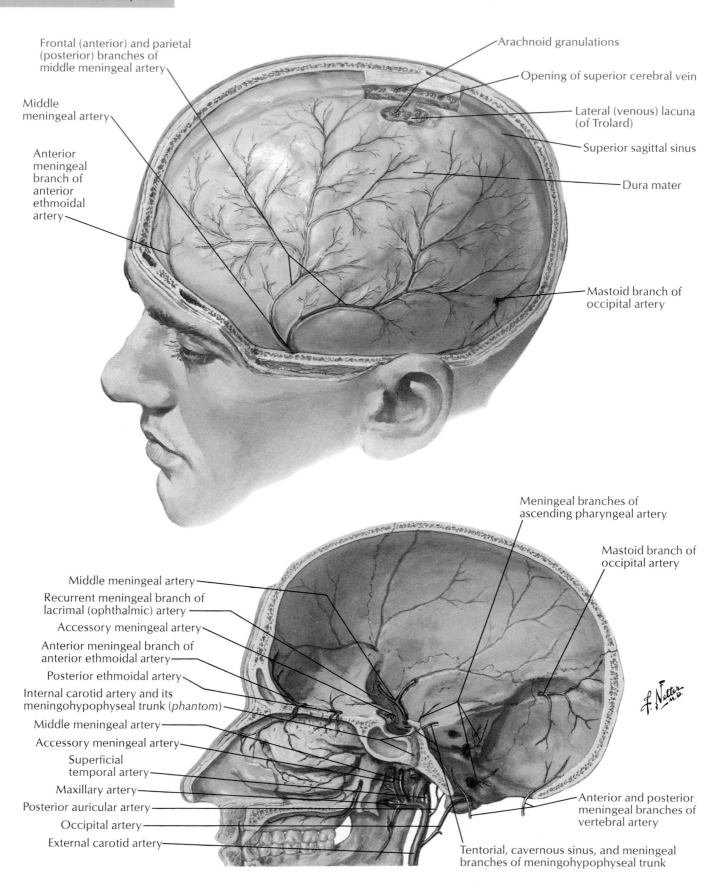

Frontal (anterior) and parietal (posterior) branches of middle meningeal artery

Middle meningeal artery

Anterior meningeal branch of anterior ethmoidal artery

Arachnoid granulations

Opening of superior cerebral vein

Lateral (venous) lacuna (of Trolard)

Superior sagittal sinus

Dura mater

Mastoid branch of occipital artery

Meningeal branches of ascending pharyngeal artery

Mastoid branch of occipital artery

Middle meningeal artery

Recurrent meningeal branch of lacrimal (ophthalmic) artery

Accessory meningeal artery

Anterior meningeal branch of anterior ethmoidal artery

Posterior ethmoidal artery

Internal carotid artery and its meningohypophyseal trunk (*phantom*)

Middle meningeal artery

Accessory meningeal artery

Superficial temporal artery

Maxillary artery

Posterior auricular artery

Occipital artery

External carotid artery

Anterior and posterior meningeal branches of vertebral artery

Tentorial, cavernous sinus, and meningeal branches of meningohypophyseal trunk

f. Netter M.D.

Plate 100

Meninges and Brain

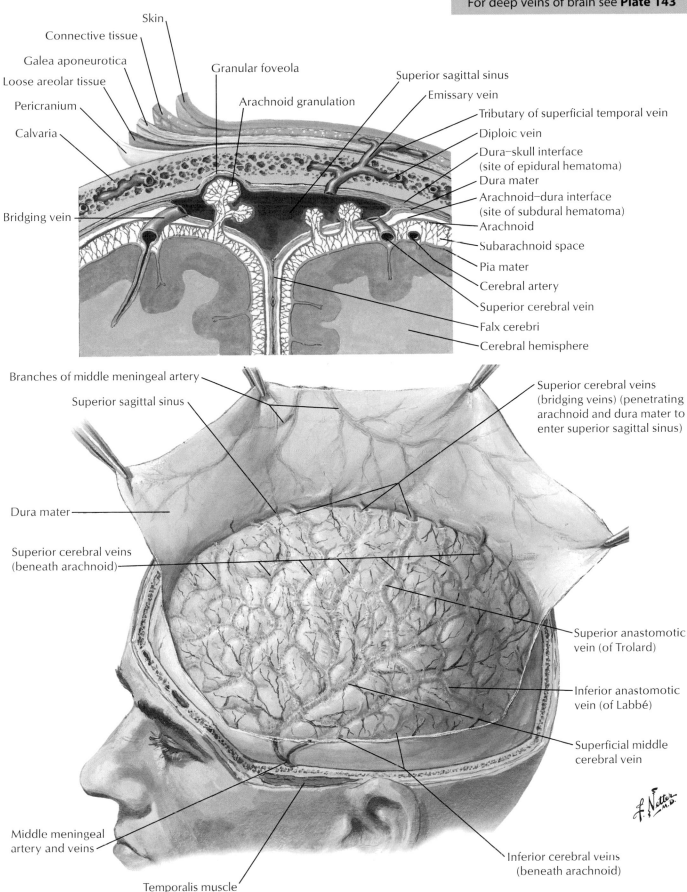

Skin

Connective tissue

Galea aponeurotica

Loose areolar tissue

Pericranium

Calvaria

Granular foveola

Arachnoid granulation

Superior sagittal sinus

Emissary vein

Tributary of superficial temporal vein

Diploic vein

Dura–skull interface (site of epidural hematoma)

Dura mater

Arachnoid–dura interface (site of subdural hematoma)

Arachnoid

Bridging vein

Subarachnoid space

Pia mater

Cerebral artery

Superior cerebral vein

Falx cerebri

Cerebral hemisphere

Branches of middle meningeal artery

Superior sagittal sinus

Superior cerebral veins (bridging veins) (penetrating arachnoid and dura mater to enter superior sagittal sinus)

Dura mater

Superior cerebral veins (beneath arachnoid)

Superior anastomotic vein (of Trolard)

Inferior anastomotic vein (of Labbé)

Superficial middle cerebral vein

Middle meningeal artery and veins

Temporalis muscle

Inferior cerebral veins (beneath arachnoid)

Meninges and Brain

Plate 101

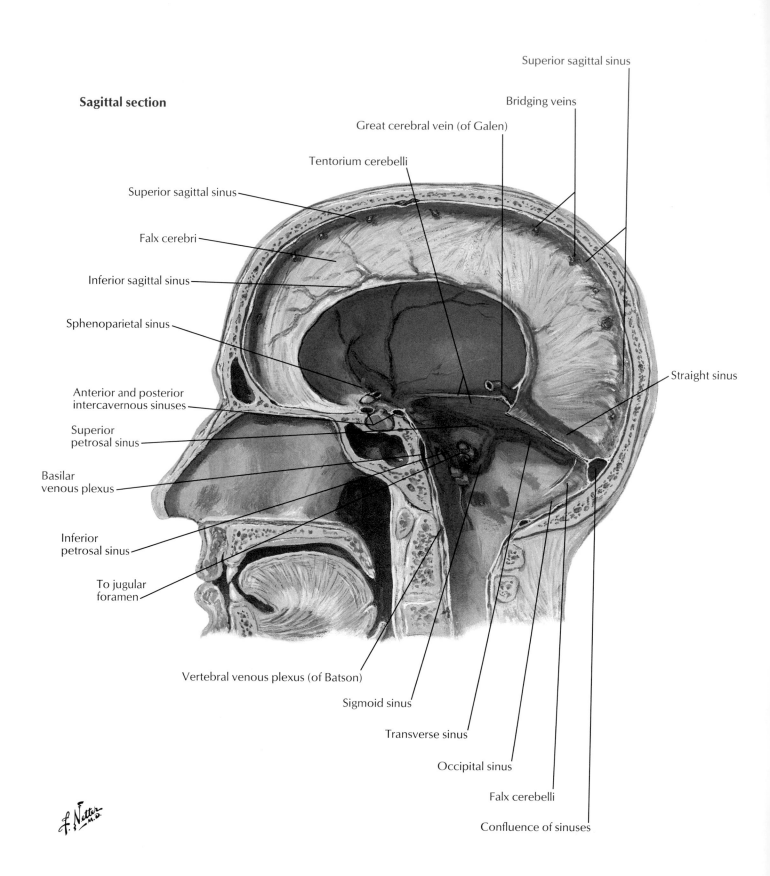

Sagittal section

Superior sagittal sinus

Bridging veins

Great cerebral vein (of Galen)

Tentorium cerebelli

Superior sagittal sinus

Falx cerebri

Inferior sagittal sinus

Sphenoparietal sinus

Straight sinus

Anterior and posterior intercavernous sinuses

Superior petrosal sinus

Basilar venous plexus

Inferior petrosal sinus

To jugular foramen

Vertebral venous plexus (of Batson)

Sigmoid sinus

Transverse sinus

Occipital sinus

Falx cerebelli

Confluence of sinuses

Plate 102

Meninges and Brain

Skull sectioned horizontally: superior view

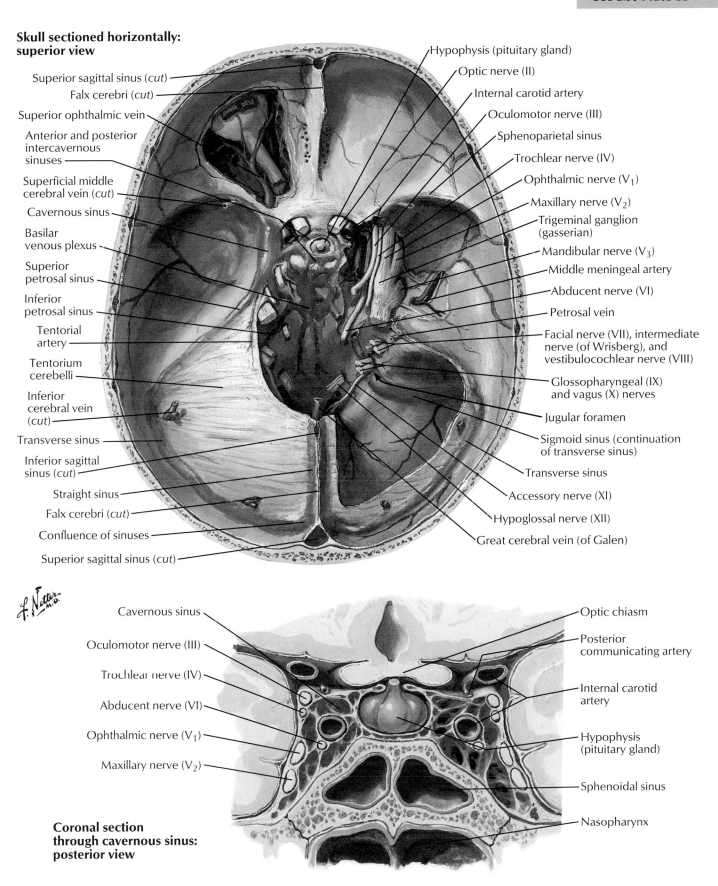

Superior sagittal sinus (*cut*)

Falx cerebri (*cut*)

Superior ophthalmic vein

Anterior and posterior intercavernous sinuses

Superficial middle cerebral vein (*cut*)

Cavernous sinus

Basilar venous plexus

Superior petrosal sinus

Inferior petrosal sinus

Tentorial artery

Tentorium cerebelli

Inferior cerebral vein (*cut*)

Transverse sinus

Inferior sagittal sinus (*cut*)

Straight sinus

Falx cerebri (*cut*)

Confluence of sinuses

Superior sagittal sinus (*cut*)

Hypophysis (pituitary gland)

Optic nerve (II)

Internal carotid artery

Oculomotor nerve (III)

Sphenoparietal sinus

Trochlear nerve (IV)

Ophthalmic nerve (V₁)

Maxillary nerve (V₂)

Trigeminal ganglion (gasserian)

Mandibular nerve (V₃)

Middle meningeal artery

Abducent nerve (VI)

Petrosal vein

Facial nerve (VII), intermediate nerve (of Wrisberg), and vestibulocochlear nerve (VIII)

Glossopharyngeal (IX) and vagus (X) nerves

Jugular foramen

Sigmoid sinus (continuation of transverse sinus)

Transverse sinus

Accessory nerve (XI)

Hypoglossal nerve (XII)

Great cerebral vein (of Galen)

Cavernous sinus

Oculomotor nerve (III)

Trochlear nerve (IV)

Abducent nerve (VI)

Ophthalmic nerve (V₁)

Maxillary nerve (V₂)

Optic chiasm

Posterior communicating artery

Internal carotid artery

Hypophysis (pituitary gland)

Sphenoidal sinus

Nasopharynx

Coronal section through cavernous sinus: posterior view

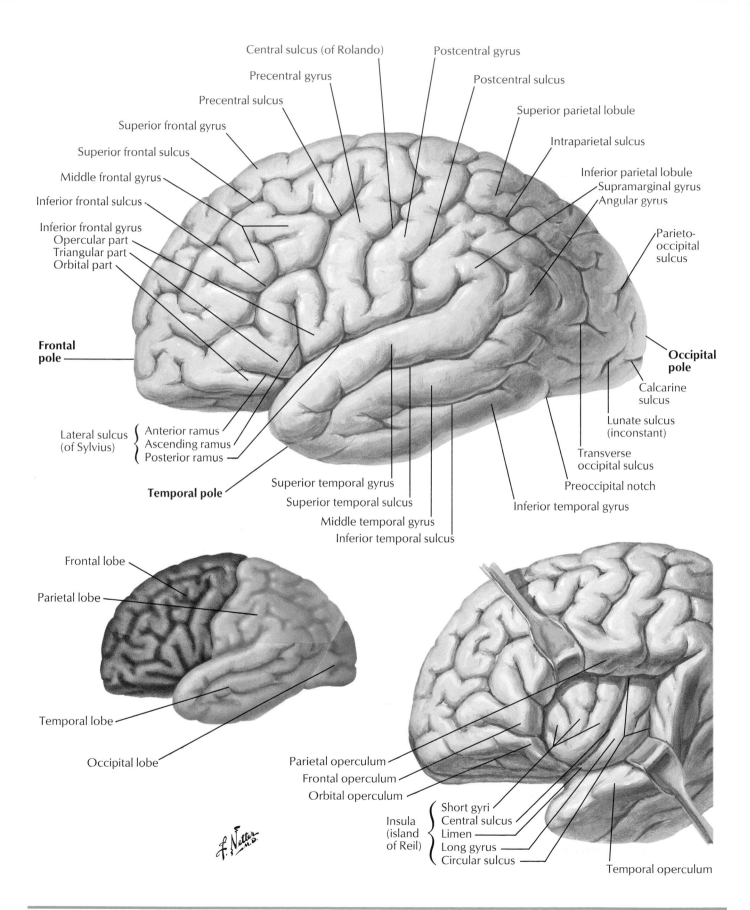

Central sulcus (of Rolando)
Precentral gyrus
Precentral sulcus
Superior frontal gyrus
Superior frontal sulcus
Middle frontal gyrus
Inferior frontal sulcus
Inferior frontal gyrus
Opercular part
Triangular part
Orbital part
Frontal pole
Postcentral gyrus
Postcentral sulcus
Superior parietal lobule
Intraparietal sulcus
Inferior parietal lobule
Supramarginal gyrus
Angular gyrus
Parieto-occipital sulcus
Occipital pole
Calcarine sulcus
Lunate sulcus (inconstant)
Transverse occipital sulcus
Preoccipital notch
Inferior temporal gyrus
Lateral sulcus (of Sylvius)
Anterior ramus
Ascending ramus
Posterior ramus
Temporal pole
Superior temporal gyrus
Superior temporal sulcus
Middle temporal gyrus
Inferior temporal sulcus

Frontal lobe
Parietal lobe
Temporal lobe
Occipital lobe

Parietal operculum
Frontal operculum
Orbital operculum
Insula (island of Reil)
Short gyri
Central sulcus
Limen
Long gyrus
Circular sulcus
Temporal operculum

Plate 104   **Meninges and Brain**

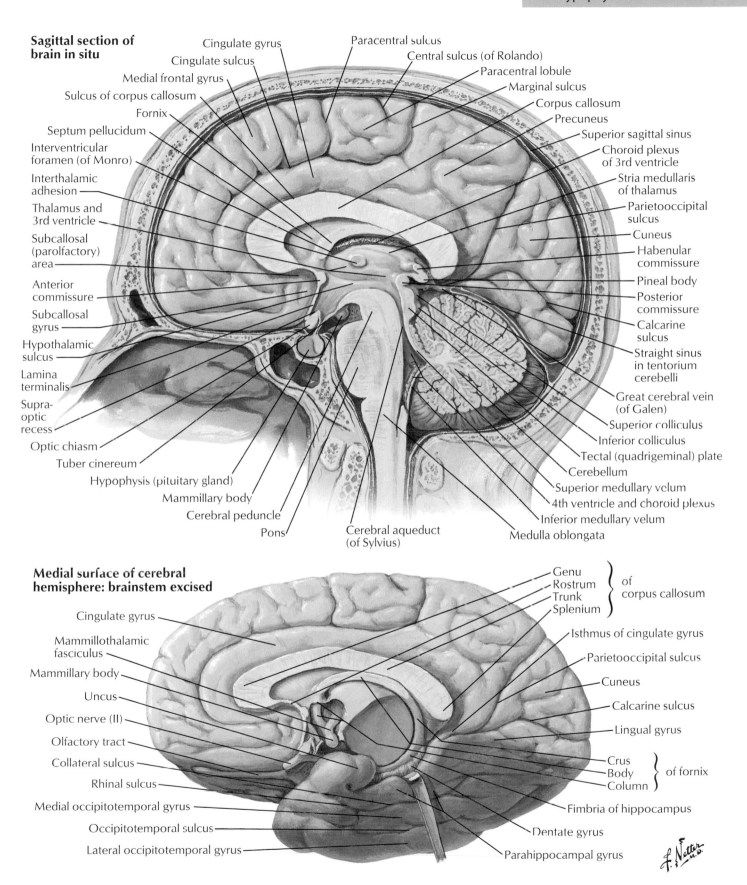

Sagittal section of brain in situ

Cingulate gyrus
Cingulate sulcus
Medial frontal gyrus
Sulcus of corpus callosum
Fornix
Septum pellucidum
Interventricular foramen (of Monro)
Interthalamic adhesion
Thalamus and 3rd ventricle
Subcallosal (parolfactory) area
Anterior commissure
Subcallosal gyrus
Hypothalamic sulcus
Lamina terminalis
Supra-optic recess
Optic chiasm
Tuber cinereum
Hypophysis (pituitary gland)
Mammillary body
Cerebral peduncle
Pons
Cerebral aqueduct (of Sylvius)

Paracentral sulcus
Central sulcus (of Rolando)
Paracentral lobule
Marginal sulcus
Corpus callosum
Precuneus
Superior sagittal sinus
Choroid plexus of 3rd ventricle
Stria medullaris of thalamus
Parietooccipital sulcus
Cuneus
Habenular commissure
Pineal body
Posterior commissure
Calcarine sulcus
Straight sinus in tentorium cerebelli
Great cerebral vein (of Galen)
Superior colliculus
Inferior colliculus
Tectal (quadrigeminal) plate
Cerebellum
Superior medullary velum
4th ventricle and choroid plexus
Inferior medullary velum
Medulla oblongata

Medial surface of cerebral hemisphere: brainstem excised

Cingulate gyrus
Mammillothalamic fasciculus
Mammillary body
Uncus
Optic nerve (II)
Olfactory tract
Collateral sulcus
Rhinal sulcus
Medial occipitotemporal gyrus
Occipitotemporal sulcus
Lateral occipitotemporal gyrus

Genu
Rostrum
Trunk
Splenium
} of corpus callosum

Isthmus of cingulate gyrus
Parietooccipital sulcus
Cuneus
Calcarine sulcus
Lingual gyrus
Crus
Body
Column
} of fornix
Fimbria of hippocampus
Dentate gyrus
Parahippocampal gyrus

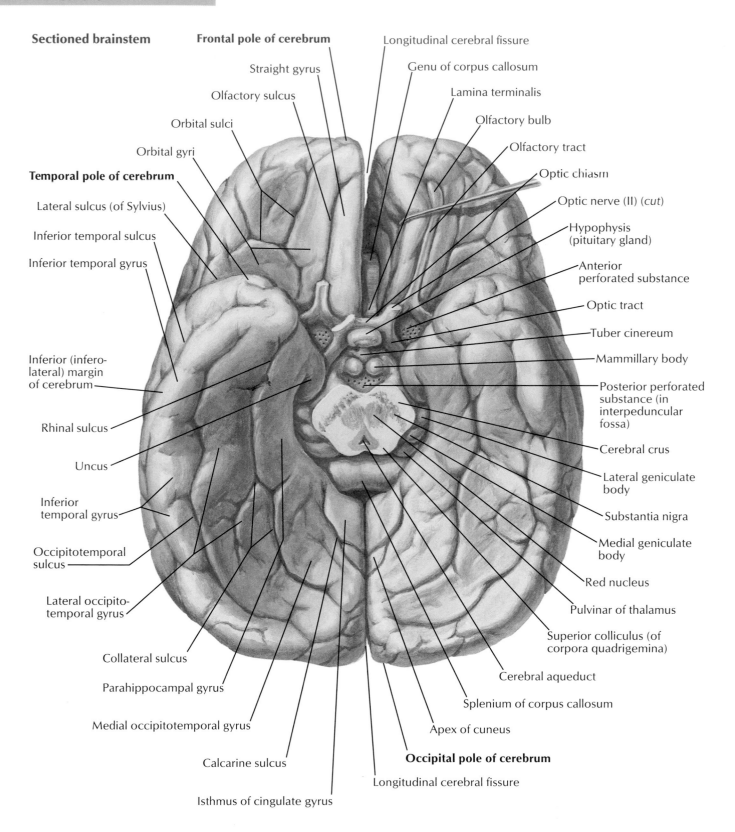

Sectioned brainstem   Frontal pole of cerebrum   Longitudinal cerebral fissure

Straight gyrus   Genu of corpus callosum

Olfactory sulcus   Lamina terminalis

Orbital sulci   Olfactory bulb

Orbital gyri   Olfactory tract

Temporal pole of cerebrum   Optic chiasm

Lateral sulcus (of Sylvius)   Optic nerve (II) *(cut)*

Inferior temporal sulcus   Hypophysis (pituitary gland)

Inferior temporal gyrus   Anterior perforated substance

Optic tract

Tuber cinereum

Mammillary body

Inferior (infero-lateral) margin of cerebrum   Posterior perforated substance (in interpeduncular fossa)

Rhinal sulcus   Cerebral crus

Uncus   Lateral geniculate body

Inferior temporal gyrus   Substantia nigra

Medial geniculate body

Occipitotemporal sulcus   Red nucleus

Lateral occipito-temporal gyrus   Pulvinar of thalamus

Superior colliculus (of corpora quadrigemina)

Collateral sulcus   Cerebral aqueduct

Parahippocampal gyrus   Splenium of corpus callosum

Medial occipitotemporal gyrus   Apex of cuneus

Calcarine sulcus   **Occipital pole of cerebrum**

Longitudinal cerebral fissure

Isthmus of cingulate gyrus

Plate 106   **Meninges and Brain**

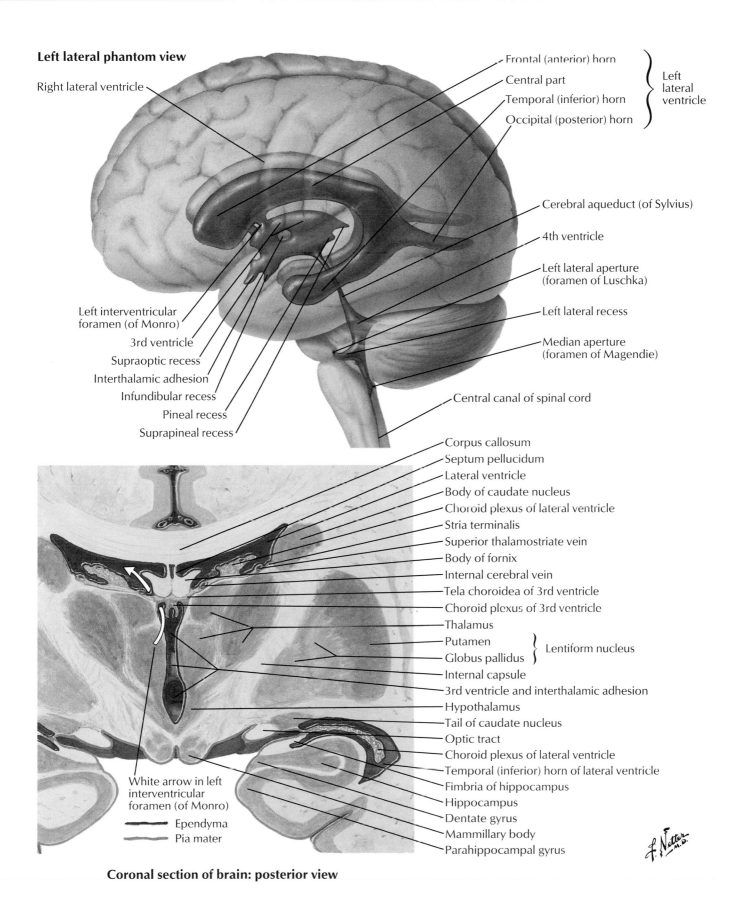

Left lateral phantom view

Right lateral ventricle

Frontal (anterior) horn
Central part
Temporal (inferior) horn
Occipital (posterior) horn
} Left lateral ventricle

Cerebral aqueduct (of Sylvius)

4th ventricle

Left lateral aperture (foramen of Luschka)

Left lateral recess

Median aperture (foramen of Magendie)

Left interventricular foramen (of Monro)

3rd ventricle

Supraoptic recess

Interthalamic adhesion

Infundibular recess

Pineal recess

Suprapineal recess

Central canal of spinal cord

Corpus callosum
Septum pellucidum
Lateral ventricle
Body of caudate nucleus
Choroid plexus of lateral ventricle
Stria terminalis
Superior thalamostriate vein
Body of fornix
Internal cerebral vein
Tela choroidea of 3rd ventricle
Choroid plexus of 3rd ventricle
Thalamus
Putamen
Globus pallidus
} Lentiform nucleus
Internal capsule
3rd ventricle and interthalamic adhesion
Hypothalamus
Tail of caudate nucleus
Optic tract
Choroid plexus of lateral ventricle
Temporal (inferior) horn of lateral ventricle
Fimbria of hippocampus
Hippocampus
Dentate gyrus
Mammillary body
Parahippocampal gyrus

White arrow in left interventricular foramen (of Monro)

— Ependyma
— Pia mater

Coronal section of brain: posterior view

Meninges and Brain

Plate 107

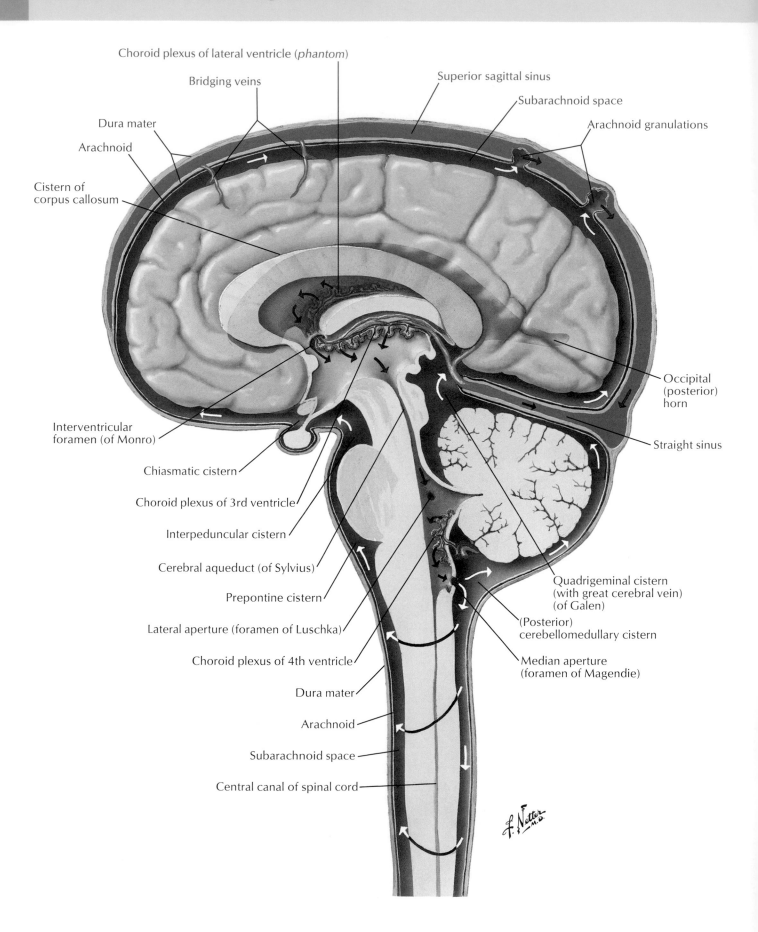

Choroid plexus of lateral ventricle (*phantom*)

Bridging veins

Dura mater

Arachnoid

Cistern of corpus callosum

Superior sagittal sinus

Subarachnoid space

Arachnoid granulations

Occipital (posterior) horn

Straight sinus

Quadrigeminal cistern (with great cerebral vein) (of Galen)

(Posterior) cerebellomedullary cistern

Median aperture (foramen of Magendie)

Interventricular foramen (of Monro)

Chiasmatic cistern

Choroid plexus of 3rd ventricle

Interpeduncular cistern

Cerebral aqueduct (of Sylvius)

Prepontine cistern

Lateral aperture (foramen of Luschka)

Choroid plexus of 4th ventricle

Dura mater

Arachnoid

Subarachnoid space

Central canal of spinal cord

Plate 108

Meninges and Brain

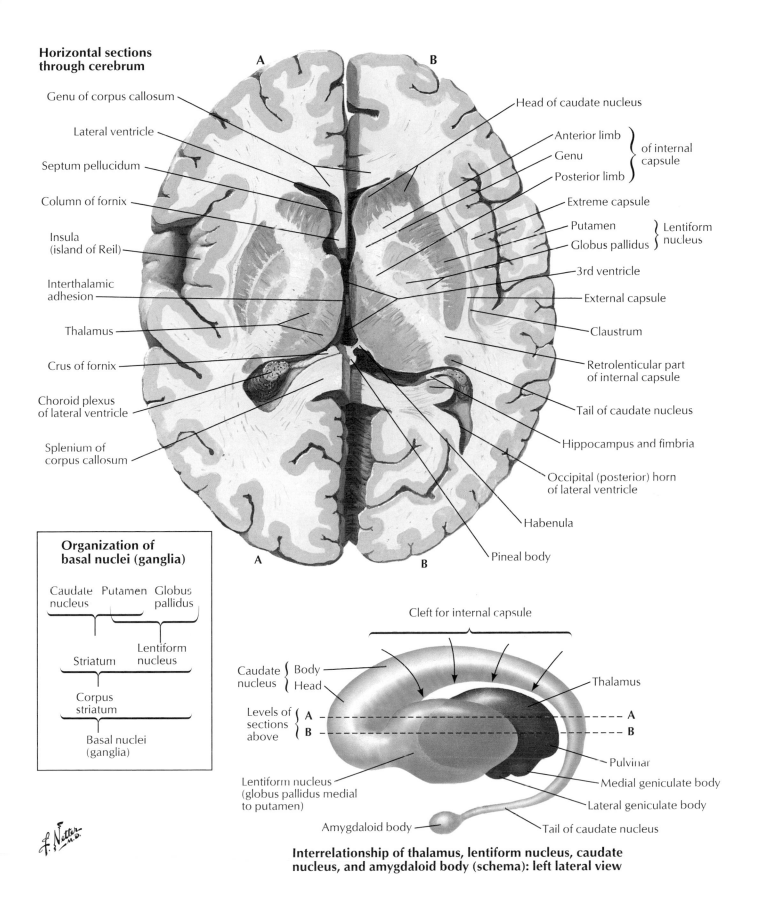

Horizontal sections through cerebrum

Genu of corpus callosum

Lateral ventricle

Septum pellucidum

Column of fornix

Insula (island of Reil)

Interthalamic adhesion

Thalamus

Crus of fornix

Choroid plexus of lateral ventricle

Splenium of corpus callosum

Head of caudate nucleus

Anterior limb
Genu
Posterior limb
} of internal capsule

Extreme capsule

Putamen
Globus pallidus
} Lentiform nucleus

3rd ventricle

External capsule

Claustrum

Retrolenticular part of internal capsule

Tail of caudate nucleus

Hippocampus and fimbria

Occipital (posterior) horn of lateral ventricle

Habenula

Pineal body

A   B

Organization of basal nuclei (ganglia)

Caudate nucleus   Putamen   Globus pallidus

Lentiform nucleus

Striatum

Corpus striatum

Basal nuclei (ganglia)

Cleft for internal capsule

Caudate nucleus { Body, Head

Levels of sections above { A, B

Thalamus

A

B

Pulvinar

Medial geniculate body

Lateral geniculate body

Lentiform nucleus (globus pallidus medial to putamen)

Amygdaloid body

Tail of caudate nucleus

Interrelationship of thalamus, lentiform nucleus, caudate nucleus, and amygdaloid body (schema): left lateral view

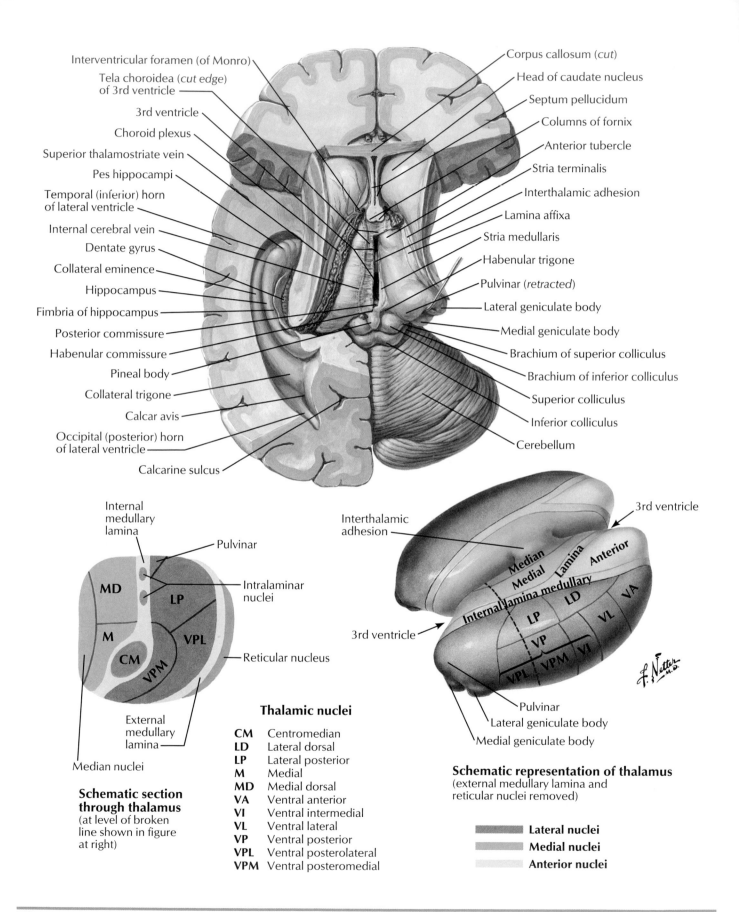

Thalamic nuclei

CM	Centromedian
LD	Lateral dorsal
LP	Lateral posterior
M	Medial
MD	Medial dorsal
VA	Ventral anterior
VI	Ventral intermedial
VL	Ventral lateral
VP	Ventral posterior
VPL	Ventral posterolateral
VPM	Ventral posteromedial

Schematic section through thalamus (at level of broken line shown in figure at right)

Schematic representation of thalamus (external medullary lamina and reticular nuclei removed)

Lateral nuclei
Medial nuclei
Anterior nuclei

Plate 110   **Meninges and Brain**

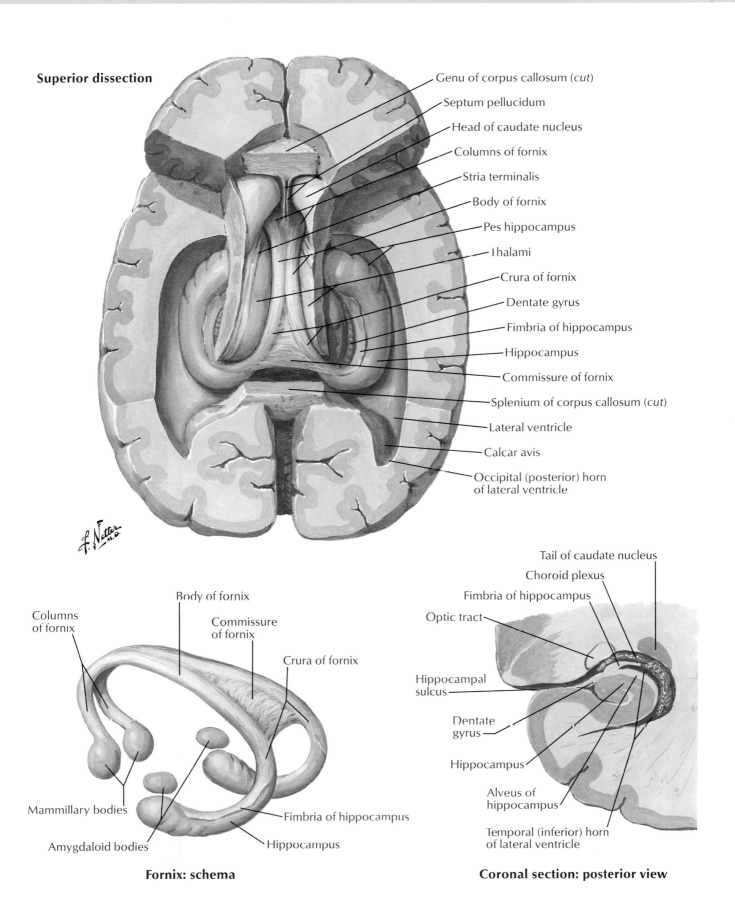

Superior dissection

Genu of corpus callosum (*cut*)

Septum pellucidum

Head of caudate nucleus

Columns of fornix

Stria terminalis

Body of fornix

Pes hippocampus

Thalami

Crura of fornix

Dentate gyrus

Fimbria of hippocampus

Hippocampus

Commissure of fornix

Splenium of corpus callosum (*cut*)

Lateral ventricle

Calcar avis

Occipital (posterior) horn
of lateral ventricle

Columns
of fornix

Body of fornix

Commissure
of fornix

Crura of fornix

Mammillary bodies

Amygdaloid bodies

Fimbria of hippocampus

Hippocampus

Fornix: schema

Tail of caudate nucleus

Choroid plexus

Fimbria of hippocampus

Optic tract

Hippocampal
sulcus

Dentate
gyrus

Hippocampus

Alveus of
hippocampus

Temporal (inferior) horn
of lateral ventricle

Coronal section: posterior view

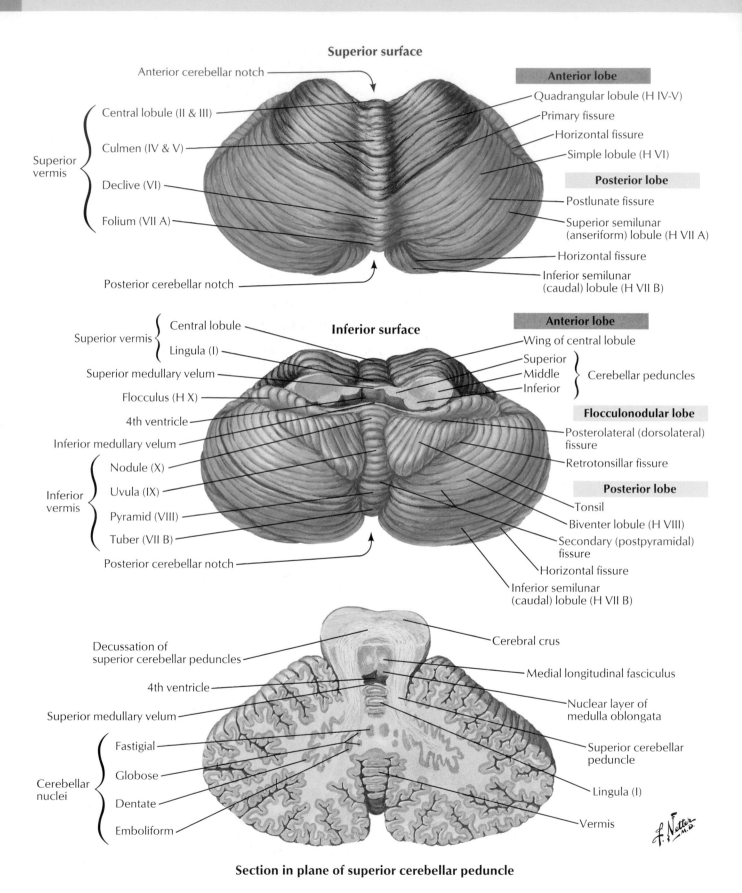

Superior surface

Anterior cerebellar notch

Central lobule (II & III)

Culmen (IV & V)

Superior vermis

Declive (VI)

Folium (VII A)

Posterior cerebellar notch

Anterior lobe

Quadrangular lobule (H IV-V)

Primary fissure

Horizontal fissure

Simple lobule (H VI)

Posterior lobe

Postlunate fissure

Superior semilunar (anseriform) lobule (H VII A)

Horizontal fissure

Inferior semilunar (caudal) lobule (H VII B)

Inferior surface

Superior vermis
Central lobule
Lingula (I)

Superior medullary velum

Flocculus (H X)

4th ventricle

Inferior medullary velum

Inferior vermis
Nodule (X)
Uvula (IX)
Pyramid (VIII)
Tuber (VII B)

Posterior cerebellar notch

Anterior lobe

Wing of central lobule

Superior
Middle
Inferior
Cerebellar peduncles

Flocculonodular lobe

Posterolateral (dorsolateral) fissure

Retrotonsillar fissure

Posterior lobe

Tonsil

Biventer lobule (H VIII)

Secondary (postpyramidal) fissure

Horizontal fissure

Inferior semilunar (caudal) lobule (H VII B)

Decussation of superior cerebellar peduncles

4th ventricle

Superior medullary velum

Cerebellar nuclei
Fastigial
Globose
Dentate
Emboliform

Cerebral crus

Medial longitudinal fasciculus

Nuclear layer of medulla oblongata

Superior cerebellar peduncle

Lingula (I)

Vermis

Section in plane of superior cerebellar peduncle

Plate 112

Meninges and Brain

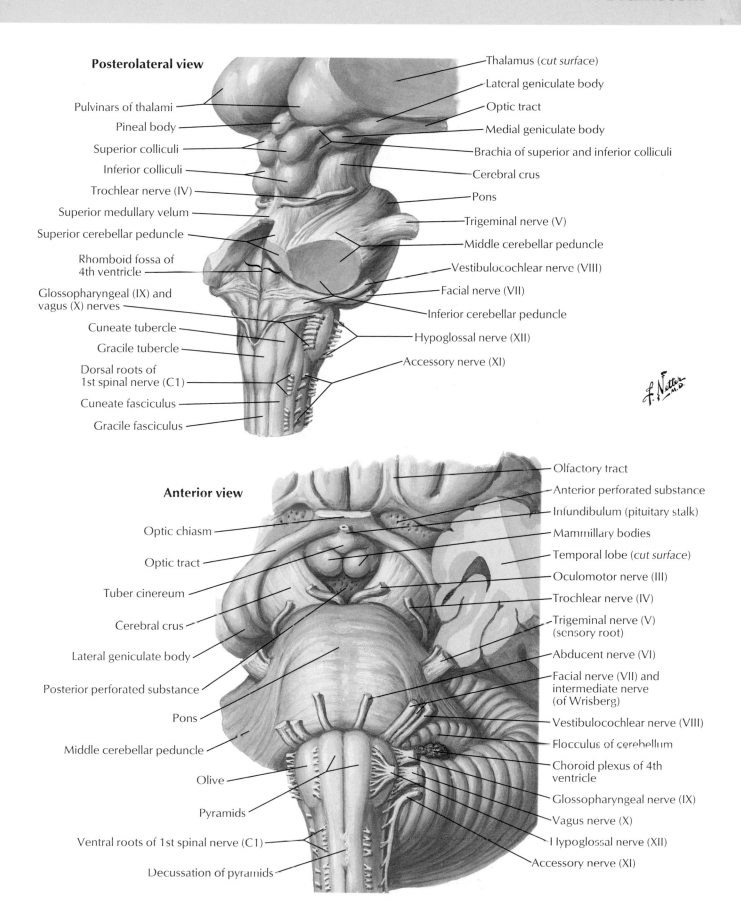

Posterolateral view

Pulvinars of thalami

Pineal body

Superior colliculi

Inferior colliculi

Trochlear nerve (IV)

Superior medullary velum

Superior cerebellar peduncle

Rhomboid fossa of 4th ventricle

Glossopharyngeal (IX) and vagus (X) nerves

Cuneate tubercle

Gracile tubercle

Dorsal roots of 1st spinal nerve (C1)

Cuneate fasciculus

Gracile fasciculus

Thalamus (cut surface)

Lateral geniculate body

Optic tract

Medial geniculate body

Brachia of superior and inferior colliculi

Cerebral crus

Pons

Trigeminal nerve (V)

Middle cerebellar peduncle

Vestibulocochlear nerve (VIII)

Facial nerve (VII)

Inferior cerebellar peduncle

Hypoglossal nerve (XII)

Accessory nerve (XI)

Anterior view

Optic chiasm

Optic tract

Tuber cinereum

Cerebral crus

Lateral geniculate body

Posterior perforated substance

Pons

Middle cerebellar peduncle

Olive

Pyramids

Ventral roots of 1st spinal nerve (C1)

Decussation of pyramids

Olfactory tract

Anterior perforated substance

Infundibulum (pituitary stalk)

Mammillary bodies

Temporal lobe (cut surface)

Oculomotor nerve (III)

Trochlear nerve (IV)

Trigeminal nerve (V) (sensory root)

Abducent nerve (VI)

Facial nerve (VII) and intermediate nerve (of Wrisberg)

Vestibulocochlear nerve (VIII)

Flocculus of cerebellum

Choroid plexus of 4th ventricle

Glossopharyngeal nerve (IX)

Vagus nerve (X)

Hypoglossal nerve (XII)

Accessory nerve (XI)

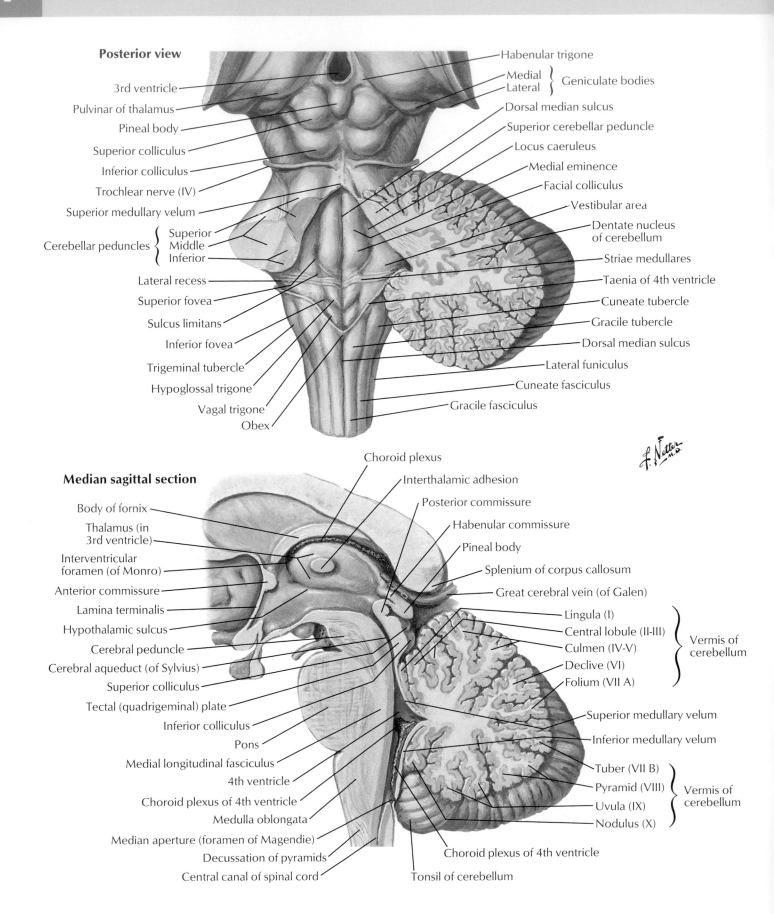

Posterior view

3rd ventricle

Pulvinar of thalamus

Pineal body

Superior colliculus

Inferior colliculus

Trochlear nerve (IV)

Superior medullary velum

Cerebellar peduncles { Superior
Middle
Inferior

Lateral recess

Superior fovea

Sulcus limitans

Inferior fovea

Trigeminal tubercle

Hypoglossal trigone

Vagal trigone

Obex

Habenular trigone

Medial } Geniculate bodies
Lateral

Dorsal median sulcus

Superior cerebellar peduncle

Locus caeruleus

Medial eminence

Facial colliculus

Vestibular area

Dentate nucleus of cerebellum

Striae medullares

Taenia of 4th ventricle

Cuneate tubercle

Gracile tubercle

Dorsal median sulcus

Lateral funiculus

Cuneate fasciculus

Gracile fasciculus

Median sagittal section

Body of fornix

Thalamus (in 3rd ventricle)

Interventricular foramen (of Monro)

Anterior commissure

Lamina terminalis

Hypothalamic sulcus

Cerebral peduncle

Cerebral aqueduct (of Sylvius)

Superior colliculus

Tectal (quadrigeminal) plate

Inferior colliculus

Pons

Medial longitudinal fasciculus

4th ventricle

Choroid plexus of 4th ventricle

Medulla oblongata

Median aperture (foramen of Magendie)

Decussation of pyramids

Central canal of spinal cord

Choroid plexus

Interthalamic adhesion

Posterior commissure

Habenular commissure

Pineal body

Splenium of corpus callosum

Great cerebral vein (of Galen)

Lingula (I)

Central lobule (II-III)

Culmen (IV-V)

Declive (VI)

Folium (VII A)

Vermis of cerebellum

Superior medullary velum

Inferior medullary velum

Tuber (VII B)

Pyramid (VIII)

Uvula (IX)

Nodulus (X)

Vermis of cerebellum

Choroid plexus of 4th ventricle

Tonsil of cerebellum

Plate 114   **Meninges and Brain**

Posterior phantom view

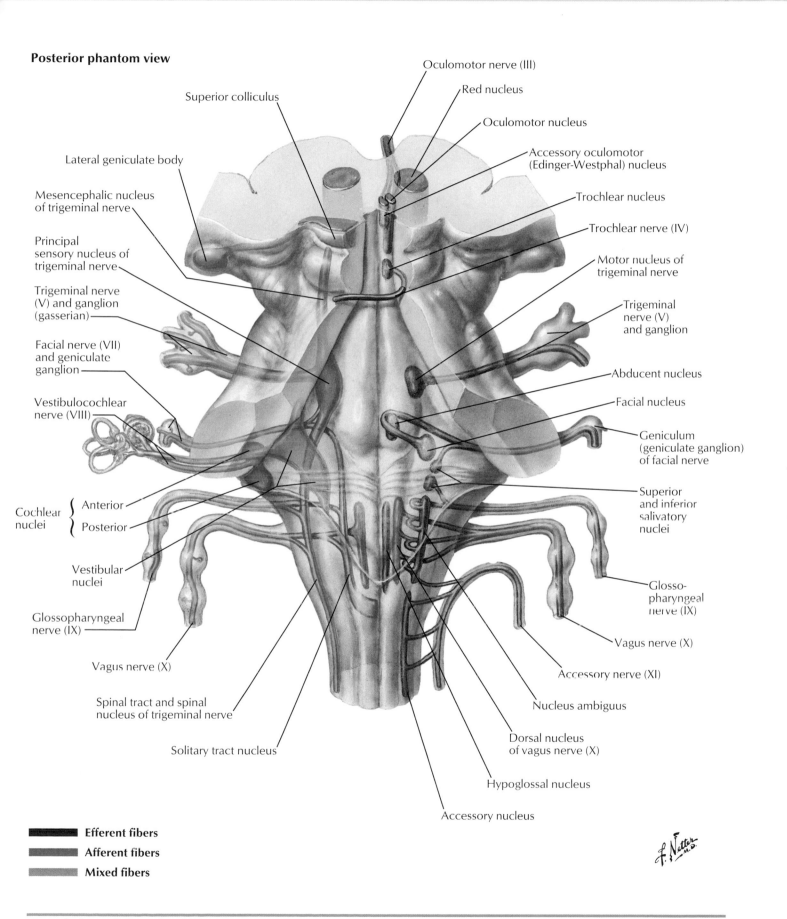

Superior colliculus

Oculomotor nerve (III)

Red nucleus

Oculomotor nucleus

Accessory oculomotor
(Edinger-Westphal) nucleus

Lateral geniculate body

Mesencephalic nucleus
of trigeminal nerve

Trochlear nucleus

Trochlear nerve (IV)

Principal
sensory nucleus of
trigeminal nerve

Motor nucleus of
trigeminal nerve

Trigeminal nerve
(V) and ganglion
(gasserian)

Trigeminal
nerve (V)
and ganglion

Facial nerve (VII)
and geniculate
ganglion

Abducent nucleus

Facial nucleus

Vestibulocochlear
nerve (VIII)

Geniculum
(geniculate ganglion)
of facial nerve

Cochlear
nuclei { Anterior
Posterior

Superior
and inferior
salivatory
nuclei

Vestibular
nuclei

Glosso-
pharyngeal
nerve (IX)

Glossopharyngeal
nerve (IX)

Vagus nerve (X)

Vagus nerve (X)

Accessory nerve (XI)

Spinal tract and spinal
nucleus of trigeminal nerve

Nucleus ambiguus

Dorsal nucleus
of vagus nerve (X)

Solitary tract nucleus

Hypoglossal nucleus

Accessory nucleus

Efferent fibers
Afferent fibers
Mixed fibers

Medial dissection

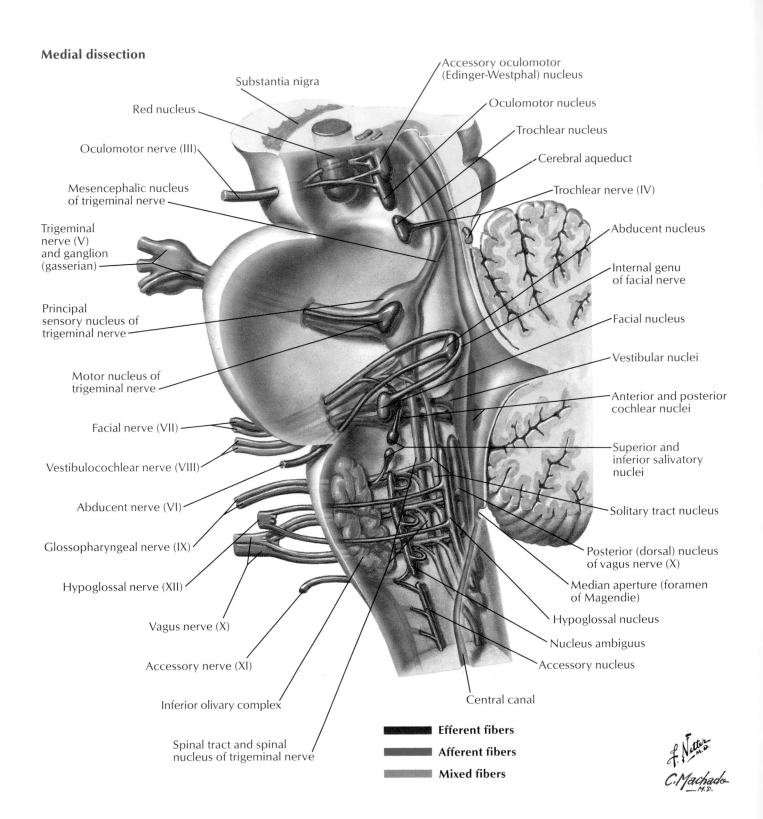

Substantia nigra

Red nucleus

Oculomotor nerve (III)

Mesencephalic nucleus of trigeminal nerve

Trigeminal nerve (V) and ganglion (gasserian)

Principal sensory nucleus of trigeminal nerve

Motor nucleus of trigeminal nerve

Facial nerve (VII)

Vestibulocochlear nerve (VIII)

Abducent nerve (VI)

Glossopharyngeal nerve (IX)

Hypoglossal nerve (XII)

Vagus nerve (X)

Accessory nerve (XI)

Inferior olivary complex

Spinal tract and spinal nucleus of trigeminal nerve

Accessory oculomotor (Edinger-Westphal) nucleus

Oculomotor nucleus

Trochlear nucleus

Cerebral aqueduct

Trochlear nerve (IV)

Abducent nucleus

Internal genu of facial nerve

Facial nucleus

Vestibular nuclei

Anterior and posterior cochlear nuclei

Superior and inferior salivatory nuclei

Solitary tract nucleus

Posterior (dorsal) nucleus of vagus nerve (X)

Median aperture (foramen of Magendie)

Hypoglossal nucleus

Nucleus ambiguus

Accessory nucleus

Central canal

Efferent fibers

Afferent fibers

Mixed fibers

Plate 116

Cranial and Cervical Nerves

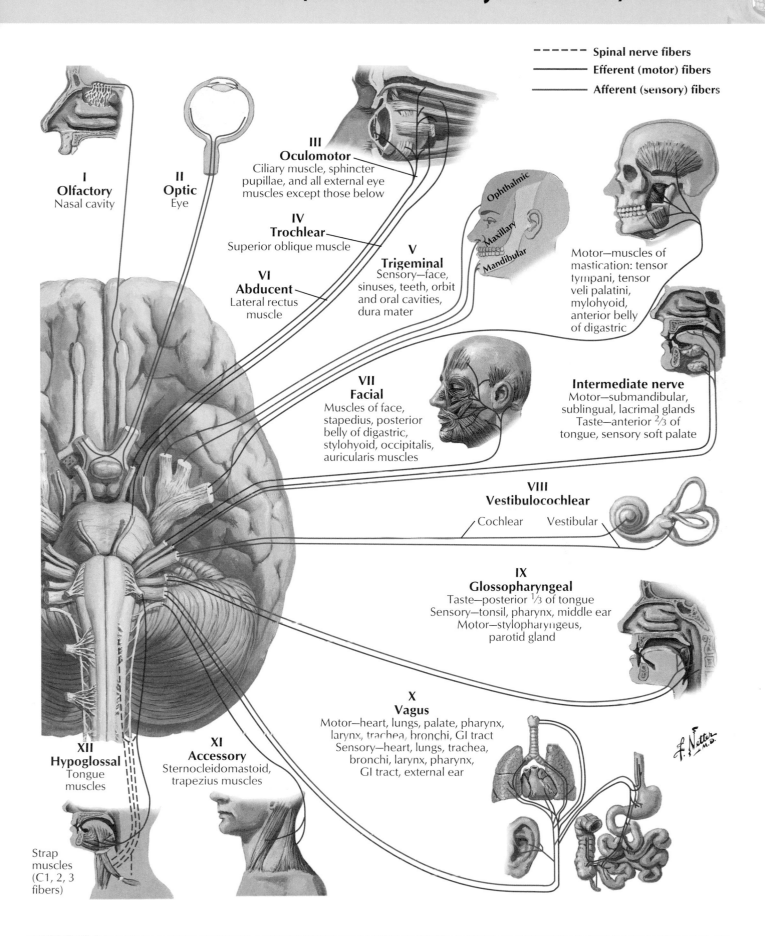

- - - - - Spinal nerve fibers
───── Efferent (motor) fibers
───── Afferent (sensory) fibers

I
Olfactory
Nasal cavity

II
Optic
Eye

III
Oculomotor
Ciliary muscle, sphincter pupillae, and all external eye muscles except those below

IV
Trochlear
Superior oblique muscle

VI
Abducent
Lateral rectus muscle

V
Trigeminal
Sensory—face, sinuses, teeth, orbit and oral cavities, dura mater

Ophthalmic
Maxillary
Mandibular

Motor—muscles of mastication: tensor tympani, tensor veli palatini, mylohyoid, anterior belly of digastric

VII
Facial
Muscles of face, stapedius, posterior belly of digastric, stylohyoid, occipitalis, auricularis muscles

Intermediate nerve
Motor—submandibular, sublingual, lacrimal glands
Taste—anterior 2/3 of tongue, sensory soft palate

VIII
Vestibulocochlear
Cochlear   Vestibular

IX
Glossopharyngeal
Taste—posterior 1/3 of tongue
Sensory—tonsil, pharynx, middle ear
Motor—stylopharyngeus, parotid gland

X
Vagus
Motor—heart, lungs, palate, pharynx, larynx, trachea, bronchi, GI tract
Sensory—heart, lungs, trachea, bronchi, larynx, pharynx, GI tract, external ear

XII
Hypoglossal
Tongue muscles

XI
Accessory
Sternocleidomastoid, trapezius muscles

Strap muscles (C1, 2, 3 fibers)

F. Netter M.D.

Olfactory Nerve (I): Schema

See also **Plate 42**

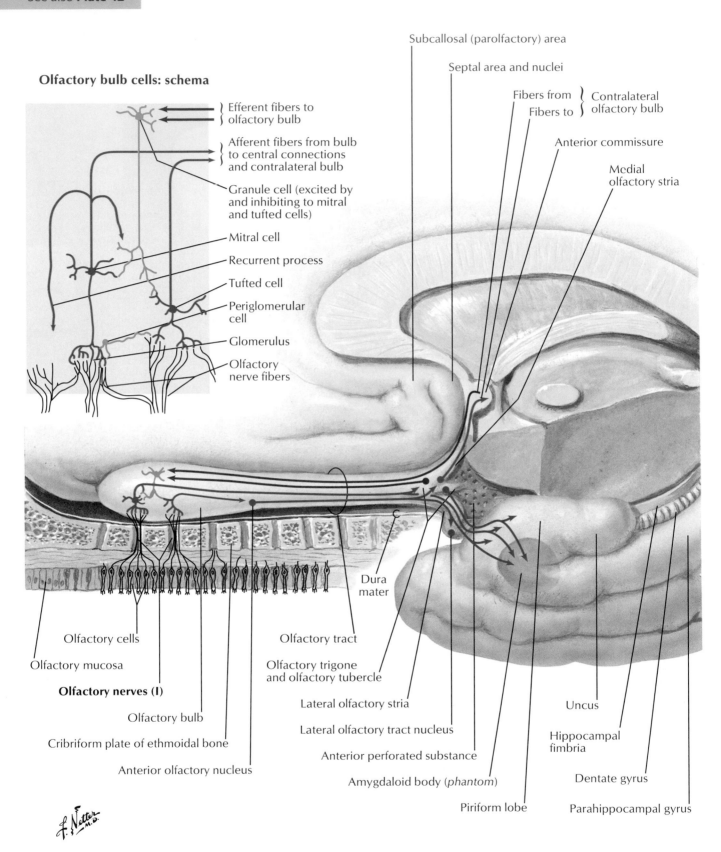

Olfactory bulb cells: schema

Efferent fibers to olfactory bulb

Afferent fibers from bulb to central connections and contralateral bulb

Granule cell (excited by and inhibiting to mitral and tufted cells)

Mitral cell

Recurrent process

Tufted cell

Periglomerular cell

Glomerulus

Olfactory nerve fibers

Subcallosal (parolfactory) area

Septal area and nuclei

Fibers from } Contralateral
Fibers to   } olfactory bulb

Anterior commissure

Medial olfactory stria

Olfactory cells

Olfactory mucosa

Olfactory nerves (I)

Olfactory bulb

Cribriform plate of ethmoidal bone

Anterior olfactory nucleus

Olfactory tract

Olfactory trigone and olfactory tubercle

Lateral olfactory stria

Lateral olfactory tract nucleus

Anterior perforated substance

Amygdaloid body (*phantom*)

Piriform lobe

Dura mater

Uncus

Hippocampal fimbria

Dentate gyrus

Parahippocampal gyrus

Plate 118

Cranial and Cervical Nerves

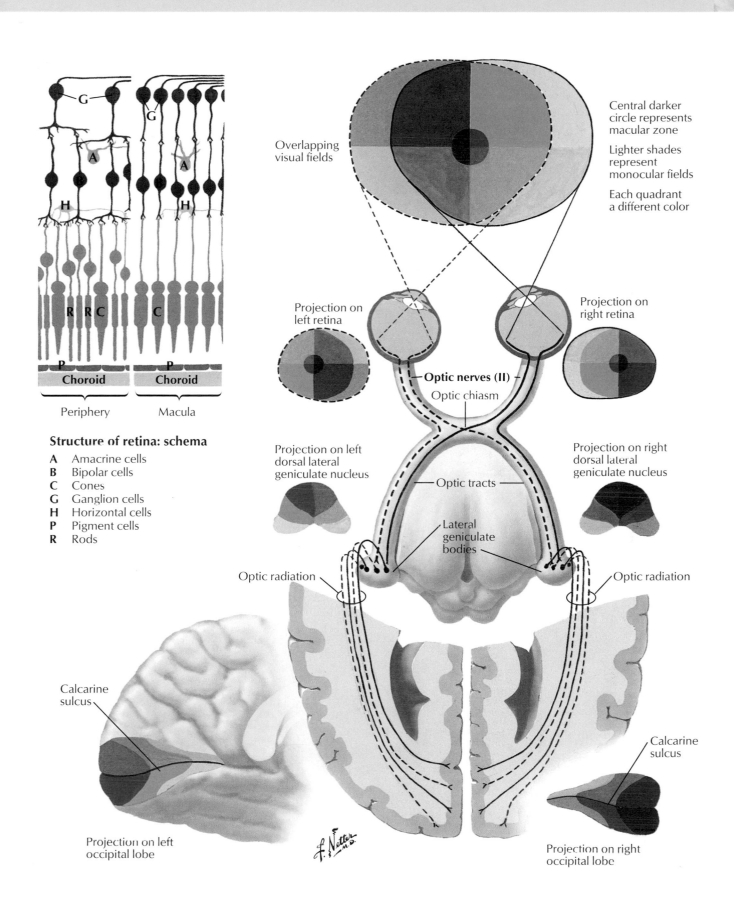

Overlapping visual fields

Central darker circle represents macular zone

Lighter shades represent monocular fields

Each quadrant a different color

Projection on left retina

Projection on right retina

Optic nerves (II)

Optic chiasm

Projection on left dorsal lateral geniculate nucleus

Projection on right dorsal lateral geniculate nucleus

Optic tracts

Lateral geniculate bodies

Optic radiation

Optic radiation

Calcarine sulcus

Calcarine sulcus

Projection on left occipital lobe

Projection on right occipital lobe

Structure of retina: schema

- **A** Amacrine cells
- **B** Bipolar cells
- **C** Cones
- **G** Ganglion cells
- **H** Horizontal cells
- **P** Pigment cells
- **R** Rods

Periphery

Macula

Choroid

Choroid

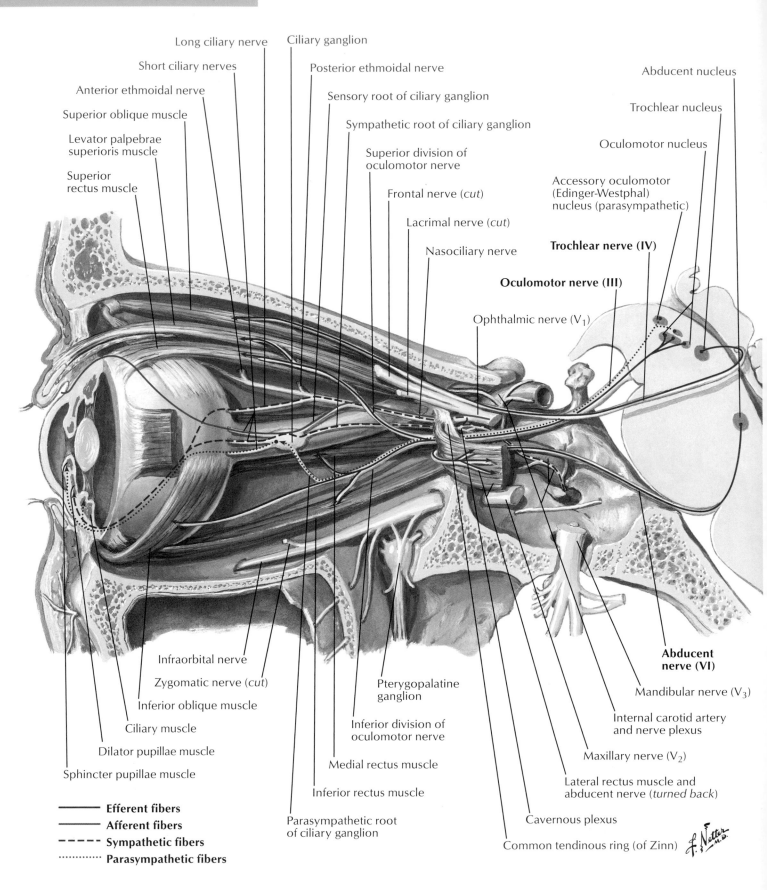

Long ciliary nerve

Short ciliary nerves

Anterior ethmoidal nerve

Superior oblique muscle

Levator palpebrae superioris muscle

Superior rectus muscle

Ciliary ganglion

Posterior ethmoidal nerve

Sensory root of ciliary ganglion

Sympathetic root of ciliary ganglion

Superior division of oculomotor nerve

Frontal nerve (*cut*)

Lacrimal nerve (*cut*)

Nasociliary nerve

Abducent nucleus

Trochlear nucleus

Oculomotor nucleus

Accessory oculomotor (Edinger-Westphal) nucleus (parasympathetic)

Trochlear nerve (IV)

Oculomotor nerve (III)

Ophthalmic nerve (V$_1$)

Infraorbital nerve

Zygomatic nerve (*cut*)

Inferior oblique muscle

Ciliary muscle

Dilator pupillae muscle

Sphincter pupillae muscle

Pterygopalatine ganglion

Inferior division of oculomotor nerve

Medial rectus muscle

Inferior rectus muscle

Parasympathetic root of ciliary ganglion

Abducent nerve (VI)

Mandibular nerve (V$_3$)

Internal carotid artery and nerve plexus

Maxillary nerve (V$_2$)

Lateral rectus muscle and abducent nerve (*turned back*)

Cavernous plexus

Common tendinous ring (of Zinn)

——— **Efferent fibers**

——— **Afferent fibers**

- - - **Sympathetic fibers**

·········· **Parasympathetic fibers**

Plate 120

Cranial and Cervical Nerves

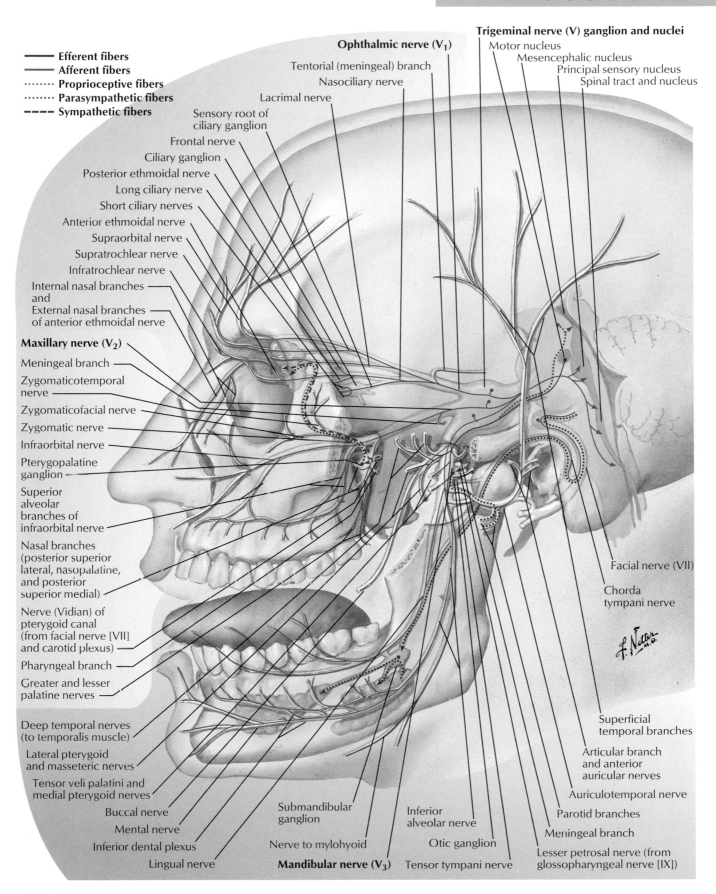

Efferent fibers
Afferent fibers
Proprioceptive fibers
Parasympathetic fibers
Sympathetic fibers

Ophthalmic nerve (V₁)

Tentorial (meningeal) branch
Nasociliary nerve
Lacrimal nerve

Trigeminal nerve (V) ganglion and nuclei
Motor nucleus
Mesencephalic nucleus
Principal sensory nucleus
Spinal tract and nucleus

Sensory root of ciliary ganglion
Frontal nerve
Ciliary ganglion
Posterior ethmoidal nerve
Long ciliary nerve
Short ciliary nerves
Anterior ethmoidal nerve
Supraorbital nerve
Supratrochlear nerve
Infratrochlear nerve
Internal nasal branches and
External nasal branches of anterior ethmoidal nerve

Maxillary nerve (V₂)

Meningeal branch
Zygomaticotemporal nerve
Zygomaticofacial nerve
Zygomatic nerve
Infraorbital nerve
Pterygopalatine ganglion
Superior alveolar branches of infraorbital nerve
Nasal branches (posterior superior lateral, nasopalatine, and posterior superior medial)
Nerve (Vidian) of pterygoid canal (from facial nerve [VII] and carotid plexus)
Pharyngeal branch
Greater and lesser palatine nerves

Deep temporal nerves (to temporalis muscle)
Lateral pterygoid and masseteric nerves
Tensor veli palatini and medial pterygoid nerves
Buccal nerve
Mental nerve
Inferior dental plexus
Lingual nerve

Submandibular ganglion
Nerve to mylohyoid
Mandibular nerve (V₃)

Inferior alveolar nerve
Otic ganglion
Tensor tympani nerve

Facial nerve (VII)
Chorda tympani nerve

Superficial temporal branches
Articular branch and anterior auricular nerves
Auriculotemporal nerve
Parotid branches
Meningeal branch
Lesser petrosal nerve (from glossopharyngeal nerve [IX])

f. Netter

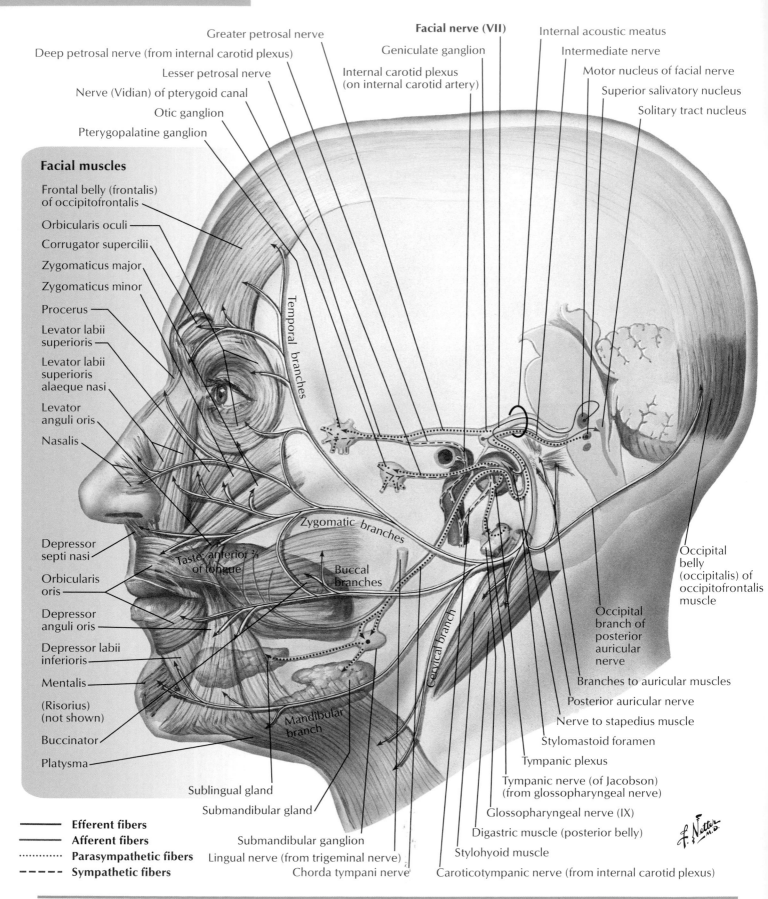

Greater petrosal nerve

Deep petrosal nerve (from internal carotid plexus)

Lesser petrosal nerve

Nerve (Vidian) of pterygoid canal

Otic ganglion

Pterygopalatine ganglion

Facial nerve (VII)

Geniculate ganglion

Internal carotid plexus (on internal carotid artery)

Internal acoustic meatus

Intermediate nerve

Motor nucleus of facial nerve

Superior salivatory nucleus

Solitary tract nucleus

Facial muscles

Frontal belly (frontalis) of occipitofrontalis

Orbicularis oculi

Corrugator supercilii

Zygomaticus major

Zygomaticus minor

Procerus

Levator labii superioris

Levator labii superioris alaeque nasi

Levator anguli oris

Nasalis

Depressor septi nasi

Orbicularis oris

Depressor anguli oris

Depressor labii inferioris

Mentalis

(Risorius) (not shown)

Buccinator

Platysma

Temporal branches

Zygomatic branches

Taste anterior ⅔ of tongue

Buccal branches

Cervical branch

Mandibular branch

Sublingual gland

Submandibular gland

Submandibular ganglion

Lingual nerve (from trigeminal nerve)

Chorda tympani nerve

Occipital belly (occipitalis) of occipitofrontalis muscle

Occipital branch of posterior auricular nerve

Branches to auricular muscles

Posterior auricular nerve

Nerve to stapedius muscle

Stylomastoid foramen

Tympanic plexus

Tympanic nerve (of Jacobson) (from glossopharyngeal nerve)

Glossopharyngeal nerve (IX)

Digastric muscle (posterior belly)

Stylohyoid muscle

Caroticotympanic nerve (from internal carotid plexus)

——— **Efferent fibers**
——— **Afferent fibers**
·········· **Parasympathetic fibers**
- - - - **Sympathetic fibers**

Plate 122

Cranial and Cervical Nerves

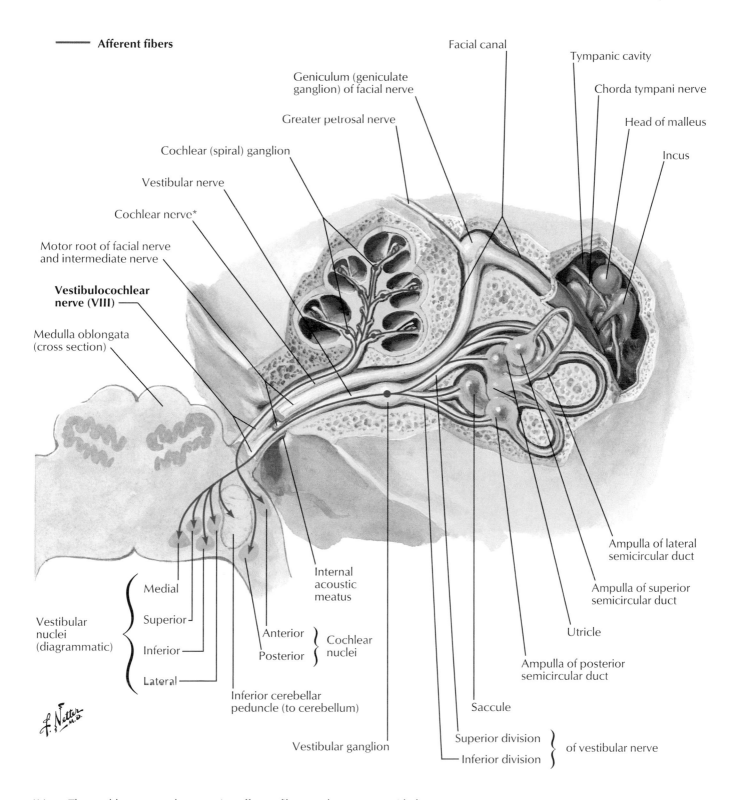

Afferent fibers

Geniculum (geniculate ganglion) of facial nerve

Greater petrosal nerve

Cochlear (spiral) ganglion

Vestibular nerve

Cochlear nerve*

Motor root of facial nerve and intermediate nerve

Vestibulocochlear nerve (VIII)

Medulla oblongata (cross section)

Facial canal

Tympanic cavity

Chorda tympani nerve

Head of malleus

Incus

Ampulla of lateral semicircular duct

Ampulla of superior semicircular duct

Utricle

Ampulla of posterior semicircular duct

Saccule

Superior division } of vestibular nerve
Inferior division }

Vestibular ganglion

Internal acoustic meatus

Inferior cerebellar peduncle (to cerebellum)

Medial
Superior
Inferior
Lateral

Anterior
Posterior
} Cochlear nuclei

Vestibular nuclei (diagrammatic)

*Note: The cochlear nerve also contains efferent fibers to the sensory epithelium. These fibers are derived from the vestibular nerve while in the internal auditory meatus.

Glosssopharyngeal Nerve (IX): Schema

See also **Plates 160, 161**

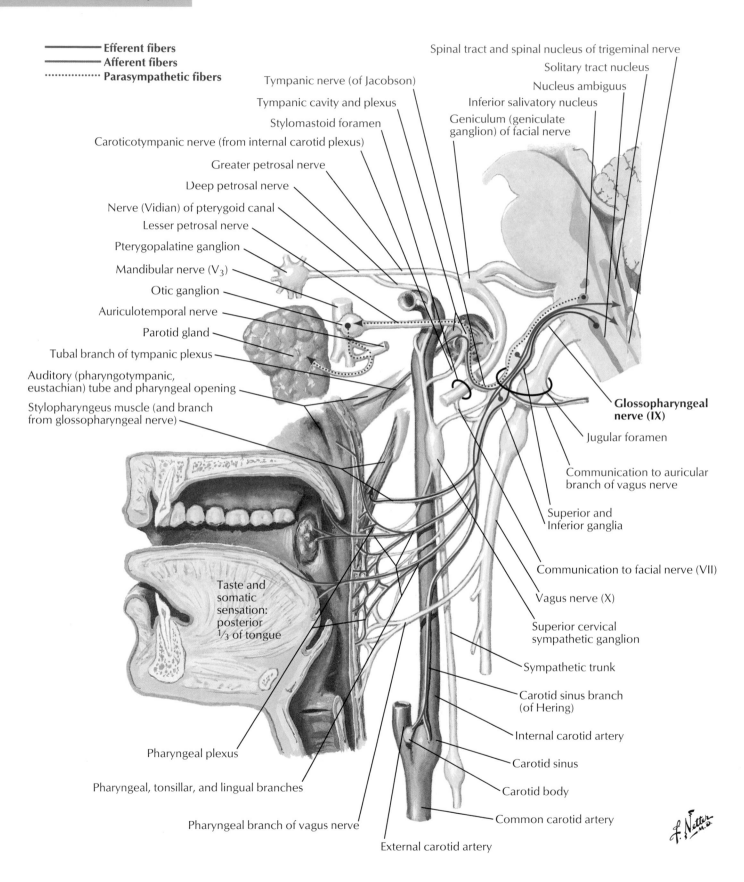

—— Efferent fibers
—— Afferent fibers
·············· Parasympathetic fibers

Spinal tract and spinal nucleus of trigeminal nerve

Solitary tract nucleus

Tympanic nerve (of Jacobson)

Nucleus ambiguus

Tympanic cavity and plexus

Inferior salivatory nucleus

Stylomastoid foramen

Geniculum (geniculate ganglion) of facial nerve

Caroticotympanic nerve (from internal carotid plexus)

Greater petrosal nerve

Deep petrosal nerve

Nerve (Vidian) of pterygoid canal

Lesser petrosal nerve

Pterygopalatine ganglion

Mandibular nerve (V₃)

Glossopharyngeal nerve (IX)

Otic ganglion

Jugular foramen

Auriculotemporal nerve

Parotid gland

Communication to auricular branch of vagus nerve

Tubal branch of tympanic plexus

Auditory (pharyngotympanic, eustachian) tube and pharyngeal opening

Superior and Inferior ganglia

Stylopharyngeus muscle (and branch from glossopharyngeal nerve)

Communication to facial nerve (VII)

Vagus nerve (X)

Superior cervical sympathetic ganglion

Taste and somatic sensation: posterior ⅓ of tongue

Sympathetic trunk

Carotid sinus branch (of Hering)

Internal carotid artery

Carotid sinus

Pharyngeal plexus

Carotid body

Pharyngeal, tonsillar, and lingual branches

Common carotid artery

Pharyngeal branch of vagus nerve

External carotid artery

Plate 124

Cranial and Cervical Nerves

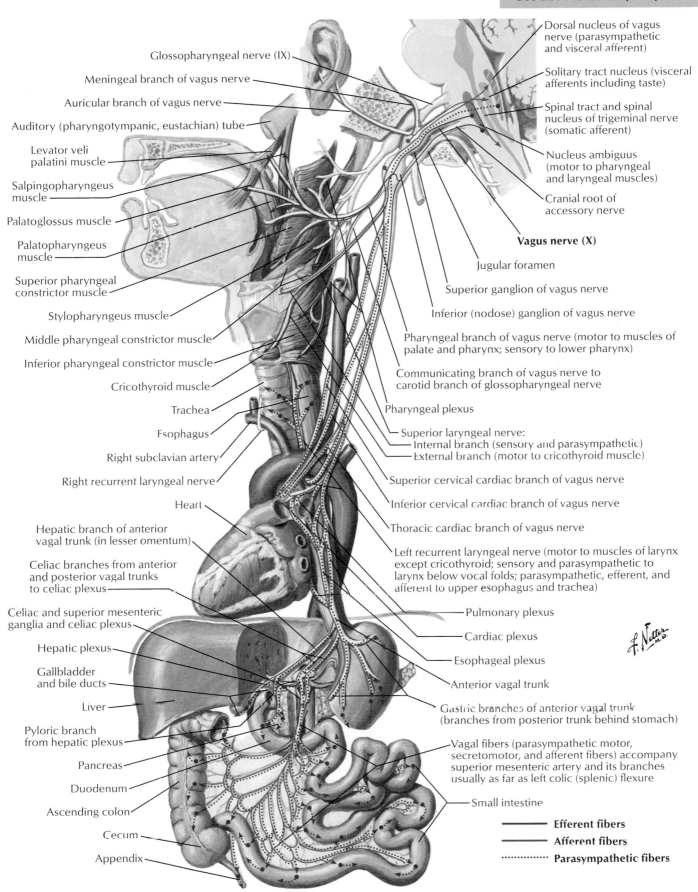

Glossopharyngeal nerve (IX)

Meningeal branch of vagus nerve

Auricular branch of vagus nerve

Auditory (pharyngotympanic, eustachian) tube

Levator veli palatini muscle

Salpingopharyngeus muscle

Palatoglossus muscle

Palatopharyngeus muscle

Superior pharyngeal constrictor muscle

Stylopharyngeus muscle

Middle pharyngeal constrictor muscle

Inferior pharyngeal constrictor muscle

Cricothyroid muscle

Trachea

Esophagus

Right subclavian artery

Right recurrent laryngeal nerve

Heart

Hepatic branch of anterior vagal trunk (in lesser omentum)

Celiac branches from anterior and posterior vagal trunks to celiac plexus

Celiac and superior mesenteric ganglia and celiac plexus

Hepatic plexus

Gallbladder and bile ducts

Liver

Pyloric branch from hepatic plexus

Pancreas

Duodenum

Ascending colon

Cecum

Appendix

Dorsal nucleus of vagus nerve (parasympathetic and visceral afferent)

Solitary tract nucleus (visceral afferents including taste)

Spinal tract and spinal nucleus of trigeminal nerve (somatic afferent)

Nucleus ambiguus (motor to pharyngeal and laryngeal muscles)

Cranial root of accessory nerve

Vagus nerve (X)

Jugular foramen

Superior ganglion of vagus nerve

Inferior (nodose) ganglion of vagus nerve

Pharyngeal branch of vagus nerve (motor to muscles of palate and pharynx; sensory to lower pharynx)

Communicating branch of vagus nerve to carotid branch of glossopharyngeal nerve

Pharyngeal plexus

Superior laryngeal nerve:
Internal branch (sensory and parasympathetic)
External branch (motor to cricothyroid muscle)

Superior cervical cardiac branch of vagus nerve

Inferior cervical cardiac branch of vagus nerve

Thoracic cardiac branch of vagus nerve

Left recurrent laryngeal nerve (motor to muscles of larynx except cricothyroid; sensory and parasympathetic to larynx below vocal folds; parasympathetic, efferent, and afferent to upper esophagus and trachea)

Pulmonary plexus

Cardiac plexus

Esophageal plexus

Anterior vagal trunk

Gastric branches of anterior vagal trunk (branches from posterior trunk behind stomach)

Vagal fibers (parasympathetic motor, secretomotor, and afferent fibers) accompany superior mesenteric artery and its branches usually as far as left colic (splenic) flexure

Small intestine

——— **Efferent fibers**

——— **Afferent fibers**

··········· **Parasympathetic fibers**

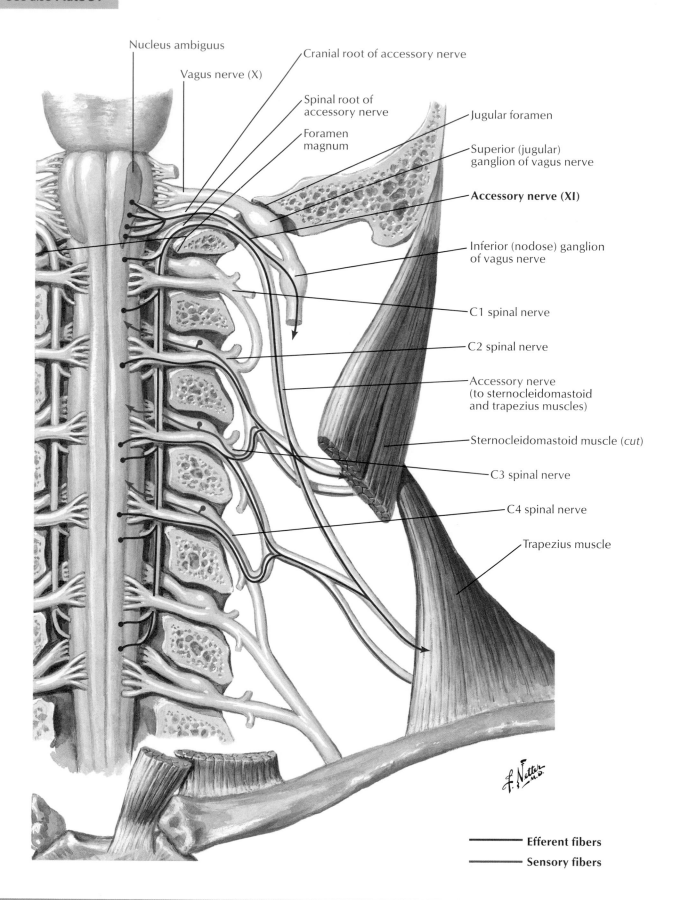

Nucleus ambiguus

Vagus nerve (X)

Cranial root of accessory nerve

Spinal root of accessory nerve

Foramen magnum

Jugular foramen

Superior (jugular) ganglion of vagus nerve

Accessory nerve (XI)

Inferior (nodose) ganglion of vagus nerve

C1 spinal nerve

C2 spinal nerve

Accessory nerve (to sternocleidomastoid and trapezius muscles)

Sternocleidomastoid muscle (*cut*)

C3 spinal nerve

C4 spinal nerve

Trapezius muscle

—— **Efferent fibers**

—— **Sensory fibers**

Plate 126

Cranial and Cervical Nerves

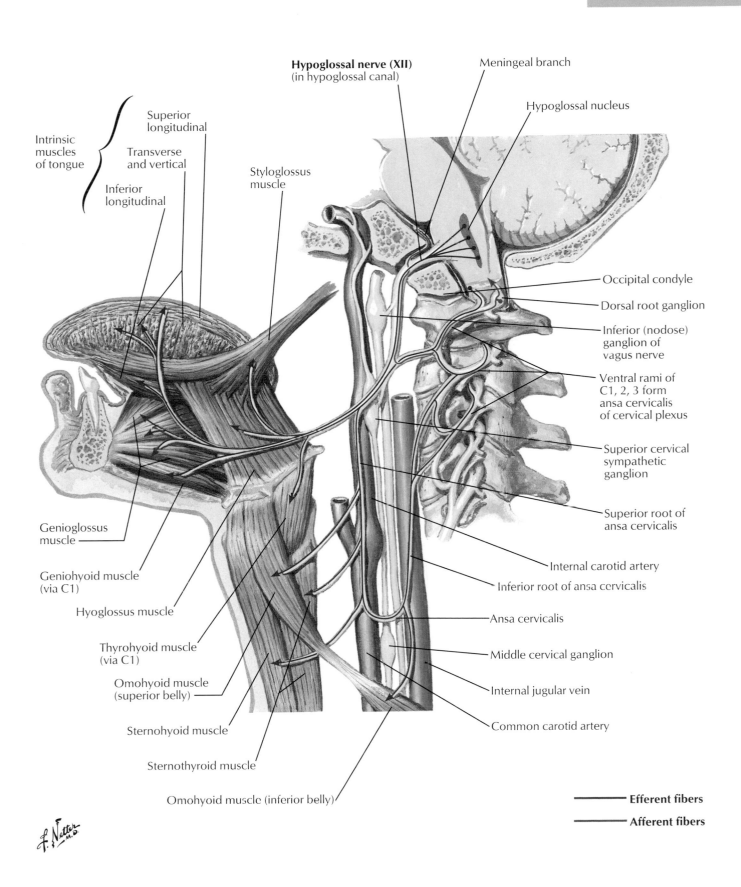

Hypoglossal nerve (XII)
(in hypoglossal canal)

Meningeal branch

Hypoglossal nucleus

Intrinsic muscles of tongue

Superior longitudinal

Transverse and vertical

Inferior longitudinal

Styloglossus muscle

Occipital condyle

Dorsal root ganglion

Inferior (nodose) ganglion of vagus nerve

Ventral rami of C1, 2, 3 form ansa cervicalis of cervical plexus

Superior cervical sympathetic ganglion

Superior root of ansa cervicalis

Genioglossus muscle

Geniohyoid muscle (via C1)

Hyoglossus muscle

Thyrohyoid muscle (via C1)

Omohyoid muscle (superior belly)

Sternohyoid muscle

Sternothyroid muscle

Omohyoid muscle (inferior belly)

Internal carotid artery

Inferior root of ansa cervicalis

Ansa cervicalis

Middle cervical ganglion

Internal jugular vein

Common carotid artery

——— Efferent fibers
——— Afferent fibers

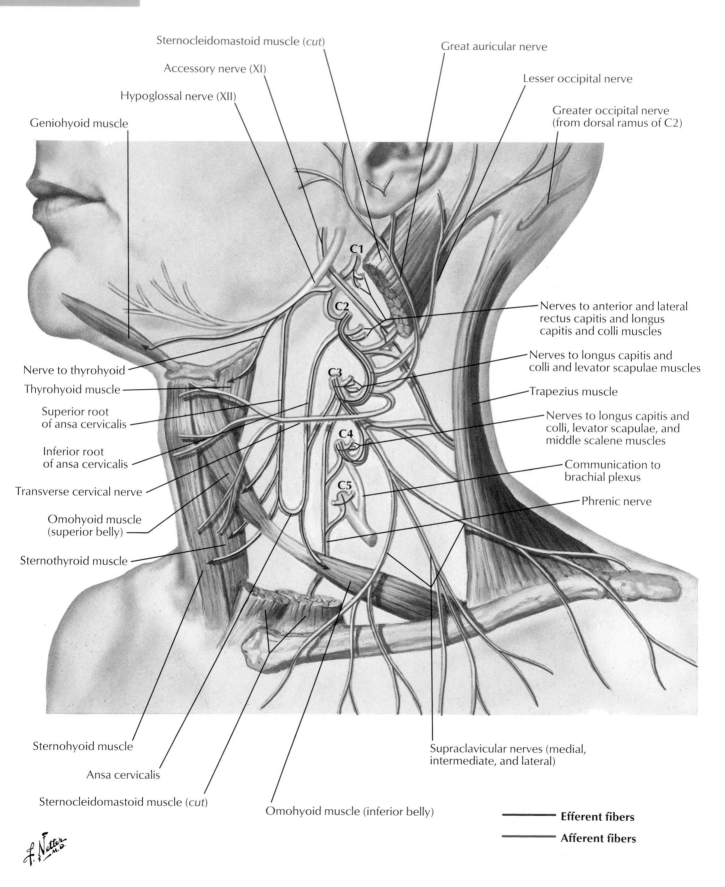

Sternocleidomastoid muscle (*cut*)

Accessory nerve (XI)

Hypoglossal nerve (XII)

Geniohyoid muscle

Great auricular nerve

Lesser occipital nerve

Greater occipital nerve (from dorsal ramus of C2)

C1

C2

Nerves to anterior and lateral rectus capitis and longus capitis and colli muscles

Nerve to thyrohyoid

Thyrohyoid muscle

Superior root of ansa cervicalis

Inferior root of ansa cervicalis

Transverse cervical nerve

Omohyoid muscle (superior belly)

Sternothyroid muscle

C3

C4

C5

Nerves to longus capitis and colli and levator scapulae muscles

Trapezius muscle

Nerves to longus capitis and colli, levator scapulae, and middle scalene muscles

Communication to brachial plexus

Phrenic nerve

Sternohyoid muscle

Ansa cervicalis

Sternocleidomastoid muscle (*cut*)

Omohyoid muscle (inferior belly)

Supraclavicular nerves (medial, intermediate, and lateral)

———— **Efferent fibers**

———— **Afferent fibers**

Plate 128

Cranial and Cervical Nerves

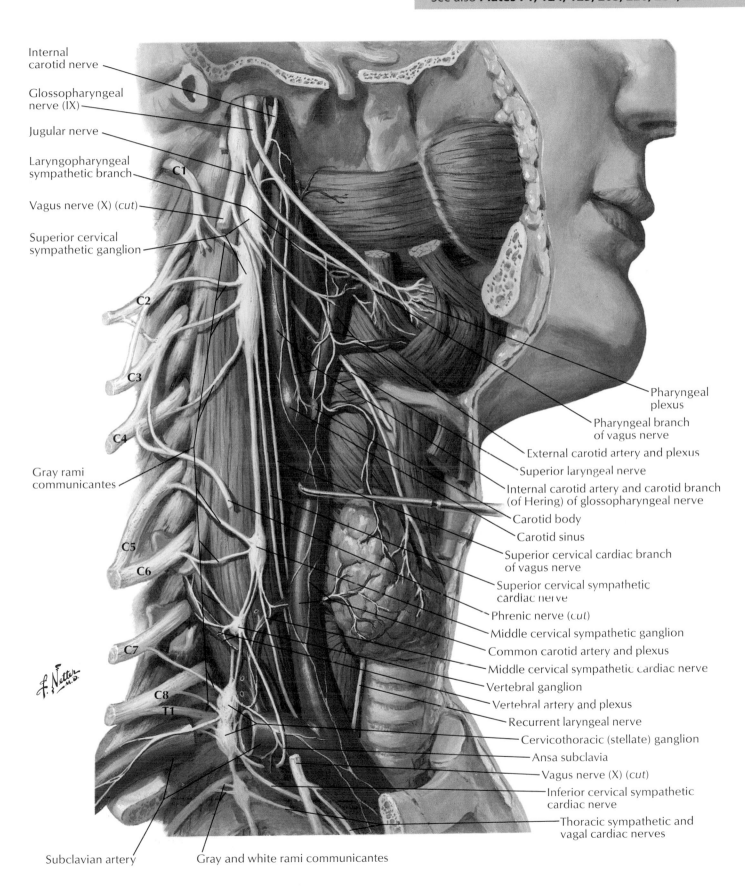

Internal carotid nerve

Glossopharyngeal nerve (IX)

Jugular nerve

Laryngopharyngeal sympathetic branch

Vagus nerve (X) (cut)

Superior cervical sympathetic ganglion

C1

C2

C3

C4

Gray rami communicantes

C5

C6

C7

C8

T1

Subclavian artery

Gray and white rami communicantes

Pharyngeal plexus

Pharyngeal branch of vagus nerve

External carotid artery and plexus

Superior laryngeal nerve

Internal carotid artery and carotid branch (of Hering) of glossopharyngeal nerve

Carotid body

Carotid sinus

Superior cervical cardiac branch of vagus nerve

Superior cervical sympathetic cardiac nerve

Phrenic nerve (cut)

Middle cervical sympathetic ganglion

Common carotid artery and plexus

Middle cervical sympathetic cardiac nerve

Vertebral ganglion

Vertebral artery and plexus

Recurrent laryngeal nerve

Cervicothoracic (stellate) ganglion

Ansa subclavia

Vagus nerve (X) (cut)

Inferior cervical sympathetic cardiac nerve

Thoracic sympathetic and vagal cardiac nerves

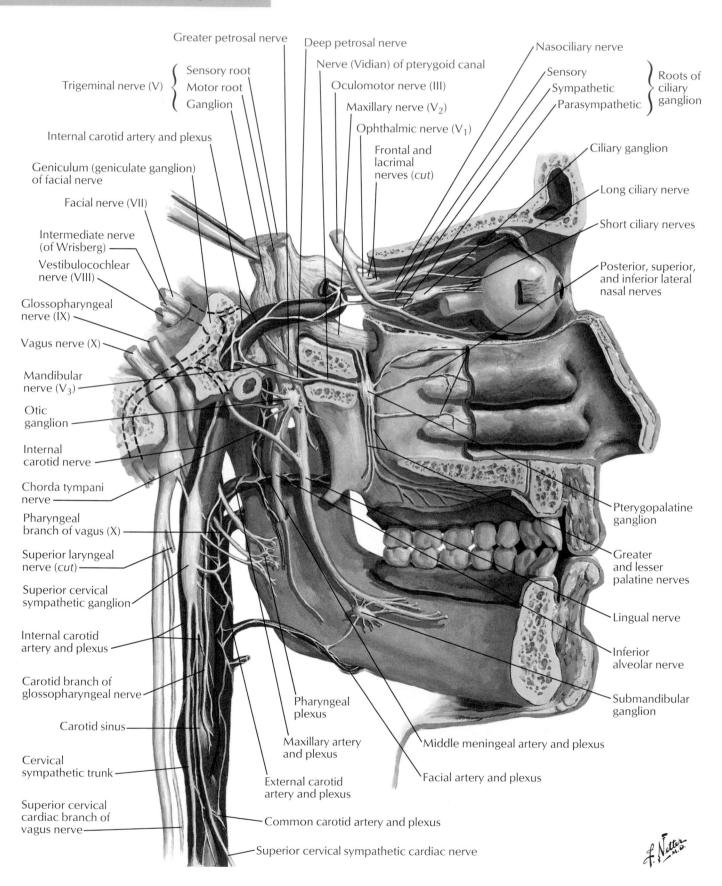

Greater petrosal nerve

Deep petrosal nerve

Nerve (Vidian) of pterygoid canal

Nasociliary nerve

Trigeminal nerve (V) { Sensory root / Motor root / Ganglion }

Oculomotor nerve (III)

Maxillary nerve (V₂)

Ophthalmic nerve (V₁)

Sensory / Sympathetic / Parasympathetic } Roots of ciliary ganglion

Internal carotid artery and plexus

Frontal and lacrimal nerves (*cut*)

Ciliary ganglion

Geniculum (geniculate ganglion) of facial nerve

Long ciliary nerve

Facial nerve (VII)

Short ciliary nerves

Intermediate nerve (of Wrisberg)

Posterior, superior, and inferior lateral nasal nerves

Vestibulocochlear nerve (VIII)

Glossopharyngeal nerve (IX)

Vagus nerve (X)

Mandibular nerve (V₃)

Otic ganglion

Pterygopalatine ganglion

Internal carotid nerve

Chorda tympani nerve

Pharyngeal branch of vagus (X)

Greater and lesser palatine nerves

Superior laryngeal nerve (*cut*)

Lingual nerve

Superior cervical sympathetic ganglion

Internal carotid artery and plexus

Inferior alveolar nerve

Carotid branch of glossopharyngeal nerve

Submandibular ganglion

Carotid sinus

Pharyngeal plexus

Cervical sympathetic trunk

Middle meningeal artery and plexus

Maxillary artery and plexus

Superior cervical cardiac branch of vagus nerve

External carotid artery and plexus

Facial artery and plexus

Common carotid artery and plexus

Superior cervical sympathetic cardiac nerve

Plate 130

Cranial and Cervical Nerves

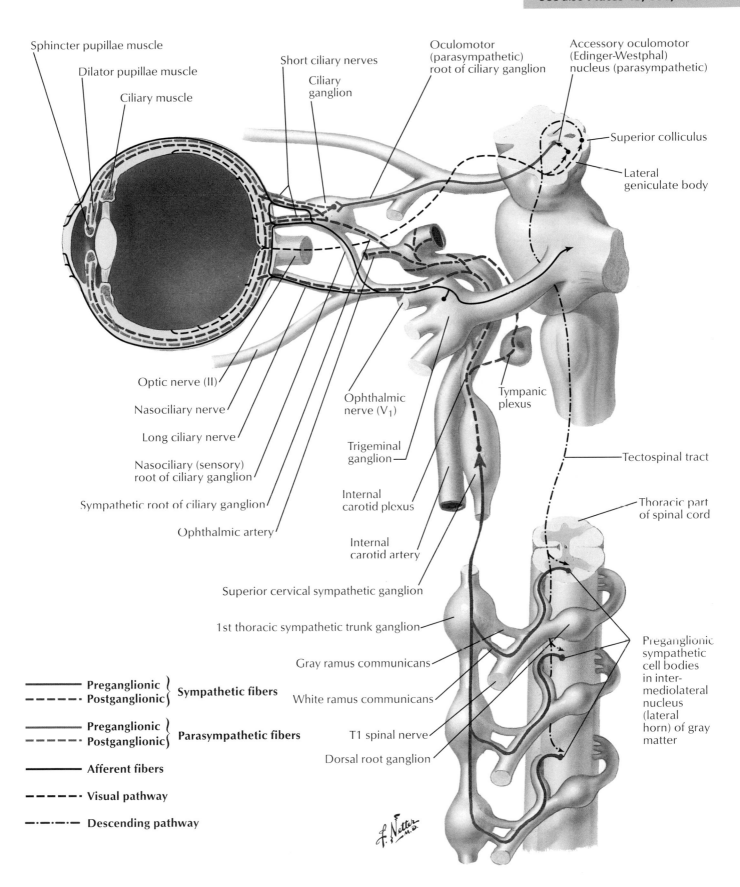

Sphincter pupillae muscle

Dilator pupillae muscle

Ciliary muscle

Short ciliary nerves

Ciliary ganglion

Oculomotor (parasympathetic) root of ciliary ganglion

Accessory oculomotor (Edinger-Westphal) nucleus (parasympathetic)

Superior colliculus

Lateral geniculate body

Optic nerve (II)

Nasociliary nerve

Long ciliary nerve

Nasociliary (sensory) root of ciliary ganglion

Sympathetic root of ciliary ganglion

Ophthalmic artery

Ophthalmic nerve (V₁)

Trigeminal ganglion

Internal carotid plexus

Internal carotid artery

Tympanic plexus

Tectospinal tract

Thoracic part of spinal cord

Superior cervical sympathetic ganglion

1st thoracic sympathetic trunk ganglion

Gray ramus communicans

White ramus communicans

T1 spinal nerve

Dorsal root ganglion

Preganglionic sympathetic cell bodies in inter-mediolateral nucleus (lateral horn) of gray matter

———— **Preganglionic** }
- - - - - · **Postganglionic** } **Sympathetic fibers**

———— **Preganglionic** }
- - - - - · **Postganglionic** } **Parasympathetic fibers**

———— **Afferent fibers**

- - - - - · **Visual pathway**

—·—·— **Descending pathway**

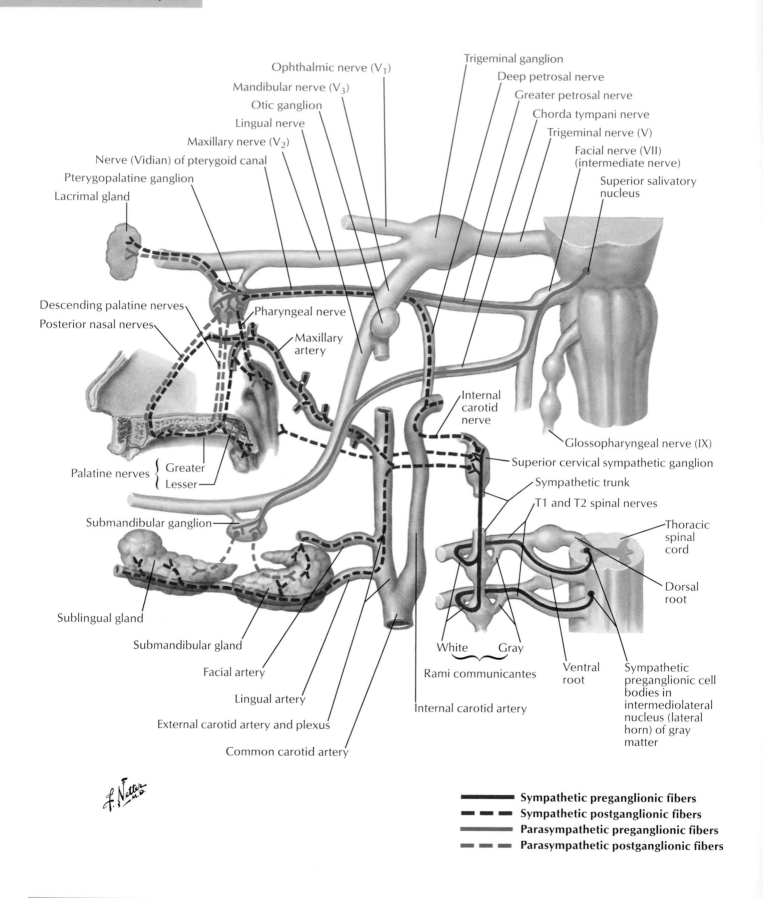

Ophthalmic nerve (V₁)

Mandibular nerve (V₃)

Otic ganglion

Lingual nerve

Maxillary nerve (V₂)

Nerve (Vidian) of pterygoid canal

Pterygopalatine ganglion

Lacrimal gland

Trigeminal ganglion

Deep petrosal nerve

Greater petrosal nerve

Chorda tympani nerve

Trigeminal nerve (V)

Facial nerve (VII) (intermediate nerve)

Superior salivatory nucleus

Descending palatine nerves

Posterior nasal nerves

Pharyngeal nerve

Maxillary artery

Internal carotid nerve

Glossopharyngeal nerve (IX)

Superior cervical sympathetic ganglion

Sympathetic trunk

T1 and T2 spinal nerves

Thoracic spinal cord

Dorsal root

Palatine nerves { Greater Lesser

Submandibular ganglion

Sublingual gland

Submandibular gland

Facial artery

Lingual artery

External carotid artery and plexus

Common carotid artery

White   Gray

Rami communicantes

Internal carotid artery

Ventral root

Sympathetic preganglionic cell bodies in intermediolateral nucleus (lateral horn) of gray matter

Sympathetic preganglionic fibers

Sympathetic postganglionic fibers

Parasympathetic preganglionic fibers

Parasympathetic postganglionic fibers

Plate 132

Cranial and Cervical Nerves

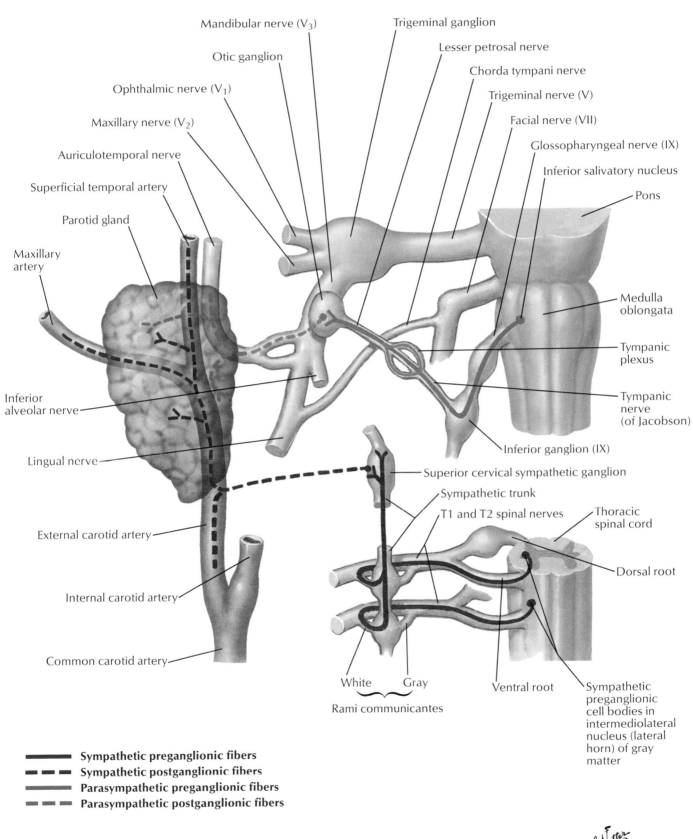

Mandibular nerve (V₃)

Trigeminal ganglion

Otic ganglion

Lesser petrosal nerve

Ophthalmic nerve (V₁)

Chorda tympani nerve

Maxillary nerve (V₂)

Trigeminal nerve (V)

Auriculotemporal nerve

Facial nerve (VII)

Superficial temporal artery

Glossopharyngeal nerve (IX)

Parotid gland

Inferior salivatory nucleus

Maxillary artery

Pons

Inferior alveolar nerve

Medulla oblongata

Lingual nerve

Tympanic plexus

Tympanic nerve (of Jacobson)

Inferior ganglion (IX)

Superior cervical sympathetic ganglion

Sympathetic trunk

T1 and T2 spinal nerves

Thoracic spinal cord

External carotid artery

Dorsal root

Internal carotid artery

Common carotid artery

White   Gray

Rami communicantes

Ventral root

Sympathetic preganglionic cell bodies in intermediolateral nucleus (lateral horn) of gray matter

————— **Sympathetic preganglionic fibers**
- - - - - **Sympathetic postganglionic fibers**
————— **Parasympathetic preganglionic fibers**
- - - - - **Parasympathetic postganglionic fibers**

f. Netter
M.D.

Cranial and Cervical Nerves

Plate 133

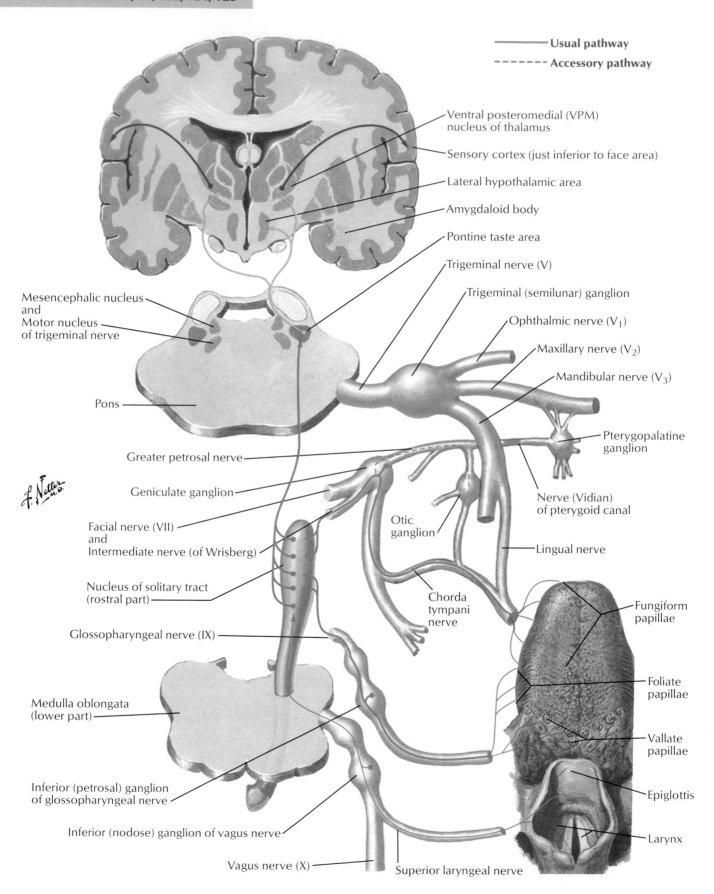

———— Usual pathway

------- Accessory pathway

Ventral posteromedial (VPM) nucleus of thalamus

Sensory cortex (just inferior to face area)

Lateral hypothalamic area

Amygdaloid body

Pontine taste area

Trigeminal nerve (V)

Trigeminal (semilunar) ganglion

Ophthalmic nerve (V₁)

Maxillary nerve (V₂)

Mandibular nerve (V₃)

Pterygopalatine ganglion

Nerve (Vidian) of pterygoid canal

Lingual nerve

Fungiform papillae

Foliate papillae

Vallate papillae

Epiglottis

Larynx

Mesencephalic nucleus and Motor nucleus of trigeminal nerve

Pons

Greater petrosal nerve

Geniculate ganglion

Facial nerve (VII) and Intermediate nerve (of Wrisberg)

Nucleus of solitary tract (rostral part)

Glossopharyngeal nerve (IX)

Medulla oblongata (lower part)

Inferior (petrosal) ganglion of glossopharyngeal nerve

Inferior (nodose) ganglion of vagus nerve

Vagus nerve (X)

Otic ganglion

Chorda tympani nerve

Superior laryngeal nerve

Plate 134

Cranial and Cervical Nerves

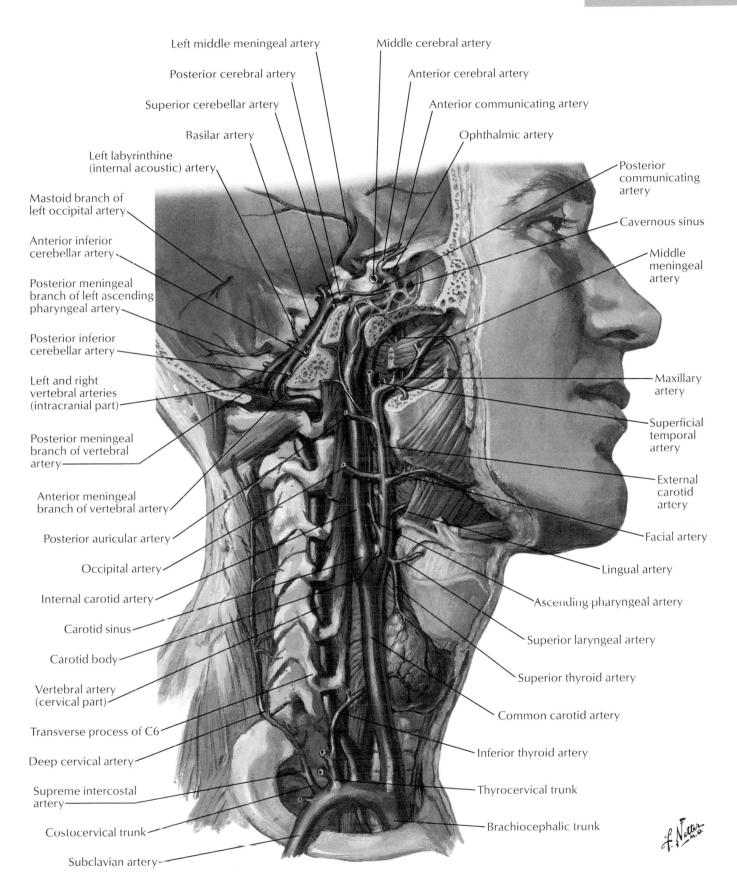

Left middle meningeal artery

Posterior cerebral artery

Superior cerebellar artery

Basilar artery

Left labyrinthine (internal acoustic) artery

Mastoid branch of left occipital artery

Anterior inferior cerebellar artery

Posterior meningeal branch of left ascending pharyngeal artery

Posterior inferior cerebellar artery

Left and right vertebral arteries (intracranial part)

Posterior meningeal branch of vertebral artery

Anterior meningeal branch of vertebral artery

Posterior auricular artery

Occipital artery

Internal carotid artery

Carotid sinus

Carotid body

Vertebral artery (cervical part)

Transverse process of C6

Deep cervical artery

Supreme intercostal artery

Costocervical trunk

Subclavian artery

Middle cerebral artery

Anterior cerebral artery

Anterior communicating artery

Ophthalmic artery

Posterior communicating artery

Cavernous sinus

Middle meningeal artery

Maxillary artery

Superficial temporal artery

External carotid artery

Facial artery

Lingual artery

Ascending pharyngeal artery

Superior laryngeal artery

Superior thyroid artery

Common carotid artery

Inferior thyroid artery

Thyrocervical trunk

Brachiocephalic trunk

f. Netter

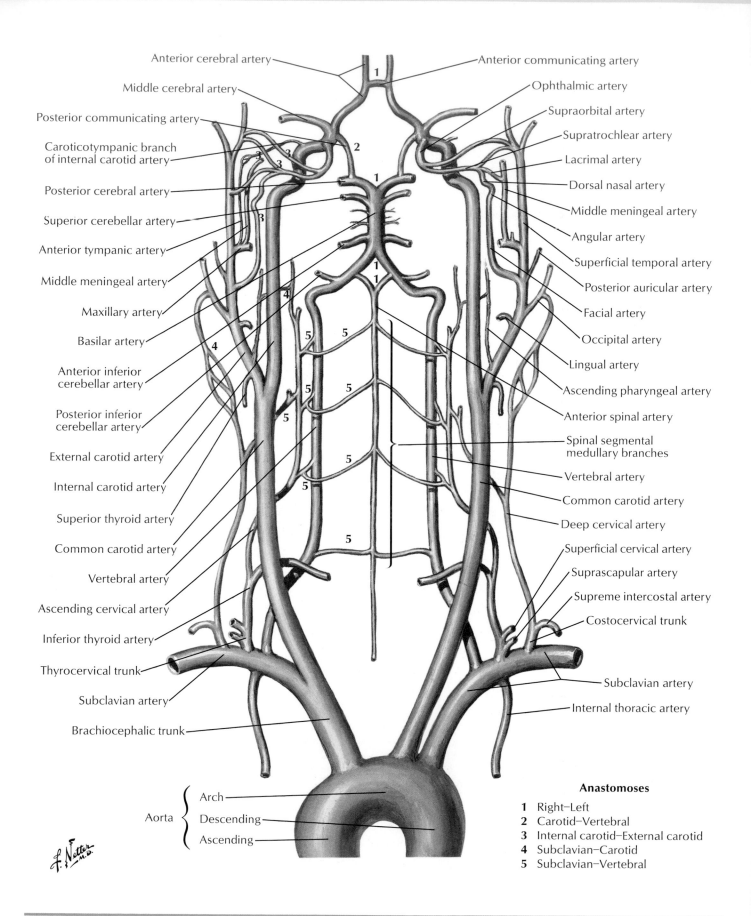

Anterior cerebral artery

Middle cerebral artery

Posterior communicating artery

Caroticotympanic branch
of internal carotid artery

Posterior cerebral artery

Superior cerebellar artery

Anterior tympanic artery

Middle meningeal artery

Maxillary artery

Basilar artery

Anterior inferior
cerebellar artery

Posterior inferior
cerebellar artery

External carotid artery

Internal carotid artery

Superior thyroid artery

Common carotid artery

Vertebral artery

Ascending cervical artery

Inferior thyroid artery

Thyrocervical trunk

Subclavian artery

Brachiocephalic trunk

Anterior communicating artery

Ophthalmic artery

Supraorbital artery

Supratrochlear artery

Lacrimal artery

Dorsal nasal artery

Middle meningeal artery

Angular artery

Superficial temporal artery

Posterior auricular artery

Facial artery

Occipital artery

Lingual artery

Ascending pharyngeal artery

Anterior spinal artery

Spinal segmental
medullary branches

Vertebral artery

Common carotid artery

Deep cervical artery

Superficial cervical artery

Suprascapular artery

Supreme intercostal artery

Costocervical trunk

Subclavian artery

Internal thoracic artery

Aorta { Arch
Descending
Ascending

Anastomoses
1 Right–Left
2 Carotid–Vertebral
3 Internal carotid–External carotid
4 Subclavian–Carotid
5 Subclavian–Vertebral

Plate 136   **Cerebral Vasculature**

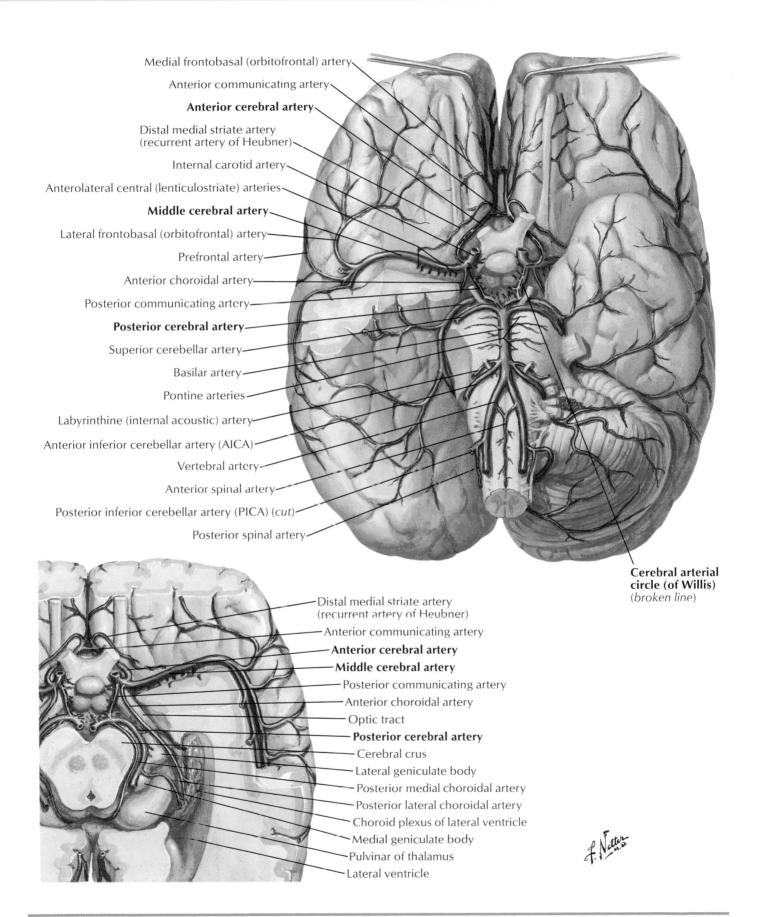

Medial frontobasal (orbitofrontal) artery

Anterior communicating artery

Anterior cerebral artery

Distal medial striate artery
(recurrent artery of Heubner)

Internal carotid artery

Anterolateral central (lenticulostriate) arteries

Middle cerebral artery

Lateral frontobasal (orbitofrontal) artery

Prefrontal artery

Anterior choroidal artery

Posterior communicating artery

Posterior cerebral artery

Superior cerebellar artery

Basilar artery

Pontine arteries

Labyrinthine (internal acoustic) artery

Anterior inferior cerebellar artery (AICA)

Vertebral artery

Anterior spinal artery

Posterior inferior cerebellar artery (PICA) (*cut*)

Posterior spinal artery

**Cerebral arterial
circle (of Willis)**
(*broken line*)

Distal medial striate artery
(recurrent artery of Heubner)

Anterior communicating artery

Anterior cerebral artery

Middle cerebral artery

Posterior communicating artery

Anterior choroidal artery

Optic tract

Posterior cerebral artery

Cerebral crus

Lateral geniculate body

Posterior medial choroidal artery

Posterior lateral choroidal artery

Choroid plexus of lateral ventricle

Medial geniculate body

Pulvinar of thalamus

Lateral ventricle

Vessels dissected out: inferior view

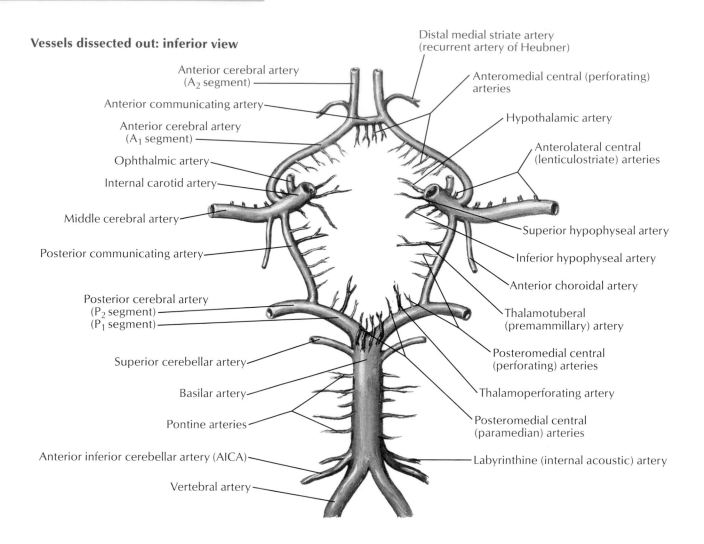

Anterior cerebral artery (A₂ segment)

Distal medial striate artery (recurrent artery of Heubner)

Anteromedial central (perforating) arteries

Anterior communicating artery

Anterior cerebral artery (A₁ segment)

Hypothalamic artery

Ophthalmic artery

Anterolateral central (lenticulostriate) arteries

Internal carotid artery

Middle cerebral artery

Posterior communicating artery

Superior hypophyseal artery

Inferior hypophyseal artery

Anterior choroidal artery

Posterior cerebral artery (P₂ segment) (P₁ segment)

Thalamotuberal (premammillary) artery

Superior cerebellar artery

Posteromedial central (perforating) arteries

Basilar artery

Thalamoperforating artery

Pontine arteries

Posteromedial central (paramedian) arteries

Anterior inferior cerebellar artery (AICA)

Labyrinthine (internal acoustic) artery

Vertebral artery

Vessels in situ: inferior view

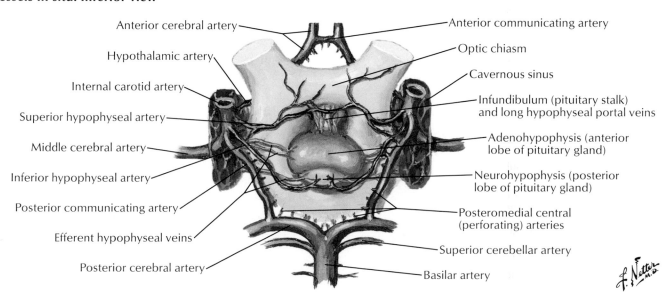

Anterior cerebral artery

Anterior communicating artery

Hypothalamic artery

Optic chiasm

Internal carotid artery

Cavernous sinus

Superior hypophyseal artery

Infundibulum (pituitary stalk) and long hypophyseal portal veins

Middle cerebral artery

Adenohypophysis (anterior lobe of pituitary gland)

Inferior hypophyseal artery

Neurohypophysis (posterior lobe of pituitary gland)

Posterior communicating artery

Posteromedial central (perforating) arteries

Efferent hypophyseal veins

Superior cerebellar artery

Posterior cerebral artery

Basilar artery

Plate 138

Cerebral Vasculature

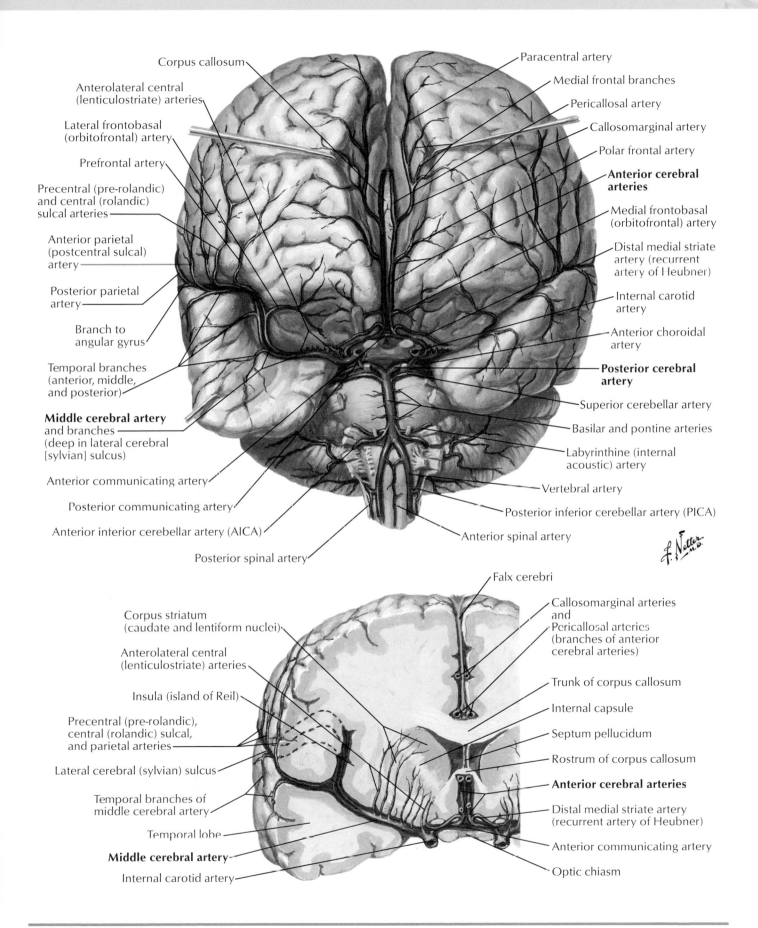

Corpus callosum

Anterolateral central (lenticulostriate) arteries

Lateral frontobasal (orbitofrontal) artery

Prefrontal artery

Precentral (pre-rolandic) and central (rolandic) sulcal arteries

Anterior parietal (postcentral sulcal) artery

Posterior parietal artery

Branch to angular gyrus

Temporal branches (anterior, middle, and posterior)

Middle cerebral artery and branches (deep in lateral cerebral [sylvian] sulcus)

Anterior communicating artery

Posterior communicating artery

Anterior interior cerebellar artery (AICA)

Posterior spinal artery

Paracentral artery

Medial frontal branches

Pericallosal artery

Callosomarginal artery

Polar frontal artery

Anterior cerebral arteries

Medial frontobasal (orbitofrontal) artery

Distal medial striate artery (recurrent artery of Heubner)

Internal carotid artery

Anterior choroidal artery

Posterior cerebral artery

Superior cerebellar artery

Basilar and pontine arteries

Labyrinthine (internal acoustic) artery

Vertebral artery

Posterior inferior cerebellar artery (PICA)

Anterior spinal artery

Corpus striatum (caudate and lentiform nuclei)

Anterolateral central (lenticulostriate) arteries

Insula (island of Reil)

Precentral (pre-rolandic), central (rolandic) sulcal, and parietal arteries

Lateral cerebral (sylvian) sulcus

Temporal branches of middle cerebral artery

Temporal lobe

Middle cerebral artery

Internal carotid artery

Falx cerebri

Callosomarginal arteries and Pericallosal arteries (branches of anterior cerebral arteries)

Trunk of corpus callosum

Internal capsule

Septum pellucidum

Rostrum of corpus callosum

Anterior cerebral arteries

Distal medial striate artery (recurrent artery of Heubner)

Anterior communicating artery

Optic chiasm

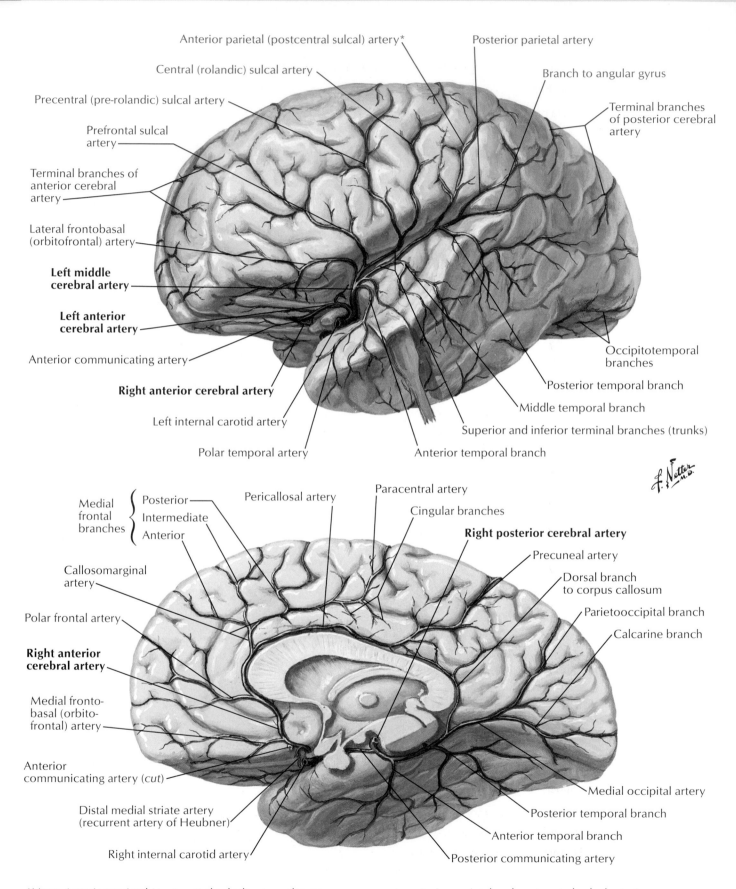

Anterior parietal (postcentral sulcal) artery*

Central (rolandic) sulcal artery

Precentral (pre-rolandic) sulcal artery

Prefrontal sulcal artery

Terminal branches of anterior cerebral artery

Lateral frontobasal (orbitofrontal) artery

Left middle cerebral artery

Left anterior cerebral artery

Anterior communicating artery

Right anterior cerebral artery

Left internal carotid artery

Polar temporal artery

Posterior parietal artery

Branch to angular gyrus

Terminal branches of posterior cerebral artery

Occipitotemporal branches

Posterior temporal branch

Middle temporal branch

Superior and inferior terminal branches (trunks)

Anterior temporal branch

Medial frontal branches { Posterior Intermediate Anterior

Pericallosal artery

Paracentral artery

Cingular branches

Right posterior cerebral artery

Precuneal artery

Dorsal branch to corpus callosum

Parietooccipital branch

Calcarine branch

Callosomarginal artery

Polar frontal artery

Right anterior cerebral artery

Medial fronto-basal (orbito-frontal) artery

Anterior communicating artery (*cut*)

Distal medial striate artery (recurrent artery of Heubner)

Right internal carotid artery

Medial occipital artery

Posterior temporal branch

Anterior temporal branch

Posterior communicating artery

*Note: Anterior parietal (postcentral sulcal) artery also occurs as separate anterior parietal and postcentral sulcal arteries.

Plate 140

Cerebral Vasculature

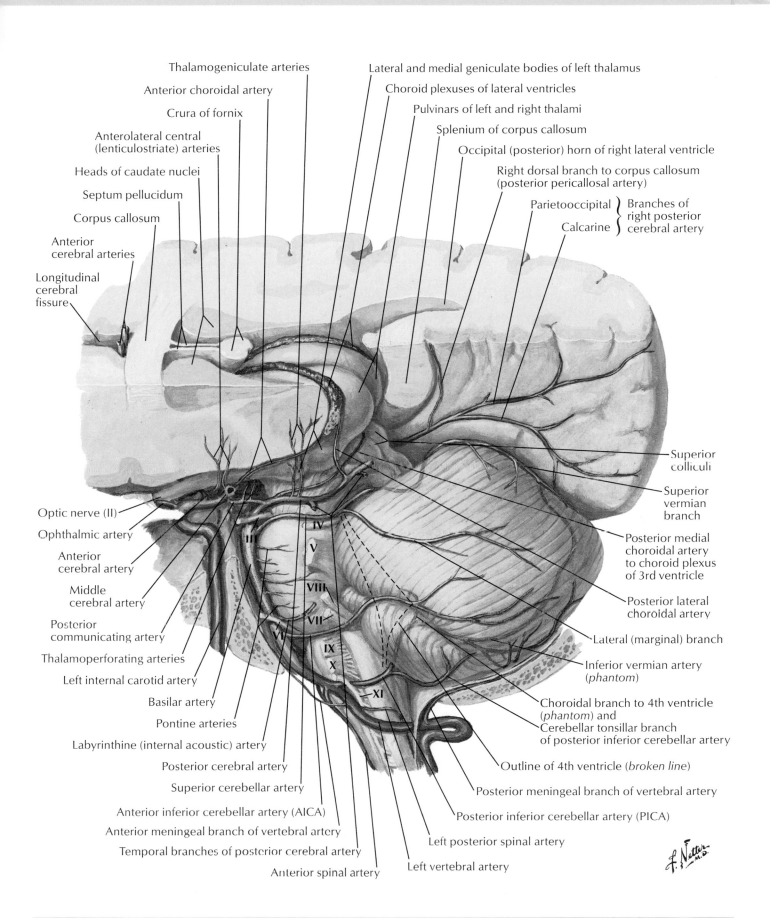

Thalamogeniculate arteries

Anterior choroidal artery

Crura of fornix

Anterolateral central (lenticulostriate) arteries

Heads of caudate nuclei

Septum pellucidum

Corpus callosum

Anterior cerebral arteries

Longitudinal cerebral fissure

Optic nerve (II)

Ophthalmic artery

Anterior cerebral artery

Middle cerebral artery

Posterior communicating artery

Thalamoperforating arteries

Left internal carotid artery

Basilar artery

Pontine arteries

Labyrinthine (internal acoustic) artery

Posterior cerebral artery

Superior cerebellar artery

Anterior inferior cerebellar artery (AICA)

Anterior meningeal branch of vertebral artery

Temporal branches of posterior cerebral artery

Anterior spinal artery

Lateral and medial geniculate bodies of left thalamus

Choroid plexuses of lateral ventricles

Pulvinars of left and right thalami

Splenium of corpus callosum

Occipital (posterior) horn of right lateral ventricle

Right dorsal branch to corpus callosum (posterior pericallosal artery)

Parietooccipital ⎫ Branches of
              ⎬ right posterior
Calcarine   ⎭ cerebral artery

Superior colliculi

Superior vermian branch

Posterior medial choroidal artery to choroid plexus of 3rd ventricle

Posterior lateral choroidal artery

Lateral (marginal) branch

Inferior vermian artery (*phantom*)

Choroidal branch to 4th ventricle (*phantom*) and Cerebellar tonsillar branch of posterior inferior cerebellar artery

Outline of 4th ventricle (*broken line*)

Posterior meningeal branch of vertebral artery

Posterior inferior cerebellar artery (PICA)

Left posterior spinal artery

Left vertebral artery

IV

V

VIII

VII

VI

IX

X

XI

III

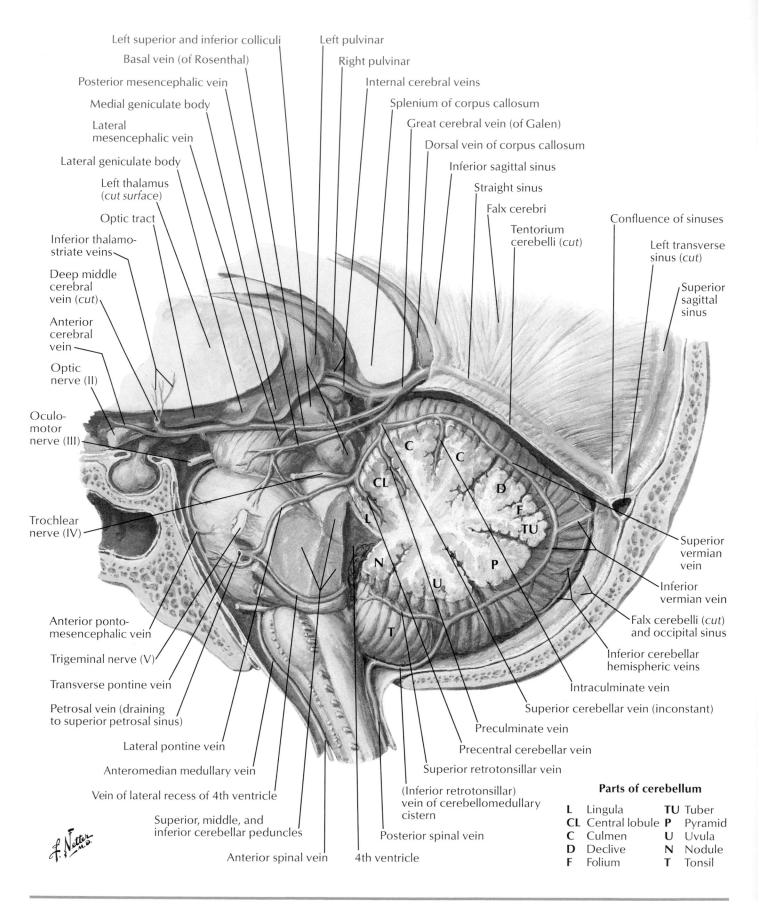

Left superior and inferior colliculi

Basal vein (of Rosenthal)

Posterior mesencephalic vein

Medial geniculate body

Lateral mesencephalic vein

Lateral geniculate body

Left thalamus (*cut surface*)

Optic tract

Inferior thalamo-striate veins

Deep middle cerebral vein (*cut*)

Anterior cerebral vein

Optic nerve (II)

Oculo-motor nerve (III)

Trochlear nerve (IV)

Anterior ponto-mesencephalic vein

Trigeminal nerve (V)

Transverse pontine vein

Petrosal vein (draining to superior petrosal sinus)

Lateral pontine vein

Anteromedian medullary vein

Vein of lateral recess of 4th ventricle

Superior, middle, and inferior cerebellar peduncles

Anterior spinal vein

Left pulvinar

Right pulvinar

Internal cerebral veins

Splenium of corpus callosum

Great cerebral vein (of Galen)

Dorsal vein of corpus callosum

Inferior sagittal sinus

Straight sinus

Falx cerebri

Tentorium cerebelli (*cut*)

Confluence of sinuses

Left transverse sinus (*cut*)

Superior sagittal sinus

Superior vermian vein

Inferior vermian vein

Falx cerebelli (*cut*) and occipital sinus

Inferior cerebellar hemispheric veins

Intraculminate vein

Superior cerebellar vein (inconstant)

Preculminate vein

Precentral cerebellar vein

Superior retrotonsillar vein

(Inferior retrotonsillar) vein of cerebellomedullary cistern

Posterior spinal vein

4th ventricle

Parts of cerebellum

L	Lingula	**TU**	Tuber
CL	Central lobule	**P**	Pyramid
C	Culmen	**U**	Uvula
D	Declive	**N**	Nodule
F	Folium	**T**	Tonsil

Plate 142

Cerebral Vasculature

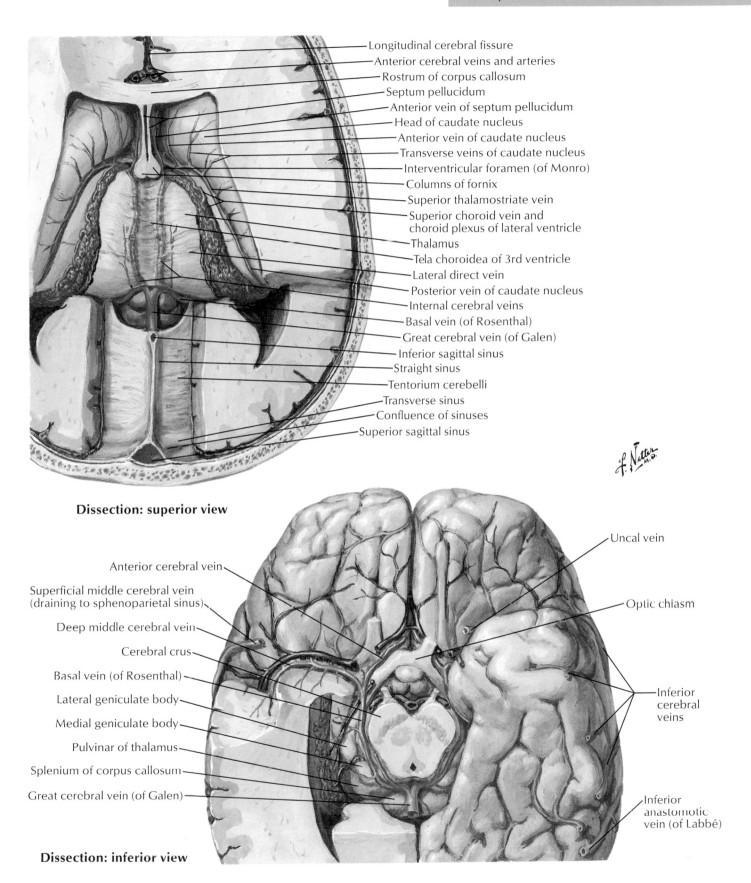

Longitudinal cerebral fissure
Anterior cerebral veins and arteries
Rostrum of corpus callosum
Septum pellucidum
Anterior vein of septum pellucidum
Head of caudate nucleus
Anterior vein of caudate nucleus
Transverse veins of caudate nucleus
Interventricular foramen (of Monro)
Columns of fornix
Superior thalamostriate vein
Superior choroid vein and choroid plexus of lateral ventricle
Thalamus
Tela choroidea of 3rd ventricle
Lateral direct vein
Posterior vein of caudate nucleus
Internal cerebral veins
Basal vein (of Rosenthal)
Great cerebral vein (of Galen)
Inferior sagittal sinus
Straight sinus
Tentorium cerebelli
Transverse sinus
Confluence of sinuses
Superior sagittal sinus

Dissection: superior view

Uncal vein

Anterior cerebral vein
Superficial middle cerebral vein (draining to sphenoparietal sinus)
Deep middle cerebral vein
Cerebral crus
Basal vein (of Rosenthal)
Lateral geniculate body
Medial geniculate body
Pulvinar of thalamus
Splenium of corpus callosum
Great cerebral vein (of Galen)

Optic chiasm

Inferior cerebral veins

Inferior anastomotic vein (of Labbé)

Dissection: inferior view

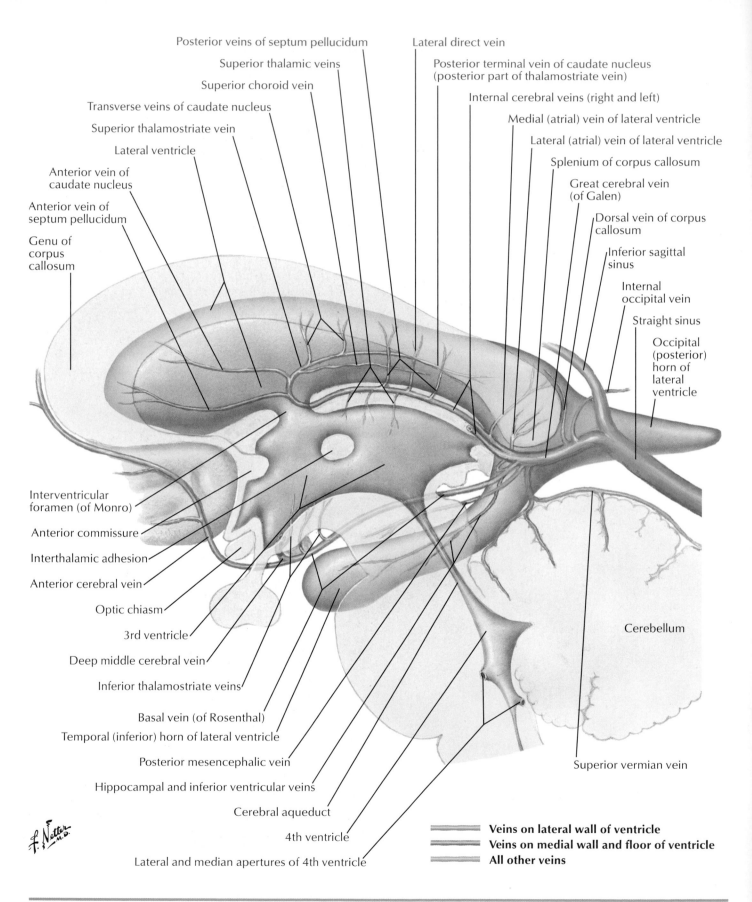

Posterior veins of septum pellucidum

Superior thalamic veins

Superior choroid vein

Transverse veins of caudate nucleus

Superior thalamostriate vein

Lateral ventricle

Anterior vein of caudate nucleus

Anterior vein of septum pellucidum

Genu of corpus callosum

Lateral direct vein

Posterior terminal vein of caudate nucleus (posterior part of thalamostriate vein)

Internal cerebral veins (right and left)

Medial (atrial) vein of lateral ventricle

Lateral (atrial) vein of lateral ventricle

Splenium of corpus callosum

Great cerebral vein (of Galen)

Dorsal vein of corpus callosum

Inferior sagittal sinus

Internal occipital vein

Straight sinus

Occipital (posterior) horn of lateral ventricle

Interventricular foramen (of Monro)

Anterior commissure

Interthalamic adhesion

Anterior cerebral vein

Optic chiasm

3rd ventricle

Deep middle cerebral vein

Inferior thalamostriate veins

Basal vein (of Rosenthal)

Temporal (inferior) horn of lateral ventricle

Posterior mesencephalic vein

Hippocampal and inferior ventricular veins

Cerebral aqueduct

4th ventricle

Lateral and median apertures of 4th ventricle

Cerebellum

Superior vermian vein

Veins on lateral wall of ventricle
Veins on medial wall and floor of ventricle
All other veins

Plate 144

Cerebral Vasculature

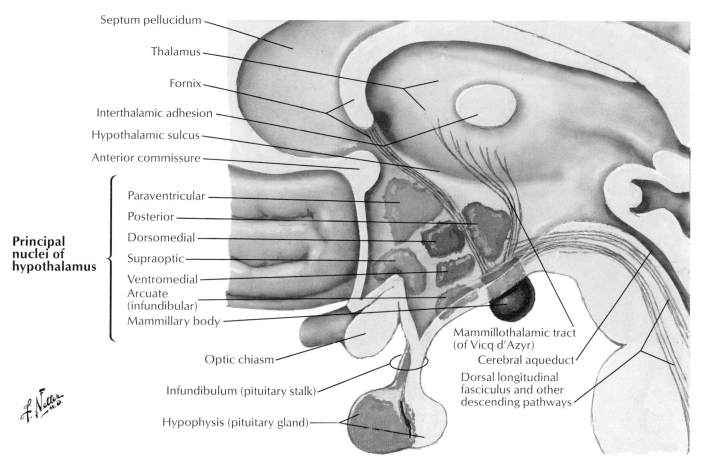

Septum pellucidum

Thalamus

Fornix

Interthalamic adhesion

Hypothalamic sulcus

Anterior commissure

Principal nuclei of hypothalamus
- Paraventricular
- Posterior
- Dorsomedial
- Supraoptic
- Ventromedial
- Arcuate (infundibular)
- Mammillary body

Optic chiasm

Infundibulum (pituitary stalk)

Hypophysis (pituitary gland)

Mammillothalamic tract (of Vicq d'Azyr)

Cerebral aqueduct

Dorsal longitudinal fasciculus and other descending pathways

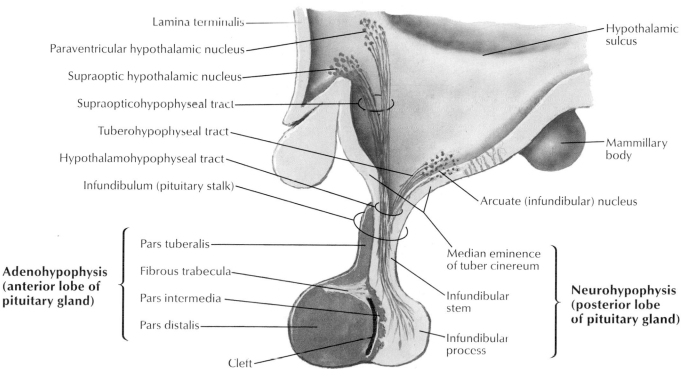

Lamina terminalis

Paraventricular hypothalamic nucleus

Supraoptic hypothalamic nucleus

Supraopticohypophyseal tract

Tuberohypophyseal tract

Hypothalamohypophyseal tract

Infundibulum (pituitary stalk)

Hypothalamic sulcus

Mammillary body

Arcuate (infundibular) nucleus

Adenohypophysis (anterior lobe of pituitary gland)
- Pars tuberalis
- Fibrous trabecula
- Pars intermedia
- Pars distalis

Clett

Median eminence of tuber cinereum

Infundibular stem

Infundibular process

Neurohypophysis (posterior lobe of pituitary gland)

Arteries and Veins of Hypothalmus and Hypophysis

See also **Plate 138**

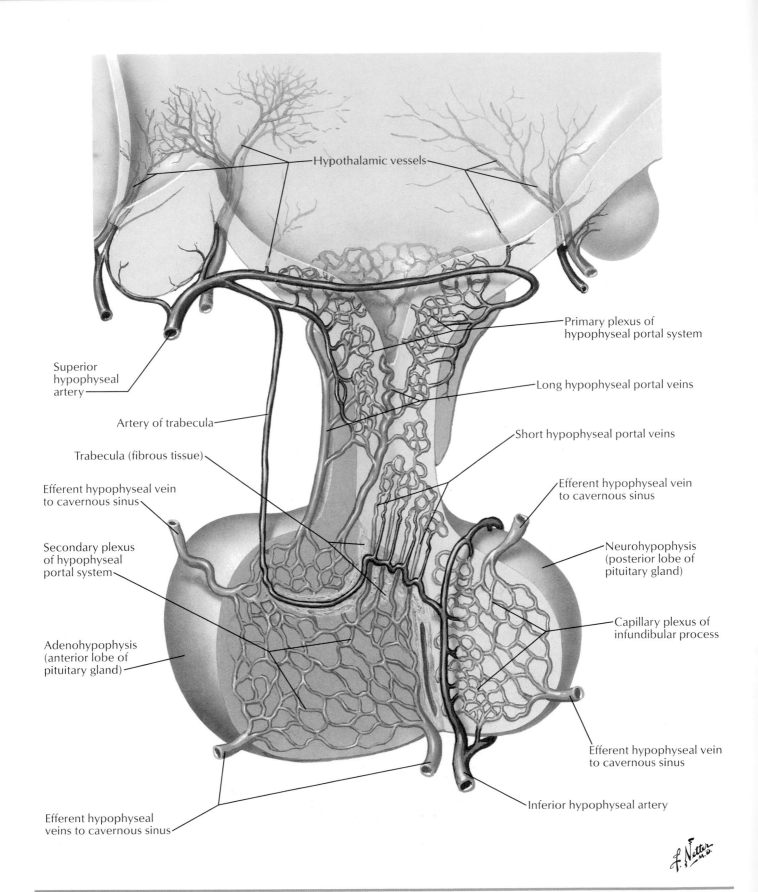

Hypothalamic vessels

Primary plexus of
hypophyseal portal system

Superior
hypophyseal
artery

Long hypophyseal portal veins

Artery of trabecula

Short hypophyseal portal veins

Trabecula (fibrous tissue)

Efferent hypophyseal vein
to cavernous sinus

Efferent hypophyseal vein
to cavernous sinus

Secondary plexus
of hypophyseal
portal system

Neurohypophysis
(posterior lobe of
pituitary gland)

Capillary plexus of
infundibular process

Adenohypophysis
(anterior lobe of
pituitary gland)

Efferent hypophyseal vein
to cavernous sinus

Efferent hypophyseal
veins to cavernous sinus

Inferior hypophyseal artery

Plate 146   **Cerebral Vasculature**

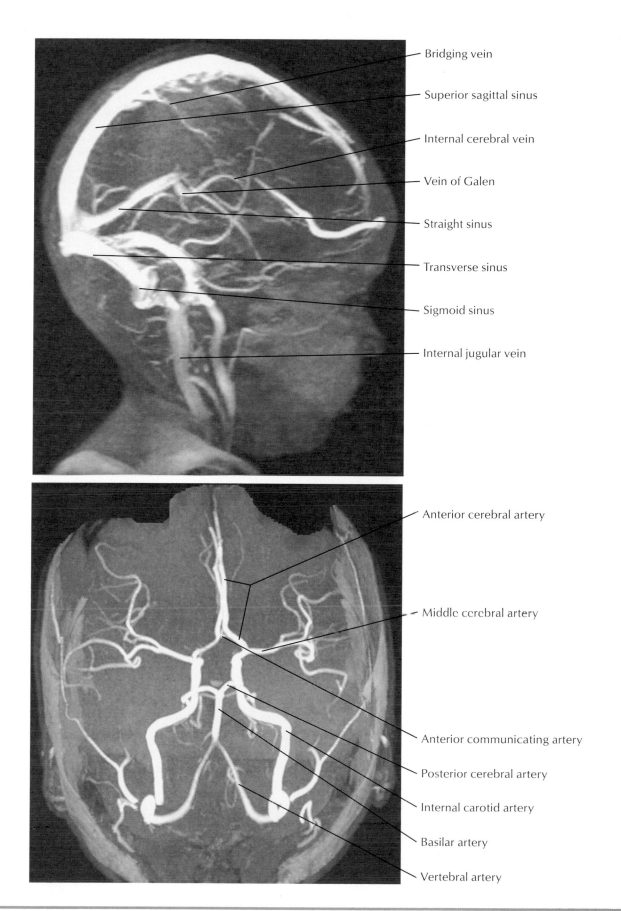

Bridging vein

Superior sagittal sinus

Internal cerebral vein

Vein of Galen

Straight sinus

Transverse sinus

Sigmoid sinus

Internal jugular vein

Anterior cerebral artery

Middle cerebral artery

Anterior communicating artery

Posterior cerebral artery

Internal carotid artery

Basilar artery

Vertebral artery

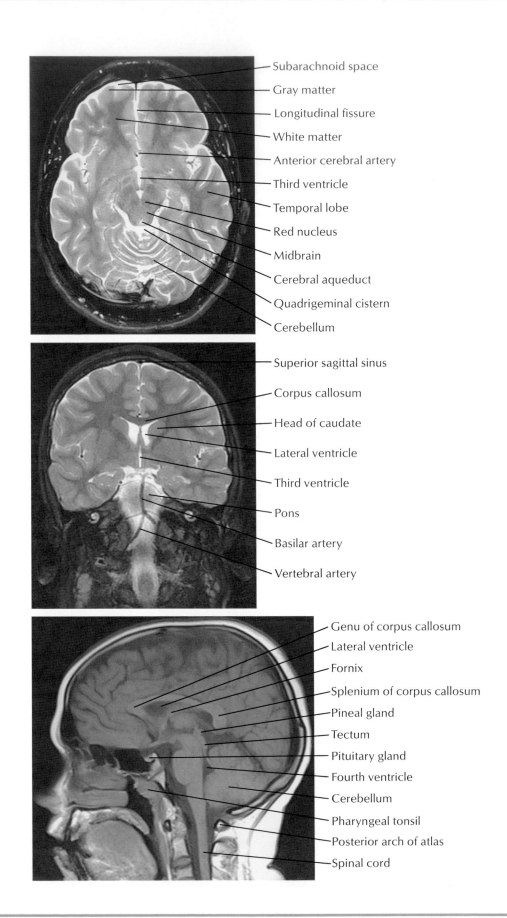

- Subarachnoid space
- Gray matter
- Longitudinal fissure
- White matter
- Anterior cerebral artery
- Third ventricle
- Temporal lobe
- Red nucleus
- Midbrain
- Cerebral aqueduct
- Quadrigeminal cistern
- Cerebellum

- Superior sagittal sinus
- Corpus callosum
- Head of caudate
- Lateral ventricle
- Third ventricle
- Pons
- Basilar artery
- Vertebral artery

- Genu of corpus callosum
- Lateral ventricle
- Fornix
- Splenium of corpus callosum
- Pineal gland
- Tectum
- Pituitary gland
- Fourth ventricle
- Cerebellum
- Pharyngeal tonsil
- Posterior arch of atlas
- Spinal cord

Plate 148

Regional Scans

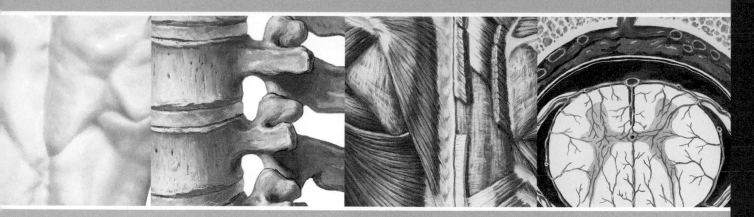

Section 2 BACK AND SPINAL CORD

2 BACK AND SPINAL CORD

Muscles and Nerves
Plates 168-172

Cross-sectional Anatomy
Plates 173-174

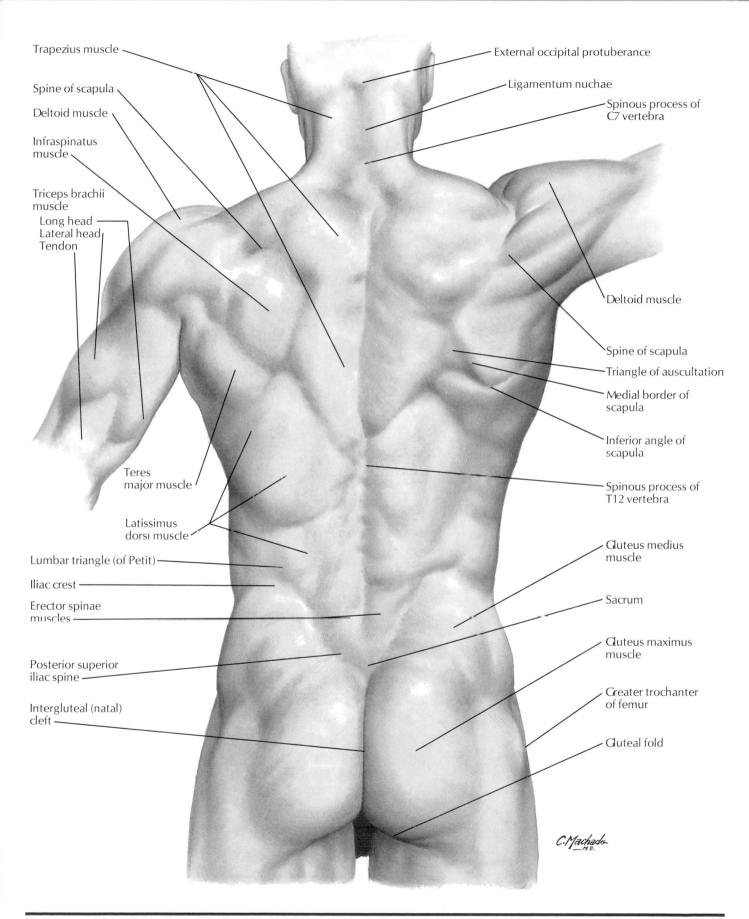

Trapezius muscle

Spine of scapula

Deltoid muscle

Infraspinatus muscle

Triceps brachii muscle

Long head
Lateral head
Tendon

Teres major muscle

Latissimus dorsi muscle

Lumbar triangle (of Petit)

Iliac crest

Erector spinae muscles

Posterior superior iliac spine

Intergluteal (natal) cleft

External occipital protuberance

Ligamentum nuchae

Spinous process of C7 vertebra

Deltoid muscle

Spine of scapula

Triangle of auscultation

Medial border of scapula

Inferior angle of scapula

Spinous process of T12 vertebra

Gluteus medius muscle

Sacrum

Gluteus maximus muscle

Greater trochanter of femur

Gluteal fold

C.Machado
_M.D.

Topographic Anatomy

Plate 149

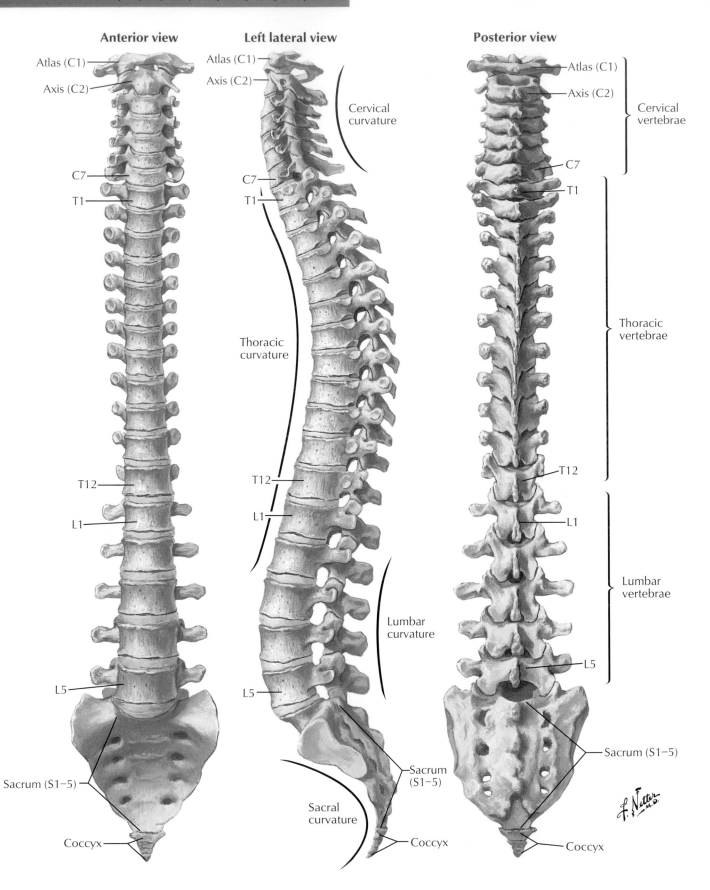

Anterior view

Atlas (C1)
Axis (C2)
C7
T1
T12
L1
L5
Sacrum (S1–5)
Coccyx

Left lateral view

Atlas (C1)
Axis (C2)
Cervical curvature
C7
T1
Thoracic curvature
T12
L1
Lumbar curvature
L5
Sacrum (S1–5)
Sacral curvature
Coccyx

Posterior view

Atlas (C1)
Axis (C2)
Cervical vertebrae
C7
T1
Thoracic vertebrae
T12
L1
Lumbar vertebrae
L5
Sacrum (S1–5)
Coccyx

Plate 150

Bones and Ligaments

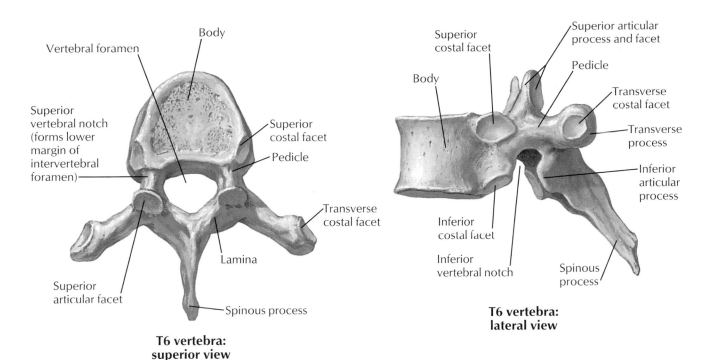

Body

Vertebral foramen

Superior vertebral notch (forms lower margin of intervertebral foramen)

Superior articular facet

Superior costal facet

Pedicle

Lamina

Spinous process

Transverse costal facet

T6 vertebra: superior view

Superior costal facet

Superior articular process and facet

Pedicle

Body

Transverse costal facet

Transverse process

Inferior costal facet

Inferior articular process

Inferior vertebral notch

Spinous process

T6 vertebra: lateral view

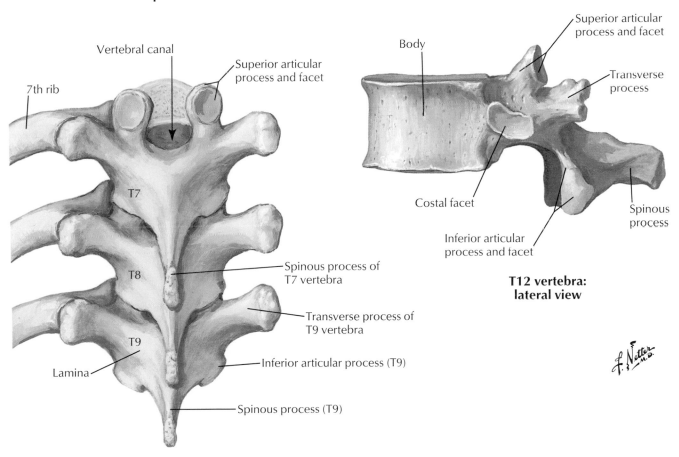

7th rib

Vertebral canal

Superior articular process and facet

T7

T8

T9

Lamina

Spinous process of T7 vertebra

Transverse process of T9 vertebra

Inferior articular process (T9)

Spinous process (T9)

T7, T8, and T9 vertebrae: posterior view

Body

Superior articular process and facet

Transverse process

Costal facet

Inferior articular process and facet

Spinous process

T12 vertebra: lateral view

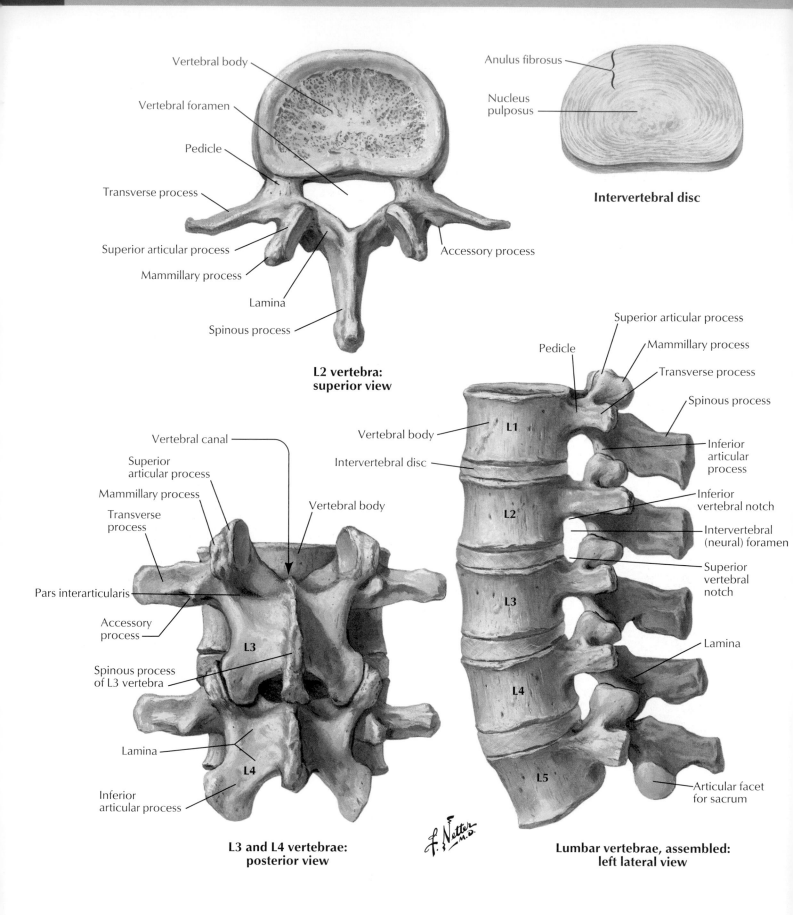

Vertebral body

Vertebral foramen

Pedicle

Transverse process

Superior articular process

Mammillary process

Lamina

Spinous process

**L2 vertebra:
superior view**

Anulus fibrosus

Nucleus pulposus

Intervertebral disc

Vertebral canal

Superior articular process

Mammillary process

Transverse process

Pars interarticularis

Accessory process

Spinous process of L3 vertebra

Vertebral body

L3

Lamina

L4

Inferior articular process

**L3 and L4 vertebrae:
posterior view**

Superior articular process

Mammillary process

Transverse process

Spinous process

Pedicle

Vertebral body

Intervertebral disc

L1

L2

L3

L4

L5

Inferior articular process

Inferior vertebral notch

Intervertebral (neural) foramen

Superior vertebral notch

Lamina

Articular facet for sacrum

**Lumbar vertebrae, assembled:
left lateral view**

Plate 152

Bones and Ligaments

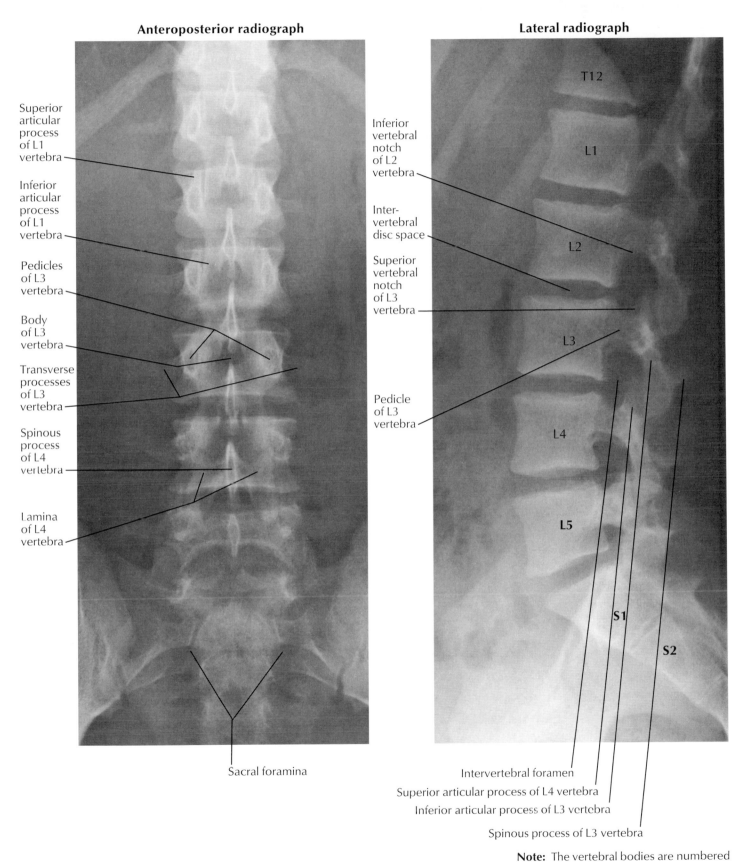

Anteroposterior radiograph

Superior articular process of L1 vertebra

Inferior articular process of L1 vertebra

Pedicles of L3 vertebra

Body of L3 vertebra

Transverse processes of L3 vertebra

Spinous process of L4 vertebra

Lamina of L4 vertebra

Sacral foramina

Lateral radiograph

T12

L1

Inferior vertebral notch of L2 vertebra

Inter-vertebral disc space

Superior vertebral notch of L3 vertebra

L2

L3

Pedicle of L3 vertebra

L4

L5

S1

S2

Intervertebral foramen

Superior articular process of L4 vertebra

Inferior articular process of L3 vertebra

Spinous process of L3 vertebra

Note: The vertebral bodies are numbered

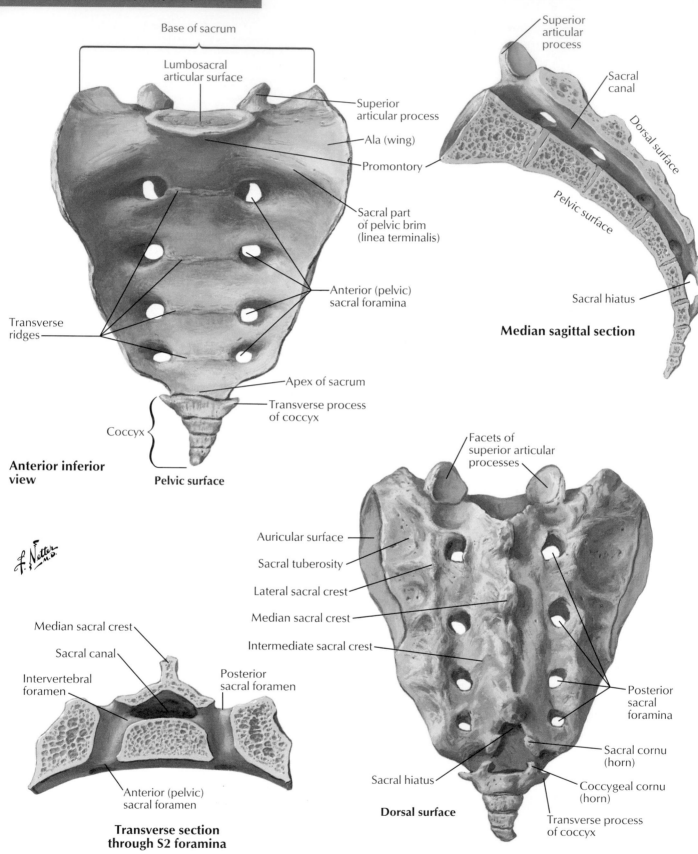

Base of sacrum

Lumbosacral articular surface

Superior articular process

Ala (wing)

Promontory

Sacral part of pelvic brim (linea terminalis)

Anterior (pelvic) sacral foramina

Transverse ridges

Apex of sacrum

Transverse process of coccyx

Coccyx

Pelvic surface

Anterior inferior view

Superior articular process

Sacral canal

Dorsal surface

Pelvic surface

Sacral hiatus

Median sagittal section

Median sacral crest

Sacral canal

Intervertebral foramen

Posterior sacral foramen

Anterior (pelvic) sacral foramen

Transverse section through S2 foramina

Facets of superior articular processes

Auricular surface

Sacral tuberosity

Lateral sacral crest

Median sacral crest

Intermediate sacral crest

Posterior sacral foramina

Sacral cornu (horn)

Sacral hiatus

Coccygeal cornu (horn)

Transverse process of coccyx

Dorsal surface

Posterior superior view

Plate 154

Bones and Ligaments

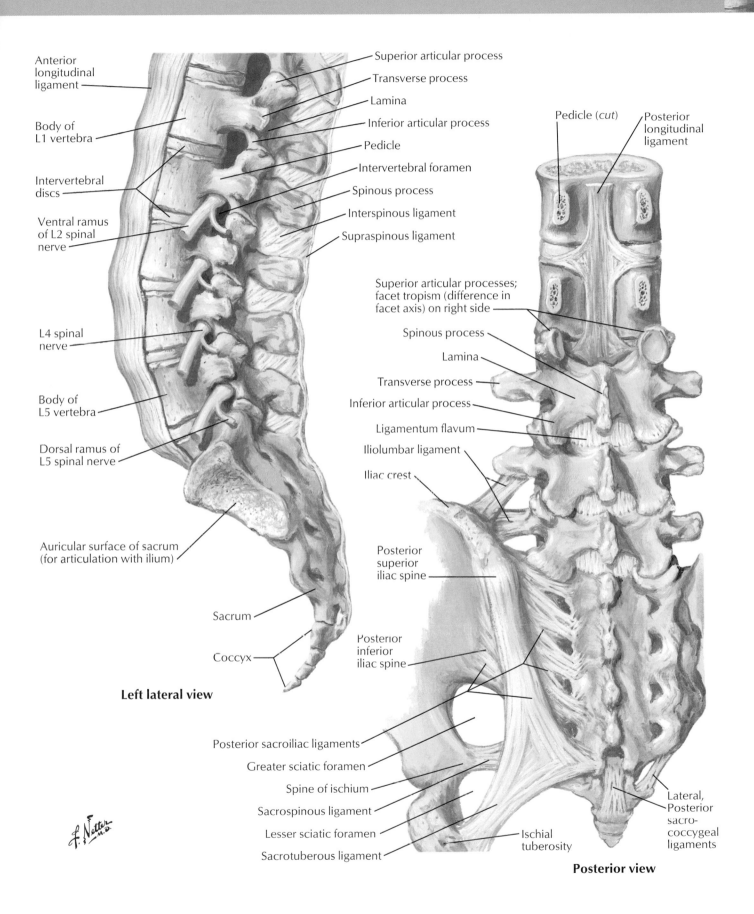

Anterior longitudinal ligament

Body of L1 vertebra

Intervertebral discs

Ventral ramus of L2 spinal nerve

L4 spinal nerve

Body of L5 vertebra

Dorsal ramus of L5 spinal nerve

Auricular surface of sacrum (for articulation with ilium)

Sacrum

Coccyx

Left lateral view

Superior articular process

Transverse process

Lamina

Inferior articular process

Pedicle

Intervertebral foramen

Spinous process

Interspinous ligament

Supraspinous ligament

Pedicle (*cut*)

Posterior longitudinal ligament

Superior articular processes; facet tropism (difference in facet axis) on right side

Spinous process

Lamina

Transverse process

Inferior articular process

Ligamentum flavum

Iliolumbar ligament

Iliac crest

Posterior superior iliac spine

Posterior inferior iliac spine

Posterior sacroiliac ligaments

Greater sciatic foramen

Spine of ischium

Sacrospinous ligament

Lesser sciatic foramen

Sacrotuberous ligament

Ischial tuberosity

Lateral, Posterior sacro-coccygeal ligaments

Posterior view

F. Netter M.D.

Left lateral view (*partially sectioned in median plane*)

Anterior longitudinal ligament

Lumbar vertebral body

Intervertebral disc

Anterior longitudinal ligament

Posterior longitudinal ligament

Inferior articular process

Capsule of zygapophyseal joint (*partially opened*)

Superior articular process

Transverse process

Spinous process

Ligamentum flavum

Interspinous ligament

Supraspinous ligament

Intervertebral foramen

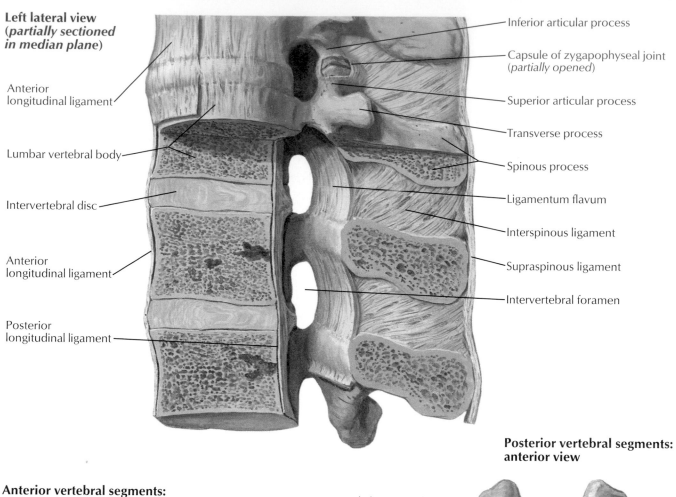

Posterior vertebral segments: anterior view

Anterior vertebral segments: posterior view (*pedicles sectioned*)

Pedicle (*cut surface*)

Posterior surface of vertebral bodies

Posterior longitudinal ligament

Intervertebral disc

Pedicle (*cut surface*)

Ligamentum flavum

Lamina

Superior articular process

Transverse process

Inferior articular facet

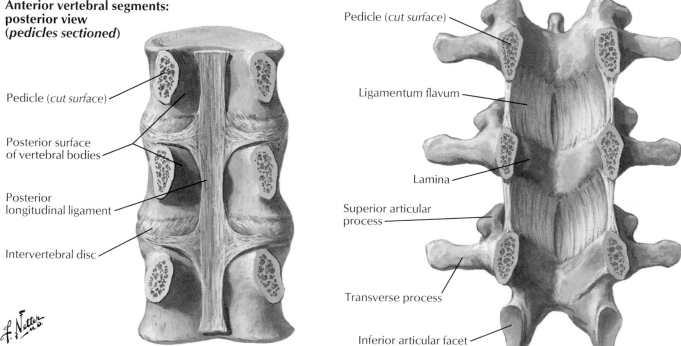

Plate 156

Bones and Ligaments

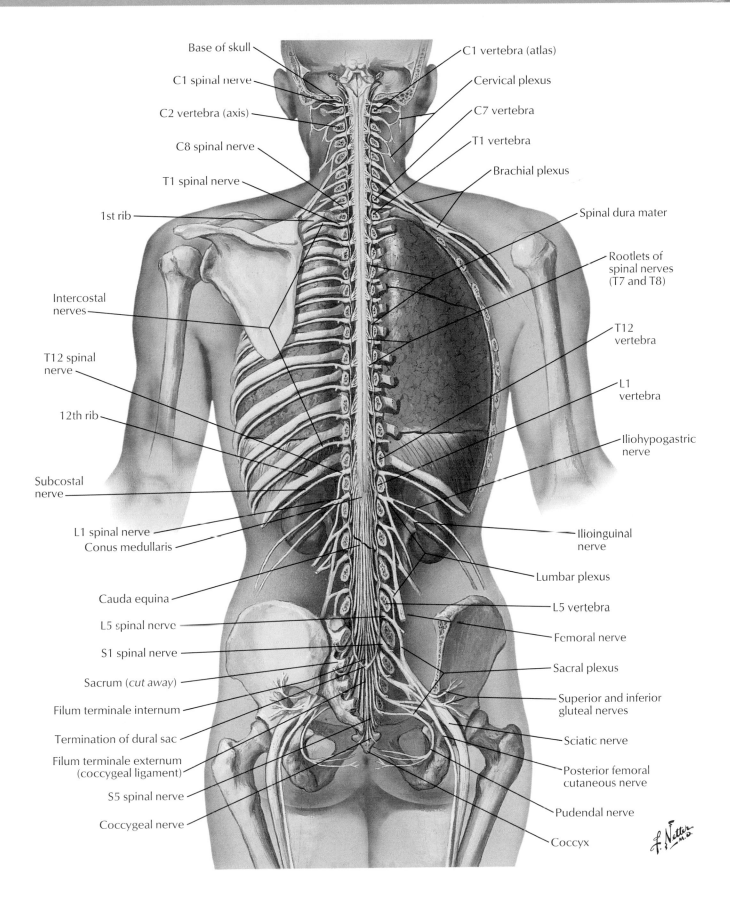

Base of skull

C1 spinal nerve

C2 vertebra (axis)

C8 spinal nerve

T1 spinal nerve

1st rib

Intercostal nerves

T12 spinal nerve

12th rib

Subcostal nerve

L1 spinal nerve

Conus medullaris

Cauda equina

L5 spinal nerve

S1 spinal nerve

Sacrum (*cut away*)

Filum terminale internum

Termination of dural sac

Filum terminale externum (coccygeal ligament)

S5 spinal nerve

Coccygeal nerve

C1 vertebra (atlas)

Cervical plexus

C7 vertebra

T1 vertebra

Brachial plexus

Spinal dura mater

Rootlets of spinal nerves (T7 and T8)

T12 vertebra

L1 vertebra

Iliohypogastric nerve

Ilioinguinal nerve

Lumbar plexus

L5 vertebra

Femoral nerve

Sacral plexus

Superior and inferior gluteal nerves

Sciatic nerve

Posterior femoral cutaneous nerve

Pudendal nerve

Coccyx

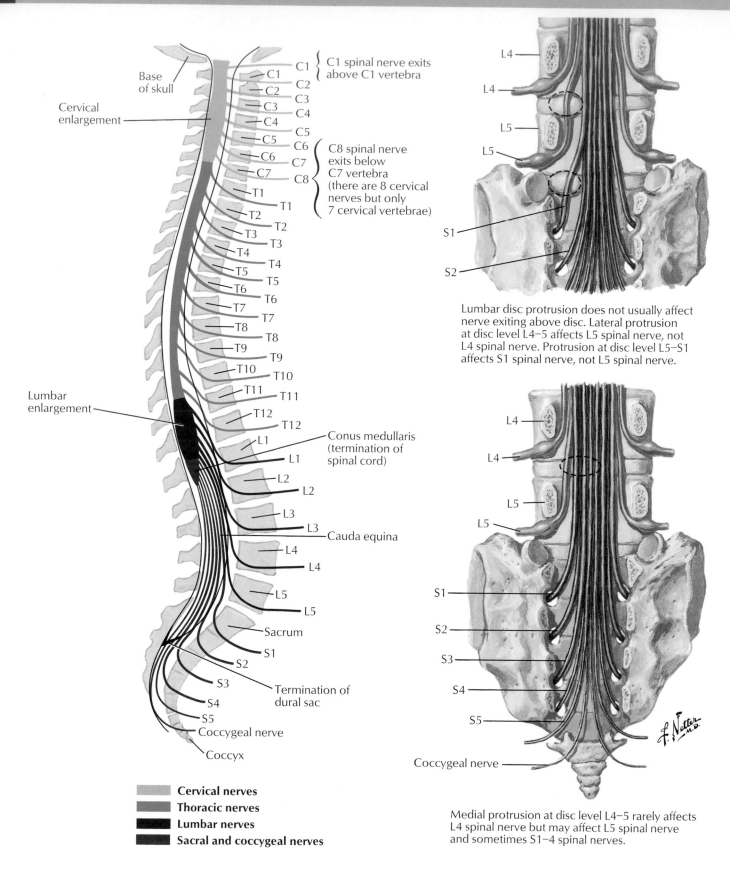

Base of skull

Cervical enlargement

C1 spinal nerve exits above C1 vertebra

C8 spinal nerve exits below C7 vertebra (there are 8 cervical nerves but only 7 cervical vertebrae)

Lumbar enlargement

Conus medullaris (termination of spinal cord)

Cauda equina

Sacrum

Termination of dural sac

Coccygeal nerve

Coccyx

Cervical nerves
Thoracic nerves
Lumbar nerves
Sacral and coccygeal nerves

Lumbar disc protrusion does not usually affect nerve exiting above disc. Lateral protrusion at disc level L4–5 affects L5 spinal nerve, not L4 spinal nerve. Protrusion at disc level L5–S1 affects S1 spinal nerve, not L5 spinal nerve.

Medial protrusion at disc level L4–5 rarely affects L4 spinal nerve but may affect L5 spinal nerve and sometimes S1–4 spinal nerves.

Plate 158

Spinal Cord

See also **Plates 401, 470;** for maps of cutaneous nerves see **Plates 2, 402, 460, 462-464, 466, 467, 526-530**

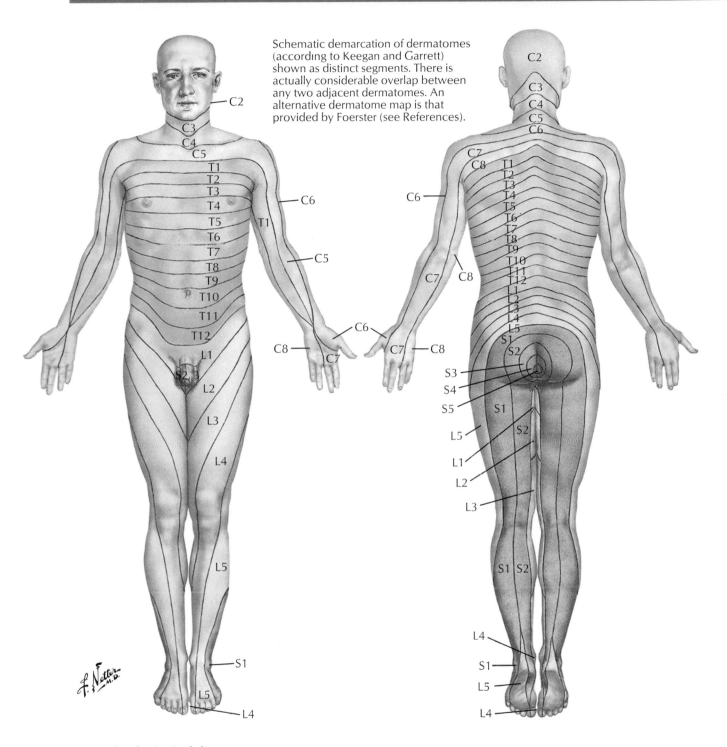

Schematic demarcation of dermatomes (according to Keegan and Garrett) shown as distinct segments. There is actually considerable overlap between any two adjacent dermatomes. An alternative dermatome map is that provided by Foerster (see References).

Levels of principal dermatomes

C5	Clavicles
C5, 6	Lateral sides of upper limbs
C8, T1	Medial sides of upper limbs
C6	Thumb
C6, 7, 8	Hand
C8	Ring and little fingers
T4	Level of nipples

T10	Level of umbilicus
L1	Inguinal or groin regions
L1, 2, 3, 4	Anterior and inner surfaces of lower limbs
L4, 5, S1	Foot
L4	Medial side of great toe
L5, S1, 2	Lateral and posterior surfaces of lower limbs
S1	Lateral margin of foot and little toe
S2, 3, 4	Perineum

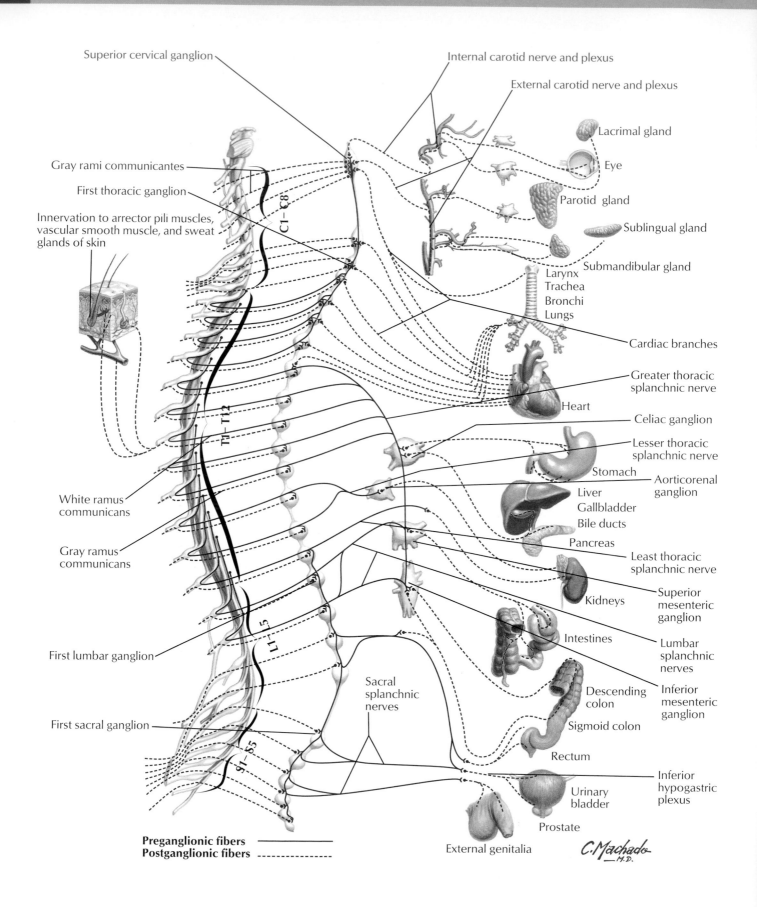

Superior cervical ganglion

Internal carotid nerve and plexus

External carotid nerve and plexus

Lacrimal gland

Gray rami communicantes

Eye

First thoracic ganglion

Parotid gland

Innervation to arrector pili muscles, vascular smooth muscle, and sweat glands of skin

Sublingual gland

Submandibular gland

Larynx
Trachea
Bronchi
Lungs

Cardiac branches

Greater thoracic splanchnic nerve

Heart

Celiac ganglion

Lesser thoracic splanchnic nerve

Stomach

Aorticorenal ganglion

Liver
Gallbladder
Bile ducts

White ramus communicans

Pancreas

Least thoracic splanchnic nerve

Gray ramus communicans

Superior mesenteric ganglion

Kidneys

Intestines

Lumbar splanchnic nerves

First lumbar ganglion

Inferior mesenteric ganglion

Descending colon

Sacral splanchnic nerves

Sigmoid colon

Rectum

First sacral ganglion

Inferior hypogastric plexus

Urinary bladder

Prostate

Preganglionic fibers ———
Postganglionic fibers --------

External genitalia

C1–C8

T1–T12

L1–L5

S1–S5

C.Machado
_M.D._

Plate 160

Spinal Cord

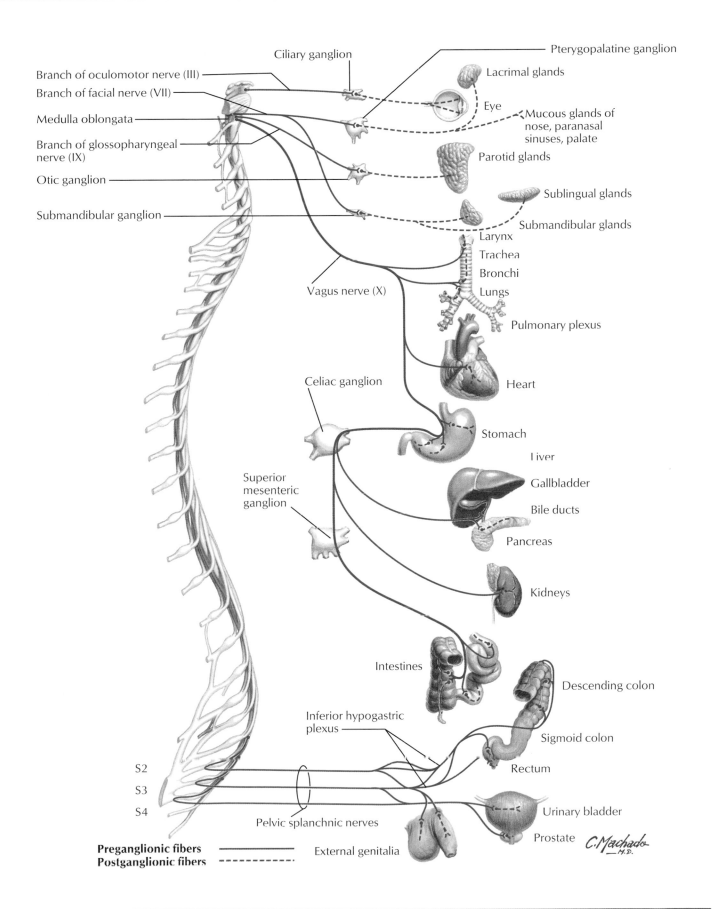

Ciliary ganglion

Pterygopalatine ganglion

Branch of oculomotor nerve (III)

Lacrimal glands

Branch of facial nerve (VII)

Eye

Medulla oblongata

Mucous glands of nose, paranasal sinuses, palate

Branch of glossopharyngeal nerve (IX)

Parotid glands

Otic ganglion

Sublingual glands

Submandibular ganglion

Submandibular glands

Larynx

Trachea

Bronchi

Vagus nerve (X)

Lungs

Pulmonary plexus

Celiac ganglion

Heart

Stomach

Liver

Gallbladder

Superior mesenteric ganglion

Bile ducts

Pancreas

Kidneys

Intestines

Descending colon

Inferior hypogastric plexus

Sigmoid colon

Rectum

S2

S3

S4

Urinary bladder

Pelvic splanchnic nerves

Prostate

Preganglionic fibers
Postganglionic fibers

External genitalia

C. Machado
—M.D.

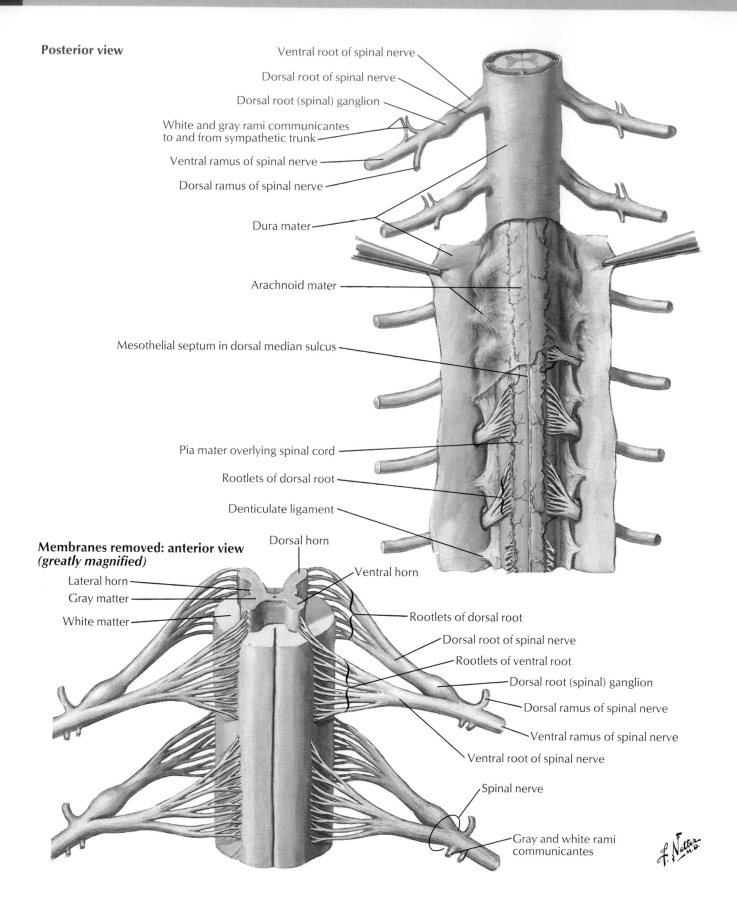

Posterior view

Ventral root of spinal nerve

Dorsal root of spinal nerve

Dorsal root (spinal) ganglion

White and gray rami communicantes
to and from sympathetic trunk

Ventral ramus of spinal nerve

Dorsal ramus of spinal nerve

Dura mater

Arachnoid mater

Mesothelial septum in dorsal median sulcus

Pia mater overlying spinal cord

Rootlets of dorsal root

Denticulate ligament

Dorsal horn

**Membranes removed: anterior view
(greatly magnified)**

Lateral horn

Gray matter

White matter

Ventral horn

Rootlets of dorsal root

Dorsal root of spinal nerve

Rootlets of ventral root

Dorsal root (spinal) ganglion

Dorsal ramus of spinal nerve

Ventral ramus of spinal nerve

Ventral root of spinal nerve

Spinal nerve

Gray and white rami
communicantes

*f. Netter
M.D.*

Plate 162

Spinal Cord

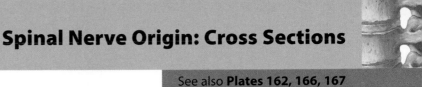

Section through thoracic vertebra

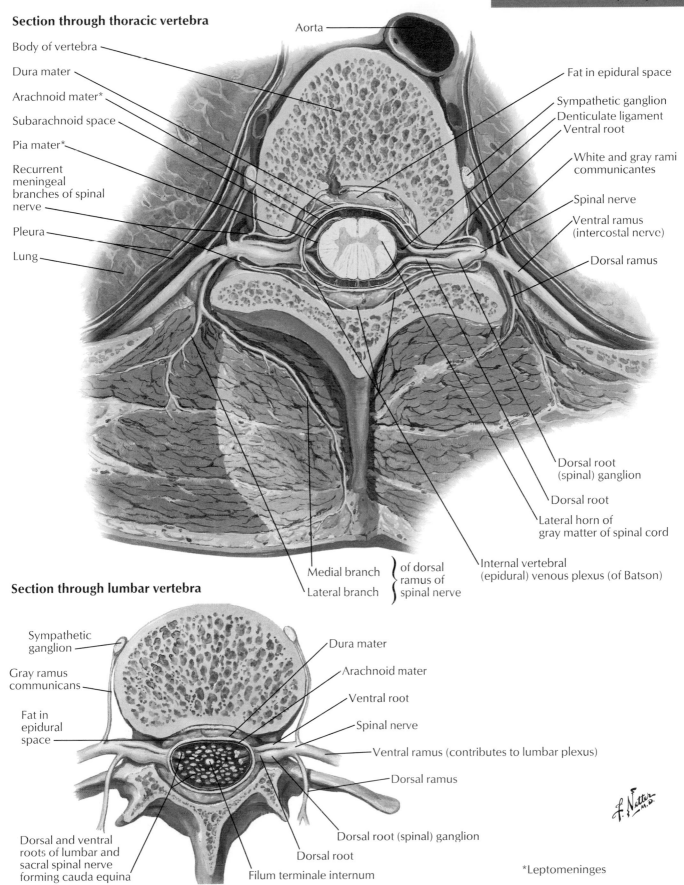

Body of vertebra

Dura mater

Arachnoid mater*

Subarachnoid space

Pia mater*

Recurrent meningeal branches of spinal nerve

Pleura

Lung

Aorta

Fat in epidural space

Sympathetic ganglion

Denticulate ligament

Ventral root

White and gray rami communicantes

Spinal nerve

Ventral ramus (intercostal nerve)

Dorsal ramus

Dorsal root (spinal) ganglion

Dorsal root

Lateral horn of gray matter of spinal cord

Internal vertebral (epidural) venous plexus (of Batson)

Medial branch ⎫
Lateral branch ⎬ of dorsal ramus of spinal nerve

Section through lumbar vertebra

Sympathetic ganglion

Gray ramus communicans

Fat in epidural space

Dura mater

Arachnoid mater

Ventral root

Spinal nerve

Ventral ramus (contributes to lumbar plexus)

Dorsal ramus

Dorsal root (spinal) ganglion

Dorsal root

Dorsal and ventral roots of lumbar and sacral spinal nerve forming cauda equina

Filum terminale internum

*Leptomeninges

Spinal Cord

Plate 163

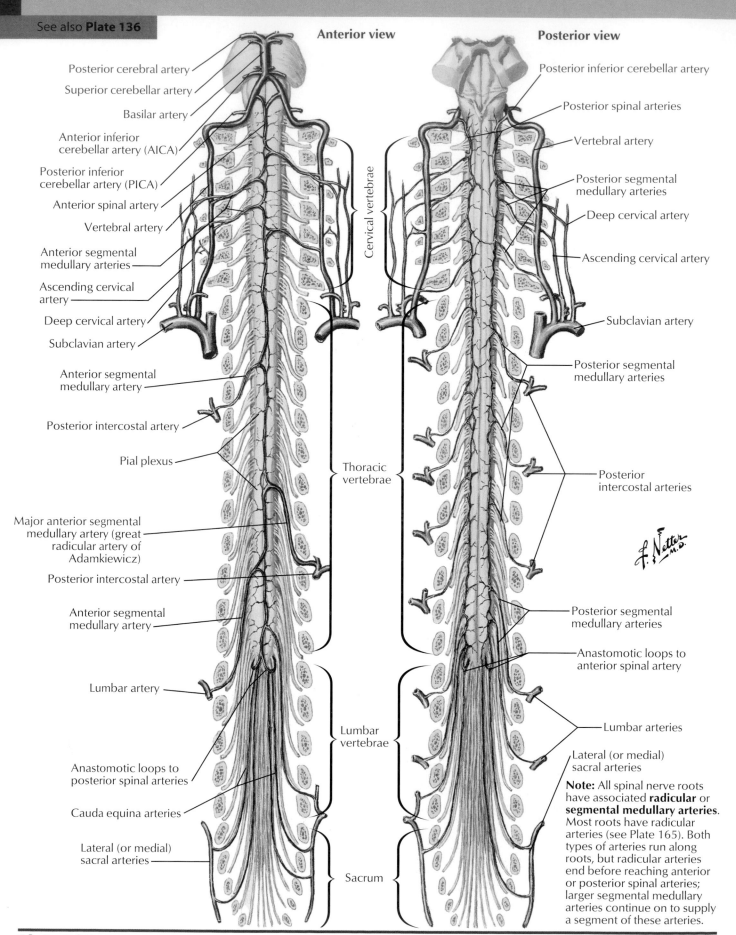

Anterior view

Posterior view

Posterior cerebral artery

Superior cerebellar artery

Basilar artery

Anterior inferior cerebellar artery (AICA)

Posterior inferior cerebellar artery (PICA)

Anterior spinal artery

Vertebral artery

Anterior segmental medullary arteries

Ascending cervical artery

Deep cervical artery

Subclavian artery

Anterior segmental medullary artery

Posterior intercostal artery

Pial plexus

Major anterior segmental medullary artery (great radicular artery of Adamkiewicz)

Posterior intercostal artery

Anterior segmental medullary artery

Lumbar artery

Anastomotic loops to posterior spinal arteries

Cauda equina arteries

Lateral (or medial) sacral arteries

Posterior inferior cerebellar artery

Posterior spinal arteries

Vertebral artery

Posterior segmental medullary arteries

Deep cervical artery

Ascending cervical artery

Subclavian artery

Posterior segmental medullary arteries

Posterior intercostal arteries

Posterior segmental medullary arteries

Anastomotic loops to anterior spinal artery

Lumbar arteries

Lateral (or medial) sacral arteries

Cervical vertebrae

Thoracic vertebrae

Lumbar vertebrae

Sacrum

Note: All spinal nerve roots have associated **radicular** or **segmental medullary arteries**. Most roots have radicular arteries (see Plate 165). Both types of arteries run along roots, but radicular arteries end before reaching anterior or posterior spinal arteries; larger segmental medullary arteries continue on to supply a segment of these arteries.

Plate 164

Spinal Cord

Arteries of Spinal Cord: Intrinsic Distribution

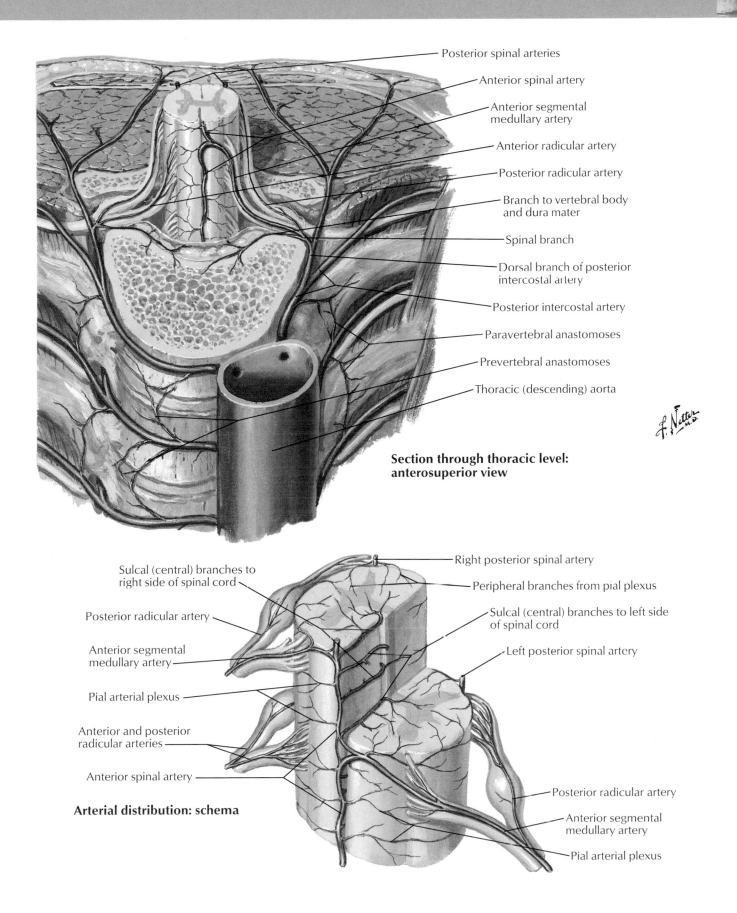

Posterior spinal arteries

Anterior spinal artery

Anterior segmental medullary artery

Anterior radicular artery

Posterior radicular artery

Branch to vertebral body and dura mater

Spinal branch

Dorsal branch of posterior intercostal artery

Posterior intercostal artery

Paravertebral anastomoses

Prevertebral anastomoses

Thoracic (descending) aorta

Section through thoracic level: anterosuperior view

Sulcal (central) branches to right side of spinal cord

Posterior radicular artery

Anterior segmental medullary artery

Pial arterial plexus

Anterior and posterior radicular arteries

Anterior spinal artery

Arterial distribution: schema

Right posterior spinal artery

Peripheral branches from pial plexus

Sulcal (central) branches to left side of spinal cord

Left posterior spinal artery

Posterior radicular artery

Anterior segmental medullary artery

Pial arterial plexus

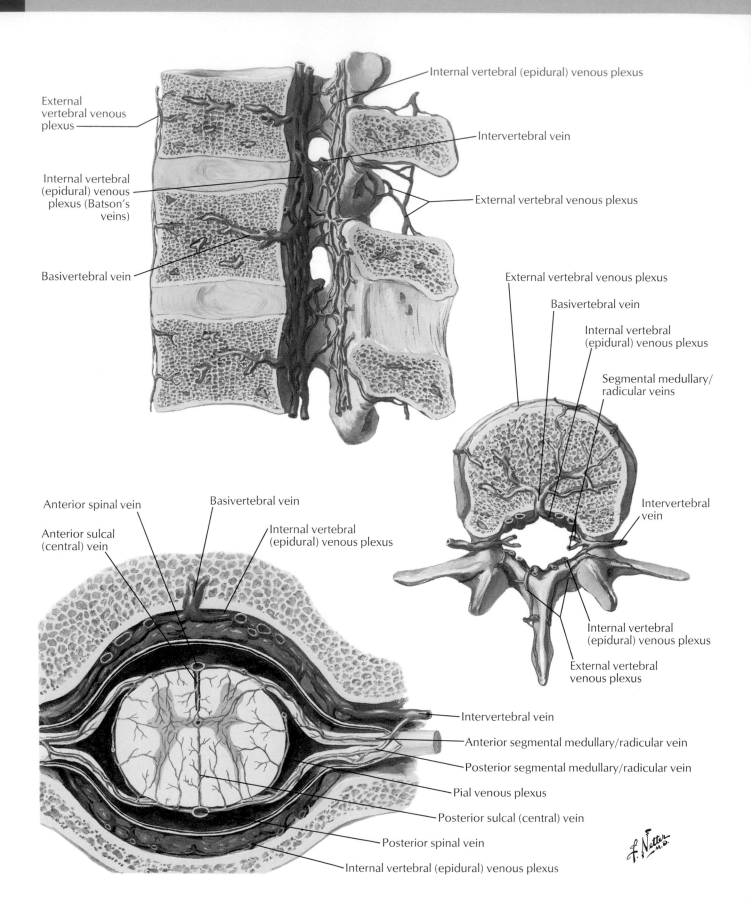

External vertebral venous plexus

Internal vertebral (epidural) venous plexus (Batson's veins)

Basivertebral vein

Internal vertebral (epidural) venous plexus

Intervertebral vein

External vertebral venous plexus

External vertebral venous plexus

Basivertebral vein

Internal vertebral (epidural) venous plexus

Segmental medullary/radicular veins

Intervertebral vein

Internal vertebral (epidural) venous plexus

External vertebral venous plexus

Anterior spinal vein

Anterior sulcal (central) vein

Basivertebral vein

Internal vertebral (epidural) venous plexus

Intervertebral vein

Anterior segmental medullary/radicular vein

Posterior segmental medullary/radicular vein

Pial venous plexus

Posterior sulcal (central) vein

Posterior spinal vein

Internal vertebral (epidural) venous plexus

Plate 166

Spinal Cord

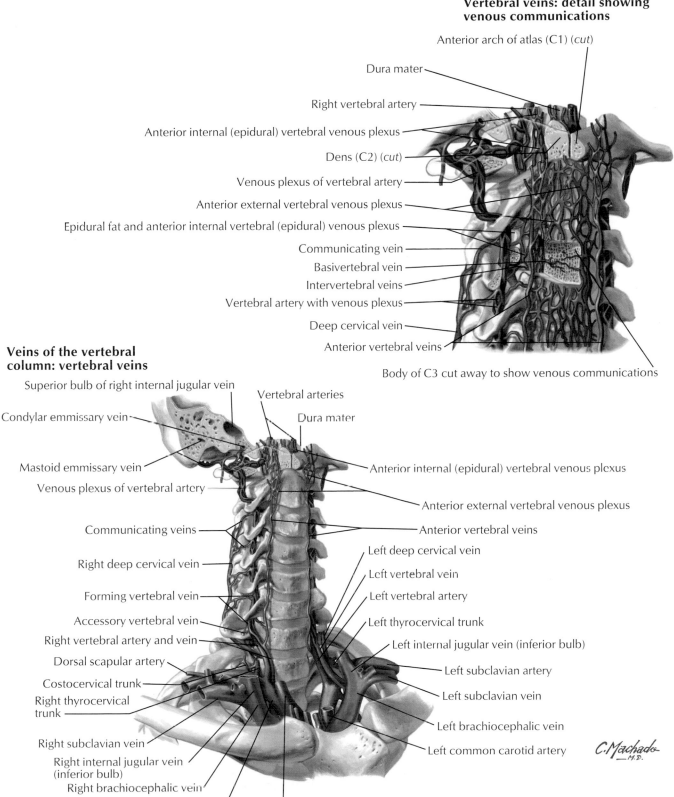

Vertebral veins: detail showing venous communications

Anterior arch of atlas (C1) (*cut*)

Dura mater

Right vertebral artery

Anterior internal (epidural) vertebral venous plexus

Dens (C2) (*cut*)

Venous plexus of vertebral artery

Anterior external vertebral venous plexus

Epidural fat and anterior internal vertebral (epidural) venous plexus

Communicating vein

Basivertebral vein

Intervertebral veins

Vertebral artery with venous plexus

Deep cervical vein

Anterior vertebral veins

Body of C3 cut away to show venous communications

Veins of the vertebral column: vertebral veins

Superior bulb of right internal jugular vein

Condylar emmissary vein

Mastoid emmissary vein

Venous plexus of vertebral artery

Communicating veins

Right deep cervical vein

Forming vertebral vein

Accessory vertebral vein

Right vertebral artery and vein

Dorsal scapular artery

Costocervical trunk

Right thyrocervical trunk

Right subclavian vein

Right internal jugular vein (inferior bulb)

Right brachiocephalic vein

Right subclavian artery

Vertebral arteries

Dura mater

Anterior internal (epidural) vertebral venous plexus

Anterior external vertebral venous plexus

Anterior vertebral veins

Left deep cervical vein

Left vertebral vein

Left vertebral artery

Left thyrocervical trunk

Left internal jugular vein (inferior bulb)

Left subclavian artery

Left subclavian vein

Left brachiocephalic vein

Left common carotid artery

Right common carotid artery

C. Machado
—M.D.

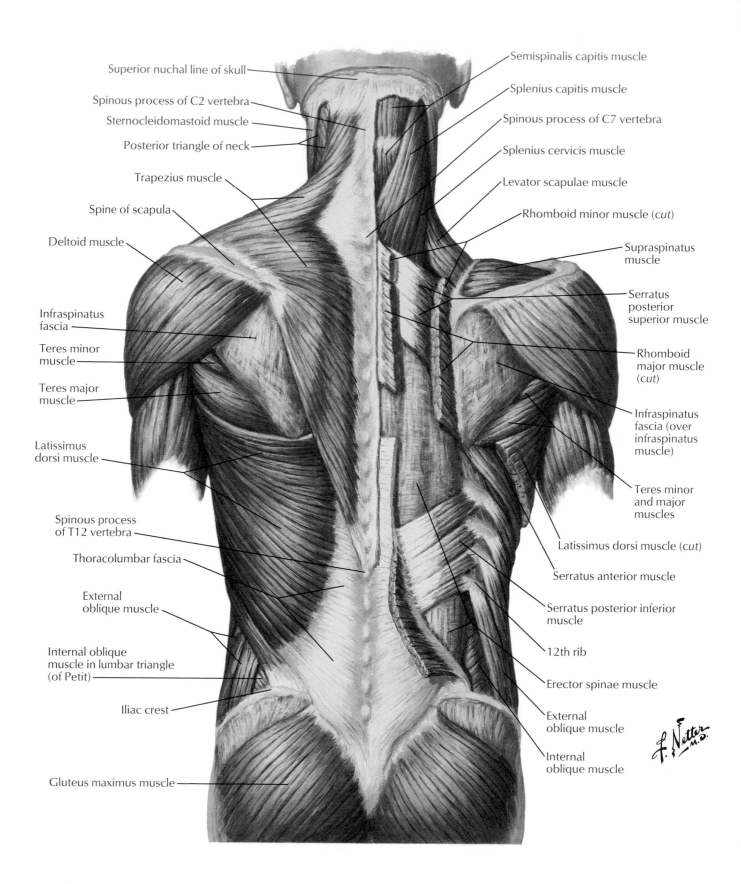

Superior nuchal line of skull

Spinous process of C2 vertebra

Sternocleidomastoid muscle

Posterior triangle of neck

Trapezius muscle

Spine of scapula

Deltoid muscle

Infraspinatus fascia

Teres minor muscle

Teres major muscle

Latissimus dorsi muscle

Spinous process of T12 vertebra

Thoracolumbar fascia

External oblique muscle

Internal oblique muscle in lumbar triangle (of Petit)

Iliac crest

Gluteus maximus muscle

Semispinalis capitis muscle

Splenius capitis muscle

Spinous process of C7 vertebra

Splenius cervicis muscle

Levator scapulae muscle

Rhomboid minor muscle (*cut*)

Supraspinatus muscle

Serratus posterior superior muscle

Rhomboid major muscle (*cut*)

Infraspinatus fascia (over infraspinatus muscle)

Teres minor and major muscles

Latissimus dorsi muscle (*cut*)

Serratus anterior muscle

Serratus posterior inferior muscle

12th rib

Erector spinae muscle

External oblique muscle

Internal oblique muscle

Plate 168

Muscles and Nerves

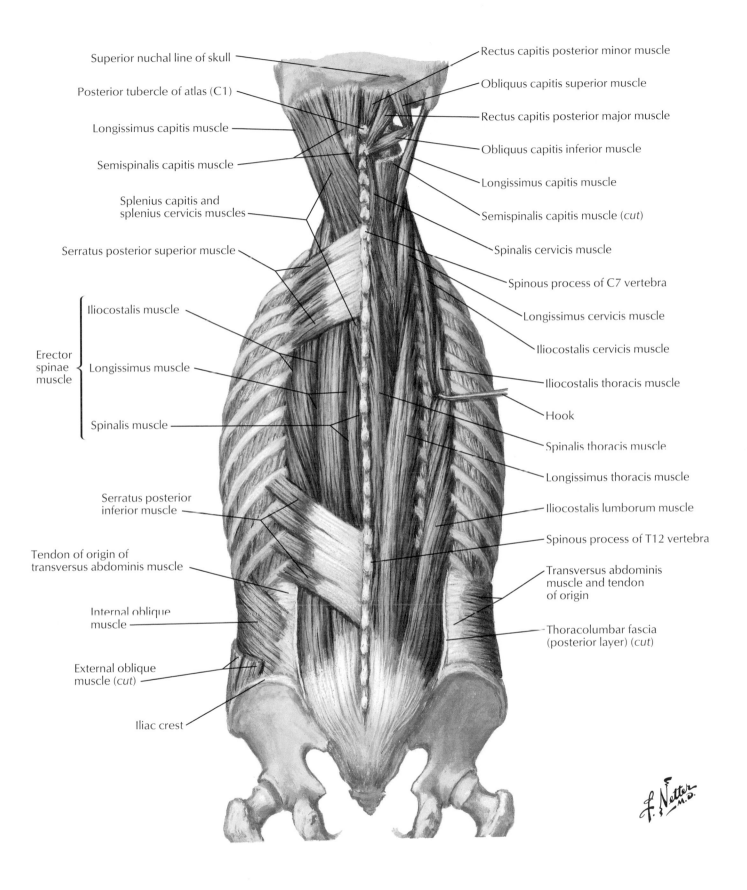

Superior nuchal line of skull

Posterior tubercle of atlas (C1)

Longissimus capitis muscle

Semispinalis capitis muscle

Splenius capitis and splenius cervicis muscles

Serratus posterior superior muscle

Erector spinae muscle
- Iliocostalis muscle
- Longissimus muscle
- Spinalis muscle

Serratus posterior inferior muscle

Tendon of origin of transversus abdominis muscle

Internal oblique muscle

External oblique muscle (cut)

Iliac crest

Rectus capitis posterior minor muscle

Obliquus capitis superior muscle

Rectus capitis posterior major muscle

Obliquus capitis inferior muscle

Longissimus capitis muscle

Semispinalis capitis muscle (cut)

Spinalis cervicis muscle

Spinous process of C7 vertebra

Longissimus cervicis muscle

Iliocostalis cervicis muscle

Iliocostalis thoracis muscle

Hook

Spinalis thoracis muscle

Longissimus thoracis muscle

Iliocostalis lumborum muscle

Spinous process of T12 vertebra

Transversus abdominis muscle and tendon of origin

Thoracolumbar fascia (posterior layer) (cut)

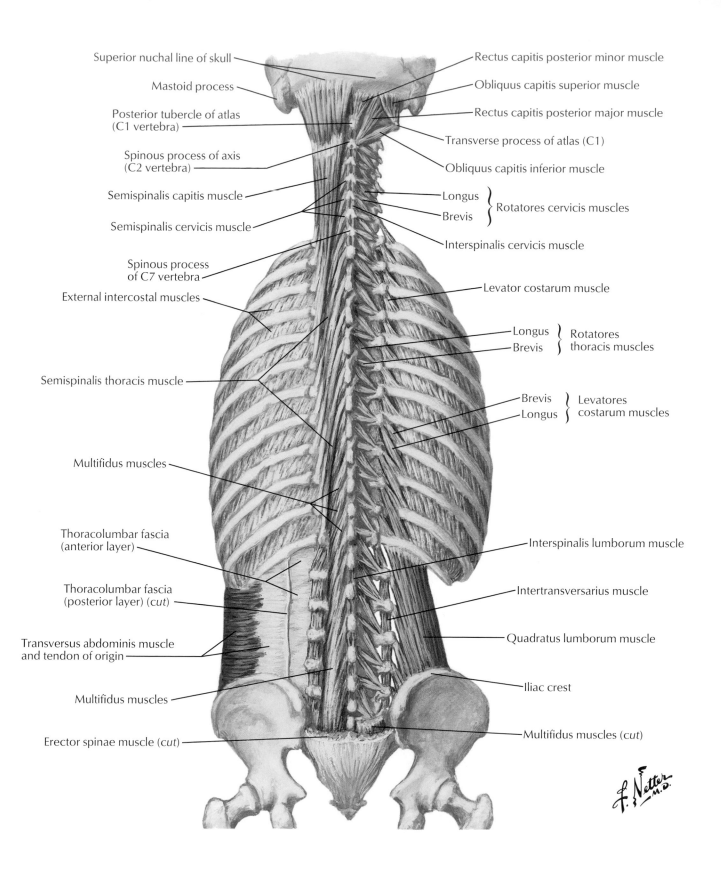

Superior nuchal line of skull

Mastoid process

Posterior tubercle of atlas
(C1 vertebra)

Spinous process of axis
(C2 vertebra)

Semispinalis capitis muscle

Semispinalis cervicis muscle

Spinous process
of C7 vertebra

External intercostal muscles

Semispinalis thoracis muscle

Multifidus muscles

Thoracolumbar fascia
(anterior layer)

Thoracolumbar fascia
(posterior layer) (cut)

Transversus abdominis muscle
and tendon of origin

Multifidus muscles

Erector spinae muscle (cut)

Rectus capitis posterior minor muscle

Obliquus capitis superior muscle

Rectus capitis posterior major muscle

Transverse process of atlas (C1)

Obliquus capitis inferior muscle

Longus
Brevis } Rotatores cervicis muscles

Interspinalis cervicis muscle

Levator costarum muscle

Longus
Brevis } Rotatores
thoracis muscles

Brevis
Longus } Levatores
costarum muscles

Interspinalis lumborum muscle

Intertransversarius muscle

Quadratus lumborum muscle

Iliac crest

Multifidus muscles (cut)

Plate 170   **Muscles and Nerves**

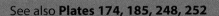

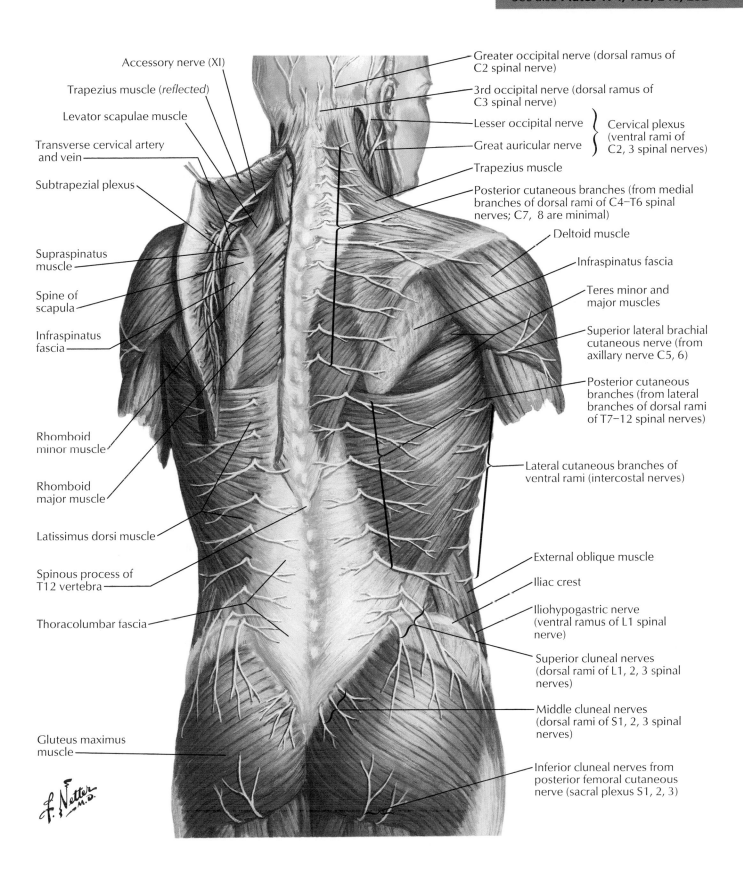

Accessory nerve (XI)

Trapezius muscle (*reflected*)

Levator scapulae muscle

Transverse cervical artery and vein

Subtrapezial plexus

Supraspinatus muscle

Spine of scapula

Infraspinatus fascia

Rhomboid minor muscle

Rhomboid major muscle

Latissimus dorsi muscle

Spinous process of T12 vertebra

Thoracolumbar fascia

Gluteus maximus muscle

Greater occipital nerve (dorsal ramus of C2 spinal nerve)

3rd occipital nerve (dorsal ramus of C3 spinal nerve)

Lesser occipital nerve

Great auricular nerve

Cervical plexus (ventral rami of C2, 3 spinal nerves)

Trapezius muscle

Posterior cutaneous branches (from medial branches of dorsal rami of C4–T6 spinal nerves; C7, 8 are minimal)

Deltoid muscle

Infraspinatus fascia

Teres minor and major muscles

Superior lateral brachial cutaneous nerve (from axillary nerve C5, 6)

Posterior cutaneous branches (from lateral branches of dorsal rami of T7–12 spinal nerves)

Lateral cutaneous branches of ventral rami (intercostal nerves)

External oblique muscle

Iliac crest

Iliohypogastric nerve (ventral ramus of L1 spinal nerve)

Superior cluneal nerves (dorsal rami of L1, 2, 3 spinal nerves)

Middle cluneal nerves (dorsal rami of S1, 2, 3 spinal nerves)

Inferior cluneal nerves from posterior femoral cutaneous nerve (sacral plexus S1, 2, 3)

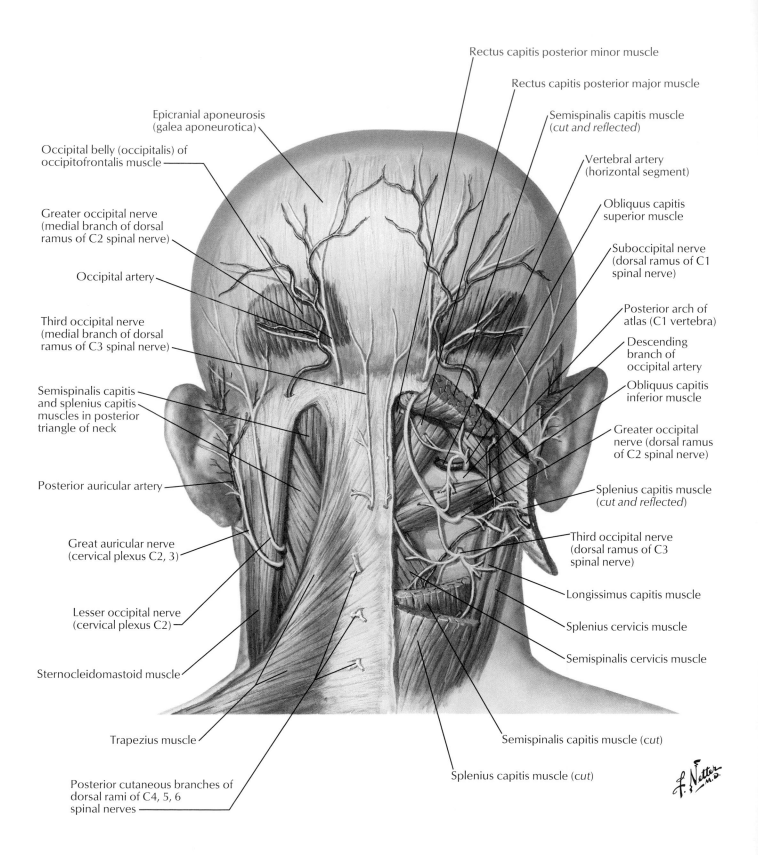

Rectus capitis posterior minor muscle

Rectus capitis posterior major muscle

Semispinalis capitis muscle (*cut and reflected*)

Vertebral artery (horizontal segment)

Obliquus capitis superior muscle

Suboccipital nerve (dorsal ramus of C1 spinal nerve)

Posterior arch of atlas (C1 vertebra)

Descending branch of occipital artery

Obliquus capitis inferior muscle

Greater occipital nerve (dorsal ramus of C2 spinal nerve)

Splenius capitis muscle (*cut and reflected*)

Third occipital nerve (dorsal ramus of C3 spinal nerve)

Longissimus capitis muscle

Splenius cervicis muscle

Semispinalis cervicis muscle

Semispinalis capitis muscle (*cut*)

Splenius capitis muscle (*cut*)

Epicranial aponeurosis (galea aponeurotica)

Occipital belly (occipitalis) of occipitofrontalis muscle

Greater occipital nerve (medial branch of dorsal ramus of C2 spinal nerve)

Occipital artery

Third occipital nerve (medial branch of dorsal ramus of C3 spinal nerve)

Semispinalis capitis and splenius capitis muscles in posterior triangle of neck

Posterior auricular artery

Great auricular nerve (cervical plexus C2, 3)

Lesser occipital nerve (cervical plexus C2)

Sternocleidomastoid muscle

Trapezius muscle

Posterior cutaneous branches of dorsal rami of C4, 5, 6 spinal nerves

Plate 172

Muscles and Nerves

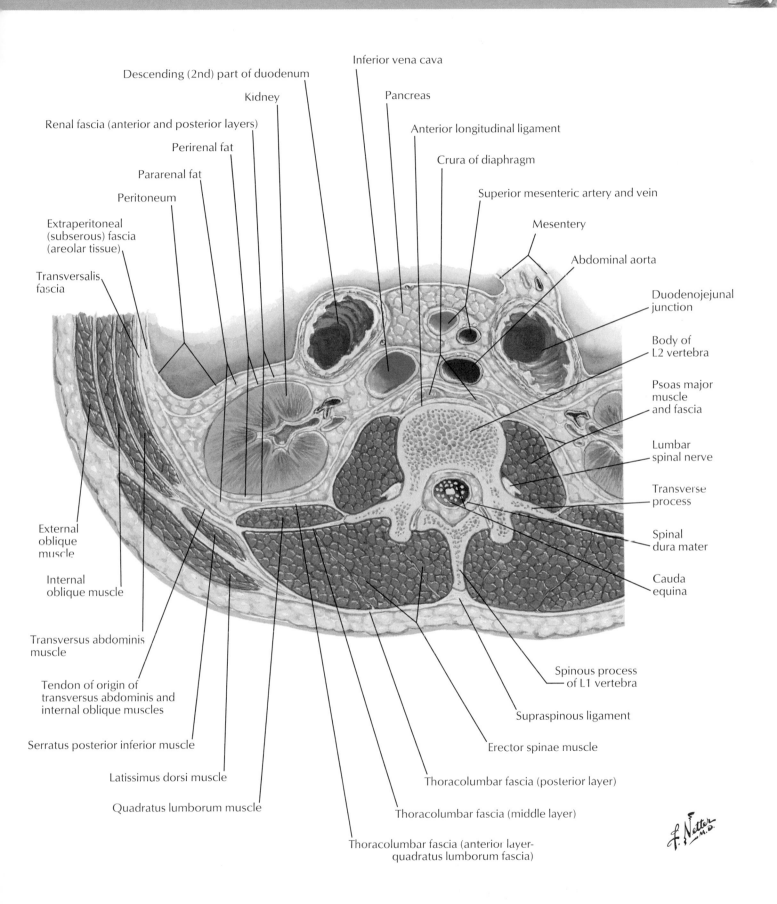

Descending (2nd) part of duodenum

Kidney

Renal fascia (anterior and posterior layers)

Perirenal fat

Pararenal fat

Peritoneum

Extraperitoneal (subserous) fascia (areolar tissue)

Transversalis fascia

External oblique muscle

Internal oblique muscle

Transversus abdominis muscle

Tendon of origin of transversus abdominis and internal oblique muscles

Serratus posterior inferior muscle

Latissimus dorsi muscle

Quadratus lumborum muscle

Inferior vena cava

Pancreas

Anterior longitudinal ligament

Crura of diaphragm

Superior mesenteric artery and vein

Mesentery

Abdominal aorta

Duodenojejunal junction

Body of L2 vertebra

Psoas major muscle and fascia

Lumbar spinal nerve

Transverse process

Spinal dura mater

Cauda equina

Spinous process of L1 vertebra

Supraspinous ligament

Erector spinae muscle

Thoracolumbar fascia (posterior layer)

Thoracolumbar fascia (middle layer)

Thoracolumbar fascia (anterior layer-quadratus lumborum fascia)

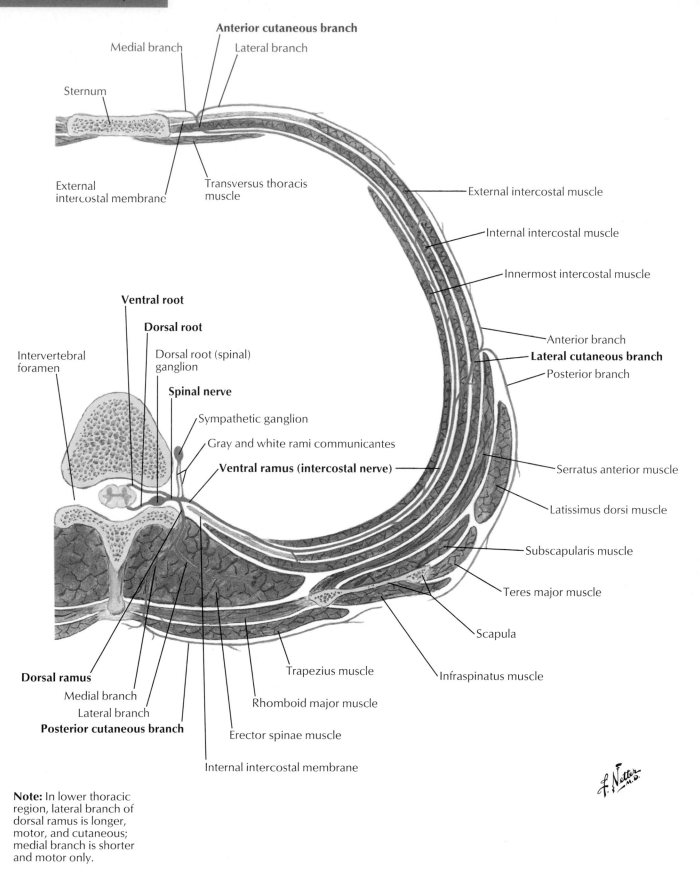

Anterior cutaneous branch

Medial branch

Lateral branch

Sternum

External intercostal muscle

External intercostal membrane

Transversus thoracis muscle

Internal intercostal muscle

Innermost intercostal muscle

Ventral root

Dorsal root

Dorsal root (spinal) ganglion

Intervertebral foramen

Spinal nerve

Anterior branch

Lateral cutaneous branch

Posterior branch

Sympathetic ganglion

Gray and white rami communicantes

Ventral ramus (intercostal nerve)

Serratus anterior muscle

Latissimus dorsi muscle

Subscapularis muscle

Teres major muscle

Scapula

Infraspinatus muscle

Dorsal ramus

Medial branch

Lateral branch

Posterior cutaneous branch

Trapezius muscle

Rhomboid major muscle

Erector spinae muscle

Internal intercostal membrane

Note: In lower thoracic region, lateral branch of dorsal ramus is longer, motor, and cutaneous; medial branch is shorter and motor only.

Plate 174

Cross-sectional Anatomy

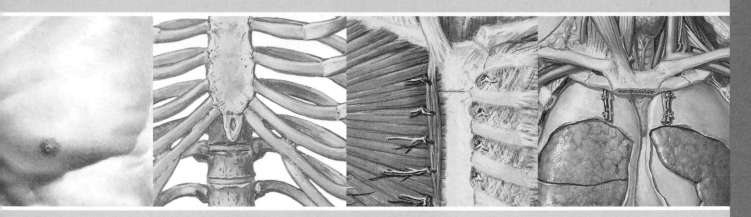

Section 3 THORAX

3 THORAX

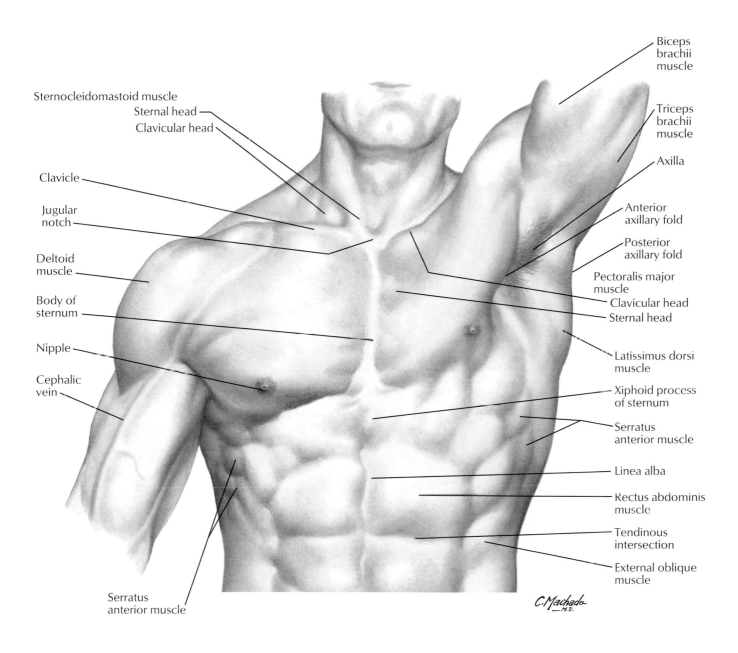

Sternocleidomastoid muscle

Sternal head

Clavicular head

Clavicle

Jugular notch

Deltoid muscle

Body of sternum

Nipple

Cephalic vein

Serratus anterior muscle

Biceps brachii muscle

Triceps brachii muscle

Axilla

Anterior axillary fold

Posterior axillary fold

Pectoralis major muscle

Clavicular head

Sternal head

Latissimus dorsi muscle

Xiphoid process of sternum

Serratus anterior muscle

Linea alba

Rectus abdominis muscle

Tendinous intersection

External oblique muscle

C.Machado
—M.D.

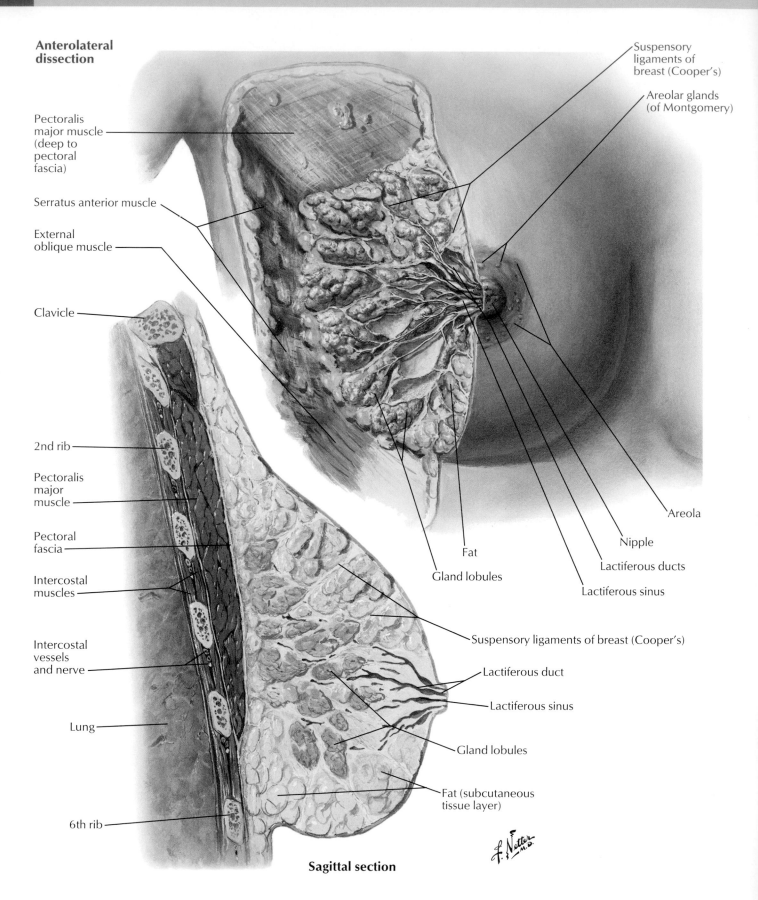

Anterolateral dissection

Pectoralis major muscle (deep to pectoral fascia)

Serratus anterior muscle

External oblique muscle

Clavicle

2nd rib

Pectoralis major muscle

Pectoral fascia

Intercostal muscles

Intercostal vessels and nerve

Lung

6th rib

Suspensory ligaments of breast (Cooper's)

Areolar glands (of Montgomery)

Areola

Nipple

Lactiferous ducts

Lactiferous sinus

Fat

Gland lobules

Suspensory ligaments of breast (Cooper's)

Lactiferous duct

Lactiferous sinus

Gland lobules

Fat (subcutaneous tissue layer)

Sagittal section

Plate 176 **Mammary Gland**

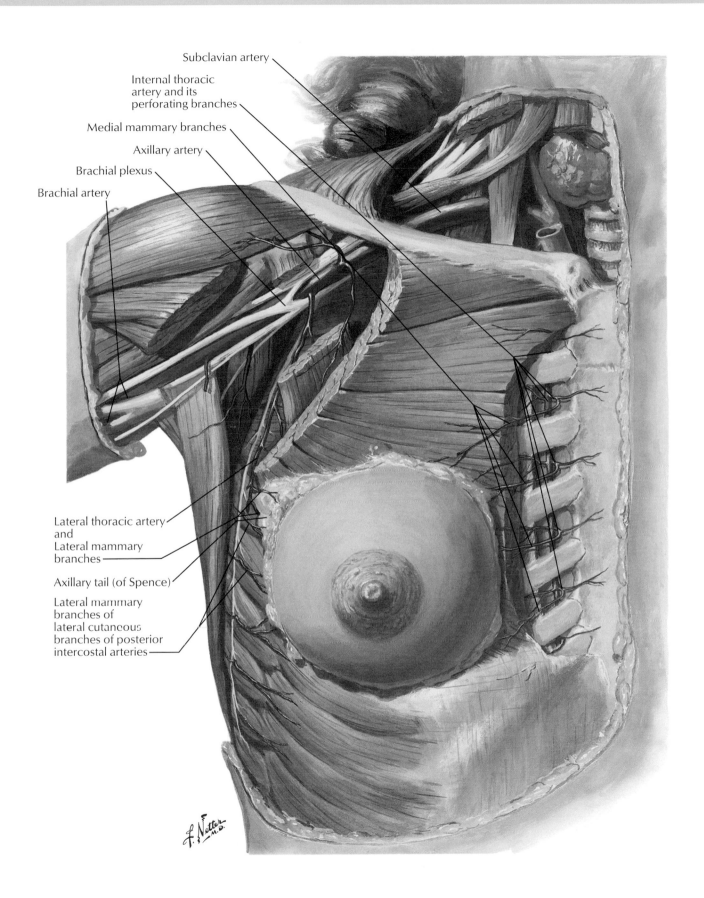

Subclavian artery

Internal thoracic artery and its perforating branches

Medial mammary branches

Axillary artery

Brachial plexus

Brachial artery

Lateral thoracic artery and Lateral mammary branches

Axillary tail (of Spence)

Lateral mammary branches of lateral cutaneous branches of posterior intercostal arteries

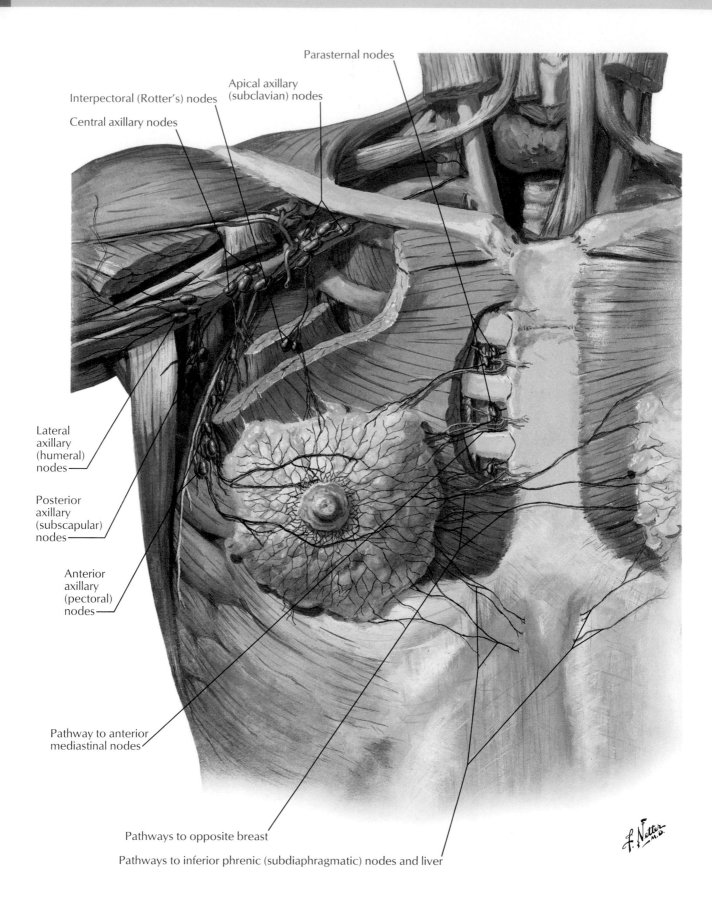

Parasternal nodes

Apical axillary
(subclavian) nodes

Interpectoral (Rotter's) nodes

Central axillary nodes

Lateral
axillary
(humeral)
nodes

Posterior
axillary
(subscapular)
nodes

Anterior
axillary
(pectoral)
nodes

Pathway to anterior
mediastinal nodes

Pathways to opposite breast

Pathways to inferior phrenic (subdiaphragmatic) nodes and liver

Plate 178

Mammary Gland

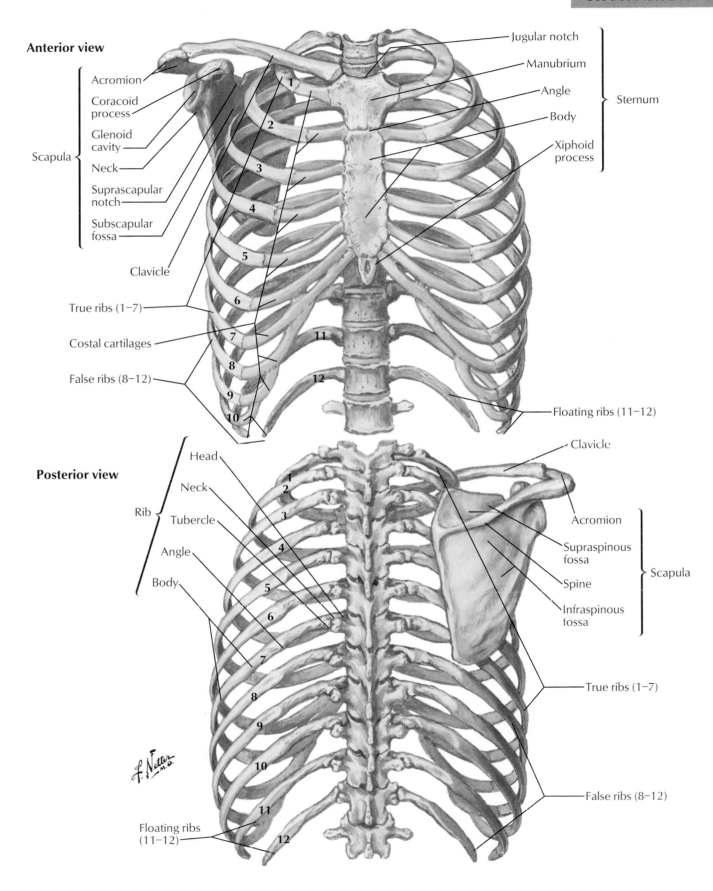

Anterior view

Scapula
- Acromion
- Coracoid process
- Glenoid cavity
- Neck
- Suprascapular notch
- Subscapular fossa

Clavicle

True ribs (1–7)

Costal cartilages

False ribs (8–12)

Jugular notch

Manubrium

Angle

Body

Xiphoid process

Sternum

1
2
3
4
5
6
7
8
9
10
11
12

Floating ribs (11–12)

Posterior view

Rib
- Head
- Neck
- Tubercle
- Angle
- Body

1
2
3
4
5
6
7
8
9
10
11
12

Clavicle

Acromion

Suprapinous fossa

Spine

Infraspinous fossa

Scapula

True ribs (1–7)

False ribs (8–12)

Floating ribs (11–12)

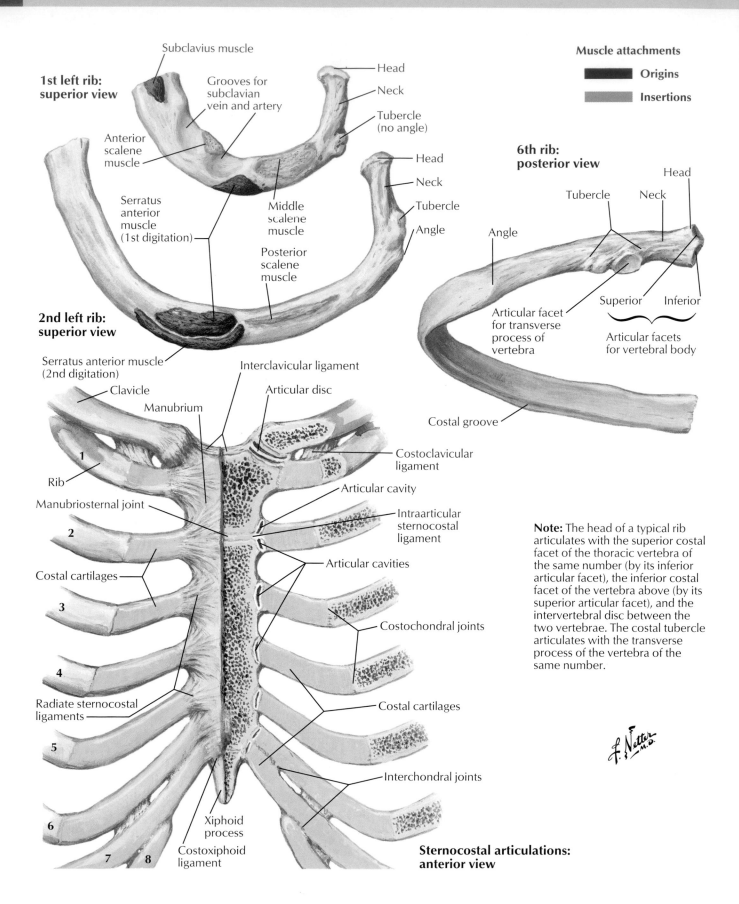

1st left rib: superior view

Subclavius muscle

Grooves for subclavian vein and artery

Anterior scalene muscle

Head

Neck

Tubercle (no angle)

Serratus anterior muscle (1st digitation)

Head

Neck

Tubercle

Angle

Middle scalene muscle

Posterior scalene muscle

2nd left rib: superior view

Serratus anterior muscle (2nd digitation)

Muscle attachments

Origins

Insertions

6th rib: posterior view

Tubercle

Neck

Head

Angle

Angle

Head

Articular facet for transverse process of vertebra

Superior

Inferior

Articular facets for vertebral body

Costal groove

Clavicle

Manubrium

Interclavicular ligament

Articular disc

Costoclavicular ligament

1

Rib

Manubriosternal joint

Articular cavity

Intraarticular sternocostal ligament

2

Articular cavities

Costal cartilages

3

Costochondral joints

4

Radiate sternocostal ligaments

Costal cartilages

5

Interchondral joints

6

Xiphoid process

7   8

Costoxiphoid ligament

Sternocostal articulations: anterior view

Note: The head of a typical rib articulates with the superior costal facet of the thoracic vertebra of the same number (by its inferior articular facet), the inferior costal facet of the vertebra above (by its superior articular facet), and the intervertebral disc between the two vertebrae. The costal tubercle articulates with the transverse process of the vertebra of the same number.

Plate 180   **Body Wall**

See also **Plate 151**

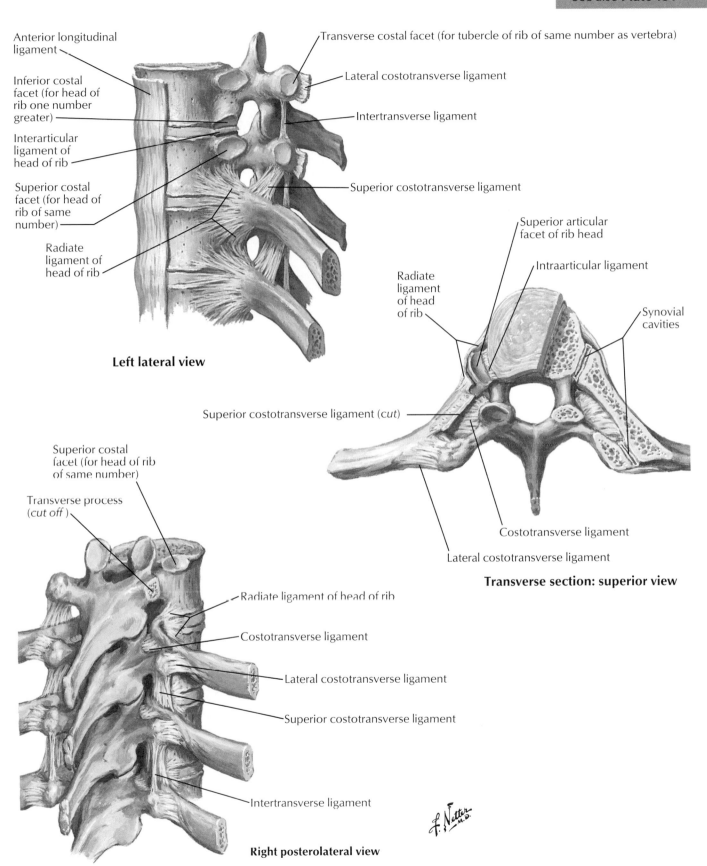

Anterior longitudinal ligament

Inferior costal facet (for head of rib one number greater)

Interarticular ligament of head of rib

Superior costal facet (for head of rib of same number)

Radiate ligament of head of rib

Transverse costal facet (for tubercle of rib of same number as vertebra)

Lateral costotransverse ligament

Intertransverse ligament

Superior costotransverse ligament

Left lateral view

Superior articular facet of rib head

Radiate ligament of head of rib

Intraarticular ligament

Synovial cavities

Superior costotransverse ligament (*cut*)

Costotransverse ligament

Lateral costotransverse ligament

Transverse section: superior view

Superior costal facet (for head of rib of same number)

Transverse process (*cut off*)

Radiate ligament of head of rib

Costotransverse ligament

Lateral costotransverse ligament

Superior costotransverse ligament

Intertransverse ligament

Right posterolateral view

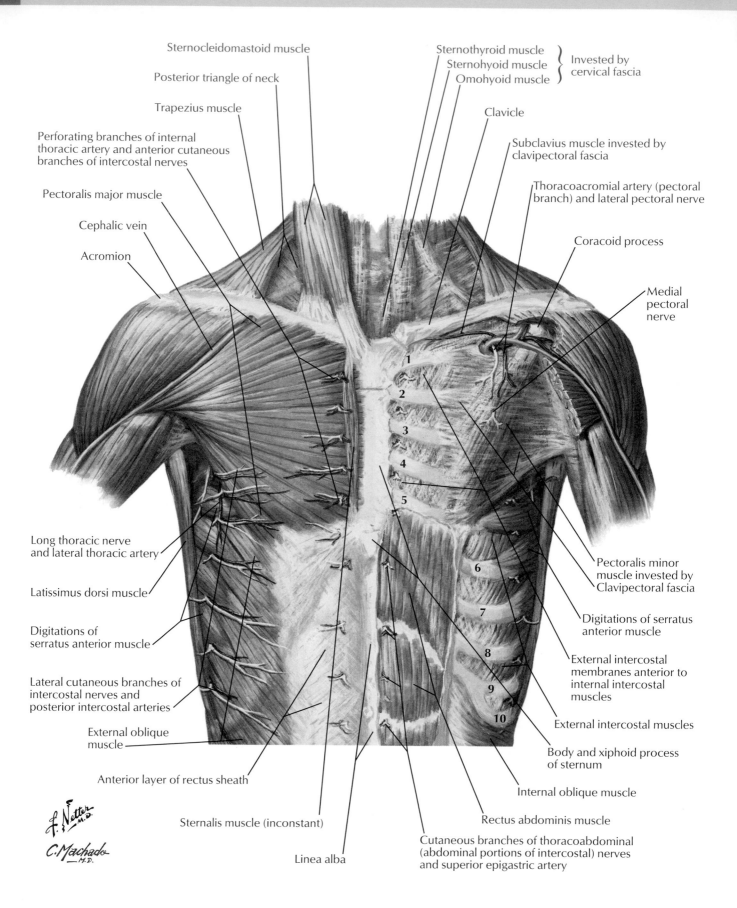

Sternocleidomastoid muscle

Posterior triangle of neck

Trapezius muscle

Perforating branches of internal thoracic artery and anterior cutaneous branches of intercostal nerves

Pectoralis major muscle

Cephalic vein

Acromion

Sternothyroid muscle
Sternohyoid muscle
Omohyoid muscle
} Invested by cervical fascia

Clavicle

Subclavius muscle invested by clavipectoral fascia

Thoracoacromial artery (pectoral branch) and lateral pectoral nerve

Coracoid process

Medial pectoral nerve

Long thoracic nerve and lateral thoracic artery

Latissimus dorsi muscle

Digitations of serratus anterior muscle

Lateral cutaneous branches of intercostal nerves and posterior intercostal arteries

External oblique muscle

Pectoralis minor muscle invested by Clavipectoral fascia

Digitations of serratus anterior muscle

External intercostal membranes anterior to internal intercostal muscles

External intercostal muscles

Body and xiphoid process of sternum

Internal oblique muscle

Rectus abdominis muscle

Anterior layer of rectus sheath

Sternalis muscle (inconstant)

Linea alba

Cutaneous branches of thoracoabdominal (abdominal portions of intercostal) nerves and superior epigastric artery

Plate 182

Body Wall

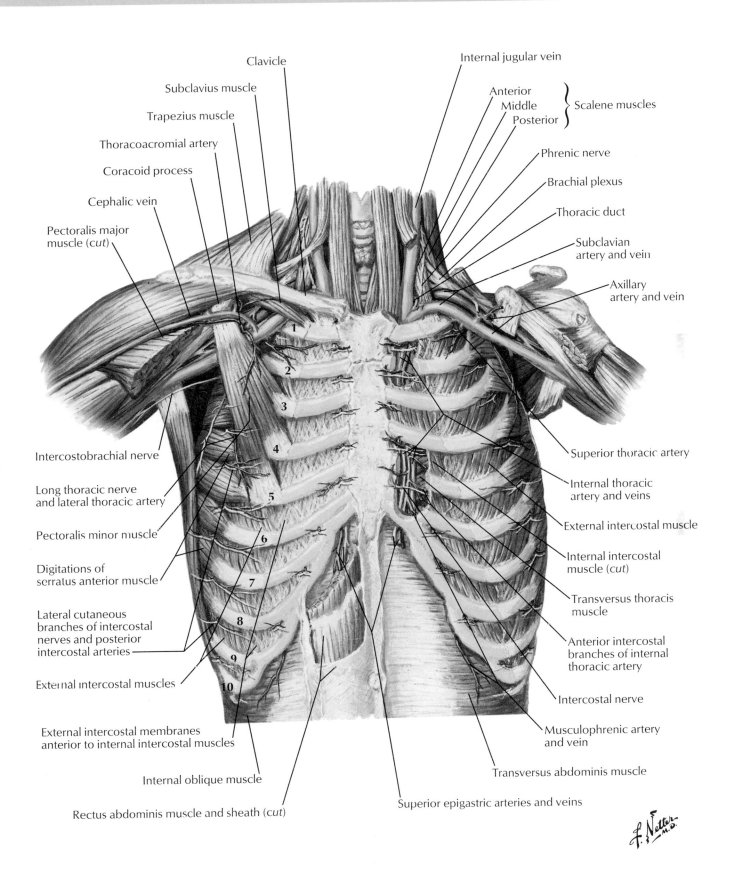

Clavicle

Subclavius muscle

Trapezius muscle

Thoracoacromial artery

Coracoid process

Cephalic vein

Pectoralis major muscle (*cut*)

Internal jugular vein

Anterior
Middle } Scalene muscles
Posterior }

Phrenic nerve

Brachial plexus

Thoracic duct

Subclavian artery and vein

Axillary artery and vein

Intercostobrachial nerve

Long thoracic nerve and lateral thoracic artery

Pectoralis minor muscle

Digitations of serratus anterior muscle

Lateral cutaneous branches of intercostal nerves and posterior intercostal arteries

External intercostal muscles

External intercostal membranes anterior to internal intercostal muscles

Internal oblique muscle

Rectus abdominis muscle and sheath (*cut*)

Superior thoracic artery

Internal thoracic artery and veins

External intercostal muscle

Internal intercostal muscle (*cut*)

Transversus thoracis muscle

Anterior intercostal branches of internal thoracic artery

Intercostal nerve

Musculophrenic artery and vein

Transversus abdominis muscle

Superior epigastric arteries and veins

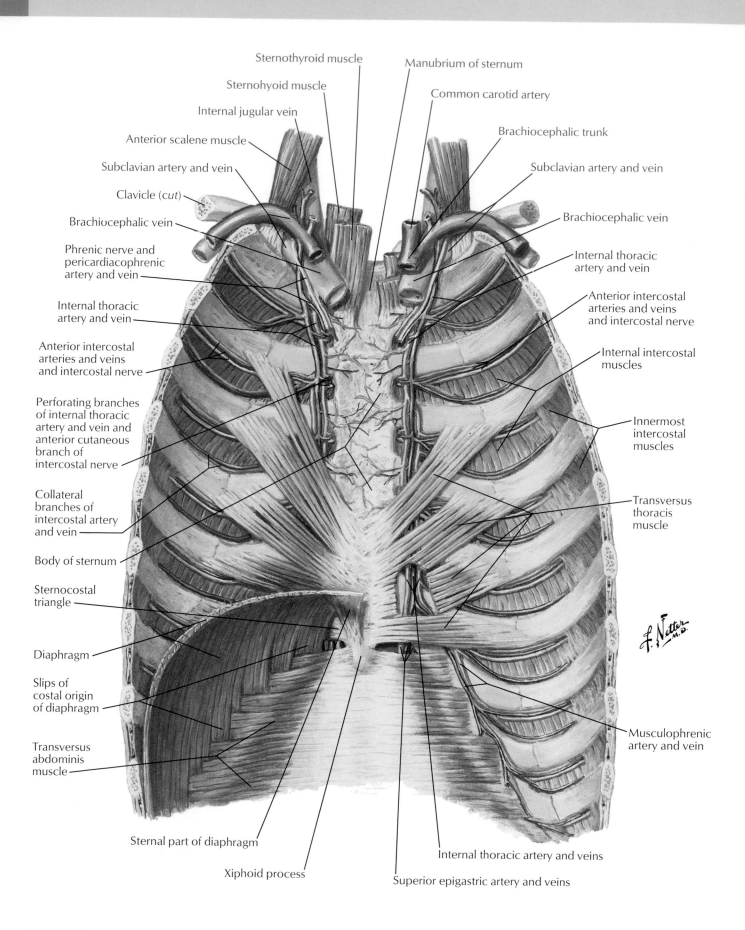

Sternothyroid muscle

Sternohyoid muscle

Internal jugular vein

Anterior scalene muscle

Subclavian artery and vein

Clavicle (*cut*)

Brachiocephalic vein

Phrenic nerve and pericardiacophrenic artery and vein

Internal thoracic artery and vein

Anterior intercostal arteries and veins and intercostal nerve

Perforating branches of internal thoracic artery and vein and anterior cutaneous branch of intercostal nerve

Collateral branches of intercostal artery and vein

Body of sternum

Sternocostal triangle

Diaphragm

Slips of costal origin of diaphragm

Transversus abdominis muscle

Manubrium of sternum

Common carotid artery

Brachiocephalic trunk

Subclavian artery and vein

Brachiocephalic vein

Internal thoracic artery and vein

Anterior intercostal arteries and veins and intercostal nerve

Internal intercostal muscles

Innermost intercostal muscles

Transversus thoracis muscle

Musculophrenic artery and vein

Sternal part of diaphragm

Xiphoid process

Internal thoracic artery and veins

Superior epigastric artery and veins

Plate 184

Body Wall

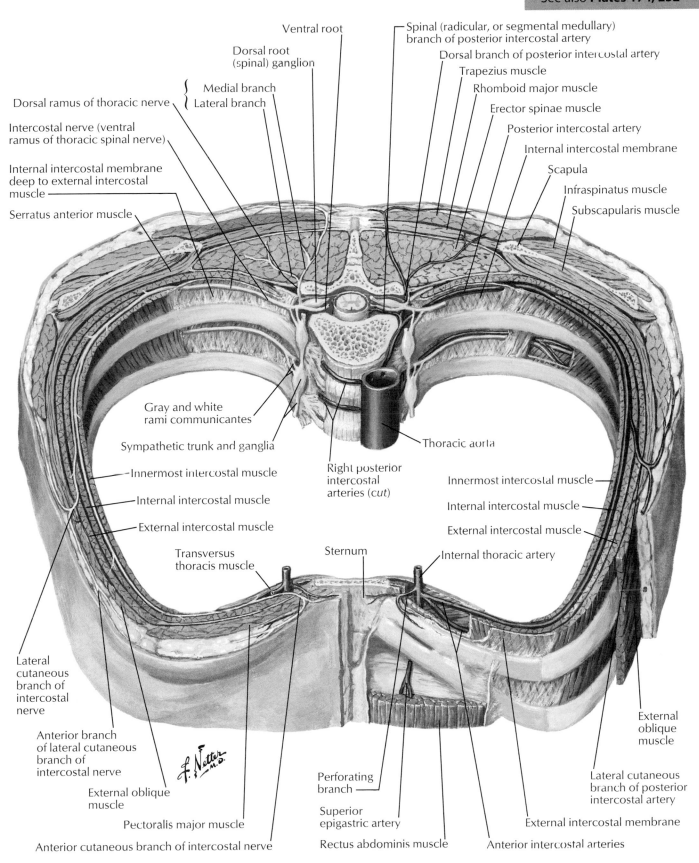

Ventral root

Dorsal root (spinal) ganglion

Spinal (radicular, or segmental medullary) branch of posterior intercostal artery

Dorsal branch of posterior intercostal artery

Trapezius muscle

Medial branch

Lateral branch

Rhomboid major muscle

Dorsal ramus of thoracic nerve

Erector spinae muscle

Intercostal nerve (ventral ramus of thoracic spinal nerve)

Posterior intercostal artery

Internal intercostal membrane

Internal intercostal membrane deep to external intercostal muscle

Scapula

Infraspinatus muscle

Serratus anterior muscle

Subscapularis muscle

Gray and white rami communicantes

Sympathetic trunk and ganglia

Innermost intercostal muscle

Internal intercostal muscle

External intercostal muscle

Right posterior intercostal arteries (cut)

Thoracic aorta

Innermost intercostal muscle

Internal intercostal muscle

External intercostal muscle

Transversus thoracis muscle

Sternum

Internal thoracic artery

Lateral cutaneous branch of intercostal nerve

Anterior branch of lateral cutaneous branch of intercostal nerve

External oblique muscle

External oblique muscle

Pectoralis major muscle

Perforating branch

Superior epigastric artery

Lateral cutaneous branch of posterior intercostal artery

External intercostal membrane

Anterior cutaneous branch of intercostal nerve

Rectus abdominis muscle

Anterior intercostal arteries

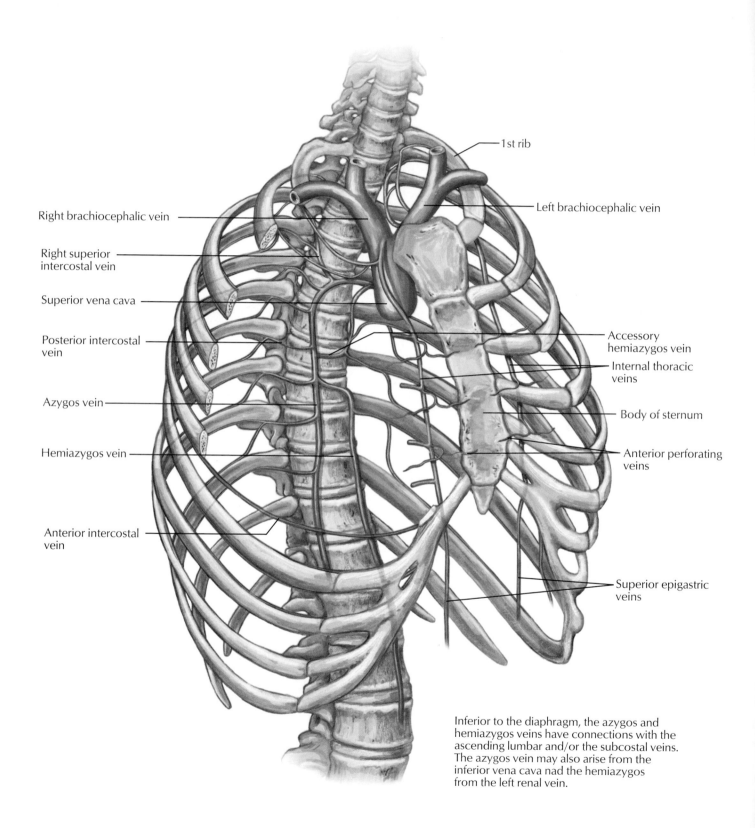

1st rib

Right brachiocephalic vein

Left brachiocephalic vein

Right superior
intercostal vein

Superior vena cava

Posterior intercostal
vein

Accessory
hemiazygos vein

Internal thoracic
veins

Azygos vein

Body of sternum

Hemiazygos vein

Anterior perforating
veins

Anterior intercostal
vein

Superior epigastric
veins

Inferior to the diaphragm, the azygos and
hemiazygos veins have connections with the
ascending lumbar and/or the subcostal veins.
The azygos vein may also arise from the
inferior vena cava nad the hemiazygos
from the left renal vein.

Plate 186

Body Wall

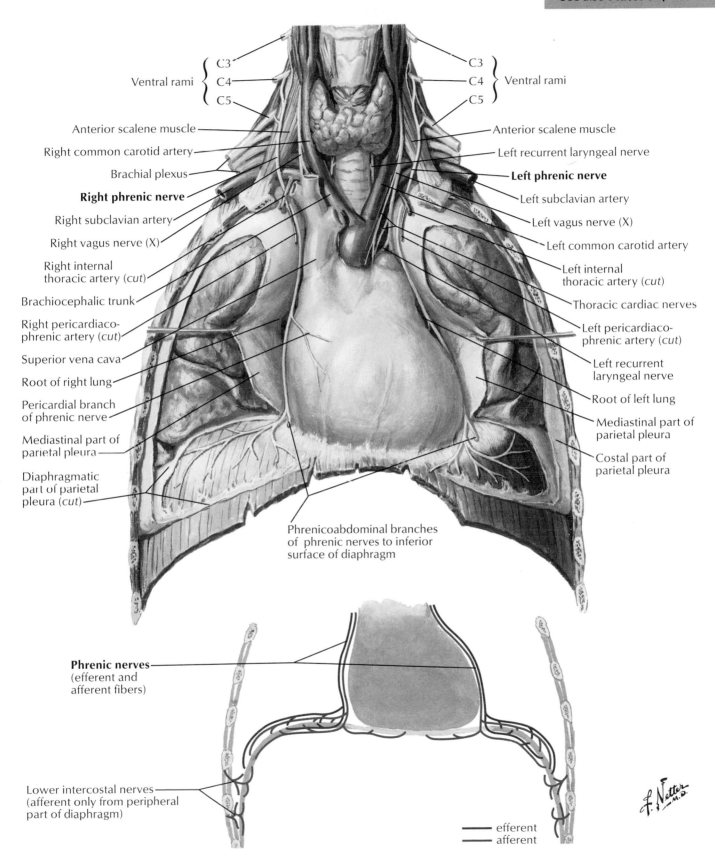

Ventral rami { C3, C4, C5 }
C3, C4, C5 } Ventral rami

Anterior scalene muscle

Right common carotid artery

Brachial plexus

Right phrenic nerve

Right subclavian artery

Right vagus nerve (X)

Right internal thoracic artery (cut)

Brachiocephalic trunk

Right pericardiaco-phrenic artery (cut)

Superior vena cava

Root of right lung

Pericardial branch of phrenic nerve

Mediastinal part of parietal pleura

Diaphragmatic part of parietal pleura (cut)

Anterior scalene muscle

Left recurrent laryngeal nerve

Left phrenic nerve

Left subclavian artery

Left vagus nerve (X)

Left common carotid artery

Left internal thoracic artery (cut)

Thoracic cardiac nerves

Left pericardiaco-phrenic artery (cut)

Left recurrent laryngeal nerve

Root of left lung

Mediastinal part of parietal pleura

Costal part of parietal pleura

Phrenicoabdominal branches of phrenic nerves to inferior surface of diaphragm

Phrenic nerves (efferent and afferent fibers)

Lower intercostal nerves (afferent only from peripheral part of diaphragm)

efferent
afferent

f. Netter M.D.

Diaphragm: Thoracic Surface

See also **Plates 224, 225**

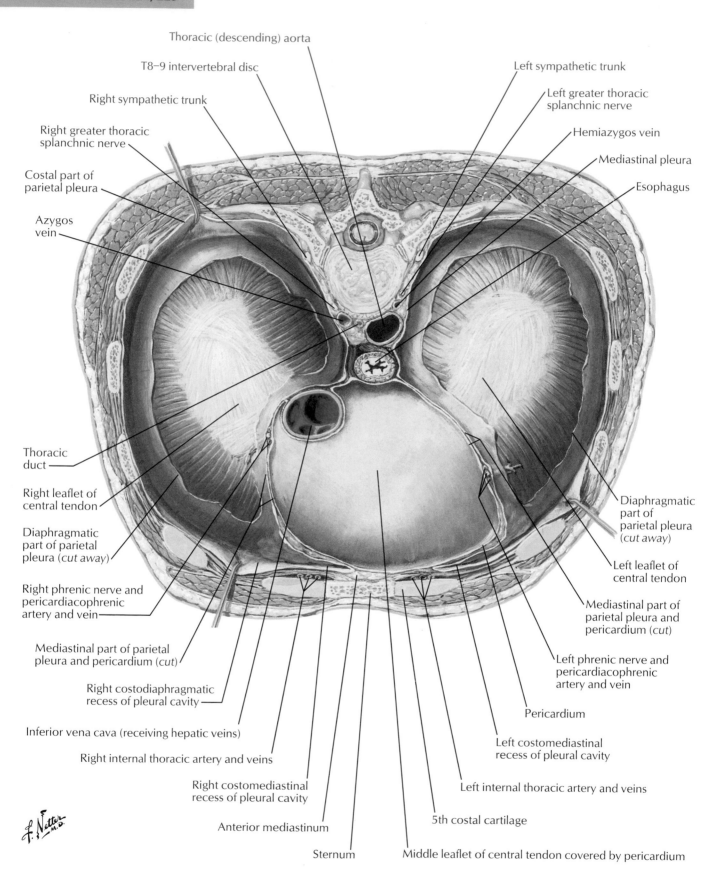

Thoracic (descending) aorta

T8–9 intervertebral disc

Right sympathetic trunk

Right greater thoracic splanchnic nerve

Costal part of parietal pleura

Azygos vein

Left sympathetic trunk

Left greater thoracic splanchnic nerve

Hemiazygos vein

Mediastinal pleura

Esophagus

Thoracic duct

Right leaflet of central tendon

Diaphragmatic part of parietal pleura (cut away)

Right phrenic nerve and pericardiacophrenic artery and vein

Mediastinal part of parietal pleura and pericardium (cut)

Right costodiaphragmatic recess of pleural cavity

Inferior vena cava (receiving hepatic veins)

Right internal thoracic artery and veins

Right costomediastinal recess of pleural cavity

Anterior mediastinum

Sternum

Diaphragmatic part of parietal pleura (cut away)

Left leaflet of central tendon

Mediastinal part of parietal pleura and pericardium (cut)

Left phrenic nerve and pericardiacophrenic artery and vein

Pericardium

Left costomediastinal recess of pleural cavity

Left internal thoracic artery and veins

5th costal cartilage

Middle leaflet of central tendon covered by pericardium

Plate 188

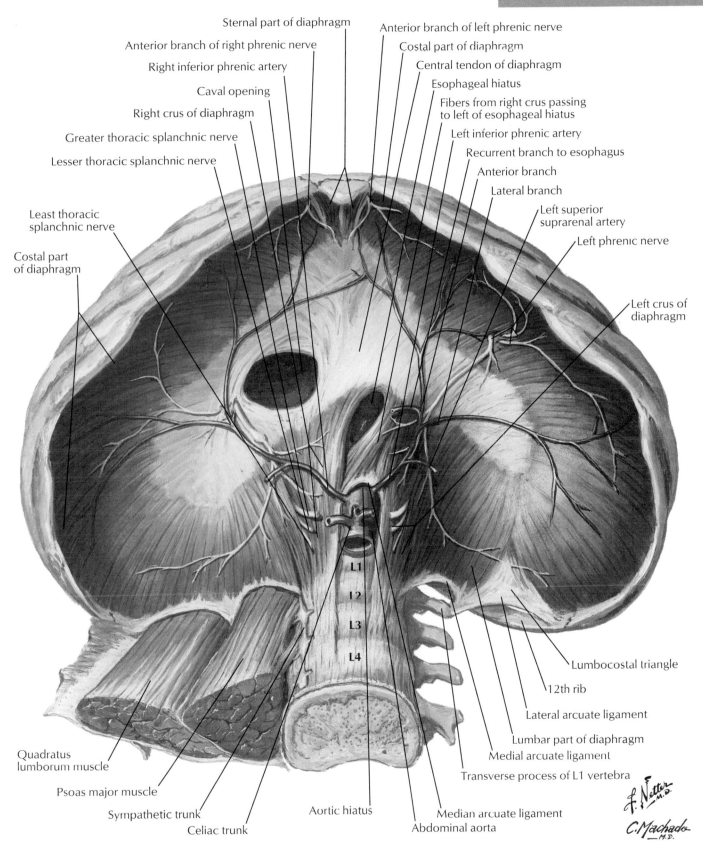

Sternal part of diaphragm

Anterior branch of right phrenic nerve

Right inferior phrenic artery

Caval opening

Right crus of diaphragm

Greater thoracic splanchnic nerve

Lesser thoracic splanchnic nerve

Least thoracic splanchnic nerve

Costal part of diaphragm

Anterior branch of left phrenic nerve

Costal part of diaphragm

Central tendon of diaphragm

Esophageal hiatus

Fibers from right crus passing to left of esophageal hiatus

Left inferior phrenic artery

Recurrent branch to esophagus

Anterior branch

Lateral branch

Left superior suprarenal artery

Left phrenic nerve

Left crus of diaphragm

L1

L2

L3

L4

Lumbocostal triangle

12th rib

Lateral arcuate ligament

Lumbar part of diaphragm

Medial arcuate ligament

Transverse process of L1 vertebra

Quadratus lumborum muscle

Psoas major muscle

Sympathetic trunk

Celiac trunk

Aortic hiatus

Median arcuate ligament

Abdominal aorta

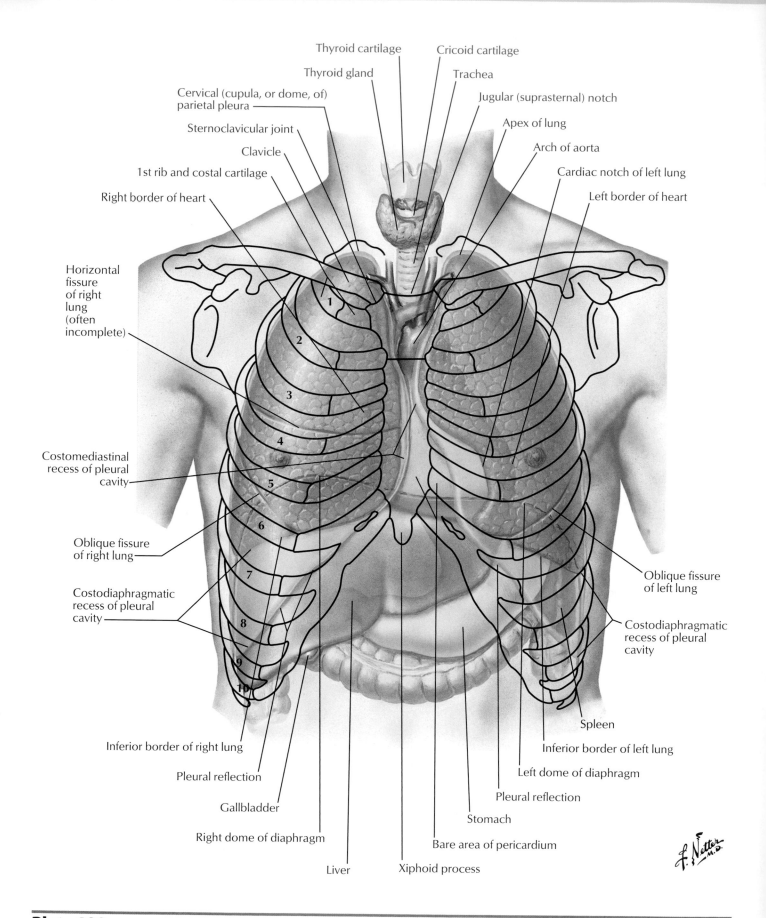

Thyroid cartilage

Cricoid cartilage

Thyroid gland

Trachea

Cervical (cupula, or dome, of) parietal pleura

Jugular (suprasternal) notch

Sternoclavicular joint

Apex of lung

Clavicle

Arch of aorta

1st rib and costal cartilage

Cardiac notch of left lung

Right border of heart

Left border of heart

Horizontal fissure of right lung (often incomplete)

Costomediastinal recess of pleural cavity

Oblique fissure of right lung

Oblique fissure of left lung

Costodiaphragmatic recess of pleural cavity

Costodiaphragmatic recess of pleural cavity

Spleen

Inferior border of right lung

Inferior border of left lung

Pleural reflection

Left dome of diaphragm

Gallbladder

Pleural reflection

Right dome of diaphragm

Stomach

Liver

Bare area of pericardium

Xiphoid process

Plate 190

Lungs

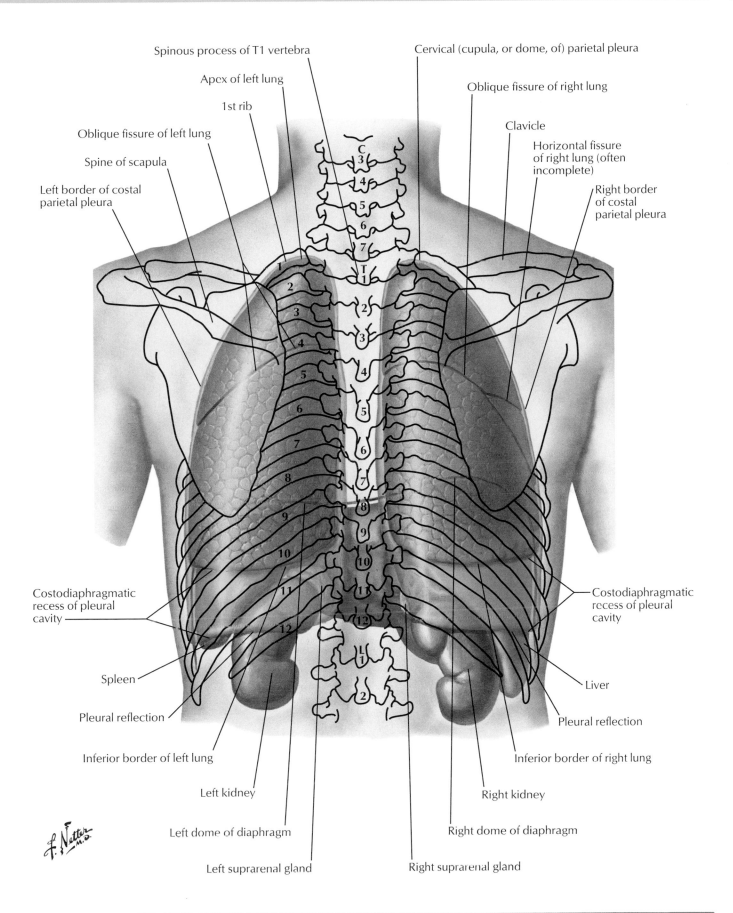

Spinous process of T1 vertebra

Apex of left lung

1st rib

Oblique fissure of left lung

Spine of scapula

Left border of costal parietal pleura

Cervical (cupula, or dome, of) parietal pleura

Oblique fissure of right lung

Clavicle

Horizontal fissure of right lung (often incomplete)

Right border of costal parietal pleura

Costodiaphragmatic recess of pleural cavity

Costodiaphragmatic recess of pleural cavity

Spleen

Pleural reflection

Inferior border of left lung

Left kidney

Left dome of diaphragm

Left suprarenal gland

Liver

Pleural reflection

Inferior border of right lung

Right kidney

Right dome of diaphragm

Right suprarenal gland

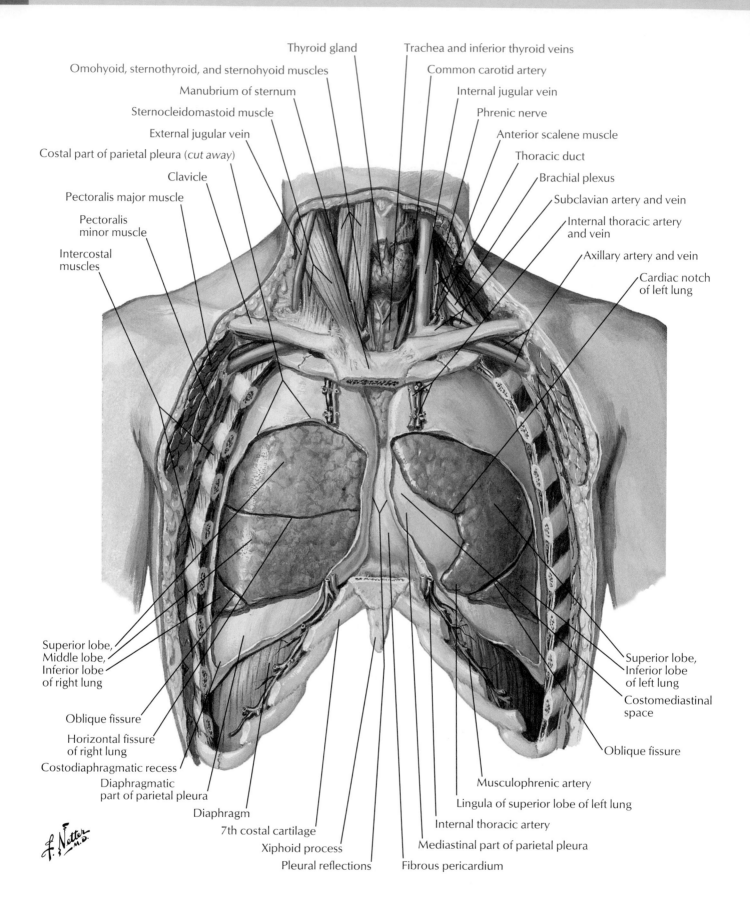

Thyroid gland

Trachea and inferior thyroid veins

Omohyoid, sternothyroid, and sternohyoid muscles

Common carotid artery

Manubrium of sternum

Internal jugular vein

Sternocleidomastoid muscle

Phrenic nerve

External jugular vein

Anterior scalene muscle

Costal part of parietal pleura (cut away)

Thoracic duct

Clavicle

Brachial plexus

Pectoralis major muscle

Subclavian artery and vein

Pectoralis minor muscle

Internal thoracic artery and vein

Intercostal muscles

Axillary artery and vein

Cardiac notch of left lung

Superior lobe, Middle lobe, Inferior lobe of right lung

Superior lobe, Inferior lobe of left lung

Oblique fissure

Costomediastinal space

Horizontal fissure of right lung

Oblique fissure

Costodiaphragmatic recess

Diaphragmatic part of parietal pleura

Musculophrenic artery

Diaphragm

Lingula of superior lobe of left lung

7th costal cartilage

Internal thoracic artery

Xiphoid process

Mediastinal part of parietal pleura

Pleural reflections

Fibrous pericardium

Plate 192

Lungs

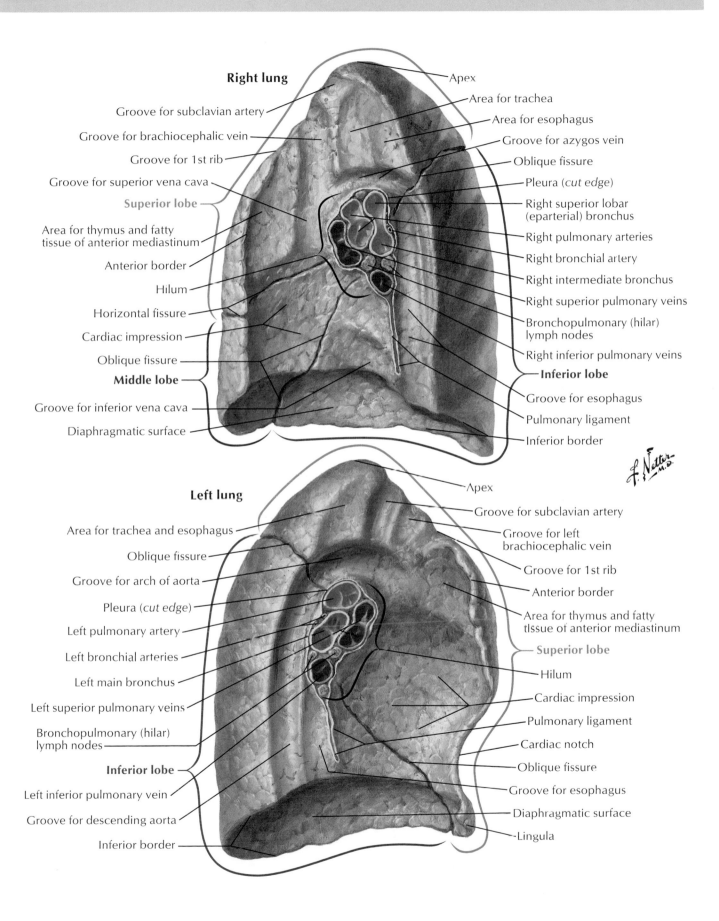

Right lung

Groove for subclavian artery
Groove for brachiocephalic vein
Groove for 1st rib
Groove for superior vena cava
Superior lobe
Area for thymus and fatty tissue of anterior mediastinum
Anterior border
Hilum
Horizontal fissure
Cardiac impression
Oblique fissure
Middle lobe
Groove for inferior vena cava
Diaphragmatic surface

Apex
Area for trachea
Area for esophagus
Groove for azygos vein
Oblique fissure
Pleura (cut edge)
Right superior lobar (eparterial) bronchus
Right pulmonary arteries
Right bronchial artery
Right intermediate bronchus
Right superior pulmonary veins
Bronchopulmonary (hilar) lymph nodes
Right inferior pulmonary veins
Inferior lobe
Groove for esophagus
Pulmonary ligament
Inferior border

Left lung

Area for trachea and esophagus
Oblique fissure
Groove for arch of aorta
Pleura (cut edge)
Left pulmonary artery
Left bronchial arteries
Left main bronchus
Left superior pulmonary veins
Bronchopulmonary (hilar) lymph nodes
Inferior lobe
Left inferior pulmonary vein
Groove for descending aorta
Inferior border

Apex
Groove for subclavian artery
Groove for left brachiocephalic vein
Groove for 1st rib
Anterior border
Area for thymus and fatty tissue of anterior mediastinum
Superior lobe
Hilum
Cardiac impression
Pulmonary ligament
Cardiac notch
Oblique fissure
Groove for esophagus
Diaphragmatic surface
Lingula

F. Netter, M.D.

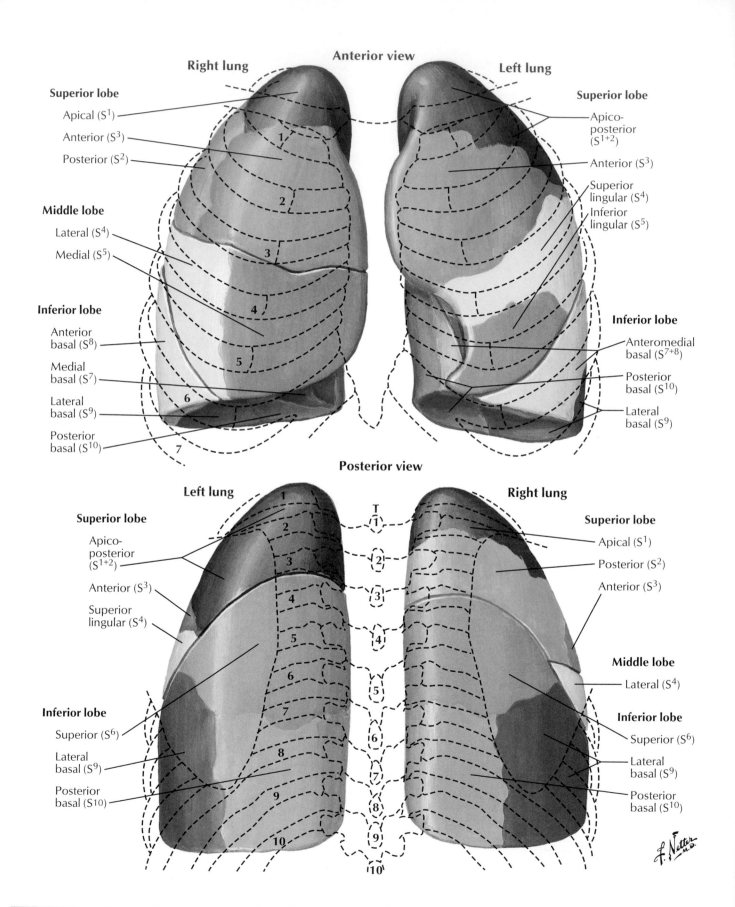

Anterior view

Right lung

Left lung

Superior lobe
Apical (S^1)
Anterior (S^3)
Posterior (S^2)

Superior lobe
Apico-posterior (S^{1+2})
Anterior (S^3)
Superior lingular (S^4)
Inferior lingular (S^5)

Middle lobe
Lateral (S^4)
Medial (S^5)

Inferior lobe
Anterior basal (S^8)
Medial basal (S^7)
Lateral basal (S^9)
Posterior basal (S^{10})

Inferior lobe
Anteromedial basal (S^{7+8})
Posterior basal (S^{10})
Lateral basal (S^9)

Posterior view

Left lung

Right lung

Superior lobe
Apico-posterior (S^{1+2})
Anterior (S^3)
Superior lingular (S^4)

Superior lobe
Apical (S^1)
Posterior (S^2)
Anterior (S^3)

Middle lobe
Lateral (S^4)

Inferior lobe
Superior (S^6)
Lateral basal (S^9)
Posterior basal (S^{10})

Inferior lobe
Superior (S^6)
Lateral basal (S^9)
Posterior basal (S^{10})

Plate 194

Lungs

Lateral views

Right lung

Superior lobe

Apical (S^1)

Posterior (S^2)

Anterior (S^3)

Middle lobe

Lateral (S^4)

Medial (S^5)

Inferior lobe

Superior (S^6)

Anterior basal (S^8)

Lateral basal (S^9)

Left lung

Superior lobe

Apico-posterior (S^{1+2})

Anterior (S^3)

Superior lingular (S^4)

Inferior lingular (S^5)

Inferior lobe

Superior (S^6)

Antero-medial basal (S^{7+8})

Lateral basal (S^9)

Medial views

Right lung

Superior lobe

Apical (S^1)

Posterior (S^2)

Anterior (S^3)

Middle lobe

Medial (S^5)

Inferior lobe

Superior (S^6)

Medial basal (S^7)

Anterior basal (S^8)

Lateral basal (S^9)

Posterior basal (S^{10})

Left lung

Superior lobe

Apico-posterior (S^{1+2})

Anterior (S^3)

Superior lingular (S^4)

Inferior lingular (S^5)

Inferior lobe

Superior (S^6)

Anteromedial basal (S^{7+8})

Lateral basal (S^9)

Posterior basal (S^{10})

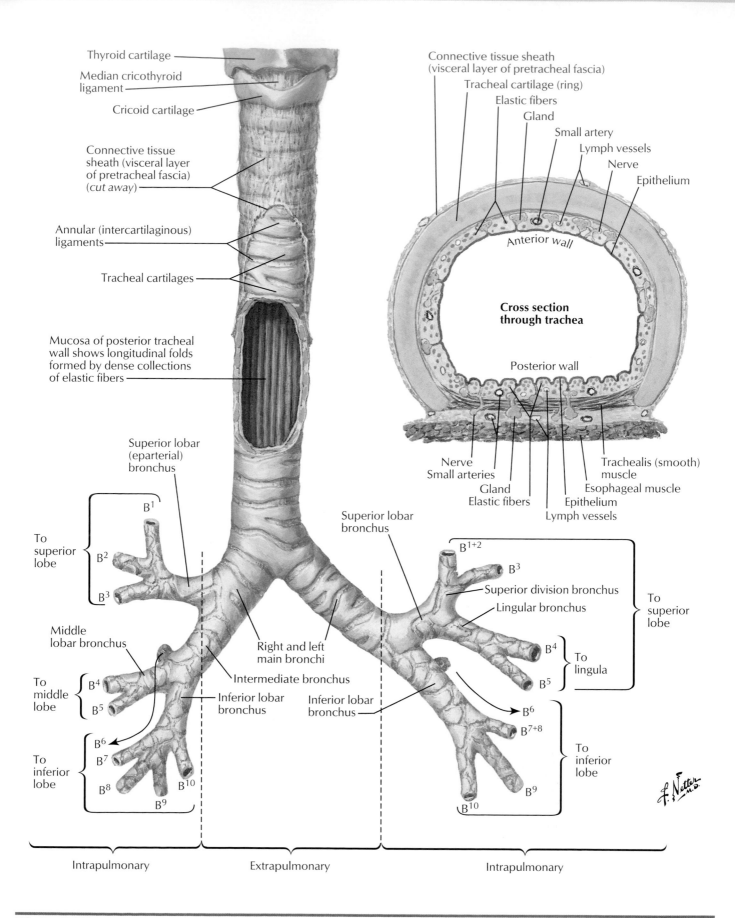

Thyroid cartilage

Median cricothyroid ligament

Cricoid cartilage

Connective tissue sheath (visceral layer of pretracheal fascia) (*cut away*)

Annular (intercartilaginous) ligaments

Tracheal cartilages

Mucosa of posterior tracheal wall shows longitudinal folds formed by dense collections of elastic fibers

Superior lobar (eparterial) bronchus

B^1

To superior lobe

B^2

B^3

Middle lobar bronchus

To middle lobe

B^4

B^5

To inferior lobe

B^6

B^7

B^8

B^9

B^{10}

Right and left main bronchi

Intermediate bronchus

Inferior lobar bronchus

Connective tissue sheath (visceral layer of pretracheal fascia)

Tracheal cartilage (ring)

Elastic fibers

Gland

Small artery

Lymph vessels

Nerve

Epithelium

Anterior *wall*

Cross section through trachea

Posterior wall

Nerve

Small arteries

Gland

Elastic fibers

Trachealis (smooth) muscle

Esophageal muscle

Epithelium

Lymph vessels

Superior lobar bronchus

B^{1+2}

B^3

Superior division bronchus

Lingular bronchus

To superior lobe

B^4

B^5

To lingula

Inferior lobar bronchus

B^6

B^{7+8}

B^9

B^{10}

To inferior lobe

Intrapulmonary

Extrapulmonary

Intrapulmonary

Plate 196

Lungs

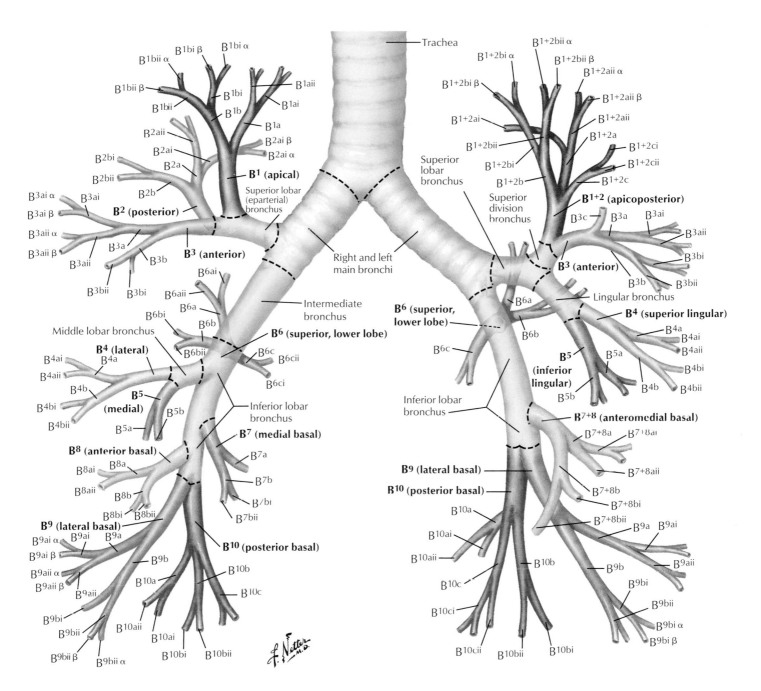

Nomenclature in common usage for bronchopulmonary segments (Plates 194 and 195) is that of Jackson and Huber, and segmental bronchi are named accordingly. Ikeda proposed nomenclature (as demonstrated here) for bronchial subdivisions as far as the 6th generation. For simplification on this illustration, only some bronchial subdivisions are labeled as far as the 5th or 6th generation. Segmental bronchi (B) are numbered from 1 to 10 in each lung, corresponding to pulmonary segments. In the left lung,

B^1 and B^2 are combined as are B^7 and B^8. Subsegmental, or 4th order, bronchi are indicated by the addition of lowercase letters a, b, or c when an additional branch is present. Fifth order bronchi are designated by Roman numerals i (anterior) or ii (posterior) and 6th order bronchi by Greek letters α or β. Several texts use alternate numbers (as proposed by Boyden) for segmental bronchi.

Variations of the standard bronchial pattern shown here are common, especially in peripheral airways.

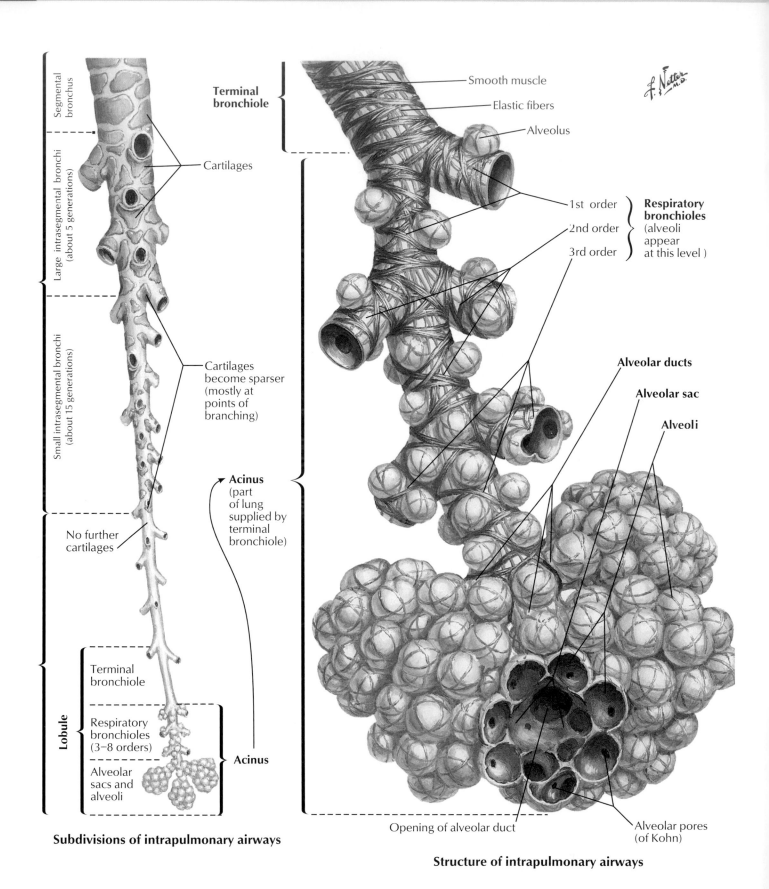

Subdivisions of intrapulmonary airways

Segmental bronchus

Large intrasegmental bronchi (about 5 generations)

Small intrasegmental bronchi (about 15 generations)

Cartilages

Cartilages become sparser (mostly at points of branching)

No further cartilages

Acinus (part of lung supplied by terminal bronchiole)

Lobule

Terminal bronchiole

Respiratory bronchioles (3–8 orders)

Alveolar sacs and alveoli

Acinus

Structure of intrapulmonary airways

Terminal bronchiole

Smooth muscle

Elastic fibers

Alveolus

1st order

2nd order

3rd order

Respiratory bronchioles (alveoli appear at this level)

Alveolar ducts

Alveolar sac

Alveoli

Opening of alveolar duct

Alveolar pores (of Kohn)

Plate 198

Lungs

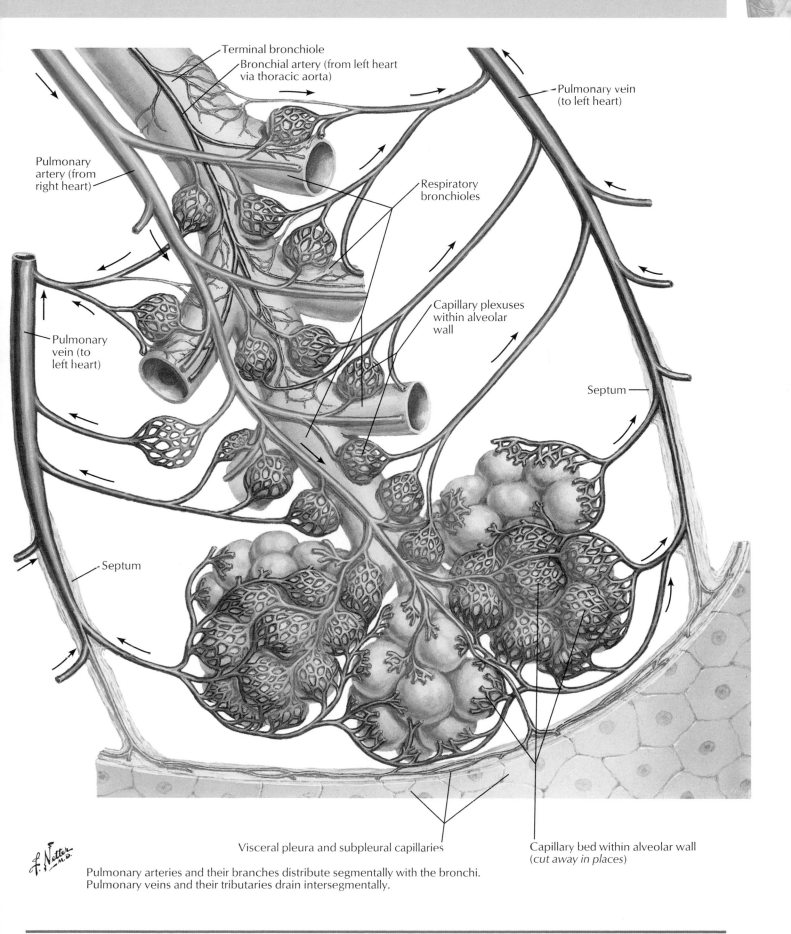

Terminal bronchiole

Bronchial artery (from left heart via thoracic aorta)

Pulmonary vein (to left heart)

Pulmonary artery (from right heart)

Respiratory bronchioles

Pulmonary vein (to left heart)

Capillary plexuses within alveolar wall

Septum

Septum

Visceral pleura and subpleural capillaries

Capillary bed within alveolar wall (*cut away in places*)

Pulmonary arteries and their branches distribute segmentally with the bronchi.
Pulmonary veins and their tributaries drain intersegmentally.

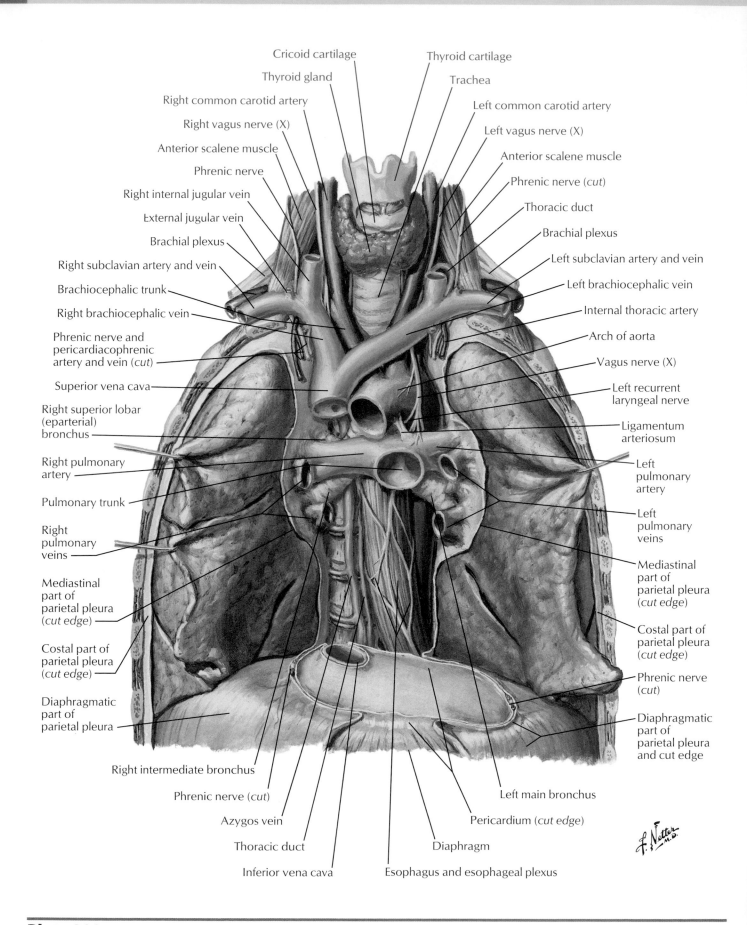

Cricoid cartilage

Thyroid gland

Right common carotid artery

Right vagus nerve (X)

Anterior scalene muscle

Phrenic nerve

Right internal jugular vein

External jugular vein

Brachial plexus

Right subclavian artery and vein

Brachiocephalic trunk

Right brachiocephalic vein

Phrenic nerve and pericardiacophrenic artery and vein (cut)

Superior vena cava

Right superior lobar (eparterial) bronchus

Right pulmonary artery

Pulmonary trunk

Right pulmonary veins

Mediastinal part of parietal pleura (cut edge)

Costal part of parietal pleura (cut edge)

Diaphragmatic part of parietal pleura

Right intermediate bronchus

Phrenic nerve (cut)

Azygos vein

Thoracic duct

Inferior vena cava

Thyroid cartilage

Trachea

Left common carotid artery

Left vagus nerve (X)

Anterior scalene muscle

Phrenic nerve (cut)

Thoracic duct

Brachial plexus

Left subclavian artery and vein

Left brachiocephalic vein

Internal thoracic artery

Arch of aorta

Vagus nerve (X)

Left recurrent laryngeal nerve

Ligamentum arteriosum

Left pulmonary artery

Left pulmonary veins

Mediastinal part of parietal pleura (cut edge)

Costal part of parietal pleura (cut edge)

Phrenic nerve (cut)

Diaphragmatic part of parietal pleura and cut edge

Left main bronchus

Pericardium (cut edge)

Diaphragm

Esophagus and esophageal plexus

Plate 200

Lungs

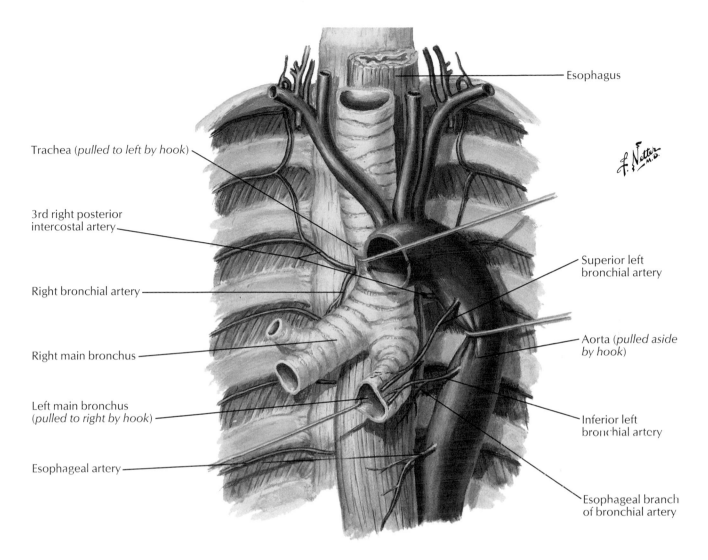

Esophagus

Trachea (*pulled to left by hook*)

3rd right posterior intercostal artery

Right bronchial artery

Right main bronchus

Left main bronchus (*pulled to right by hook*)

Esophageal artery

Superior left bronchial artery

Aorta (*pulled aside by hook*)

Inferior left bronchial artery

Esophageal branch of bronchial artery

Bronchial veins

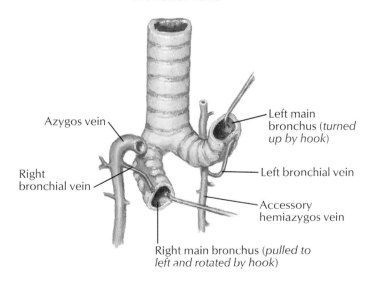

Azygos vein

Right bronchial vein

Left main bronchus (*turned up by hook*)

Left bronchial vein

Accessory hemiazygos vein

Right main bronchus (*pulled to left and rotated by hook*)

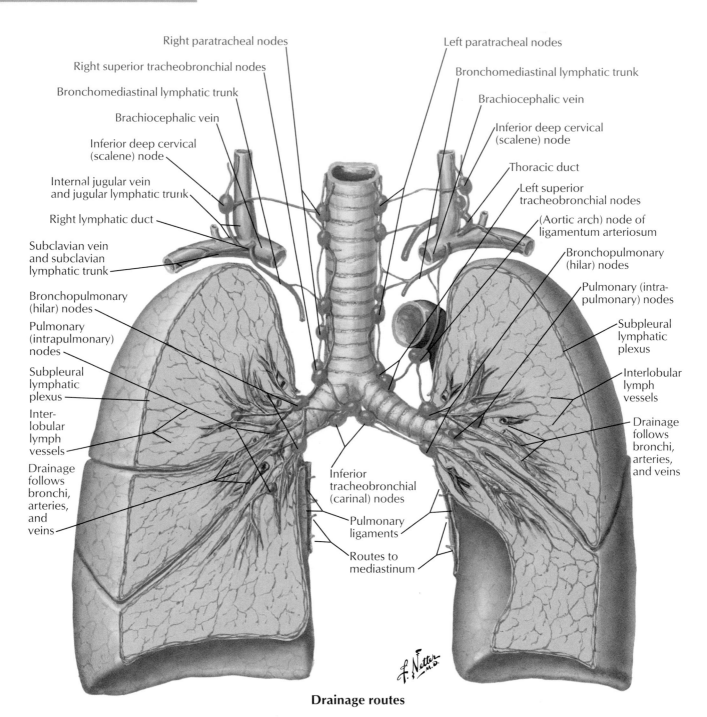

Right paratracheal nodes

Right superior tracheobronchial nodes

Bronchomediastinal lymphatic trunk

Brachiocephalic vein

Inferior deep cervical (scalene) node

Internal jugular vein and jugular lymphatic trunk

Right lymphatic duct

Subclavian vein and subclavian lymphatic trunk

Bronchopulmonary (hilar) nodes

Pulmonary (intrapulmonary) nodes

Subpleural lymphatic plexus

Interlobular lymph vessels

Drainage follows bronchi, arteries, and veins

Left paratracheal nodes

Bronchomediastinal lymphatic trunk

Brachiocephalic vein

Inferior deep cervical (scalene) node

Thoracic duct

Left superior tracheobronchial nodes

(Aortic arch) node of ligamentum arteriosum

Bronchopulmonary (hilar) nodes

Pulmonary (intra-pulmonary) nodes

Subpleural lymphatic plexus

Interlobular lymph vessels

Drainage follows bronchi, arteries, and veins

Inferior tracheobronchial (carinal) nodes

Pulmonary ligaments

Routes to mediastinum

Drainage routes

Right lung: All lobes drain to pulmonary and bronchopulmonary (hilar) nodes, then to inferior tracheobronchial (carinal) nodes, right superior tracheobronchial nodes, and right paratracheal nodes on the way to the brachiocephalic vein via the bronchomediastinal lymphatic trunk and/ or inferior deep cervical (scalene) node.

Left lung: The superior lobe drains to pulmonary and broncho-pulmonary (hilar) nodes, inferior tracheobronchial (carinal) nodes, left superior tracheobronchial nodes, left paratracheal nodes and/or (aortic arch) node of ligamentum arteriosum, then to the brachiocephalic vein via the left bronchomediastinal trunk and thoracic duct. The left inferior lobe also drains to the pulmonary and bronchopulmonary (hilar) nodes and to inferior tracheobronchial (carinal) nodes, but then mostly to right superior tracheobronchial nodes, where it follows the same route as lymph from the right lung.

Plate 202

Lungs

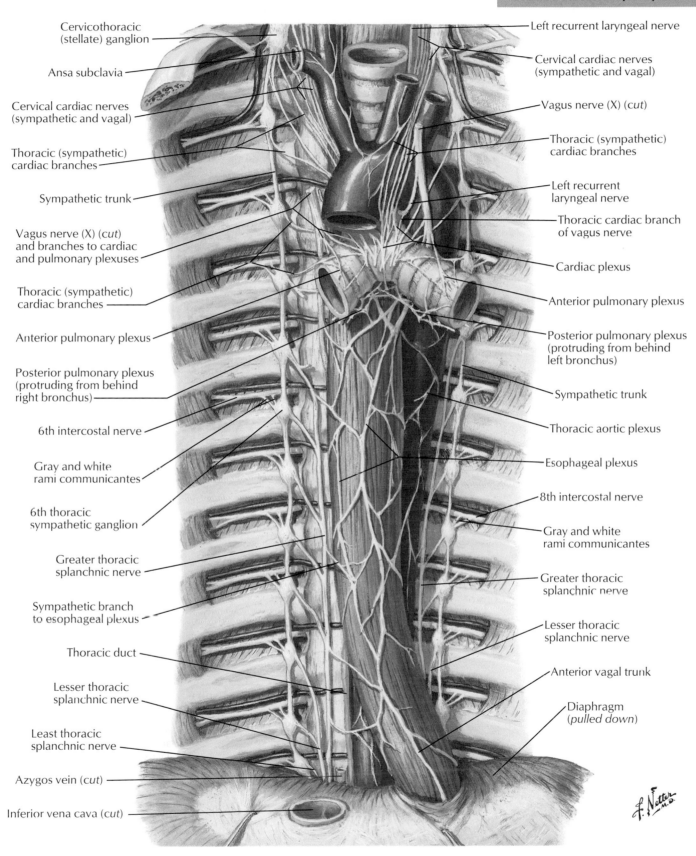

Cervicothoracic (stellate) ganglion

Ansa subclavia

Cervical cardiac nerves (sympathetic and vagal)

Thoracic (sympathetic) cardiac branches

Sympathetic trunk

Vagus nerve (X) (cut) and branches to cardiac and pulmonary plexuses

Thoracic (sympathetic) cardiac branches

Anterior pulmonary plexus

Posterior pulmonary plexus (protruding from behind right bronchus)

6th intercostal nerve

Gray and white rami communicantes

6th thoracic sympathetic ganglion

Greater thoracic splanchnic nerve

Sympathetic branch to esophageal plexus

Thoracic duct

Lesser thoracic splanchnic nerve

Least thoracic splanchnic nerve

Azygos vein (cut)

Inferior vena cava (cut)

Left recurrent laryngeal nerve

Cervical cardiac nerves (sympathetic and vagal)

Vagus nerve (X) (cut)

Thoracic (sympathetic) cardiac branches

Left recurrent laryngeal nerve

Thoracic cardiac branch of vagus nerve

Cardiac plexus

Anterior pulmonary plexus

Posterior pulmonary plexus (protruding from behind left bronchus)

Sympathetic trunk

Thoracic aortic plexus

Esophageal plexus

8th intercostal nerve

Gray and white rami communicantes

Greater thoracic splanchnic nerve

Lesser thoracic splanchnic nerve

Anterior vagal trunk

Diaphragm (pulled down)

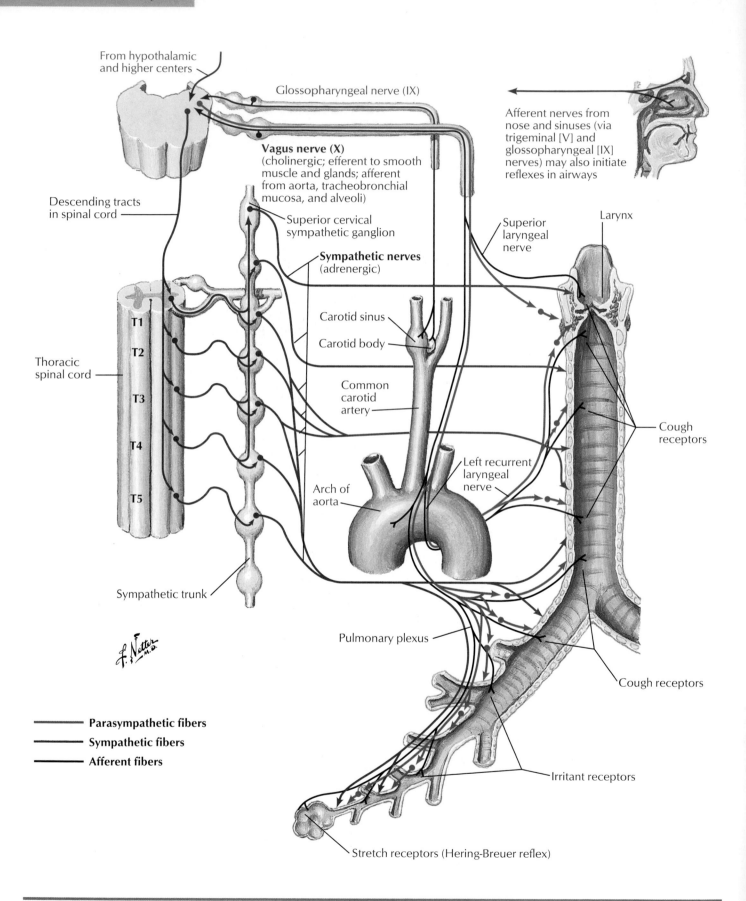

From hypothalamic and higher centers

Glossopharyngeal nerve (IX)

Afferent nerves from nose and sinuses (via trigeminal [V] and glossopharyngeal [IX] nerves) may also initiate reflexes in airways

Vagus nerve (X)
(cholinergic; efferent to smooth muscle and glands; afferent from aorta, tracheobronchial mucosa, and alveoli)

Descending tracts in spinal cord

Superior cervical sympathetic ganglion

Superior laryngeal nerve

Larynx

Sympathetic nerves
(adrenergic)

T1

T2

Carotid sinus

Carotid body

Thoracic spinal cord

T3

Common carotid artery

Cough receptors

T4

Left recurrent laryngeal nerve

T5

Arch of aorta

Sympathetic trunk

Pulmonary plexus

Cough receptors

Irritant receptors

f. Netter

Stretch receptors (Hering-Breuer reflex)

——— Parasympathetic fibers
——— Sympathetic fibers
——— Afferent fibers

Plate 204

Lungs

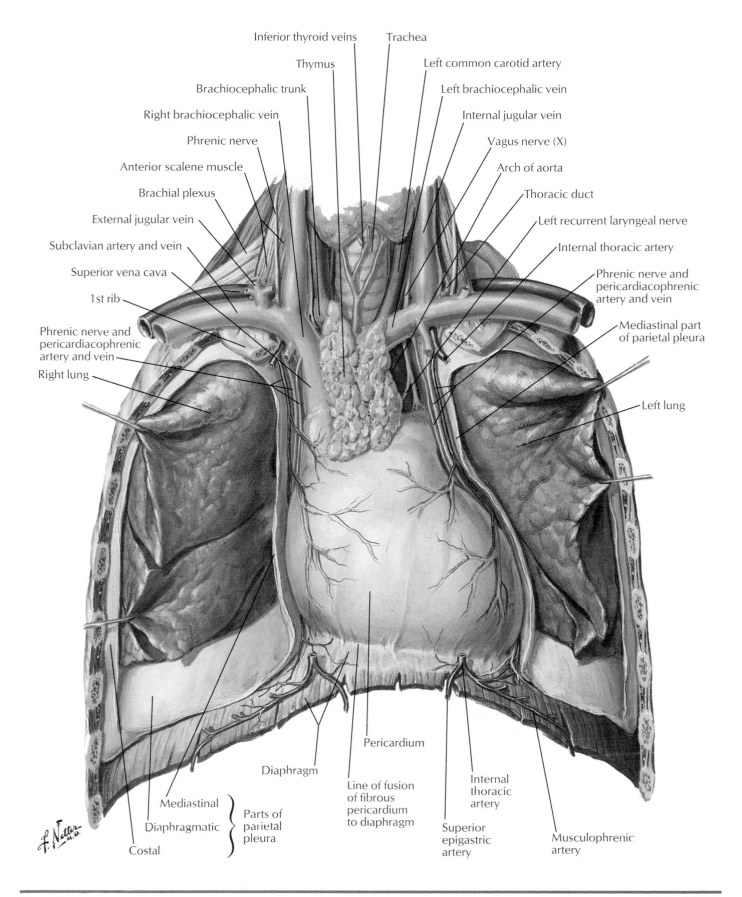

Inferior thyroid veins

Trachea

Thymus

Left common carotid artery

Brachiocephalic trunk

Left brachiocephalic vein

Right brachiocephalic vein

Internal jugular vein

Phrenic nerve

Vagus nerve (X)

Anterior scalene muscle

Arch of aorta

Brachial plexus

Thoracic duct

External jugular vein

Left recurrent laryngeal nerve

Subclavian artery and vein

Internal thoracic artery

Superior vena cava

Phrenic nerve and
pericardiacophrenic
artery and vein

1st rib

Mediastinal part
of parietal pleura

Phrenic nerve and
pericardiacophrenic
artery and vein

Right lung

Left lung

Diaphragm

Mediastinal
Diaphragmatic
Costal

} Parts of
parietal
pleura

Line of fusion
of fibrous
pericardium
to diaphragm

Pericardium

Internal
thoracic
artery

Superior
epigastric
artery

Musculophrenic
artery

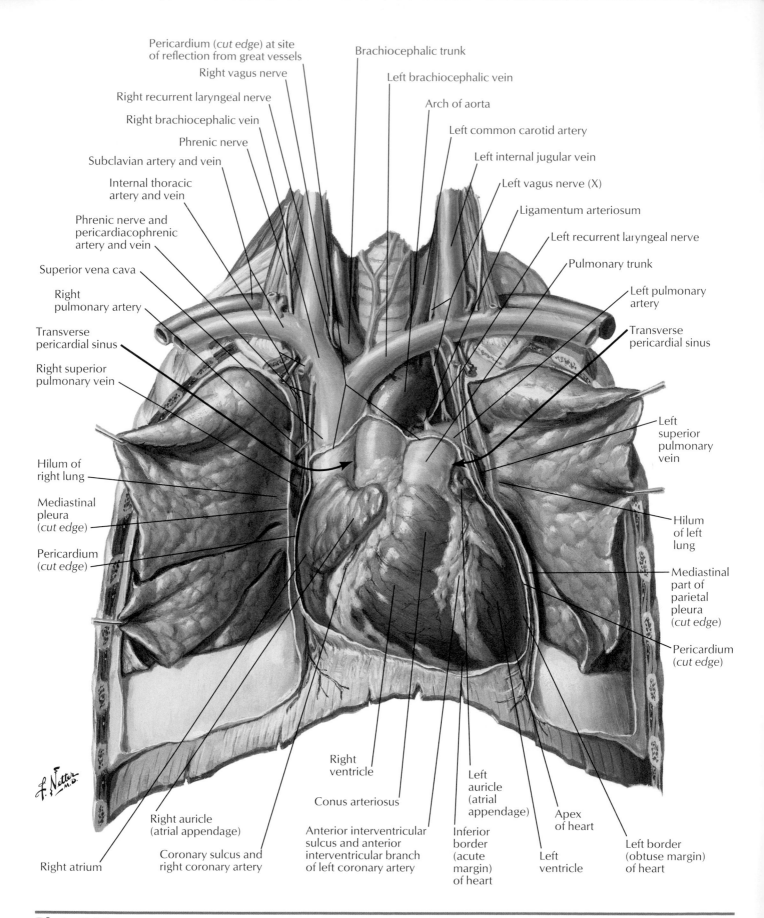

Pericardium (*cut edge*) at site of reflection from great vessels

Right vagus nerve

Right recurrent laryngeal nerve

Right brachiocephalic vein

Phrenic nerve

Subclavian artery and vein

Internal thoracic artery and vein

Phrenic nerve and pericardiacophrenic artery and vein

Superior vena cava

Right pulmonary artery

Transverse pericardial sinus

Right superior pulmonary vein

Hilum of right lung

Mediastinal pleura (*cut edge*)

Pericardium (*cut edge*)

Right atrium

Right auricle (atrial appendage)

Coronary sulcus and right coronary artery

Right ventricle

Conus arteriosus

Anterior interventricular sulcus and anterior interventricular branch of left coronary artery

Brachiocephalic trunk

Left brachiocephalic vein

Arch of aorta

Left common carotid artery

Left internal jugular vein

Left vagus nerve (X)

Ligamentum arteriosum

Left recurrent laryngeal nerve

Pulmonary trunk

Left pulmonary artery

Transverse pericardial sinus

Left superior pulmonary vein

Hilum of left lung

Mediastinal part of parietal pleura (*cut edge*)

Pericardium (*cut edge*)

Left auricle (atrial appendage)

Inferior border (acute margin) of heart

Left ventricle

Apex of heart

Left border (obtuse margin) of heart

Plate 206　　　　　　　　　　　　　　　**Heart**

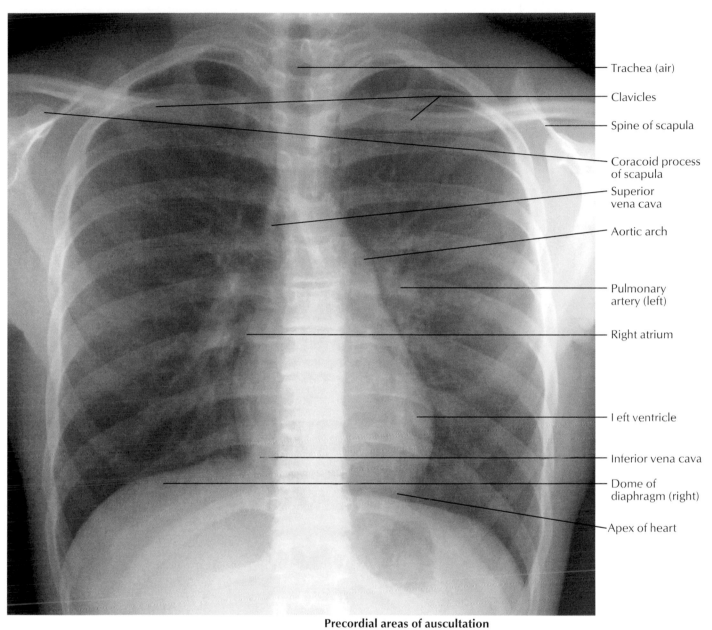

Trachea (air)

Clavicles

Spine of scapula

Coracoid process of scapula

Superior vena cava

Aortic arch

Pulmonary artery (left)

Right atrium

Left ventricle

Inferior vena cava

Dome of diaphragm (right)

Apex of heart

Precordial areas of auscultation

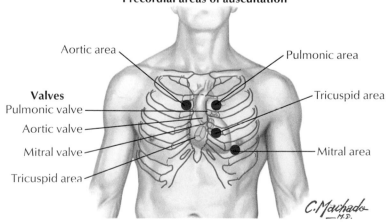

Aortic area

Pulmonic area

Valves

Pulmonic valve

Tricuspid area

Aortic valve

Mitral valve

Mitral area

Tricuspid area

C. Machado
—M.D.

Heart

Plate 207

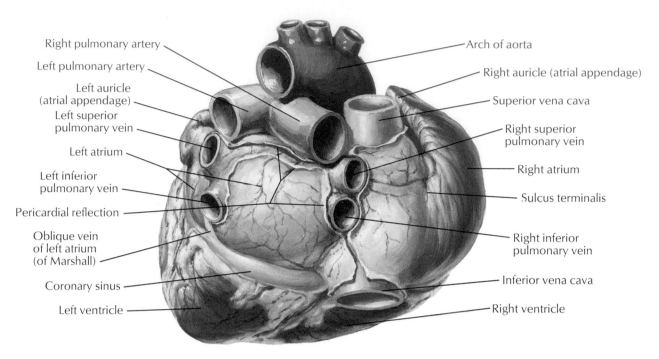

Right pulmonary artery

Left pulmonary artery

Left auricle (atrial appendage)

Left superior pulmonary vein

Left atrium

Left inferior pulmonary vein

Pericardial reflection

Oblique vein of left atrium (of Marshall)

Coronary sinus

Left ventricle

Arch of aorta

Right auricle (atrial appendage)

Superior vena cava

Right superior pulmonary vein

Right atrium

Sulcus terminalis

Right inferior pulmonary vein

Inferior vena cava

Right ventricle

Base of heart: posterior view

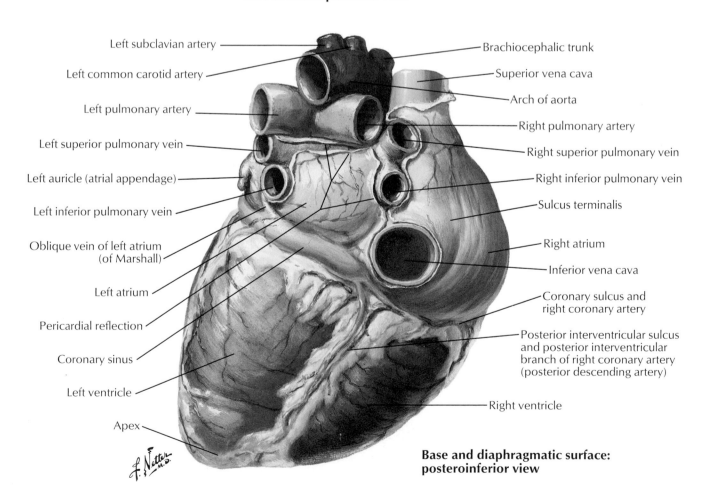

Left subclavian artery

Left common carotid artery

Left pulmonary artery

Left superior pulmonary vein

Left auricle (atrial appendage)

Left inferior pulmonary vein

Oblique vein of left atrium (of Marshall)

Left atrium

Pericardial reflection

Coronary sinus

Left ventricle

Apex

Brachiocephalic trunk

Superior vena cava

Arch of aorta

Right pulmonary artery

Right superior pulmonary vein

Right inferior pulmonary vein

Sulcus terminalis

Right atrium

Inferior vena cava

Coronary sulcus and right coronary artery

Posterior interventricular sulcus and posterior interventricular branch of right coronary artery (posterior descending artery)

Right ventricle

Base and diaphragmatic surface: posteroinferior view

Plate 208 | **Heart**

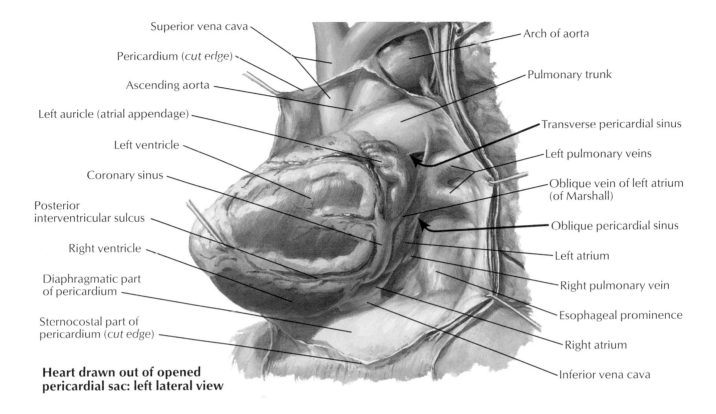

Superior vena cava

Pericardium (*cut edge*)

Ascending aorta

Left auricle (atrial appendage)

Left ventricle

Coronary sinus

Posterior interventricular sulcus

Right ventricle

Diaphragmatic part of pericardium

Sternocostal part of pericardium (*cut edge*)

Arch of aorta

Pulmonary trunk

Transverse pericardial sinus

Left pulmonary veins

Oblique vein of left atrium (of Marshall)

Oblique pericardial sinus

Left atrium

Right pulmonary vein

Esophageal prominence

Right atrium

Inferior vena cava

Heart drawn out of opened pericardial sac: left lateral view

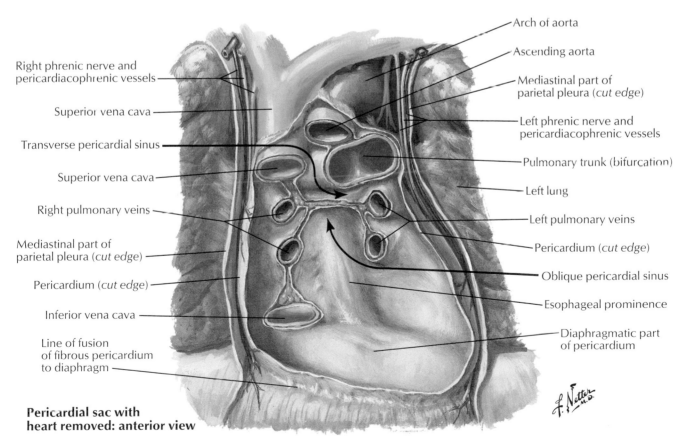

Right phrenic nerve and pericardiacophrenic vessels

Superior vena cava

Transverse pericardial sinus

Superior vena cava

Right pulmonary veins

Mediastinal part of parietal pleura (*cut edge*)

Pericardium (*cut edge*)

Inferior vena cava

Line of fusion of fibrous pericardium to diaphragm

Arch of aorta

Ascending aorta

Mediastinal part of parietal pleura (*cut edge*)

Left phrenic nerve and pericardiacophrenic vessels

Pulmonary trunk (bifurcation)

Left lung

Left pulmonary veins

Pericardium (*cut edge*)

Oblique pericardial sinus

Esophageal prominence

Diaphragmatic part of pericardium

Pericardial sac with heart removed: anterior view

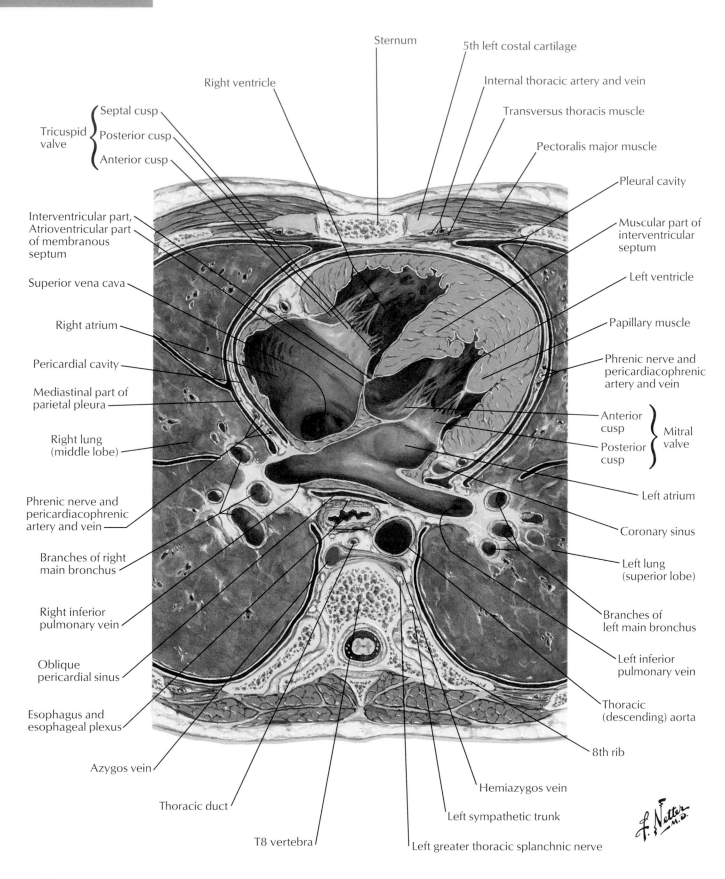

Sternum

5th left costal cartilage

Right ventricle

Internal thoracic artery and vein

Septal cusp

Transversus thoracis muscle

Tricuspid valve — Posterior cusp

Pectoralis major muscle

Anterior cusp

Pleural cavity

Interventricular part, Atrioventricular part of membranous septum

Muscular part of interventricular septum

Superior vena cava

Left ventricle

Right atrium

Papillary muscle

Pericardial cavity

Phrenic nerve and pericardiacophrenic artery and vein

Mediastinal part of parietal pleura

Anterior cusp

Right lung (middle lobe)

Posterior cusp — Mitral valve

Phrenic nerve and pericardiacophrenic artery and vein

Left atrium

Branches of right main bronchus

Coronary sinus

Right inferior pulmonary vein

Left lung (superior lobe)

Branches of left main bronchus

Oblique pericardial sinus

Left inferior pulmonary vein

Esophagus and esophageal plexus

Thoracic (descending) aorta

Azygos vein

8th rib

Thoracic duct

Hemiazygos vein

T8 vertebra

Left sympathetic trunk

Left greater thoracic splanchnic nerve

Plate 210

Heart

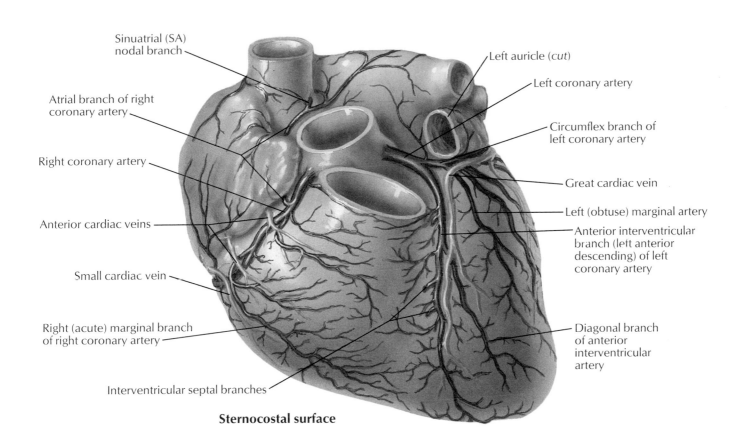

Sinuatrial (SA) nodal branch

Atrial branch of right coronary artery

Right coronary artery

Anterior cardiac veins

Small cardiac vein

Right (acute) marginal branch of right coronary artery

Interventricular septal branches

Left auricle (*cut*)

Left coronary artery

Circumflex branch of left coronary artery

Great cardiac vein

Left (obtuse) marginal artery

Anterior interventricular branch (left anterior descending) of left coronary artery

Diagonal branch of anterior interventricular artery

Sternocostal surface

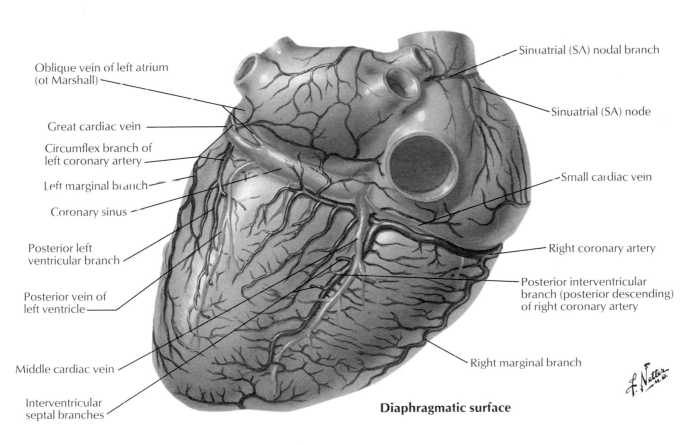

Oblique vein of left atrium (of Marshall)

Great cardiac vein

Circumflex branch of left coronary artery

Left marginal branch

Coronary sinus

Posterior left ventricular branch

Posterior vein of left ventricle

Middle cardiac vein

Interventricular septal branches

Sinuatrial (SA) nodal branch

Sinuatrial (SA) node

Small cardiac vein

Right coronary artery

Posterior interventricular branch (posterior descending) of right coronary artery

Right marginal branch

Diaphragmatic surface

Right coronary artery: left anterior oblique view

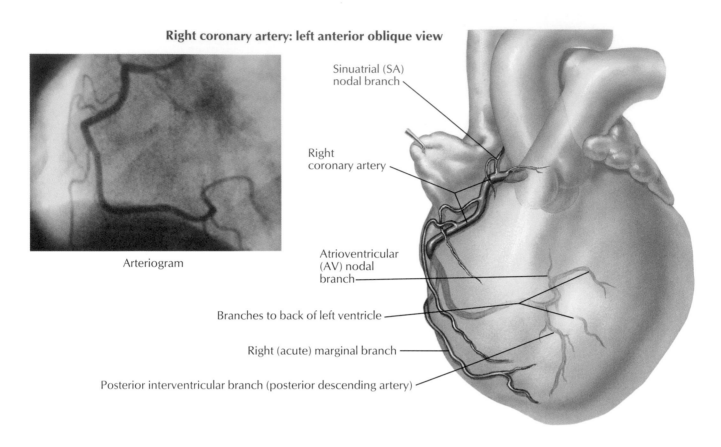

Arteriogram

Sinuatrial (SA) nodal branch

Right coronary artery

Atrioventricular (AV) nodal branch

Branches to back of left ventricle

Right (acute) marginal branch

Posterior interventricular branch (posterior descending artery)

Right coronary artery: right anterior oblique view

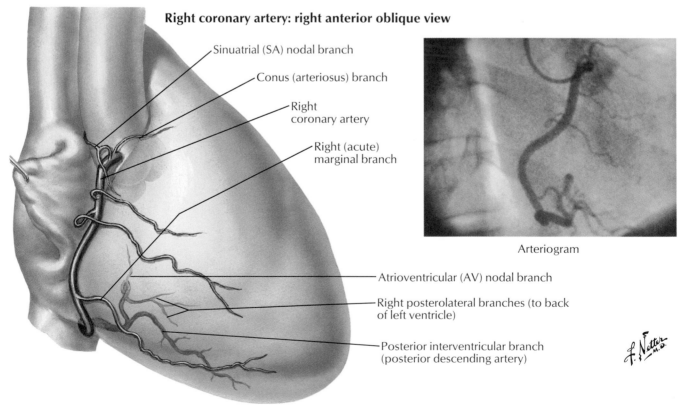

Sinuatrial (SA) nodal branch

Conus (arteriosus) branch

Right coronary artery

Right (acute) marginal branch

Arteriogram

Atrioventricular (AV) nodal branch

Right posterolateral branches (to back of left ventricle)

Posterior interventricular branch (posterior descending artery)

Plate 212 **Heart**

Left coronary artery: left anterior oblique view

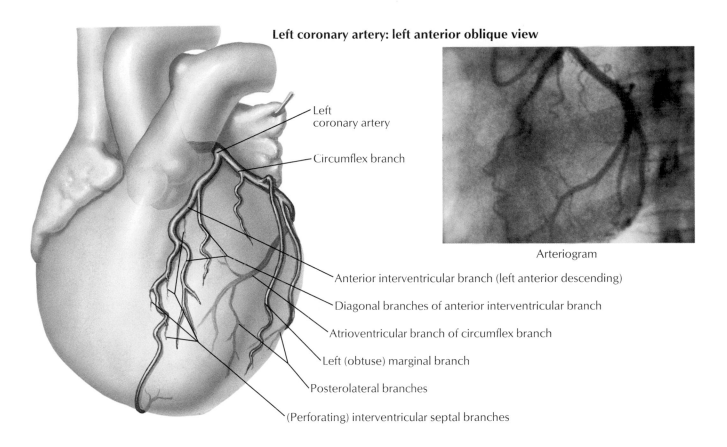

Left coronary artery

Circumflex branch

Arteriogram

Anterior interventricular branch (left anterior descending)

Diagonal branches of anterior interventricular branch

Atrioventricular branch of circumflex branch

Left (obtuse) marginal branch

Posterolateral branches

(Perforating) interventricular septal branches

Left coronary artery: right anterior oblique view

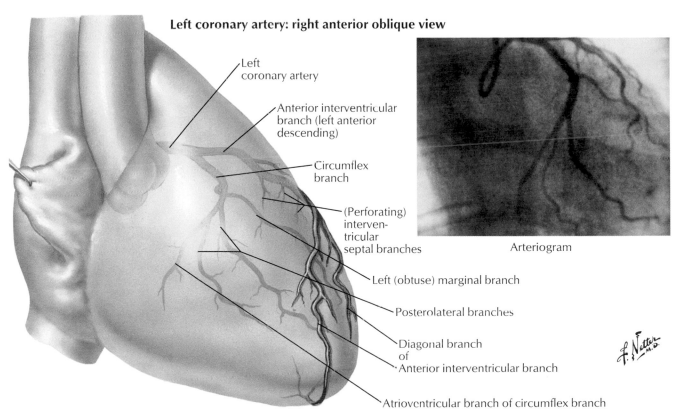

Left coronary artery

Anterior interventricular branch (left anterior descending)

Circumflex branch

(Perforating) interventricular septal branches

Arteriogram

Left (obtuse) marginal branch

Posterolateral branches

Diagonal branch of Anterior interventricular branch

Atrioventricular branch of circumflex branch

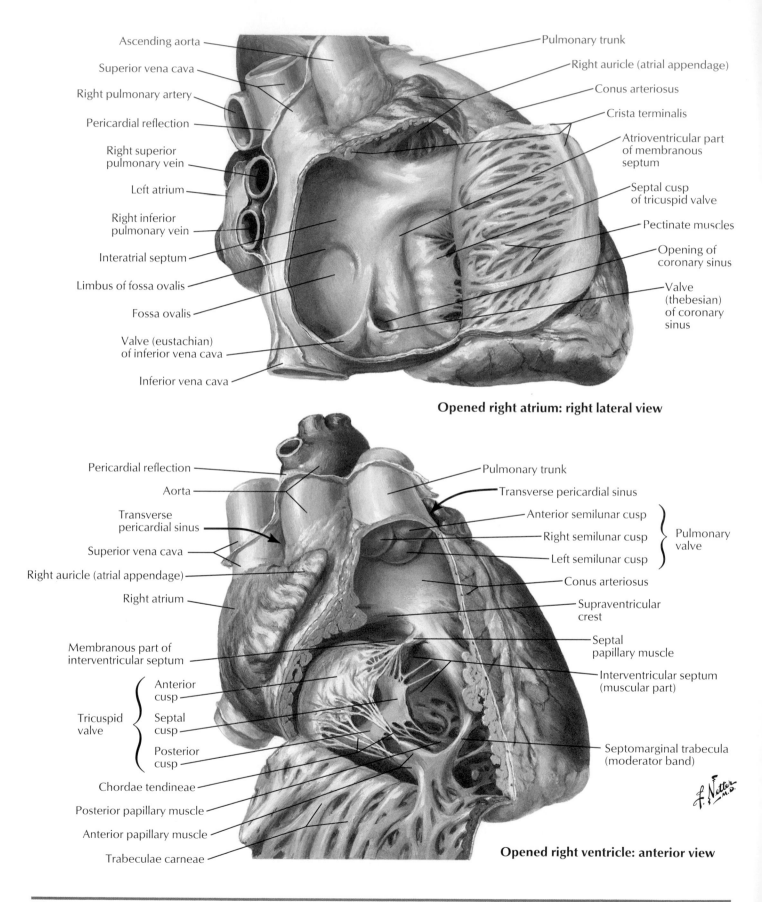

Ascending aorta

Superior vena cava

Right pulmonary artery

Pericardial reflection

Right superior
pulmonary vein

Left atrium

Right inferior
pulmonary vein

Interatrial septum

Limbus of fossa ovalis

Fossa ovalis

Valve (eustachian)
of inferior vena cava

Inferior vena cava

Pulmonary trunk

Right auricle (atrial appendage)

Conus arteriosus

Crista terminalis

Atrioventricular part
of membranous
septum

Septal cusp
of tricuspid valve

Pectinate muscles

Opening of
coronary sinus

Valve
(thebesian)
of coronary
sinus

Opened right atrium: right lateral view

Pericardial reflection

Aorta

Transverse
pericardial sinus

Superior vena cava

Right auricle (atrial appendage)

Right atrium

Membranous part of
interventricular septum

Anterior
cusp

Tricuspid
valve

Septal
cusp

Posterior
cusp

Chordae tendineae

Posterior papillary muscle

Anterior papillary muscle

Trabeculae carneae

Pulmonary trunk

Transverse pericardial sinus

Anterior semilunar cusp

Right semilunar cusp

Left semilunar cusp

Pulmonary
valve

Conus arteriosus

Supraventricular
crest

Septal
papillary muscle

Interventricular septum
(muscular part)

Septomarginal trabecula
(moderator band)

Opened right ventricle: anterior view

Plate 214   **Heart**

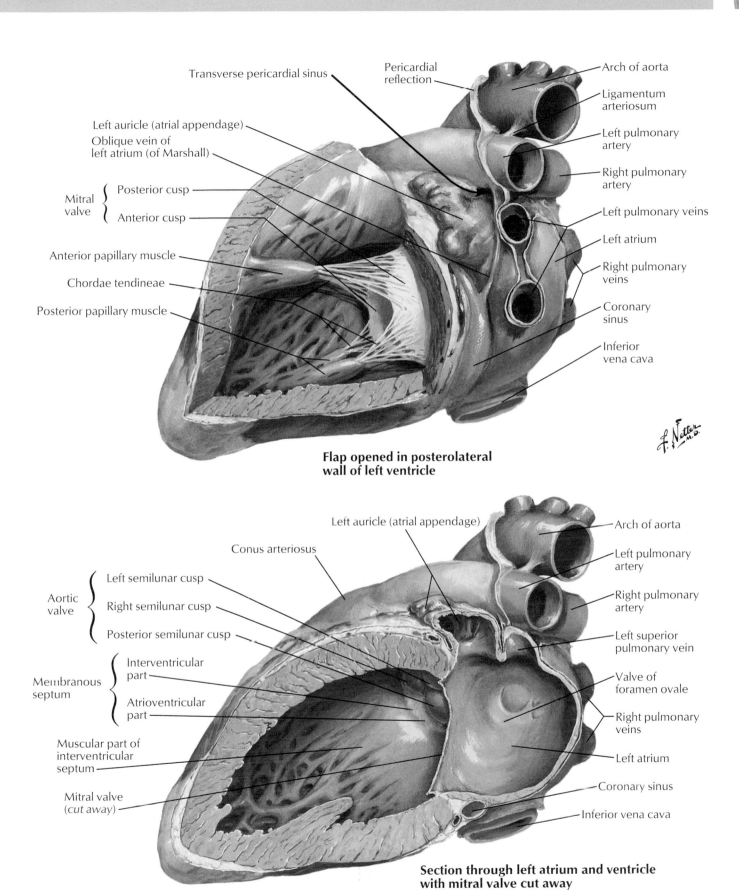

Transverse pericardial sinus

Pericardial reflection

Arch of aorta

Ligamentum arteriosum

Left pulmonary artery

Left auricle (atrial appendage)

Oblique vein of left atrium (of Marshall)

Right pulmonary artery

Mitral valve {
Posterior cusp

Anterior cusp
}

Left pulmonary veins

Left atrium

Anterior papillary muscle

Right pulmonary veins

Chordae tendineae

Coronary sinus

Posterior papillary muscle

Inferior vena cava

Flap opened in posterolateral wall of left ventricle

Left auricle (atrial appendage)

Arch of aorta

Conus arteriosus

Left pulmonary artery

Aortic valve {
Left semilunar cusp

Right semilunar cusp

Posterior semilunar cusp
}

Right pulmonary artery

Left superior pulmonary vein

Membranous septum {
Interventricular part

Atrioventricular part
}

Valve of foramen ovale

Right pulmonary veins

Muscular part of interventricular septum

Left atrium

Mitral valve (*cut away*)

Coronary sinus

Inferior vena cava

Section through left atrium and ventricle with mitral valve cut away

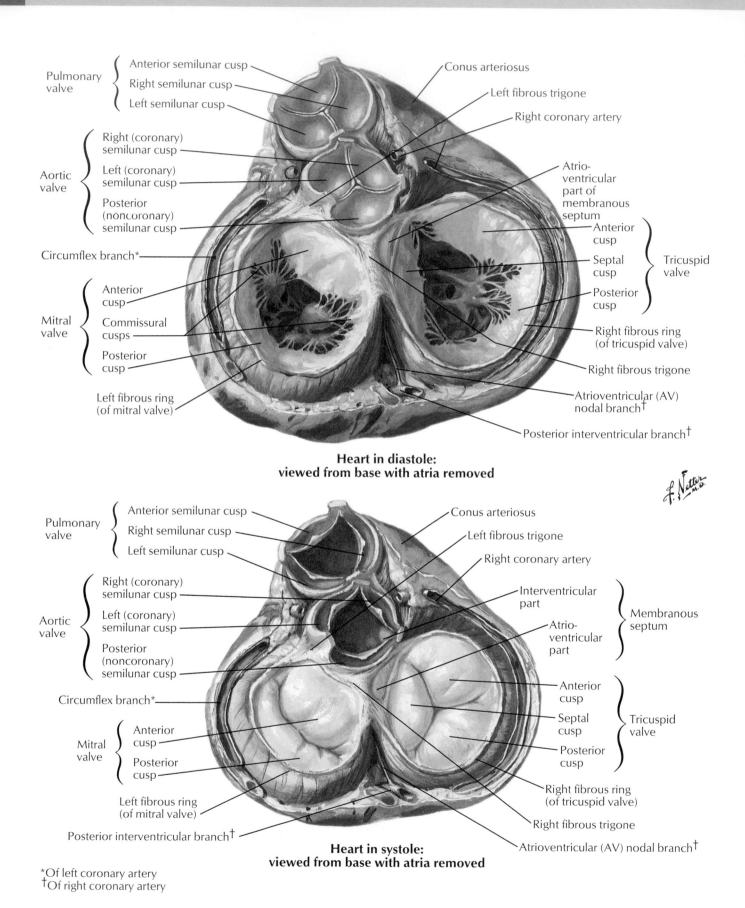

Pulmonary valve
- Anterior semilunar cusp
- Right semilunar cusp
- Left semilunar cusp

Aortic valve
- Right (coronary) semilunar cusp
- Left (coronary) semilunar cusp
- Posterior (noncoronary) semilunar cusp

Circumflex branch*

Mitral valve
- Anterior cusp
- Commissural cusps
- Posterior cusp

Left fibrous ring (of mitral valve)

Conus arteriosus

Left fibrous trigone

Right coronary artery

Atrio-ventricular part of membranous septum

Tricuspid valve
- Anterior cusp
- Septal cusp
- Posterior cusp

Right fibrous ring (of tricuspid valve)

Right fibrous trigone

Atrioventricular (AV) nodal branch†

Posterior interventricular branch†

Heart in diastole:
viewed from base with atria removed

f. Netter M.D.

Pulmonary valve
- Anterior semilunar cusp
- Right semilunar cusp
- Left semilunar cusp

Aortic valve
- Right (coronary) semilunar cusp
- Left (coronary) semilunar cusp
- Posterior (noncoronary) semilunar cusp

Circumflex branch*

Mitral valve
- Anterior cusp
- Posterior cusp

Left fibrous ring (of mitral valve)

Posterior interventricular branch†

Conus arteriosus

Left fibrous trigone

Right coronary artery

Membranous septum
- Interventricular part
- Atrio-ventricular part

Tricuspid valve
- Anterior cusp
- Septal cusp
- Posterior cusp

Right fibrous ring (of tricuspid valve)

Right fibrous trigone

Atrioventricular (AV) nodal branch†

Heart in systole:
viewed from base with atria removed

*Of left coronary artery
†Of right coronary artery

Plate 216

Heart

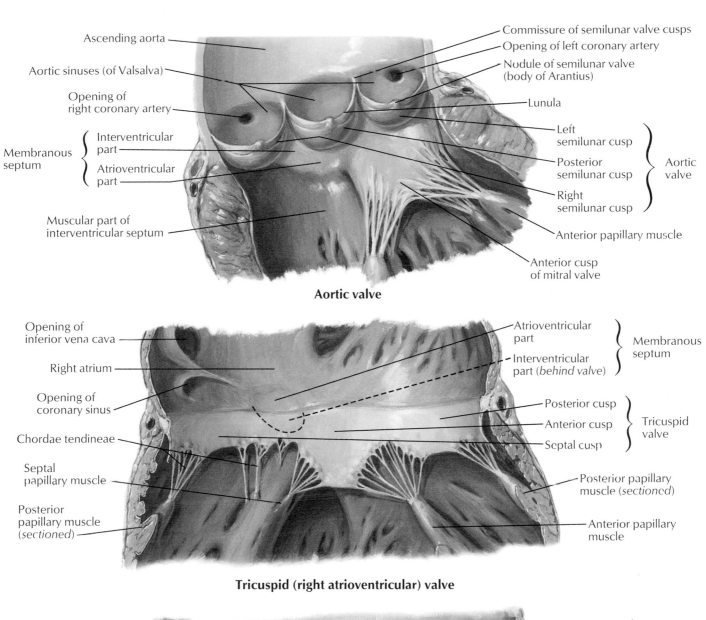

Ascending aorta

Aortic sinuses (of Valsalva)

Opening of right coronary artery

Membranous septum { Interventricular part / Atrioventricular part

Muscular part of interventricular septum

Commissure of semilunar valve cusps

Opening of left coronary artery

Nodule of semilunar valve (body of Arantius)

Lunula

Left semilunar cusp

Posterior semilunar cusp } Aortic valve

Right semilunar cusp

Anterior papillary muscle

Anterior cusp of mitral valve

Aortic valve

Opening of inferior vena cava

Right atrium

Opening of coronary sinus

Chordae tendineae

Septal papillary muscle

Posterior papillary muscle (sectioned)

Atrioventricular part } Membranous septum

Interventricular part (behind valve)

Posterior cusp

Anterior cusp } Tricuspid valve

Septal cusp

Posterior papillary muscle (sectioned)

Anterior papillary muscle

Tricuspid (right atrioventricular) valve

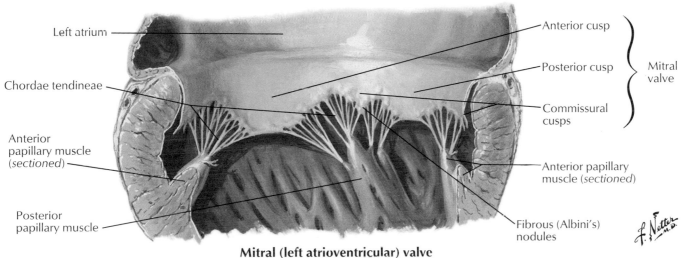

Left atrium

Chordae tendineae

Anterior papillary muscle (sectioned)

Posterior papillary muscle

Anterior cusp

Posterior cusp } Mitral valve

Commissural cusps

Anterior papillary muscle (sectioned)

Fibrous (Albini's) nodules

Mitral (left atrioventricular) valve

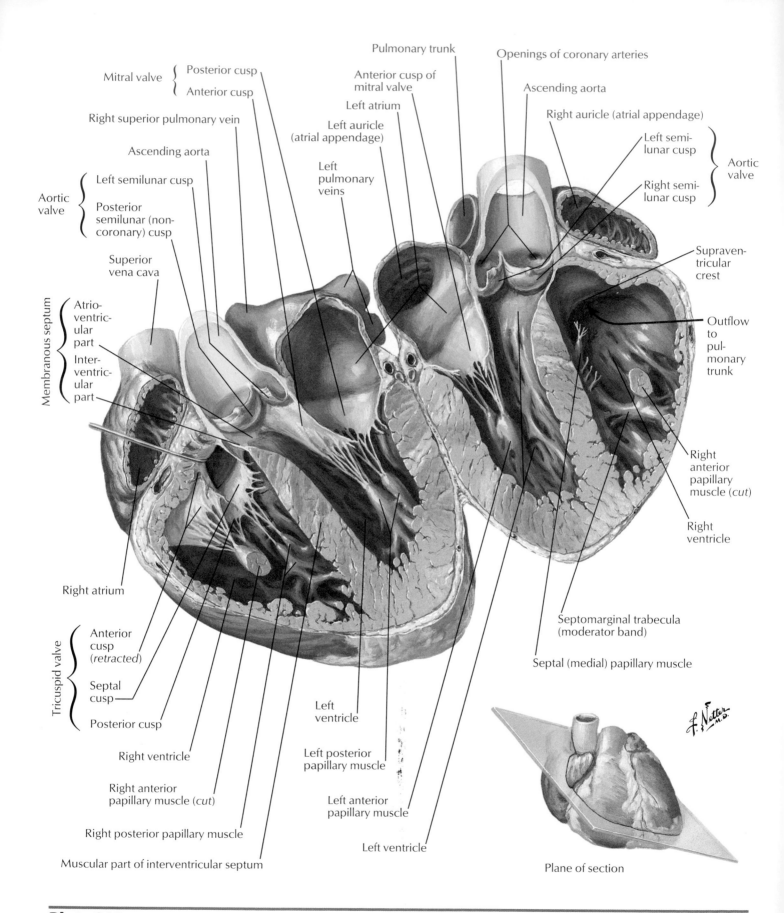

Mitral valve { Posterior cusp / Anterior cusp

Right superior pulmonary vein

Ascending aorta

Aortic valve { Left semilunar cusp / Posterior semilunar (non-coronary) cusp

Superior vena cava

Membranous septum { Atrio-ventricular part / Inter-ventricular part

Pulmonary trunk

Anterior cusp of mitral valve

Left atrium

Left auricle (atrial appendage)

Left pulmonary veins

Openings of coronary arteries

Ascending aorta

Right auricle (atrial appendage)

Left semilunar cusp

Right semilunar cusp

Aortic valve

Supraventricular crest

Outflow to pulmonary trunk

Right anterior papillary muscle (cut)

Right ventricle

Right atrium

Tricuspid valve { Anterior cusp (retracted) / Septal cusp / Posterior cusp

Right ventricle

Right anterior papillary muscle (cut)

Right posterior papillary muscle

Muscular part of interventricular septum

Left ventricle

Left posterior papillary muscle

Left anterior papillary muscle

Left ventricle

Septomarginal trabecula (moderator band)

Septal (medial) papillary muscle

Plane of section

f. Netter
M.D.

Plate 218

Heart

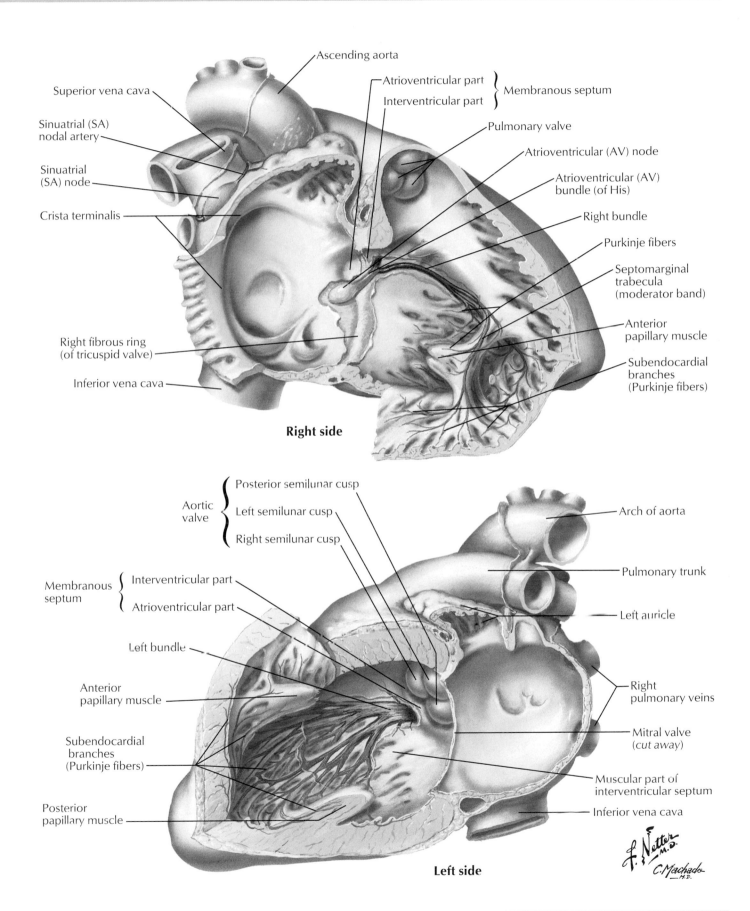

Ascending aorta

Superior vena cava

Atrioventricular part

Interventricular part

Membranous septum

Sinuatrial (SA) nodal artery

Pulmonary valve

Atrioventricular (AV) node

Sinuatrial (SA) node

Atrioventricular (AV) bundle (of His)

Crista terminalis

Right bundle

Purkinje fibers

Septomarginal trabecula (moderator band)

Right fibrous ring (of tricuspid valve)

Anterior papillary muscle

Inferior vena cava

Subendocardial branches (Purkinje fibers)

Right side

Posterior semilunar cusp

Aortic valve

Left semilunar cusp

Arch of aorta

Right semilunar cusp

Pulmonary trunk

Membranous septum

Interventricular part

Atrioventricular part

Left auricle

Left bundle

Anterior papillary muscle

Right pulmonary veins

Subendocardial branches (Purkinje fibers)

Mitral valve (*cut away*)

Muscular part of interventricular septum

Posterior papillary muscle

Inferior vena cava

Left side

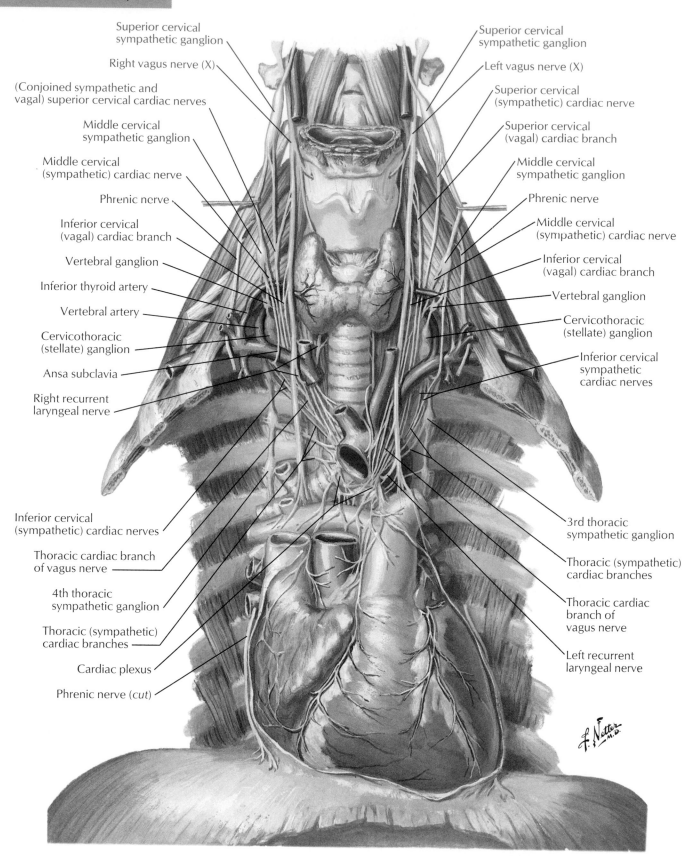

Superior cervical sympathetic ganglion

Right vagus nerve (X)

(Conjoined sympathetic and vagal) superior cervical cardiac nerves

Middle cervical sympathetic ganglion

Middle cervical (sympathetic) cardiac nerve

Phrenic nerve

Inferior cervical (vagal) cardiac branch

Vertebral ganglion

Inferior thyroid artery

Vertebral artery

Cervicothoracic (stellate) ganglion

Ansa subclavia

Right recurrent laryngeal nerve

Inferior cervical (sympathetic) cardiac nerves

Thoracic cardiac branch of vagus nerve

4th thoracic sympathetic ganglion

Thoracic (sympathetic) cardiac branches

Cardiac plexus

Phrenic nerve (cut)

Superior cervical sympathetic ganglion

Left vagus nerve (X)

Superior cervical (sympathetic) cardiac nerve

Superior cervical (vagal) cardiac branch

Middle cervical sympathetic ganglion

Phrenic nerve

Middle cervical (sympathetic) cardiac nerve

Inferior cervical (vagal) cardiac branch

Vertebral ganglion

Cervicothoracic (stellate) ganglion

Inferior cervical sympathetic cardiac nerves

3rd thoracic sympathetic ganglion

Thoracic (sympathetic) cardiac branches

Thoracic cardiac branch of vagus nerve

Left recurrent laryngeal nerve

Plate 220

Heart

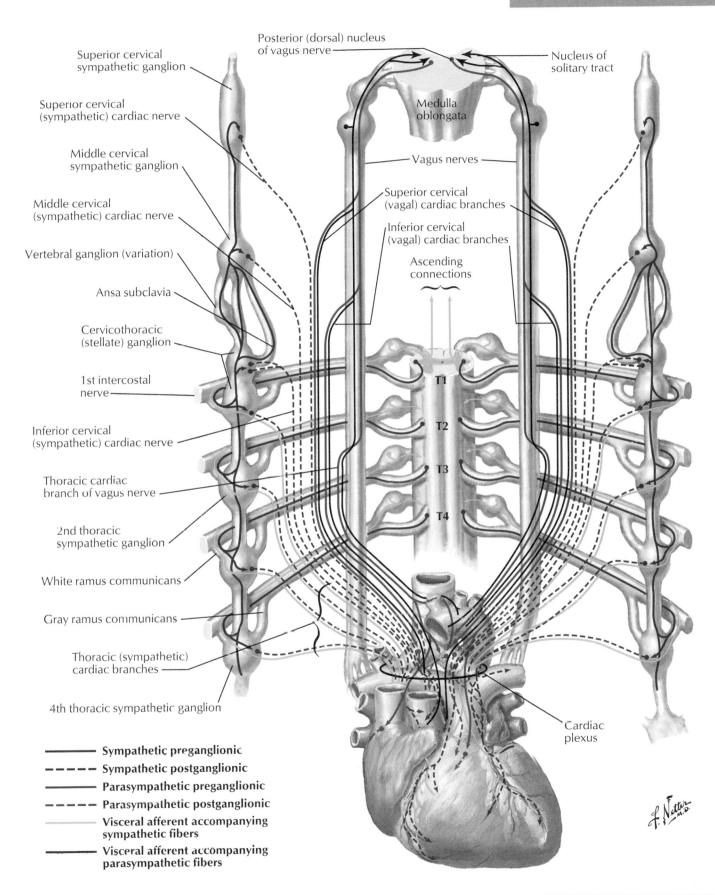

Superior cervical sympathetic ganglion

Superior cervical (sympathetic) cardiac nerve

Middle cervical sympathetic ganglion

Middle cervical (sympathetic) cardiac nerve

Vertebral ganglion (variation)

Ansa subclavia

Cervicothoracic (stellate) ganglion

1st intercostal nerve

Inferior cervical (sympathetic) cardiac nerve

Thoracic cardiac branch of vagus nerve

2nd thoracic sympathetic ganglion

White ramus communicans

Gray ramus communicans

Thoracic (sympathetic) cardiac branches

4th thoracic sympathetic ganglion

Posterior (dorsal) nucleus of vagus nerve

Nucleus of solitary tract

Medulla oblongata

Vagus nerves

Superior cervical (vagal) cardiac branches

Inferior cervical (vagal) cardiac branches

Ascending connections

T1

T2

T3

T4

Cardiac plexus

─────── Sympathetic preganglionic

- - - - - - Sympathetic postganglionic

─────── Parasympathetic preganglionic

- - - - - - Parasympathetic postganglionic

─────── Visceral afferent accompanying sympathetic fibers

─────── Visceral afferent accompanying parasympathetic fibers

F. Netter M.D.

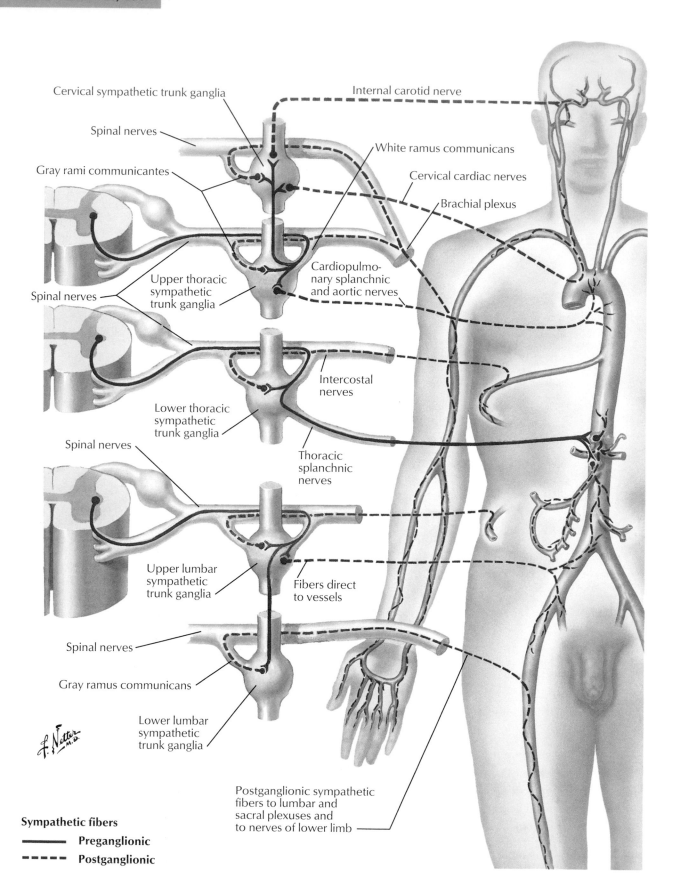

Cervical sympathetic trunk ganglia

Internal carotid nerve

Spinal nerves

White ramus communicans

Gray rami communicantes

Cervical cardiac nerves

Brachial plexus

Upper thoracic sympathetic trunk ganglia

Cardiopulmonary splanchnic and aortic nerves

Spinal nerves

Intercostal nerves

Lower thoracic sympathetic trunk ganglia

Spinal nerves

Thoracic splanchnic nerves

Upper lumbar sympathetic trunk ganglia

Fibers direct to vessels

Spinal nerves

Gray ramus communicans

Lower lumbar sympathetic trunk ganglia

Postganglionic sympathetic fibers to lumbar and sacral plexuses and to nerves of lower limb

Sympathetic fibers

———— **Preganglionic**

----- **Postganglionic**

Plate 222

Heart

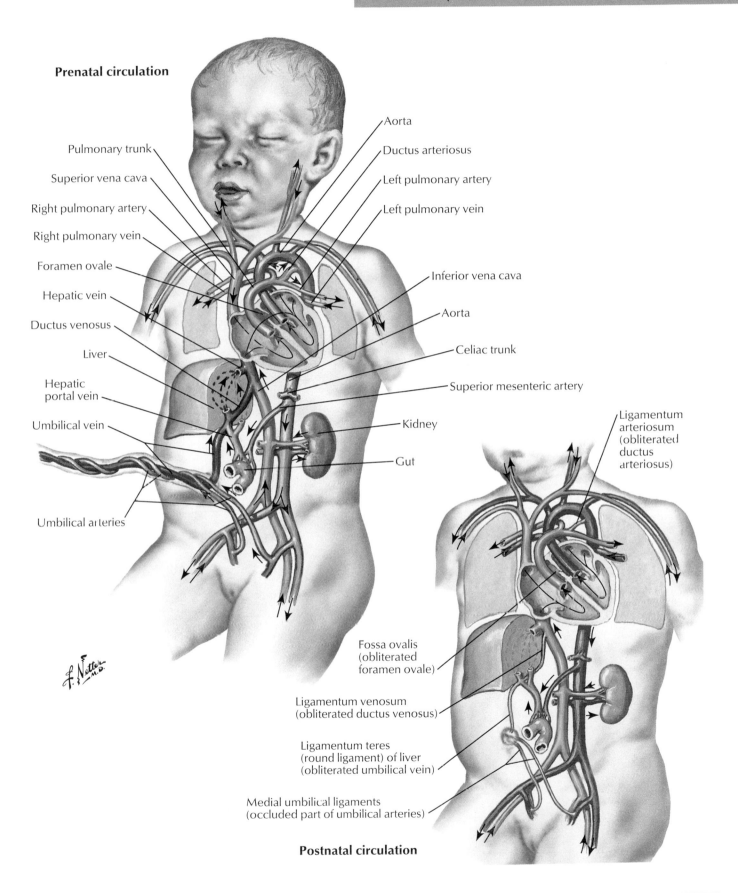

Prenatal circulation

Pulmonary trunk

Superior vena cava

Right pulmonary artery

Right pulmonary vein

Foramen ovale

Hepatic vein

Ductus venosus

Liver

Hepatic portal vein

Umbilical vein

Umbilical arteries

Aorta

Ductus arteriosus

Left pulmonary artery

Left pulmonary vein

Inferior vena cava

Aorta

Celiac trunk

Superior mesenteric artery

Kidney

Gut

Ligamentum arteriosum (obliterated ductus arteriosus)

Fossa ovalis (obliterated foramen ovale)

Ligamentum venosum (obliterated ductus venosus)

Ligamentum teres (round ligament) of liver (obliterated umbilical vein)

Medial umbilical ligaments (occluded part of umbilical arteries)

Postnatal circulation

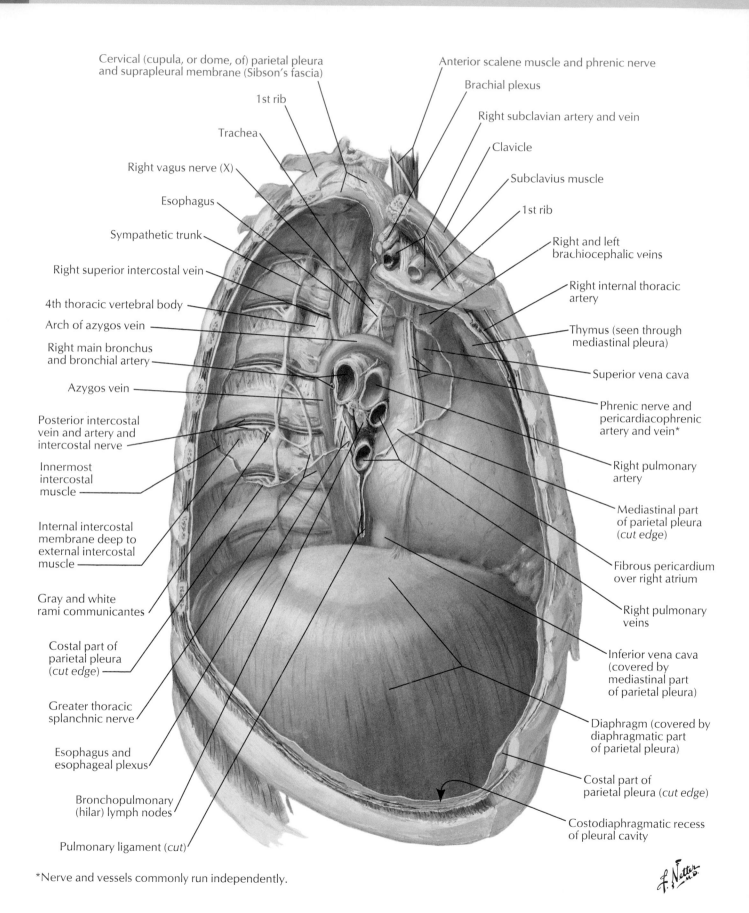

Cervical (cupula, or dome, of) parietal pleura and suprapleural membrane (Sibson's fascia)

1st rib

Trachea

Right vagus nerve (X)

Esophagus

Sympathetic trunk

Right superior intercostal vein

4th thoracic vertebral body

Arch of azygos vein

Right main bronchus and bronchial artery

Azygos vein

Posterior intercostal vein and artery and intercostal nerve

Innermost intercostal muscle

Internal intercostal membrane deep to external intercostal muscle

Gray and white rami communicantes

Costal part of parietal pleura (cut edge)

Greater thoracic splanchnic nerve

Esophagus and esophageal plexus

Bronchopulmonary (hilar) lymph nodes

Pulmonary ligament (cut)

Anterior scalene muscle and phrenic nerve

Brachial plexus

Right subclavian artery and vein

Clavicle

Subclavius muscle

1st rib

Right and left brachiocephalic veins

Right internal thoracic artery

Thymus (seen through mediastinal pleura)

Superior vena cava

Phrenic nerve and pericardiacophrenic artery and vein*

Right pulmonary artery

Mediastinal part of parietal pleura (cut edge)

Fibrous pericardium over right atrium

Right pulmonary veins

Inferior vena cava (covered by mediastinal part of parietal pleura)

Diaphragm (covered by diaphragmatic part of parietal pleura)

Costal part of parietal pleura (cut edge)

Costodiaphragmatic recess of pleural cavity

*Nerve and vessels commonly run independently.

Plate 224

Mediastinum

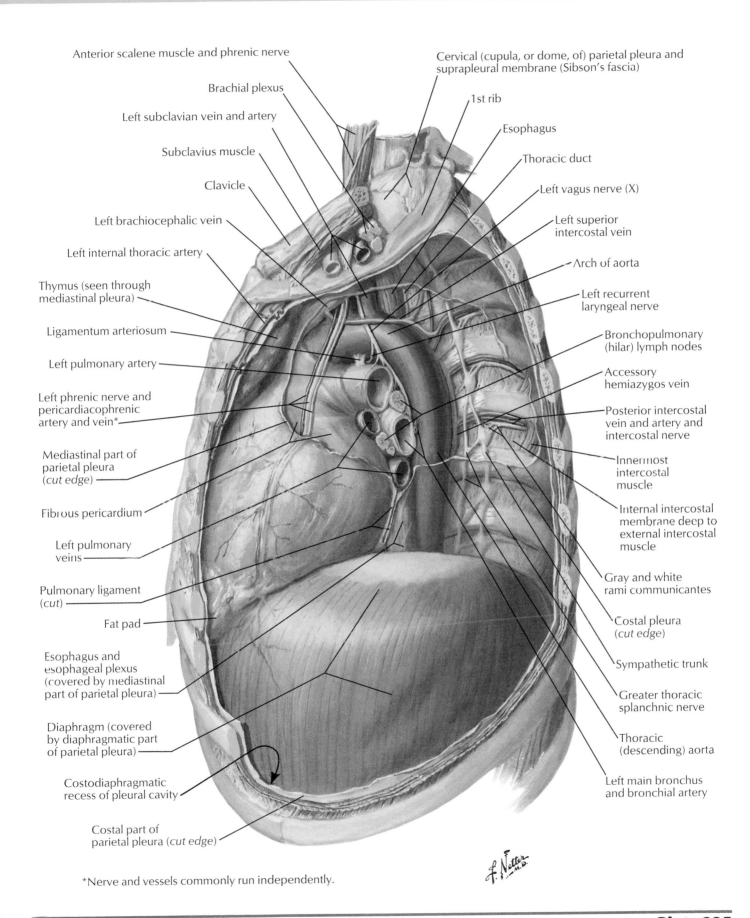

Anterior scalene muscle and phrenic nerve

Brachial plexus

Left subclavian vein and artery

Subclavius muscle

Clavicle

Left brachiocephalic vein

Left internal thoracic artery

Thymus (seen through mediastinal pleura)

Ligamentum arteriosum

Left pulmonary artery

Left phrenic nerve and pericardiacophrenic artery and vein*

Mediastinal part of parietal pleura (*cut edge*)

Fibrous pericardium

Left pulmonary veins

Pulmonary ligament (*cut*)

Fat pad

Esophagus and esophageal plexus (covered by mediastinal part of parietal pleura)

Diaphragm (covered by diaphragmatic part of parietal pleura)

Costodiaphragmatic recess of pleural cavity

Costal part of parietal pleura (*cut edge*)

Cervical (cupula, or dome, of) parietal pleura and suprapleural membrane (Sibson's fascia)

1st rib

Esophagus

Thoracic duct

Left vagus nerve (X)

Left superior intercostal vein

Arch of aorta

Left recurrent laryngeal nerve

Bronchopulmonary (hilar) lymph nodes

Accessory hemiazygos vein

Posterior intercostal vein and artery and intercostal nerve

Innermost intercostal muscle

Internal intercostal membrane deep to external intercostal muscle

Gray and white rami communicantes

Costal pleura (*cut edge*)

Sympathetic trunk

Greater thoracic splanchnic nerve

Thoracic (descending) aorta

Left main bronchus and bronchial artery

*Nerve and vessels commonly run independently.

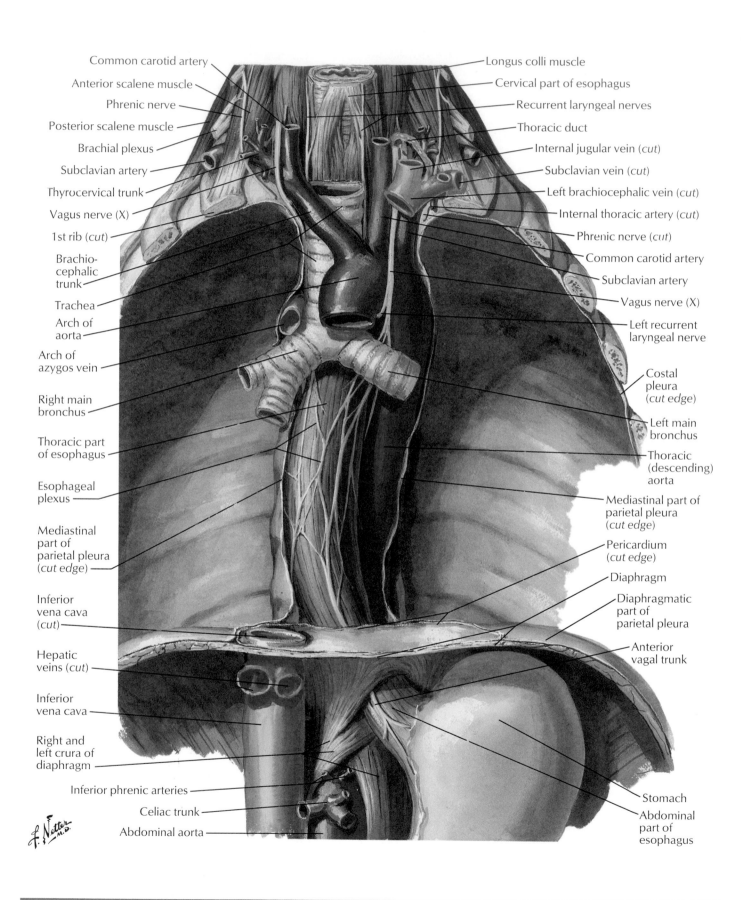

Common carotid artery

Anterior scalene muscle

Phrenic nerve

Posterior scalene muscle

Brachial plexus

Subclavian artery

Thyrocervical trunk

Vagus nerve (X)

1st rib (cut)

Brachio-
cephalic
trunk

Trachea

Arch of
aorta

Arch of
azygos vein

Right main
bronchus

Thoracic part
of esophagus

Esophageal
plexus

Mediastinal
part of
parietal pleura
(cut edge)

Inferior
vena cava
(cut)

Hepatic
veins (cut)

Inferior
vena cava

Right and
left crura of
diaphragm

Inferior phrenic arteries

Celiac trunk

Abdominal aorta

Longus colli muscle

Cervical part of esophagus

Recurrent laryngeal nerves

Thoracic duct

Internal jugular vein (cut)

Subclavian vein (cut)

Left brachiocephalic vein (cut)

Internal thoracic artery (cut)

Phrenic nerve (cut)

Common carotid artery

Subclavian artery

Vagus nerve (X)

Left recurrent
laryngeal nerve

Costal
pleura
(cut edge)

Left main
bronchus

Thoracic
(descending)
aorta

Mediastinal part of
parietal pleura
(cut edge)

Pericardium
(cut edge)

Diaphragm

Diaphragmatic
part of
parietal pleura

Anterior
vagal trunk

Stomach

Abdominal
part of
esophagus

Plate 226

Mediastinum

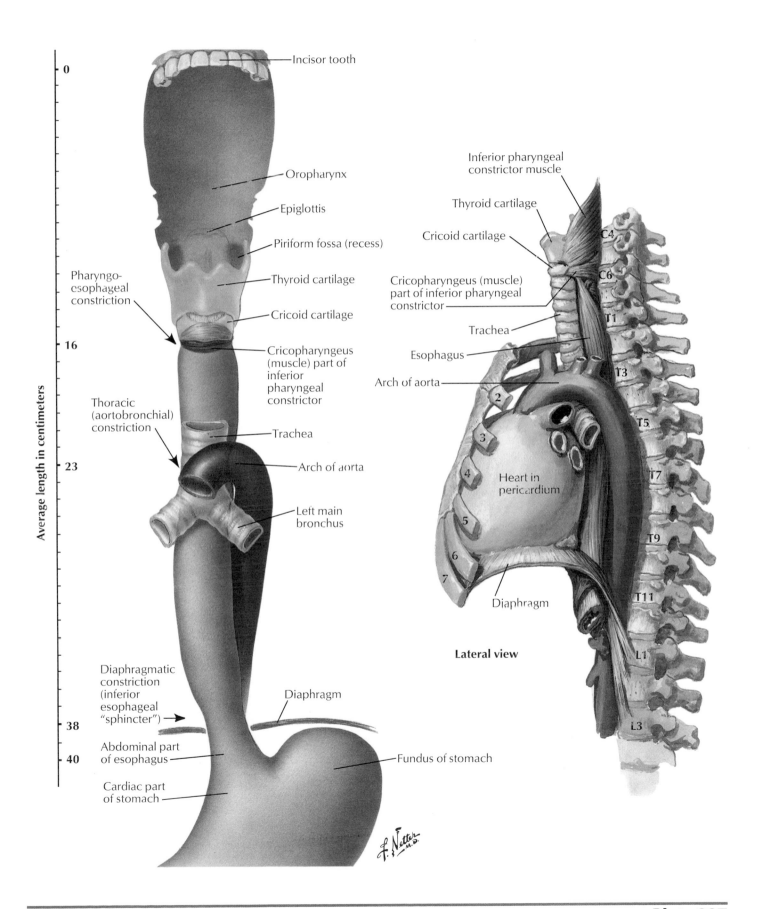

Incisor tooth

Oropharynx

Epiglottis

Piriform fossa (recess)

Pharyngo-
esophageal
constriction

Thyroid cartilage

Cricoid cartilage

Cricopharyngeus
(muscle) part of
inferior
pharyngeal
constrictor

Thoracic
(aortobronchial)
constriction

Trachea

Arch of aorta

Left main
bronchus

Diaphragmatic
constriction
(inferior
esophageal
"sphincter")

Diaphragm

Abdominal part
of esophagus

Fundus of stomach

Cardiac part
of stomach

Average length in centimeters

0

16

23

38

40

Inferior pharyngeal
constrictor muscle

Thyroid cartilage

Cricoid cartilage

Cricopharyngeus (muscle)
part of inferior pharyngeal
constrictor

Trachea

Esophagus

Arch of aorta

Heart in
pericardium

Diaphragm

Lateral view

C4

C6

T1

T3

T5

T7

T9

T11

L1

L3

2

3

4

5

6

7

f. Netter.
M.D.

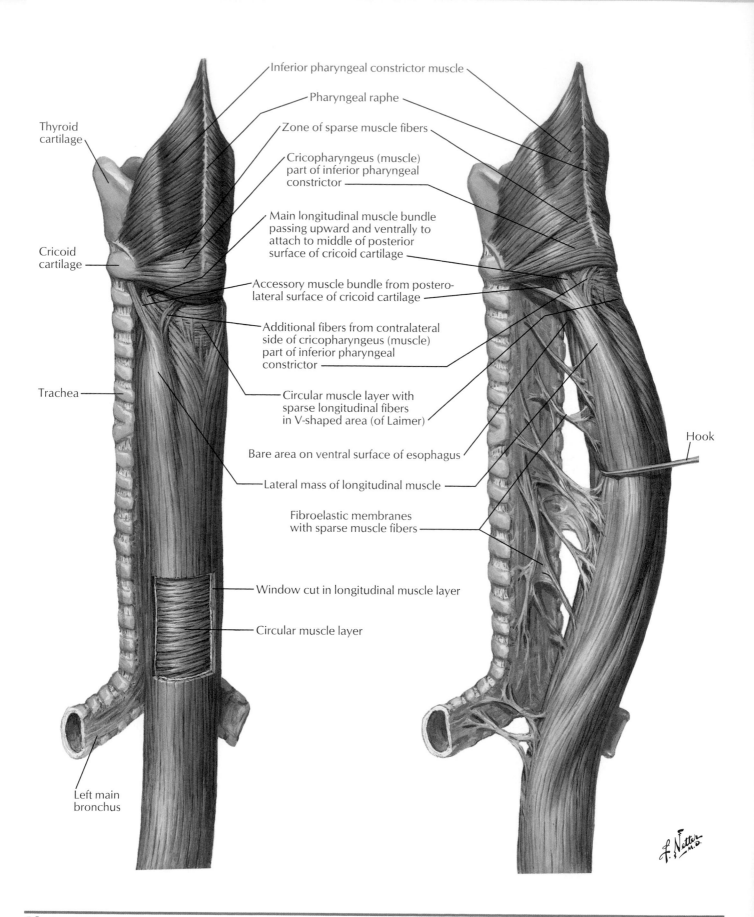

Inferior pharyngeal constrictor muscle

Pharyngeal raphe

Zone of sparse muscle fibers

Cricopharyngeus (muscle) part of inferior pharyngeal constrictor

Thyroid cartilage

Main longitudinal muscle bundle passing upward and ventrally to attach to middle of posterior surface of cricoid cartilage

Cricoid cartilage

Accessory muscle bundle from postero-lateral surface of cricoid cartilage

Additional fibers from contralateral side of cricopharyngeus (muscle) part of inferior pharyngeal constrictor

Trachea

Circular muscle layer with sparse longitudinal fibers in V-shaped area (of Laimer)

Bare area on ventral surface of esophagus

Lateral mass of longitudinal muscle

Fibroelastic membranes with sparse muscle fibers

Window cut in longitudinal muscle layer

Circular muscle layer

Hook

Left main bronchus

Plate 228

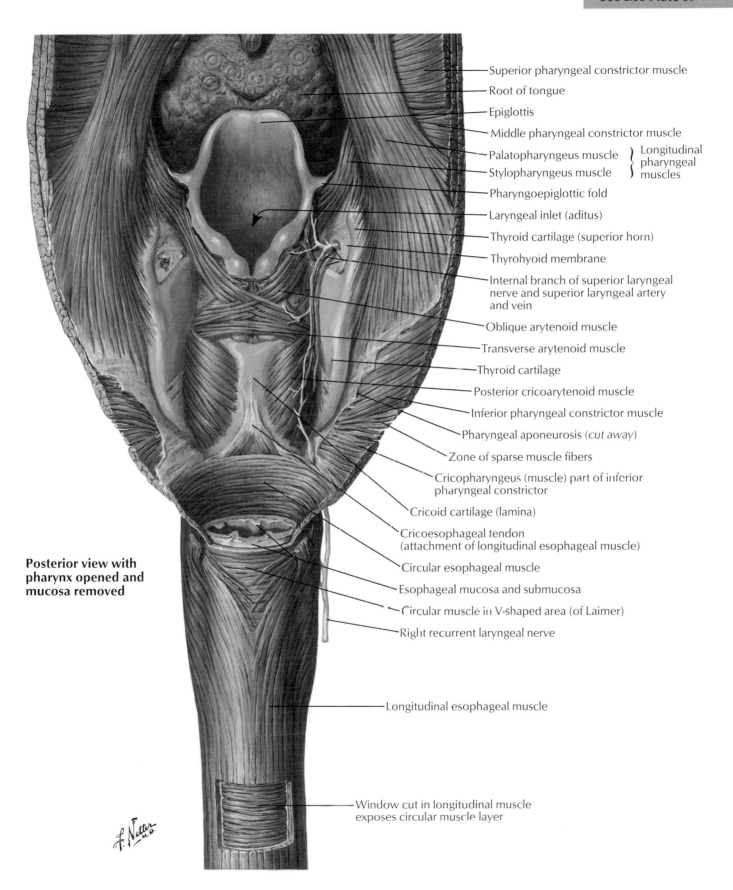

Superior pharyngeal constrictor muscle

Root of tongue

Epiglottis

Middle pharyngeal constrictor muscle

Palatopharyngeus muscle } Longitudinal pharyngeal muscles

Stylopharyngeus muscle

Pharyngoepiglottic fold

Laryngeal inlet (aditus)

Thyroid cartilage (superior horn)

Thyrohyoid membrane

Internal branch of superior laryngeal nerve and superior laryngeal artery and vein

Oblique arytenoid muscle

Transverse arytenoid muscle

Thyroid cartilage

Posterior cricoarytenoid muscle

Inferior pharyngeal constrictor muscle

Pharyngeal aponeurosis (*cut away*)

Zone of sparse muscle fibers

Cricopharyngeus (muscle) part of inferior pharyngeal constrictor

Cricoid cartilage (lamina)

Cricoesophageal tendon (attachment of longitudinal esophageal muscle)

Circular esophageal muscle

Esophageal mucosa and submucosa

Circular muscle in V-shaped area (of Laimer)

Right recurrent laryngeal nerve

Longitudinal esophageal muscle

Window cut in longitudinal muscle exposes circular muscle layer

Posterior view with pharynx opened and mucosa removed

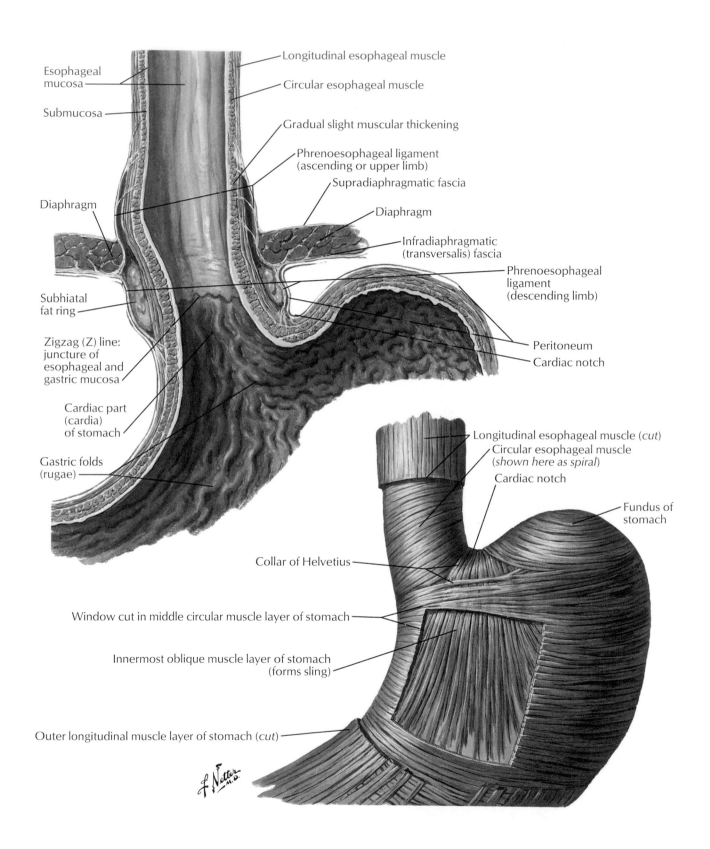

Esophageal mucosa

Submucosa

Diaphragm

Subhiatal fat ring

Zigzag (Z) line: juncture of esophageal and gastric mucosa

Cardiac part (cardia) of stomach

Gastric folds (rugae)

Longitudinal esophageal muscle

Circular esophageal muscle

Gradual slight muscular thickening

Phrenoesophageal ligament (ascending or upper limb)

Supradiaphragmatic fascia

Diaphragm

Infradiaphragmatic (transversalis) fascia

Phrenoesophageal ligament (descending limb)

Peritoneum

Cardiac notch

Longitudinal esophageal muscle (cut)

Circular esophageal muscle (shown here as spiral)

Cardiac notch

Fundus of stomach

Collar of Helvetius

Window cut in middle circular muscle layer of stomach

Innermost oblique muscle layer of stomach (forms sling)

Outer longitudinal muscle layer of stomach (cut)

Plate 230

Mediastinum

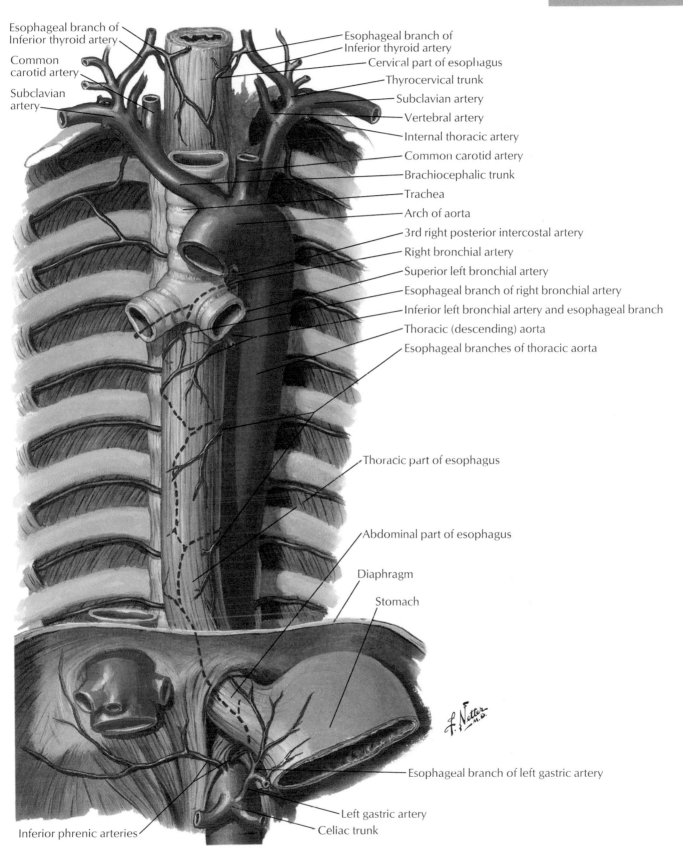

Esophageal branch of Inferior thyroid artery

Common carotid artery

Subclavian artery

Esophageal branch of Inferior thyroid artery

Cervical part of esophagus

Thyrocervical trunk

Subclavian artery

Vertebral artery

Internal thoracic artery

Common carotid artery

Brachiocephalic trunk

Trachea

Arch of aorta

3rd right posterior intercostal artery

Right bronchial artery

Superior left bronchial artery

Esophageal branch of right bronchial artery

Inferior left bronchial artery and esophageal branch

Thoracic (descending) aorta

Esophageal branches of thoracic aorta

Thoracic part of esophagus

Abdominal part of esophagus

Diaphragm

Stomach

Esophageal branch of left gastric artery

Left gastric artery

Celiac trunk

Inferior phrenic arteries

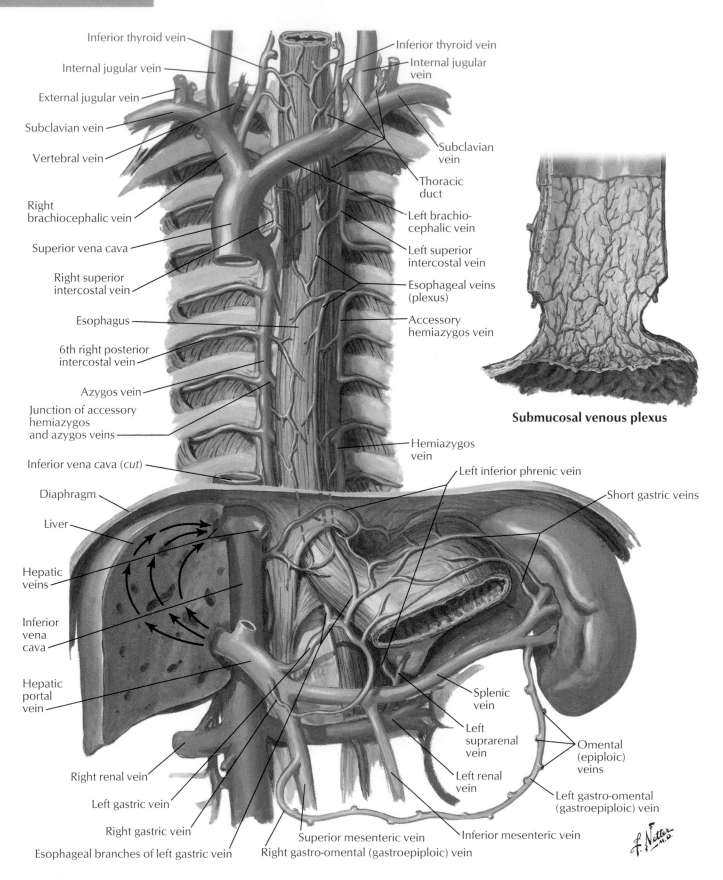

Inferior thyroid vein

Internal jugular vein

External jugular vein

Subclavian vein

Vertebral vein

Right brachiocephalic vein

Superior vena cava

Right superior intercostal vein

Esophagus

6th right posterior intercostal vein

Azygos vein

Junction of accessory hemiazygos and azygos veins

Inferior vena cava (*cut*)

Diaphragm

Liver

Hepatic veins

Inferior vena cava

Hepatic portal vein

Right renal vein

Left gastric vein

Right gastric vein

Esophageal branches of left gastric vein

Inferior thyroid vein

Internal jugular vein

Subclavian vein

Thoracic duct

Left brachio-cephalic vein

Left superior intercostal vein

Esophageal veins (plexus)

Accessory hemiazygos vein

Hemiazygos vein

Left inferior phrenic vein

Short gastric veins

Submucosal venous plexus

Splenic vein

Left suprarenal vein

Left renal vein

Omental (epiploic) veins

Left gastro-omental (gastroepiploic) vein

Superior mesenteric vein

Right gastro-omental (gastroepiploic) vein

Inferior mesenteric vein

Plate 232

Mediastinum

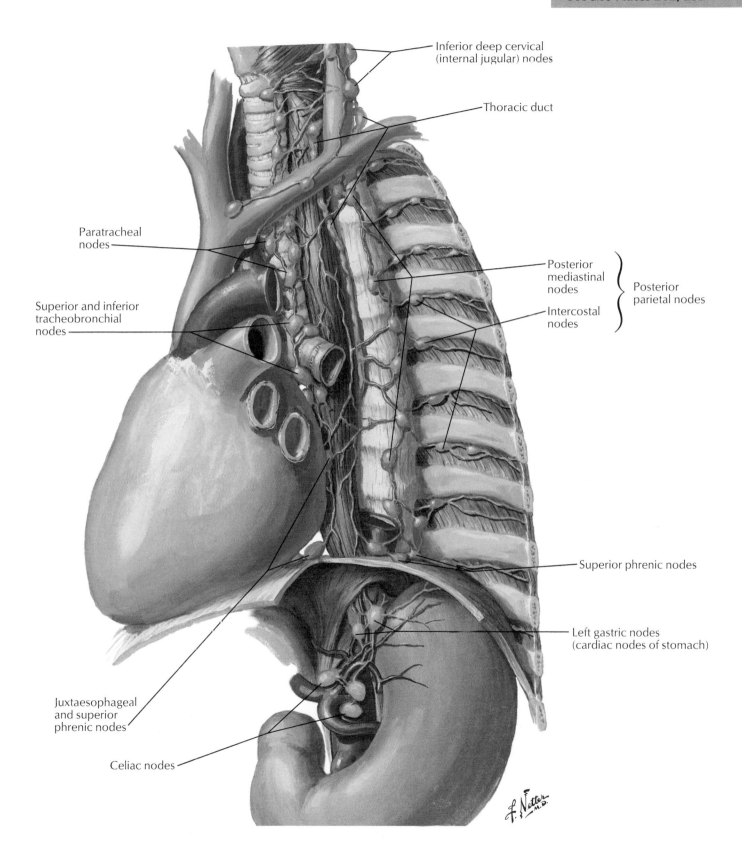

Inferior deep cervical (internal jugular) nodes

Thoracic duct

Paratracheal nodes

Posterior mediastinal nodes

Intercostal nodes

Posterior parietal nodes

Superior and inferior tracheobronchial nodes

Superior phrenic nodes

Left gastric nodes (cardiac nodes of stomach)

Juxtaesophageal and superior phrenic nodes

Celiac nodes

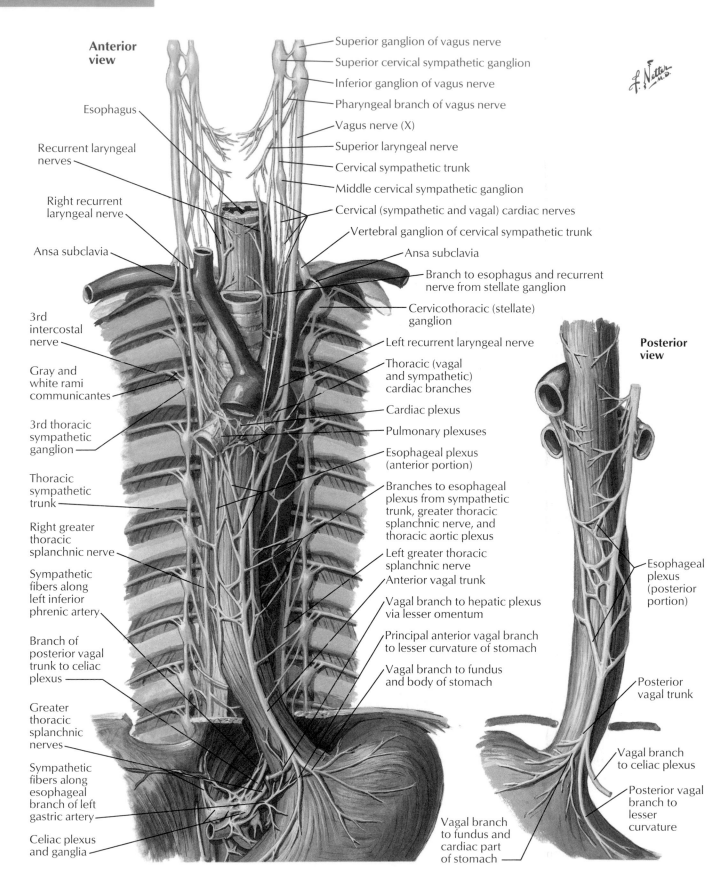

Anterior view

Esophagus

Recurrent laryngeal nerves

Right recurrent laryngeal nerve

Ansa subclavia

3rd intercostal nerve

Gray and white rami communicantes

3rd thoracic sympathetic ganglion

Thoracic sympathetic trunk

Right greater thoracic splanchnic nerve

Sympathetic fibers along left inferior phrenic artery

Branch of posterior vagal trunk to celiac plexus

Greater thoracic splanchnic nerves

Sympathetic fibers along esophageal branch of left gastric artery

Celiac plexus and ganglia

Superior ganglion of vagus nerve

Superior cervical sympathetic ganglion

Inferior ganglion of vagus nerve

Pharyngeal branch of vagus nerve

Vagus nerve (X)

Superior laryngeal nerve

Cervical sympathetic trunk

Middle cervical sympathetic ganglion

Cervical (sympathetic and vagal) cardiac nerves

Vertebral ganglion of cervical sympathetic trunk

Ansa subclavia

Branch to esophagus and recurrent nerve from stellate ganglion

Cervicothoracic (stellate) ganglion

Left recurrent laryngeal nerve

Thoracic (vagal and sympathetic) cardiac branches

Cardiac plexus

Pulmonary plexuses

Esophageal plexus (anterior portion)

Branches to esophageal plexus from sympathetic trunk, greater thoracic splanchnic nerve, and thoracic aortic plexus

Left greater thoracic splanchnic nerve

Anterior vagal trunk

Vagal branch to hepatic plexus via lesser omentum

Principal anterior vagal branch to lesser curvature of stomach

Vagal branch to fundus and body of stomach

Posterior view

Esophageal plexus (posterior portion)

Posterior vagal trunk

Vagal branch to celiac plexus

Posterior vagal branch to lesser curvature

Vagal branch to fundus and cardiac part of stomach

Plate 234

Mediastinum

Series of chest axial CT images from superior (A) to inferior (C)

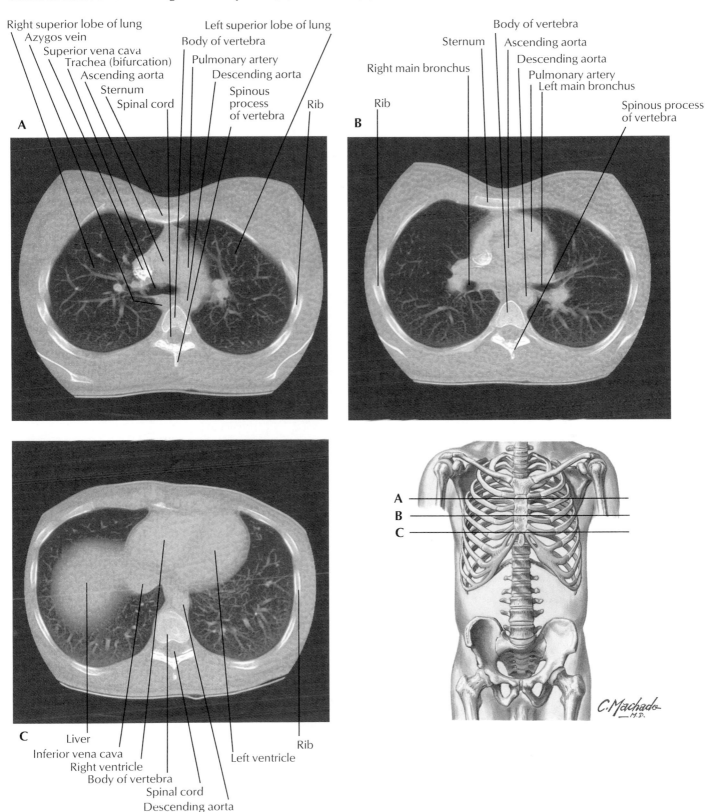

A

Right superior lobe of lung
Azygos vein
Superior vena cava
Trachea (bifurcation)
Ascending aorta
Sternum
Spinal cord

Left superior lobe of lung
Body of vertebra
Pulmonary artery
Descending aorta
Spinous process of vertebra
Rib

B

Right main bronchus
Rib

Sternum
Body of vertebra
Ascending aorta
Descending aorta
Pulmonary artery
Left main bronchus
Spinous process of vertebra

C
Liver
Inferior vena cava
Right ventricle
Body of vertebra
Spinal cord
Descending aorta
Left ventricle
Rib

A
B
C

C. Machado
—M.D.

Transverse Section: Lower Level of T3, Sternoclavicular Joint

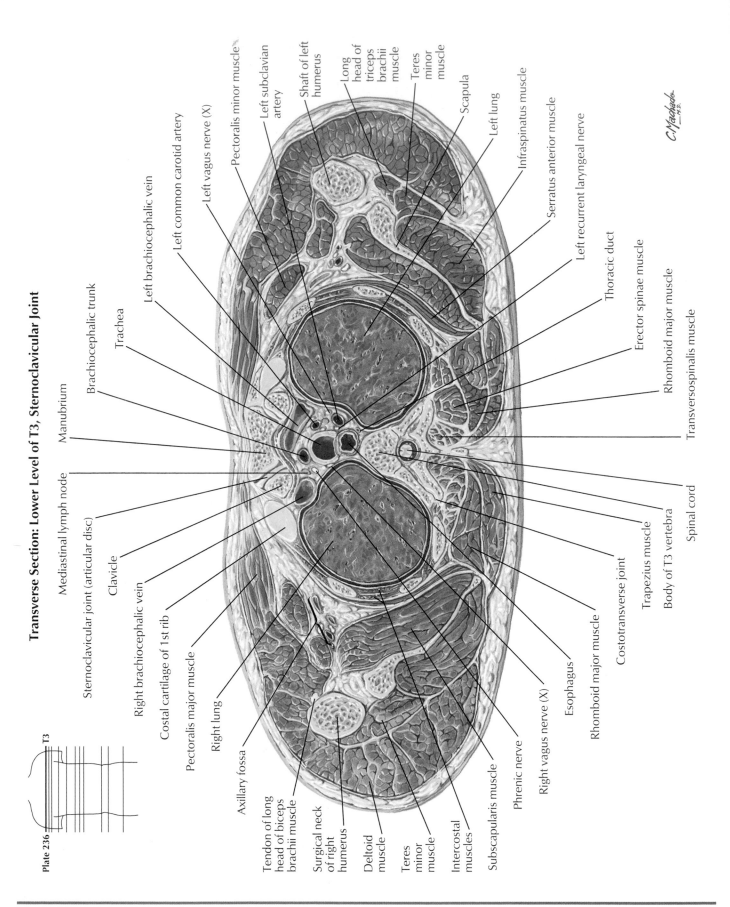

Mediastinal lymph node

Sternoclavicular joint (articular disc)

Clavicle

Right brachiocephalic vein

Costal cartilage of 1st rib

Pectoralis major muscle

Right lung

Axillary fossa

Tendon of long head of biceps brachii muscle

Surgical neck of right humerus

Deltoid muscle

Teres minor muscle

Intercostal muscles

Subscapularis muscle

Phrenic nerve

Right vagus nerve (X)

Esophagus

Rhomboid major muscle

Costotransverse joint

Trapezius muscle

Body of T3 vertebra

Spinal cord

Manubrium

Brachiocephalic trunk

Trachea

Left brachiocephalic vein

Left common carotid artery

Left vagus nerve (X)

Pectoralis minor muscle

Left subclavian artery

Shaft of left humerus

Long head of triceps brachii muscle

Teres minor muscle

Scapula

Left lung

Infraspinatus muscle

Serratus anterior muscle

Left recurrent laryngeal nerve

Thoracic duct

Erector spinae muscle

Rhomboid major muscle

Transversospinalis muscle

C. Machado
_M.D._

Transverse Section: T3–4 Intervertebral Disc, Manubrium

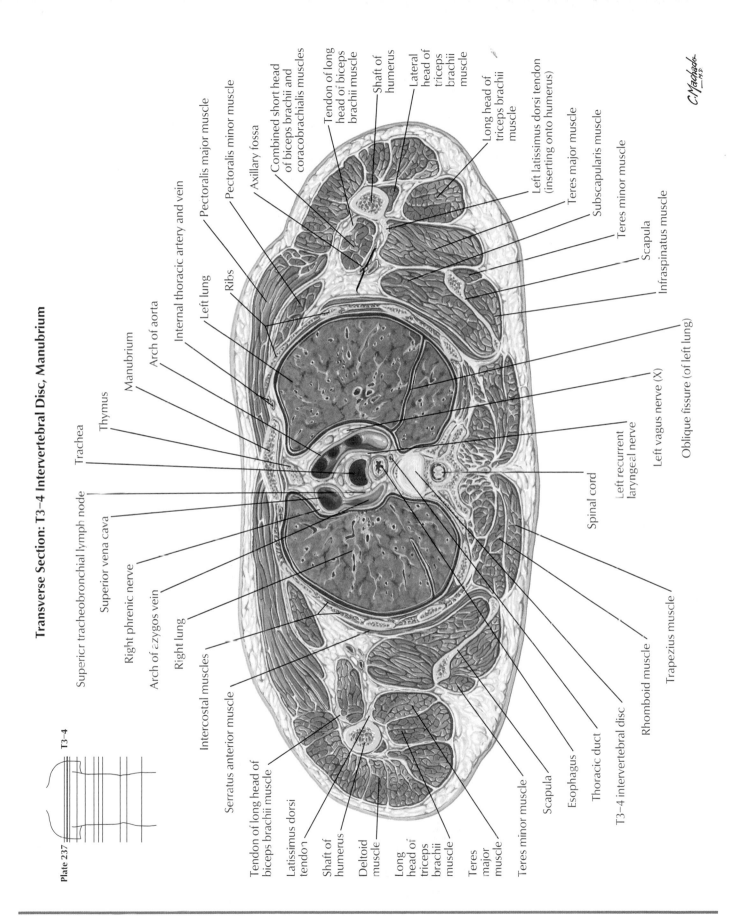

Superior tracheobronchial lymph node

Trachea

Thymus

Superior vena cava

Manubrium

Right phrenic nerve

Arch of aorta

Arch of azygos vein

Internal thoracic artery and vein

Right lung

Left lung

Ribs

Pectoralis major muscle

Pectoralis minor muscle

Axillary fossa

Combined short head of biceps brachii and coracobrachialis muscles

Tendon of long head of biceps brachii muscle

Shaft of humerus

Lateral head of triceps brachii muscle

Long head of triceps brachii muscle

Left latissimus dorsi tendon (inserting onto humerus)

Teres major muscle

Subscapularis muscle

Teres minor muscle

Scapula

Infraspinatus muscle

Oblique fissure (of left lung)

Left vagus nerve (X)

Left recurrent laryngeal nerve

Spinal cord

Trapezius muscle

Rhomboid muscle

T3–4 intervertebral disc

Thoracic duct

Esophagus

Scapula

Teres minor muscle

Teres major muscle

Long head of triceps brachii muscle

Deltoid muscle

Shaft of humerus

Latissimus dorsi tendon

Tendon of long head of biceps brachii muscle

Serratus anterior muscle

Intercostal muscles

Plate 237

T3–4

Transverse Section: T4–5 Intervertebral Disc, Sternal Angle

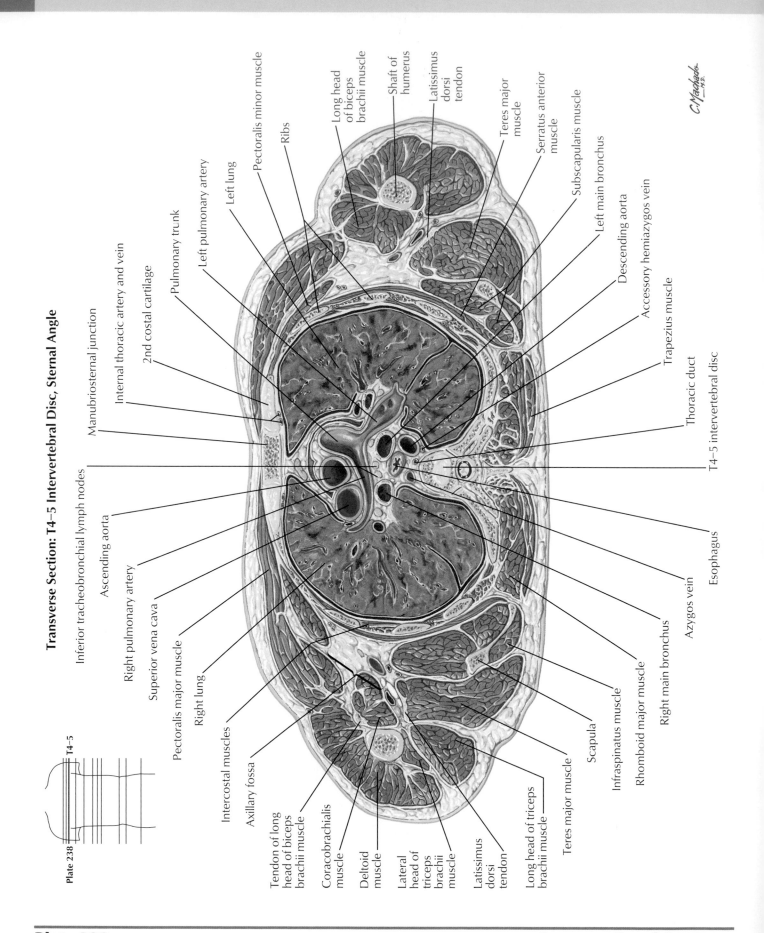

Inferior tracheobronchial lymph nodes

Ascending aorta

Right pulmonary artery

Superior vena cava

Pectoralis major muscle

Right lung

Intercostal muscles

Axillary fossa

Tendon of long head of biceps brachii muscle

Coracobrachialis muscle

Deltoid muscle

Lateral head of triceps brachii muscle

Latissimus dorsi tendon

Long head of triceps brachii muscle

Teres major muscle

Scapula

Infraspinatus muscle

Rhomboid major muscle

Right main bronchus

Azygos vein

Esophagus

Manubriosternal junction

Internal thoracic artery and vein

2nd costal cartilage

Pulmonary trunk

Left pulmonary artery

Left lung

Pectoralis minor muscle

Ribs

Long head of biceps brachii muscle

Shaft of humerus

Latissimus dorsi tendon

Teres major muscle

Serratus anterior muscle

Subscapularis muscle

Left main bronchus

Descending aorta

Accessory hemiazygos vein

Trapezius muscle

Thoracic duct

T4–5 intervertebral disc

T4–5

Plate 238

Transverse Section: Level of T7, 3rd Interchondral Space

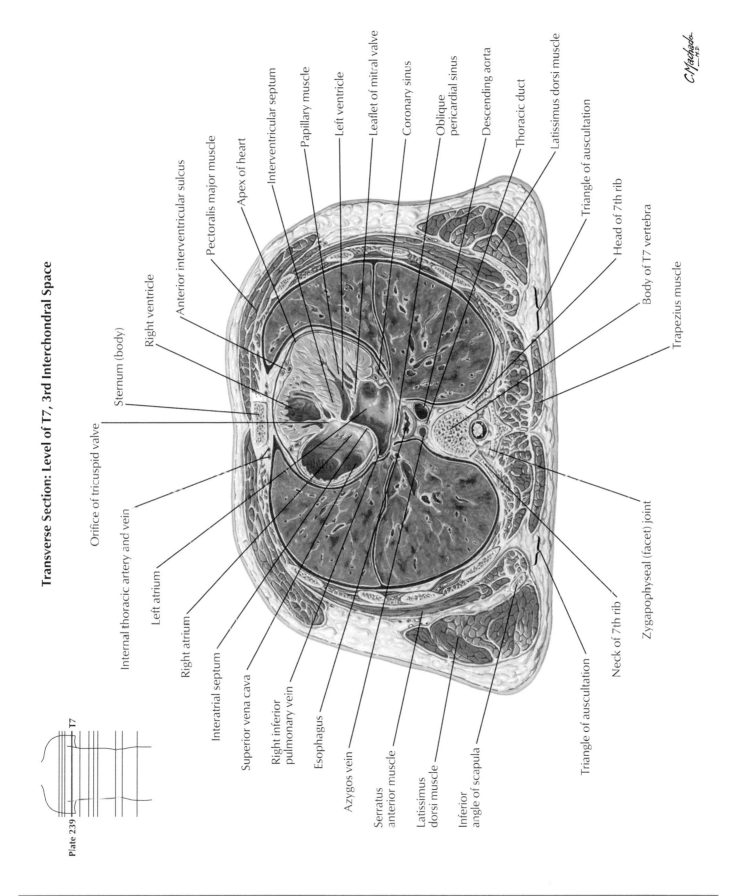

Orifice of tricuspid valve

Internal thoracic artery and vein

Sternum (body)

Right ventricle

Left atrium

Anterior interventricular sulcus

Right atrium

Pectoralis major muscle

Interatrial septum

Apex of heart

Superior vena cava

Interventricular septum

Right inferior pulmonary vein

Papillary muscle

Esophagus

Left ventricle

Azygos vein

Leaflet of mitral valve

Serratus anterior muscle

Coronary sinus

Latissimus dorsi muscle

Oblique pericardial sinus

Inferior angle of scapula

Descending aorta

Thoracic duct

Latissimus dorsi muscle

Triangle of auscultation

Triangle of auscultation

Head of 7th rib

Neck of 7th rib

Body of T7 vertebra

Zygapophyseal (facet) joint

Trapezius muscle

Plate 239

T7

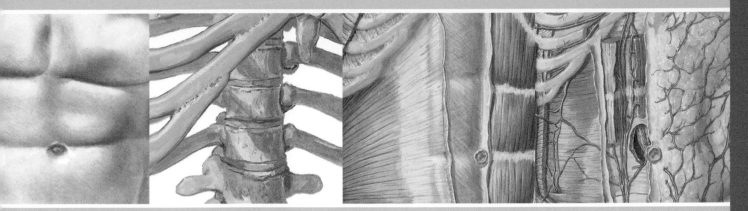

Section 4 ABDOMEN

Cross-sectional Anatomy

Plates 323-330

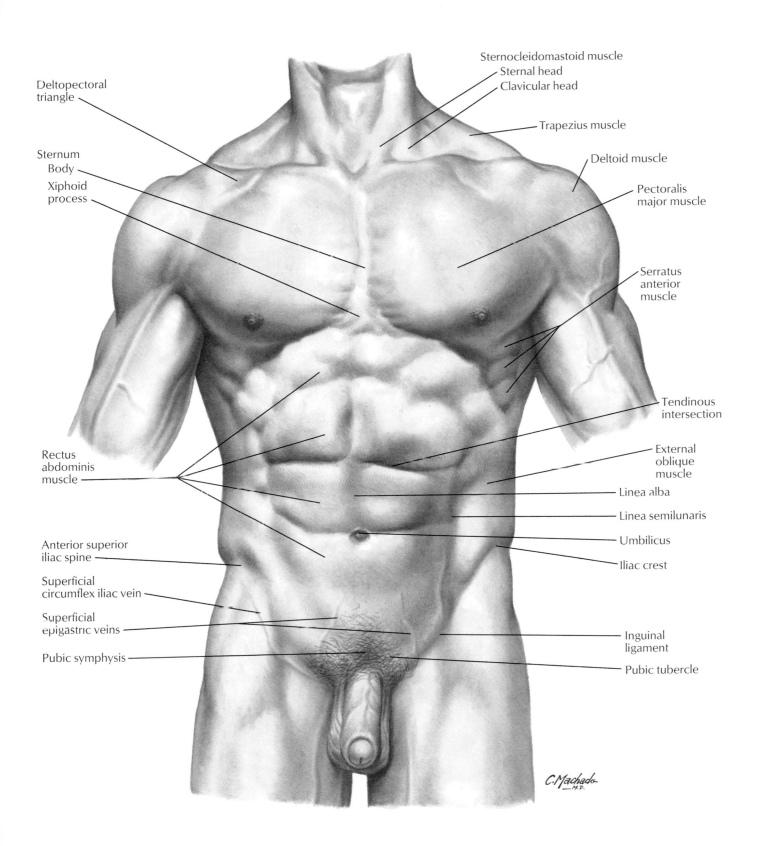

Deltopectoral triangle

Sternum
Body
Xiphoid process

Rectus abdominis muscle

Anterior superior iliac spine

Superficial circumflex iliac vein

Superficial epigastric veins

Pubic symphysis

Sternocleidomastoid muscle
Sternal head
Clavicular head

Trapezius muscle

Deltoid muscle

Pectoralis major muscle

Serratus anterior muscle

Tendinous intersection

External oblique muscle

Linea alba

Linea semilunaris

Umbilicus

Iliac crest

Inguinal ligament

Pubic tubercle

C. Machado
M.D.

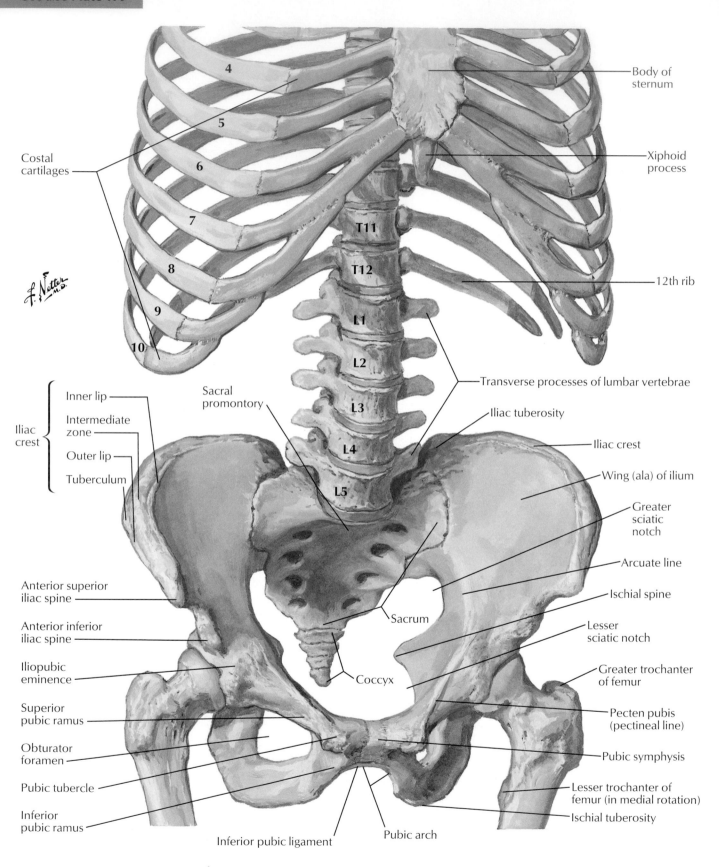

Body of
sternum

Xiphoid
process

Costal
cartilages

4

5

6

7

T11

T12

8

12th rib

9

10

Transverse processes of lumbar vertebrae

L1

L2

Inner lip

Sacral
promontory

Iliac tuberosity

Intermediate
zone

L3

Iliac crest

Iliac
crest

Outer lip

L4

Wing (ala) of ilium

Tuberculum

L5

Greater
sciatic
notch

Arcuate line

Anterior superior
iliac spine

Ischial spine

Anterior inferior
iliac spine

Sacrum

Lesser
sciatic
notch

Iliopubic
eminence

Coccyx

Greater trochanter
of femur

Superior
pubic ramus

Pecten pubis
(pectineal line)

Obturator
foramen

Pubic symphysis

Pubic tubercle

Lesser trochanter of
femur (in medial rotation)

Inferior
pubic ramus

Ischial tuberosity

Inferior pubic ligament

Pubic arch

Plate 241

Body Wall

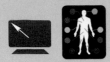

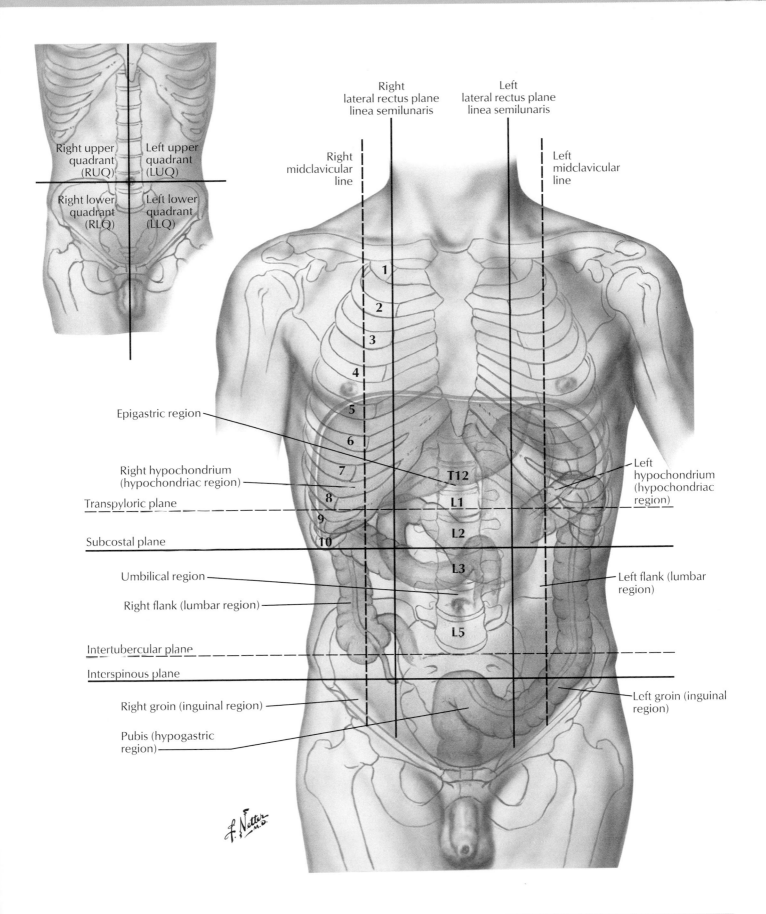

Right upper quadrant (RUQ)

Left upper quadrant (LUQ)

Right lower quadrant (RLQ)

Left lower quadrant (LLQ)

Right lateral rectus plane linea semilunaris

Left lateral rectus plane linea semilunaris

Right midclavicular line

Left midclavicular line

1

2

3

4

5

6

7

8

9

10

T12

L1

L2

L3

L5

Epigastric region

Right hypochondrium (hypochondriac region)

Transpyloric plane

Subcostal plane

Umbilical region

Right flank (lumbar region)

Intertubercular plane

Interspinous plane

Right groin (inguinal region)

Pubis (hypogastric region)

Left hypochondrium (hypochondriac region)

Left flank (lumbar region)

Left groin (inguinal region)

F. Netter M.D.

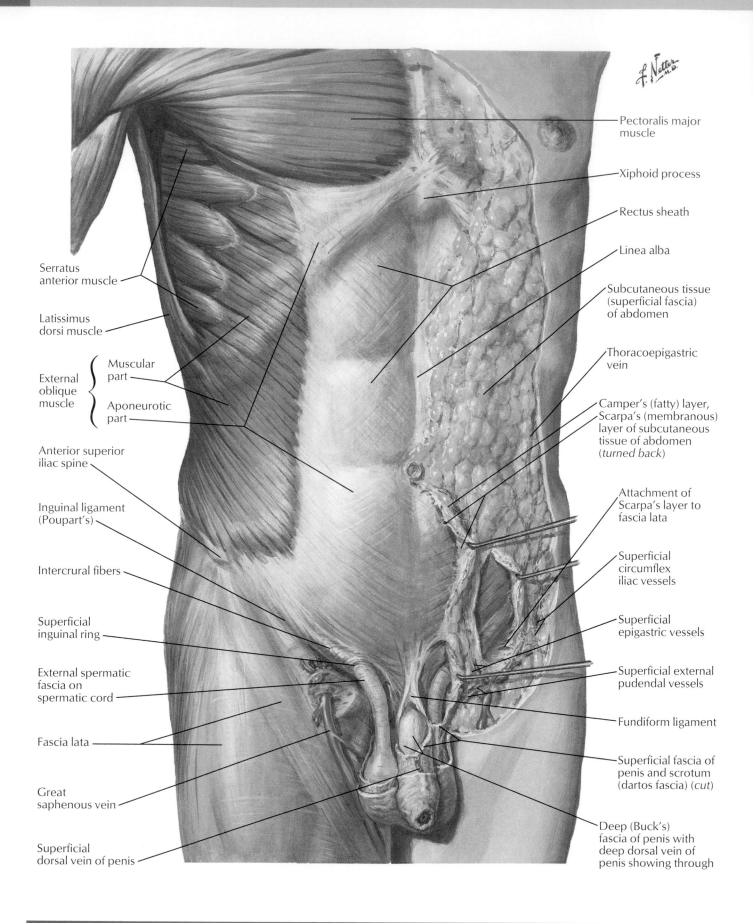

Pectoralis major muscle

Xiphoid process

Rectus sheath

Linea alba

Subcutaneous tissue (superficial fascia) of abdomen

Thoracoepigastric vein

Camper's (fatty) layer, Scarpa's (membranous) layer of subcutaneous tissue of abdomen (*turned back*)

Attachment of Scarpa's layer to fascia lata

Superficial circumflex iliac vessels

Superficial epigastric vessels

Superficial external pudendal vessels

Fundiform ligament

Superficial fascia of penis and scrotum (dartos fascia) (*cut*)

Deep (Buck's) fascia of penis with deep dorsal vein of penis showing through

Serratus anterior muscle

Latissimus dorsi muscle

External oblique muscle { Muscular part / Aponeurotic part

Anterior superior iliac spine

Inguinal ligament (Poupart's)

Intercrural fibers

Superficial inguinal ring

External spermatic fascia on spermatic cord

Fascia lata

Great saphenous vein

Superficial dorsal vein of penis

Plate 243   **Body Wall**

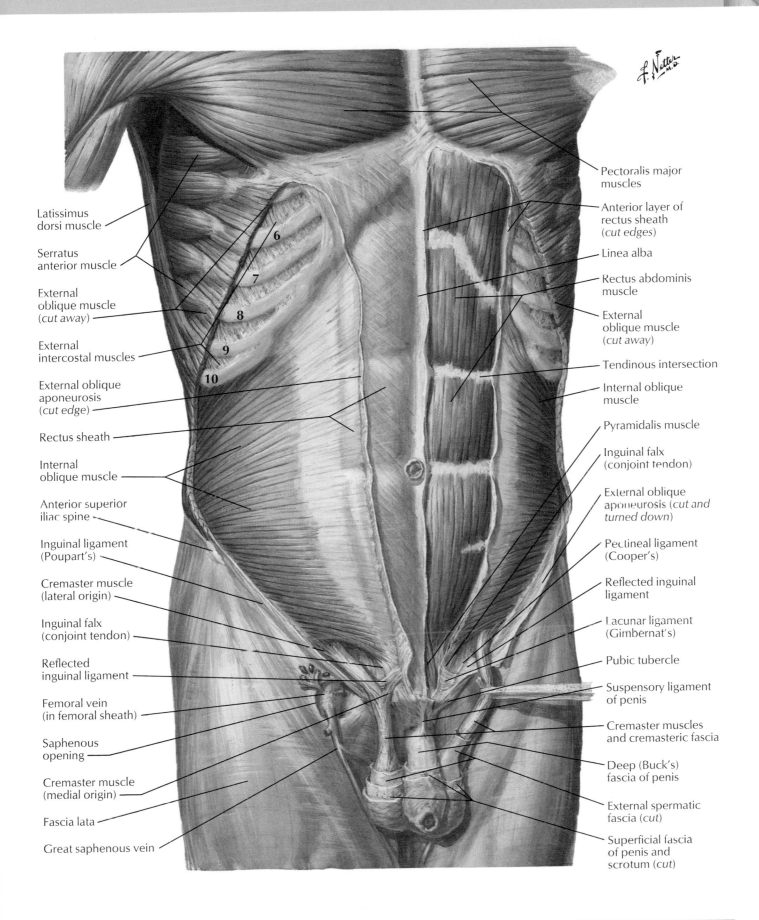

Latissimus
dorsi muscle

Serratus
anterior muscle

External
oblique muscle
(cut away)

External
intercostal muscles

External oblique
aponeurosis
(cut edge)

Rectus sheath

Internal
oblique muscle

Anterior superior
iliac spine

Inguinal ligament
(Poupart's)

Cremaster muscle
(lateral origin)

Inguinal falx
(conjoint tendon)

Reflected
inguinal ligament

Femoral vein
(in femoral sheath)

Saphenous
opening

Cremaster muscle
(medial origin)

Fascia lata

Great saphenous vein

6

7

8

9

10

Pectoralis major
muscles

Anterior layer of
rectus sheath
(cut edges)

Linea alba

Rectus abdominis
muscle

External
oblique muscle
(cut away)

Tendinous intersection

Internal oblique
muscle

Pyramidalis muscle

Inguinal falx
(conjoint tendon)

External oblique
aponeurosis (cut and
turned down)

Pectineal ligament
(Cooper's)

Reflected inguinal
ligament

Lacunar ligament
(Gimbernat's)

Pubic tubercle

Suspensory ligament
of penis

Cremaster muscles
and cremasteric fascia

Deep (Buck's)
fascia of penis

External spermatic
fascia (cut)

Superficial fascia
of penis and
scrotum (cut)

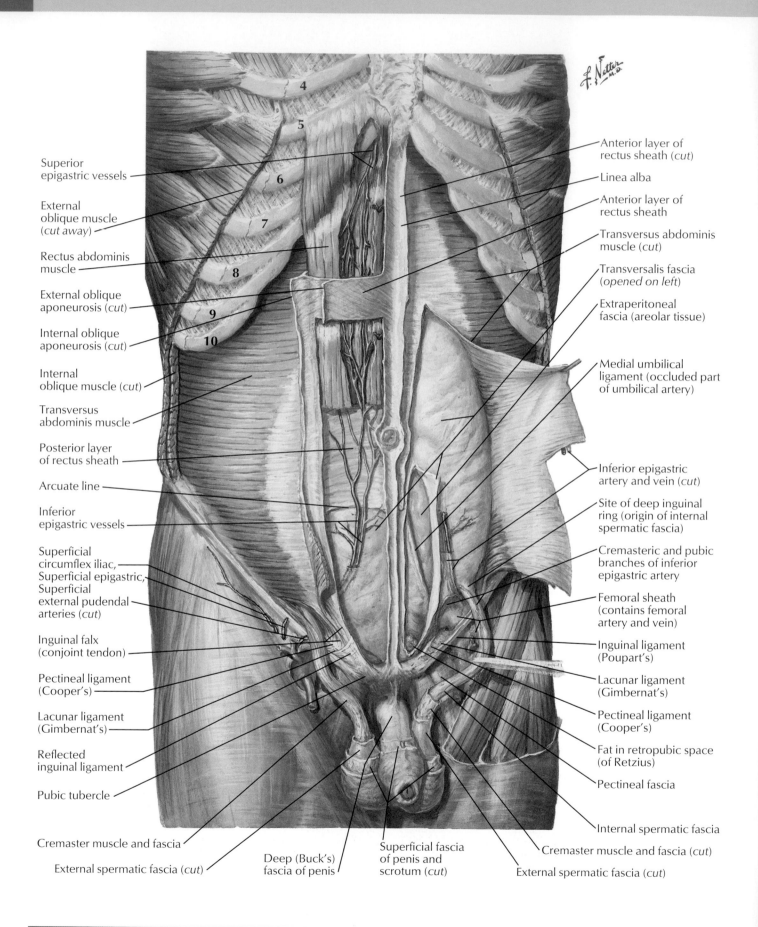

Superior epigastric vessels

External oblique muscle (*cut away*)

Rectus abdominis muscle

External oblique aponeurosis (*cut*)

Internal oblique aponeurosis (*cut*)

Internal oblique muscle (*cut*)

Transversus abdominis muscle

Posterior layer of rectus sheath

Arcuate line

Inferior epigastric vessels

Superficial circumflex iliac, Superficial epigastric, Superficial external pudendal arteries (*cut*)

Inguinal falx (conjoint tendon)

Pectineal ligament (Cooper's)

Lacunar ligament (Gimbernat's)

Reflected inguinal ligament

Pubic tubercle

Cremaster muscle and fascia

External spermatic fascia (*cut*)

Deep (Buck's) fascia of penis

Superficial fascia of penis and scrotum (*cut*)

Anterior layer of rectus sheath (*cut*)

Linea alba

Anterior layer of rectus sheath

Transversus abdominis muscle (*cut*)

Transversalis fascia (*opened on left*)

Extraperitoneal fascia (areolar tissue)

Medial umbilical ligament (occluded part of umbilical artery)

Inferior epigastric artery and vein (*cut*)

Site of deep inguinal ring (origin of internal spermatic fascia)

Cremasteric and pubic branches of inferior epigastric artery

Femoral sheath (contains femoral artery and vein)

Inguinal ligament (Poupart's)

Lacunar ligament (Gimbernat's)

Pectineal ligament (Cooper's)

Fat in retropubic space (of Retzius)

Pectineal fascia

Internal spermatic fascia

Cremaster muscle and fascia (*cut*)

External spermatic fascia (*cut*)

Plate 245

Body Wall

Section above arcuate line

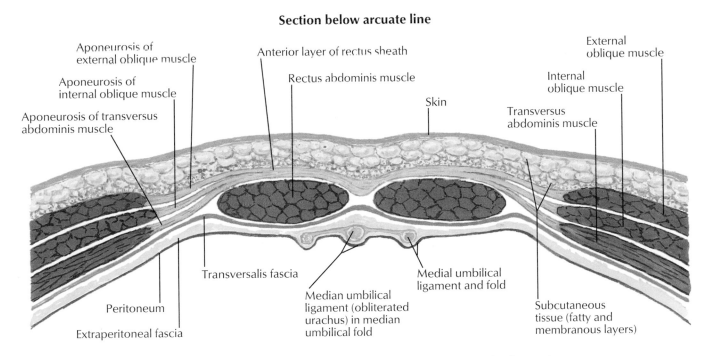

Aponeurosis of external oblique muscle

Aponeurosis of internal oblique muscle

Aponeurosis of transversus abdominis muscle

Anterior layer of rectus sheath

Rectus abdominis muscle

Linea alba

Skin

External oblique muscle

Internal oblique muscle

Transversus abdominis muscle

Posterior layer of rectus sheath

Falciform ligament

Subcutaneous tissue (fatty layer)

Peritoneum

Extraperitoneal fascia

Transversalis fascia

Aponeurosis of internal oblique muscle splits to form anterior and posterior layers of rectus sheath. Aponeurosis of external oblique muscle joins anterior layer of sheath; aponeurosis of transversus abdominis muscle joins posterior layer. Anterior and posterior layers of rectus sheath unite medially to form linea alba.

Section below arcuate line

Aponeurosis of external oblique muscle

Aponeurosis of internal oblique muscle

Aponeurosis of transversus abdominis muscle

Anterior layer of rectus sheath

Rectus abdominis muscle

Skin

External oblique muscle

Internal oblique muscle

Transversus abdominis muscle

Transversalis fascia

Medial umbilical ligament and fold

Median umbilical ligament (obliterated urachus) in median umbilical fold

Peritoneum

Extraperitoneal fascia

Subcutaneous tissue (fatty and membranous layers)

Aponeurosis of internal oblique muscle does not split at this level but passes completely anterior to rectus abdominis muscle and is fused there with both aponeurosis of external oblique muscle and that of transversus abdominis muscle. Thus, posterior wall of rectus sheath is absent below arcuate line and is composed of only transversalis fascia.

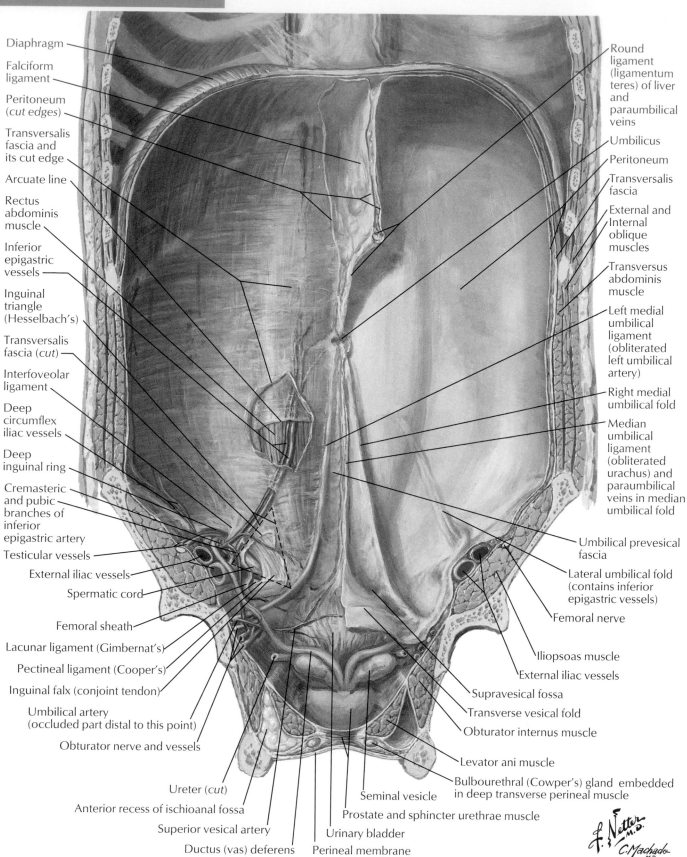

Diaphragm

Falciform ligament

Peritoneum (*cut edges*)

Transversalis fascia and its cut edge

Arcuate line

Rectus abdominis muscle

Inferior epigastric vessels

Inguinal triangle (Hesselbach's)

Transversalis fascia (*cut*)

Interfoveolar ligament

Deep circumflex iliac vessels

Deep inguinal ring

Cremasteric and pubic branches of inferior epigastric artery

Testicular vessels

External iliac vessels

Spermatic cord

Femoral sheath

Lacunar ligament (Gimbernat's)

Pectineal ligament (Cooper's)

Inguinal falx (conjoint tendon)

Umbilical artery (occluded part distal to this point)

Obturator nerve and vessels

Ureter (*cut*)

Anterior recess of ischioanal fossa

Superior vesical artery

Ductus (vas) deferens

Round ligament (ligamentum teres) of liver and paraumbilical veins

Umbilicus

Peritoneum

Transversalis fascia

External and Internal oblique muscles

Transversus abdominis muscle

Left medial umbilical ligament (obliterated left umbilical artery)

Right medial umbilical fold

Median umbilical ligament (obliterated urachus) and paraumbilical veins in median umbilical fold

Umbilical prevesical fascia

Lateral umbilical fold (contains inferior epigastric vessels)

Femoral nerve

Iliopsoas muscle

External iliac vessels

Supravesical fossa

Transverse vesical fold

Obturator internus muscle

Levator ani muscle

Bulbourethral (Cowper's) gland embedded in deep transverse perineal muscle

Seminal vesicle

Prostate and sphincter urethrae muscle

Urinary bladder

Perineal membrane

Plate 247

Body Wall

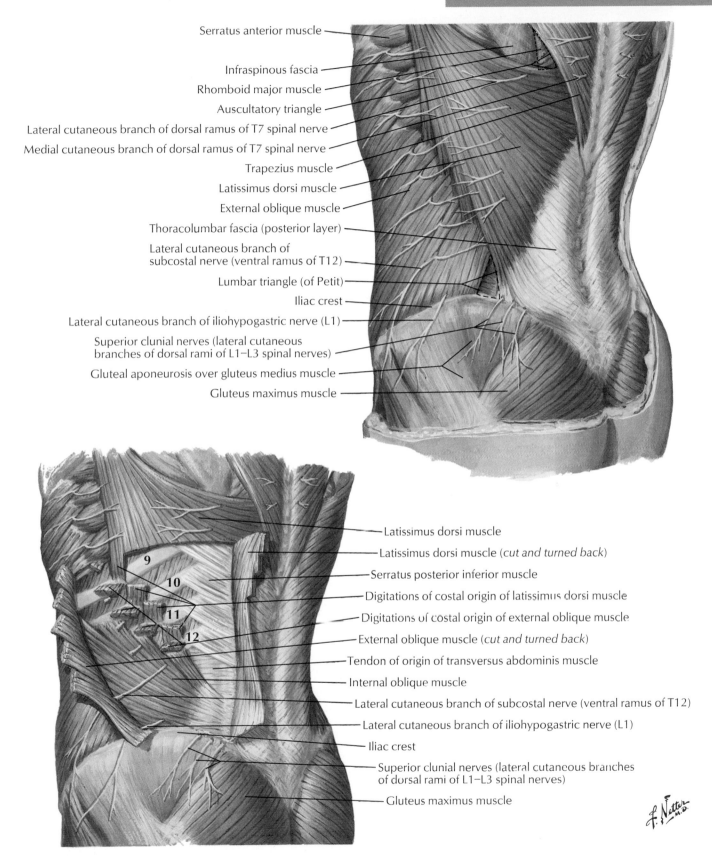

Serratus anterior muscle

Infraspinous fascia

Rhomboid major muscle

Auscultatory triangle

Lateral cutaneous branch of dorsal ramus of T7 spinal nerve

Medial cutaneous branch of dorsal ramus of T7 spinal nerve

Trapezius muscle

Latissimus dorsi muscle

External oblique muscle

Thoracolumbar fascia (posterior layer)

Lateral cutaneous branch of subcostal nerve (ventral ramus of T12)

Lumbar triangle (of Petit)

Iliac crest

Lateral cutaneous branch of iliohypogastric nerve (L1)

Superior clunial nerves (lateral cutaneous branches of dorsal rami of L1–L3 spinal nerves)

Gluteal aponeurosis over gluteus medius muscle

Gluteus maximus muscle

Latissimus dorsi muscle

Latissimus dorsi muscle (*cut and turned back*)

Serratus posterior inferior muscle

Digitations of costal origin of latissimus dorsi muscle

Digitations of costal origin of external oblique muscle

External oblique muscle (*cut and turned back*)

Tendon of origin of transversus abdominis muscle

Internal oblique muscle

Lateral cutaneous branch of subcostal nerve (ventral ramus of T12)

Lateral cutaneous branch of iliohypogastric nerve (L1)

Iliac crest

Superior clunial nerves (lateral cutaneous branches of dorsal rami of L1–L3 spinal nerves)

Gluteus maximus muscle

9

10

11

12

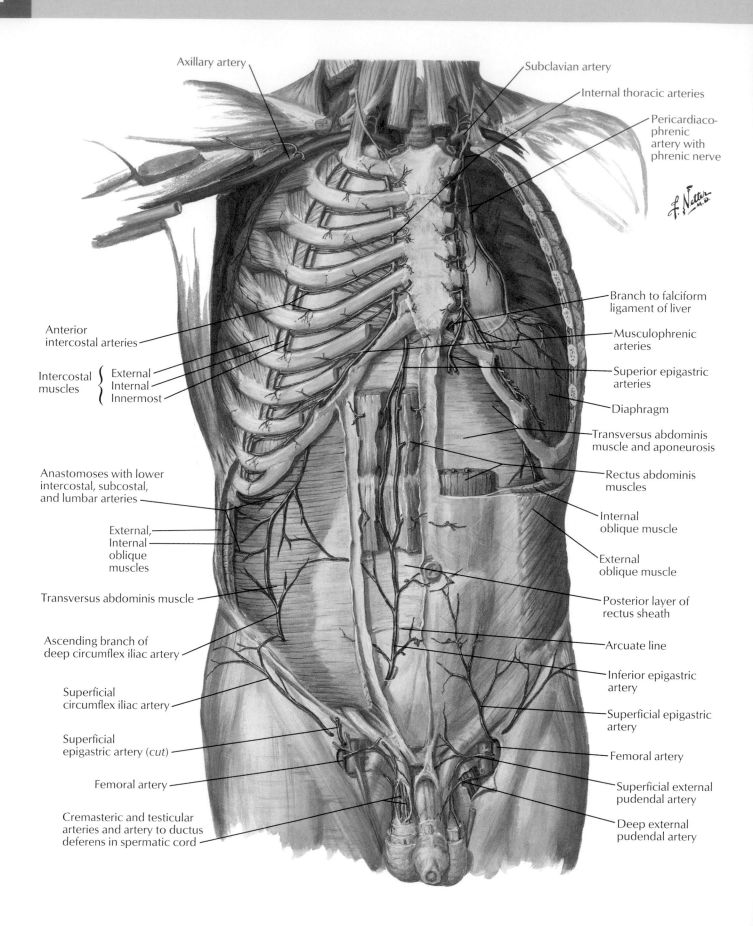

Axillary artery

Subclavian artery

Internal thoracic arteries

Pericardiaco-phrenic artery with phrenic nerve

Anterior intercostal arteries

Intercostal muscles { External Internal Innermost

Branch to falciform ligament of liver

Musculophrenic arteries

Superior epigastric arteries

Diaphragm

Transversus abdominis muscle and aponeurosis

Rectus abdominis muscles

Anastomoses with lower intercostal, subcostal, and lumbar arteries

Internal oblique muscle

External, Internal oblique muscles

External oblique muscle

Transversus abdominis muscle

Posterior layer of rectus sheath

Ascending branch of deep circumflex iliac artery

Arcuate line

Inferior epigastric artery

Superficial circumflex iliac artery

Superficial epigastric artery

Superficial epigastric artery (cut)

Femoral artery

Femoral artery

Superficial external pudendal artery

Cremasteric and testicular arteries and artery to ductus deferens in spermatic cord

Deep external pudendal artery

Plate 249

Body Wall

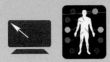

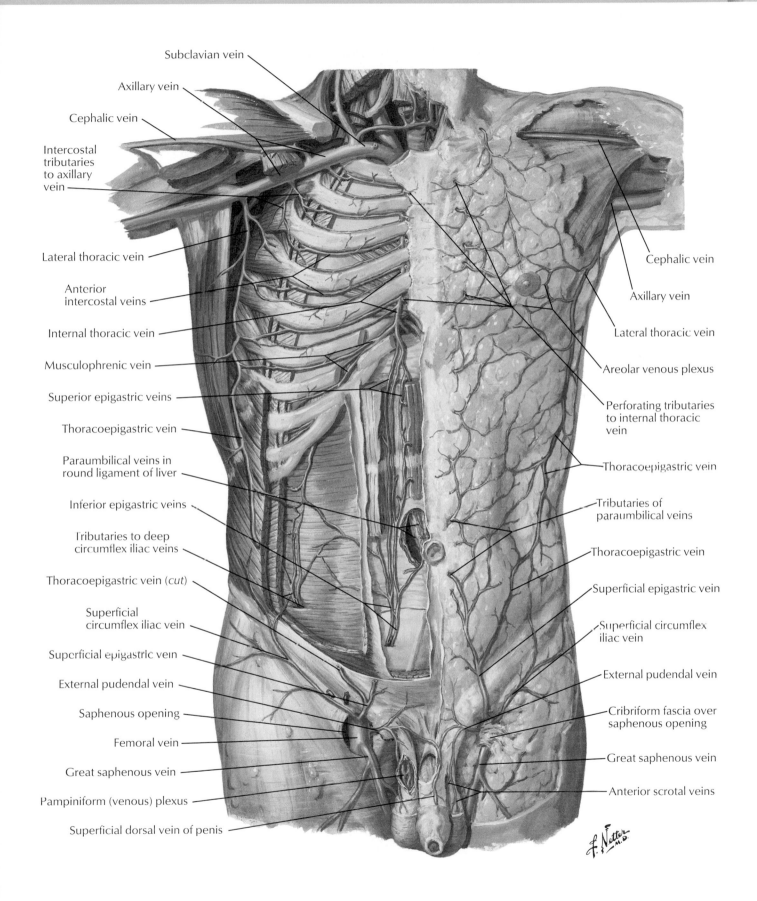

Subclavian vein

Axillary vein

Cephalic vein

Intercostal tributaries to axillary vein

Lateral thoracic vein

Anterior intercostal veins

Internal thoracic vein

Musculophrenic vein

Superior epigastric veins

Thoracoepigastric vein

Paraumbilical veins in round ligament of liver

Inferior epigastric veins

Tributaries to deep circumflex iliac veins

Thoracoepigastric vein (cut)

Superficial circumflex iliac vein

Superficial epigastric vein

External pudendal vein

Saphenous opening

Femoral vein

Great saphenous vein

Pampiniform (venous) plexus

Superficial dorsal vein of penis

Cephalic vein

Axillary vein

Lateral thoracic vein

Areolar venous plexus

Perforating tributaries to internal thoracic vein

Thoracoepigastric vein

Tributaries of paraumbilical veins

Thoracoepigastric vein

Superficial epigastric vein

Superficial circumflex iliac vein

External pudendal vein

Cribriform fascia over saphenous opening

Great saphenous vein

Anterior scrotal veins

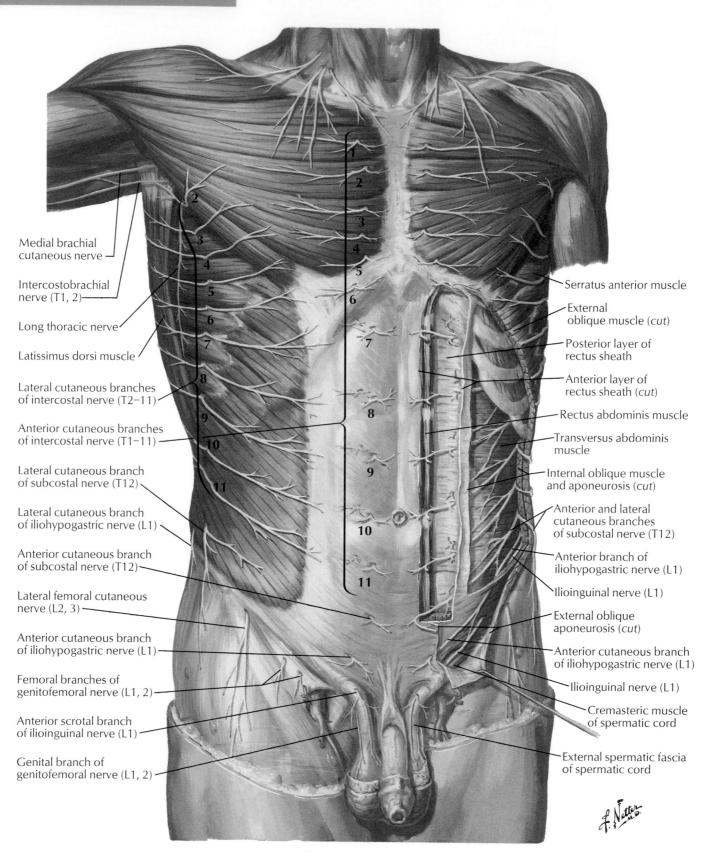

Medial brachial cutaneous nerve

Intercostobrachial nerve (T1, 2)

Long thoracic nerve

Latissimus dorsi muscle

Lateral cutaneous branches of intercostal nerve (T2–11)

Anterior cutaneous branches of intercostal nerve (T1–11)

Lateral cutaneous branch of subcostal nerve (T12)

Lateral cutaneous branch of iliohypogastric nerve (L1)

Anterior cutaneous branch of subcostal nerve (T12)

Lateral femoral cutaneous nerve (L2, 3)

Anterior cutaneous branch of iliohypogastric nerve (L1)

Femoral branches of genitofemoral nerve (L1, 2)

Anterior scrotal branch of ilioinguinal nerve (L1)

Genital branch of genitofemoral nerve (L1, 2)

Serratus anterior muscle

External oblique muscle (cut)

Posterior layer of rectus sheath

Anterior layer of rectus sheath (cut)

Rectus abdominis muscle

Transversus abdominis muscle

Internal oblique muscle and aponeurosis (cut)

Anterior and lateral cutaneous branches of subcostal nerve (T12)

Anterior branch of iliohypogastric nerve (L1)

Ilioinguinal nerve (L1)

External oblique aponeurosis (cut)

Anterior cutaneous branch of iliohypogastric nerve (L1)

Ilioinguinal nerve (L1)

Cremasteric muscle of spermatic cord

External spermatic fascia of spermatic cord

Plate 251

Body Wall

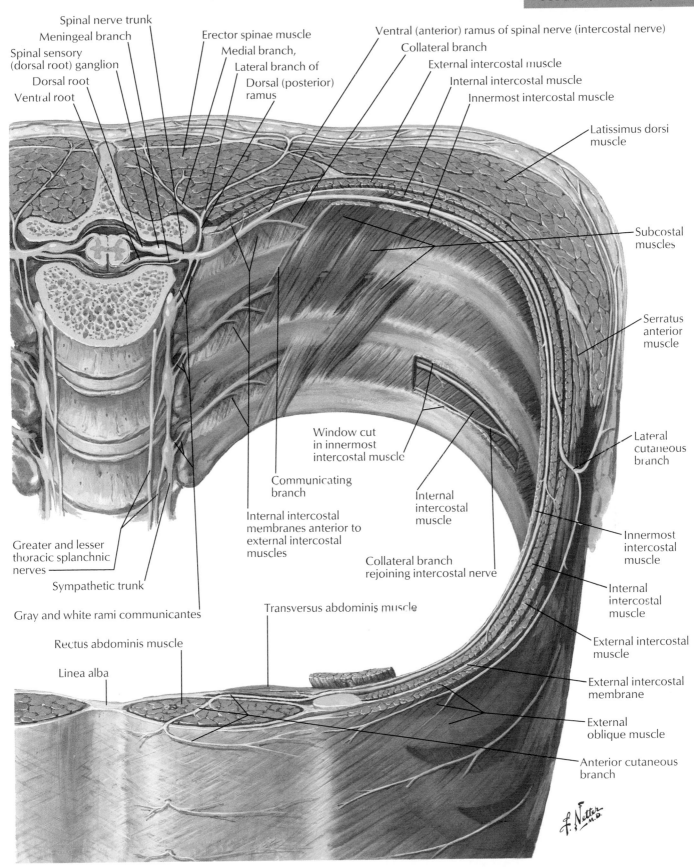

Spinal nerve trunk

Meningeal branch

Spinal sensory
(dorsal root) ganglion

Dorsal root

Ventral root

Erector spinae muscle

Medial branch,

Lateral branch of

Dorsal (posterior)
ramus

Ventral (anterior) ramus of spinal nerve (intercostal nerve)

Collateral branch

External intercostal muscle

Internal intercostal muscle

Innermost intercostal muscle

Latissimus dorsi
muscle

Subcostal
muscles

Serratus
anterior
muscle

Lateral
cutaneous
branch

Window cut
in innermost
intercostal muscle

Communicating
branch

Internal intercostal
membranes anterior to
external intercostal
muscles

Internal
intercostal
muscle

Collateral branch
rejoining intercostal nerve

Innermost
intercostal
muscle

Internal
intercostal
muscle

External intercostal
muscle

Greater and lesser
thoracic splanchnic
nerves

Sympathetic trunk

Gray and white rami communicantes

Rectus abdominis muscle

Linea alba

Transversus abdominis muscle

External intercostal
membrane

External
oblique muscle

Anterior cutaneous
branch

F. Netter M.D.

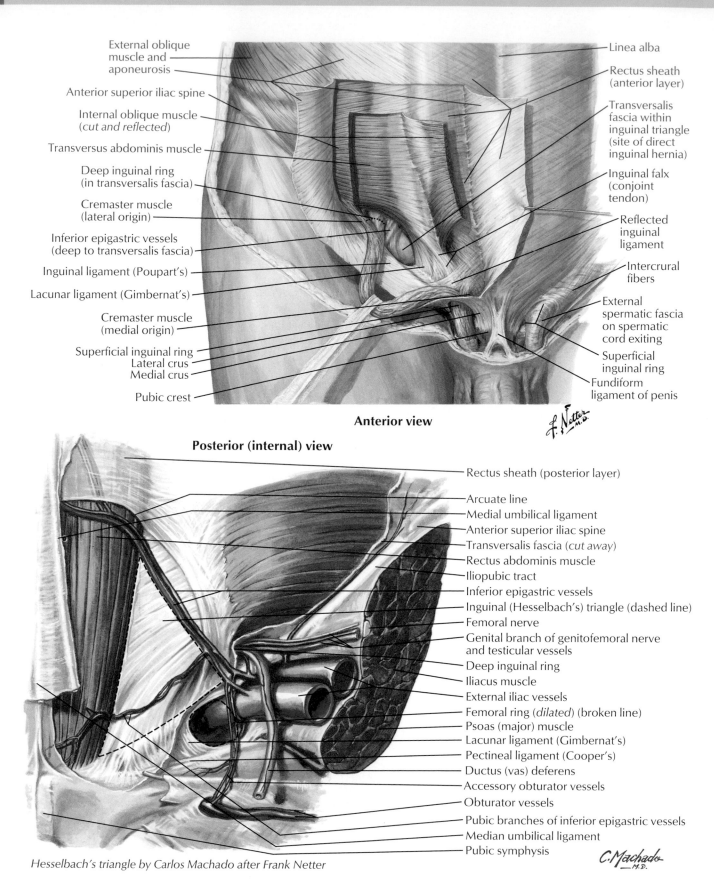

External oblique muscle and aponeurosis

Anterior superior iliac spine

Internal oblique muscle (cut and reflected)

Transversus abdominis muscle

Deep inguinal ring (in transversalis fascia)

Cremaster muscle (lateral origin)

Inferior epigastric vessels (deep to transversalis fascia)

Inguinal ligament (Poupart's)

Lacunar ligament (Gimbernat's)

Cremaster muscle (medial origin)

Superficial inguinal ring
Lateral crus
Medial crus

Pubic crest

Linea alba

Rectus sheath (anterior layer)

Transversalis fascia within inguinal triangle (site of direct inguinal hernia)

Inguinal falx (conjoint tendon)

Reflected inguinal ligament

Intercrural fibers

External spermatic fascia on spermatic cord exiting

Superficial inguinal ring

Fundiform ligament of penis

Anterior view

Posterior (internal) view

Rectus sheath (posterior layer)

Arcuate line

Medial umbilical ligament

Anterior superior iliac spine

Transversalis fascia (cut away)

Rectus abdominis muscle

Iliopubic tract

Inferior epigastric vessels

Inguinal (Hesselbach's) triangle (dashed line)

Femoral nerve

Genital branch of genitofemoral nerve and testicular vessels

Deep inguinal ring

Iliacus muscle

External iliac vessels

Femoral ring (dilated) (broken line)

Psoas (major) muscle

Lacunar ligament (Gimbernat's)

Pectineal ligament (Cooper's)

Ductus (vas) deferens

Accessory obturator vessels

Obturator vessels

Pubic branches of inferior epigastric vessels

Median umbilical ligament

Pubic symphysis

Hesselbach's triangle by Carlos Machado after Frank Netter

Plate 253   **Body Wall**

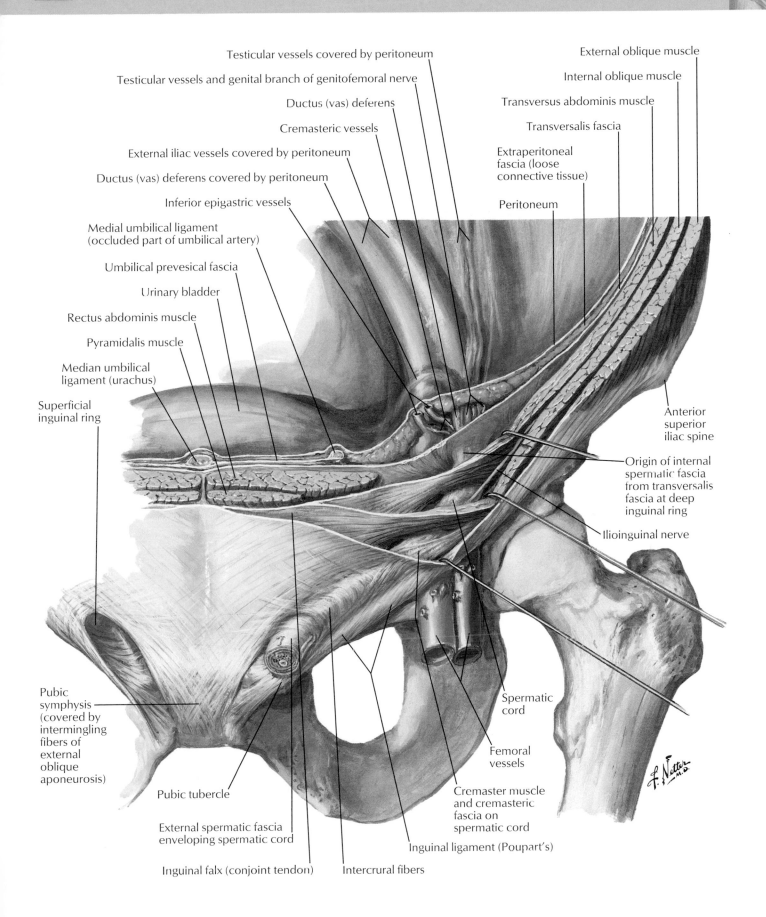

Testicular vessels covered by peritoneum

Testicular vessels and genital branch of genitofemoral nerve

Ductus (vas) deferens

Cremasteric vessels

External iliac vessels covered by peritoneum

Ductus (vas) deferens covered by peritoneum

Inferior epigastric vessels

Medial umbilical ligament (occluded part of umbilical artery)

Umbilical prevesical fascia

Urinary bladder

Rectus abdominis muscle

Pyramidalis muscle

Median umbilical ligament (urachus)

Superficial inguinal ring

External oblique muscle

Internal oblique muscle

Transversus abdominis muscle

Transversalis fascia

Extraperitoneal fascia (loose connective tissue)

Peritoneum

Anterior superior iliac spine

Origin of internal spermatic fascia from transversalis fascia at deep inguinal ring

Ilioinguinal nerve

Spermatic cord

Femoral vessels

Cremaster muscle and cremasteric fascia on spermatic cord

Inguinal ligament (Poupart's)

Pubic symphysis (covered by intermingling fibers of external oblique aponeurosis)

Pubic tubercle

External spermatic fascia enveloping spermatic cord

Inguinal falx (conjoint tendon)

Intercrural fibers

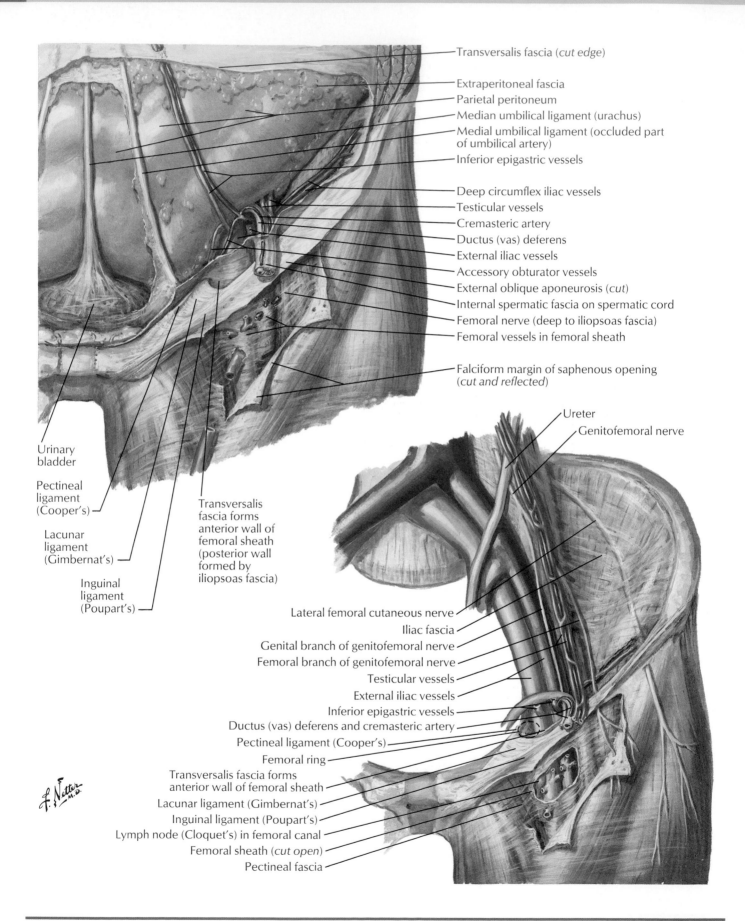

Transversalis fascia (*cut edge*)

Extraperitoneal fascia

Parietal peritoneum

Median umbilical ligament (urachus)

Medial umbilical ligament (occluded part of umbilical artery)

Inferior epigastric vessels

Deep circumflex iliac vessels

Testicular vessels

Cremasteric artery

Ductus (vas) deferens

External iliac vessels

Accessory obturator vessels

External oblique aponeurosis (*cut*)

Internal spermatic fascia on spermatic cord

Femoral nerve (deep to iliopsoas fascia)

Femoral vessels in femoral sheath

Falciform margin of saphenous opening (*cut and reflected*)

Ureter

Genitofemoral nerve

Urinary bladder

Pectineal ligament (Cooper's)

Lacunar ligament (Gimbernat's)

Inguinal ligament (Poupart's)

Transversalis fascia forms anterior wall of femoral sheath (posterior wall formed by iliopsoas fascia)

Lateral femoral cutaneous nerve

Iliac fascia

Genital branch of genitofemoral nerve

Femoral branch of genitofemoral nerve

Testicular vessels

External iliac vessels

Inferior epigastric vessels

Ductus (vas) deferens and cremasteric artery

Pectineal ligament (Cooper's)

Femoral ring

Transversalis fascia forms anterior wall of femoral sheath

Lacunar ligament (Gimbernat's)

Inguinal ligament (Poupart's)

Lymph node (Cloquet's) in femoral canal

Femoral sheath (*cut open*)

Pectineal fascia

Plate 255

Body Wall

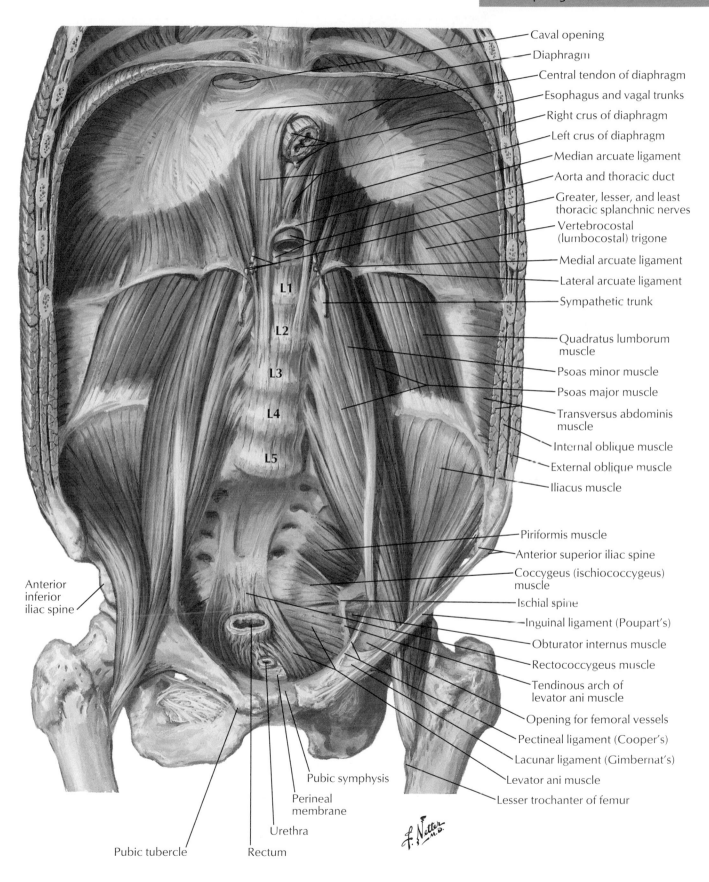

Caval opening

Diaphragm

Central tendon of diaphragm

Esophagus and vagal trunks

Right crus of diaphragm

Left crus of diaphragm

Median arcuate ligament

Aorta and thoracic duct

Greater, lesser, and least thoracic splanchnic nerves

Vertebrocostal (lumbocostal) trigone

Medial arcuate ligament

Lateral arcuate ligament

Sympathetic trunk

Quadratus lumborum muscle

Psoas minor muscle

Psoas major muscle

Transversus abdominis muscle

Internal oblique muscle

External oblique muscle

Iliacus muscle

Piriformis muscle

Anterior superior iliac spine

Coccygeus (ischiococcygeus) muscle

Ischial spine

Inguinal ligament (Poupart's)

Obturator internus muscle

Rectococcygeus muscle

Tendinous arch of levator ani muscle

Opening for femoral vessels

Pectineal ligament (Cooper's)

Lacunar ligament (Gimbernat's)

Levator ani muscle

Lesser trochanter of femur

L1
L2
L3
L4
L5

Anterior inferior iliac spine

Pubic symphysis

Perineal membrane

Urethra

Pubic tubercle

Rectum

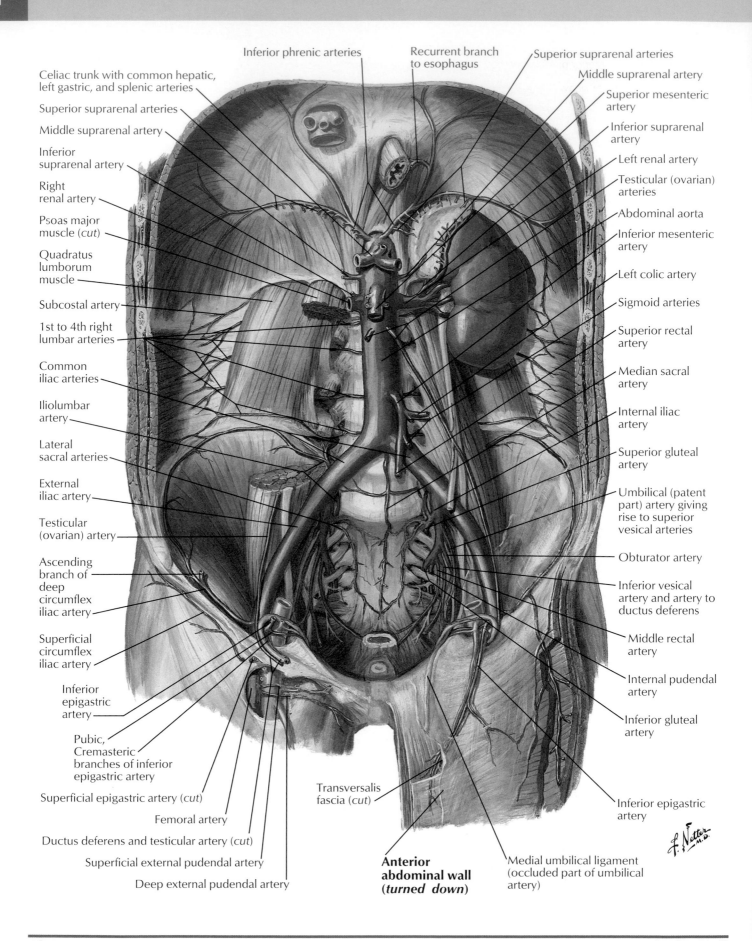

Inferior phrenic arteries

Recurrent branch to esophagus

Superior suprarenal arteries

Middle suprarenal artery

Superior mesenteric artery

Inferior suprarenal artery

Left renal artery

Testicular (ovarian) arteries

Abdominal aorta

Inferior mesenteric artery

Left colic artery

Sigmoid arteries

Superior rectal artery

Median sacral artery

Internal iliac artery

Superior gluteal artery

Umbilical (patent part) artery giving rise to superior vesical arteries

Obturator artery

Inferior vesical artery and artery to ductus deferens

Middle rectal artery

Internal pudendal artery

Inferior gluteal artery

Inferior epigastric artery

Medial umbilical ligament (occluded part of umbilical artery)

Anterior abdominal wall (_turned down_)

Transversalis fascia (cut)

Deep external pudendal artery

Superficial external pudendal artery

Ductus deferens and testicular artery (cut)

Femoral artery

Superficial epigastric artery (cut)

Pubic, Cremasteric branches of inferior epigastric artery

Inferior epigastric artery

Superficial circumflex iliac artery

Ascending branch of deep circumflex iliac artery

Testicular (ovarian) artery

External iliac artery

Lateral sacral arteries

Iliolumbar artery

Common iliac arteries

1st to 4th right lumbar arteries

Subcostal artery

Quadratus lumborum muscle

Psoas major muscle (cut)

Right renal artery

Inferior suprarenal artery

Middle suprarenal artery

Superior suprarenal arteries

Celiac trunk with common hepatic, left gastric, and splenic arteries

F. Netter M.D.

Plate 257 **Body Wall**

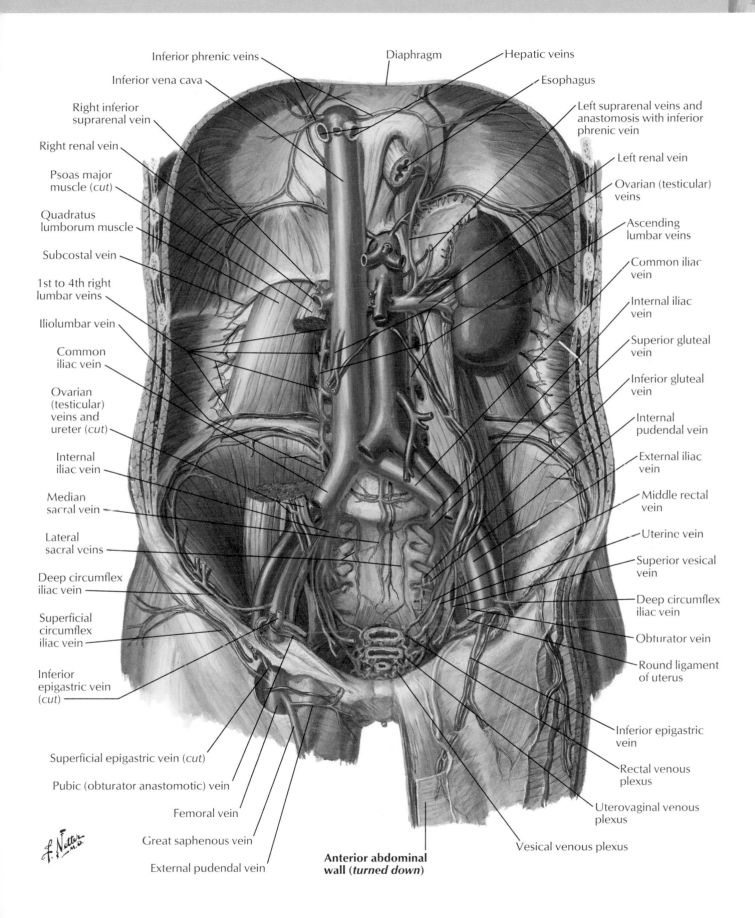

Inferior phrenic veins

Diaphragm

Hepatic veins

Inferior vena cava

Esophagus

Right inferior suprarenal vein

Left suprarenal veins and anastomosis with inferior phrenic vein

Right renal vein

Left renal vein

Psoas major muscle (cut)

Ovarian (testicular) veins

Quadratus lumborum muscle

Ascending lumbar veins

Subcostal vein

Common iliac vein

1st to 4th right lumbar veins

Internal iliac vein

Iliolumbar vein

Superior gluteal vein

Common iliac vein

Inferior gluteal vein

Ovarian (testicular) veins and ureter (cut)

Internal pudendal vein

Internal iliac vein

External iliac vein

Median sacral vein

Middle rectal vein

Lateral sacral veins

Uterine vein

Deep circumflex iliac vein

Superior vesical vein

Superficial circumflex iliac vein

Deep circumflex iliac vein

Inferior epigastric vein (cut)

Obturator vein

Round ligament of uterus

Inferior epigastric vein

Superficial epigastric vein (cut)

Rectal venous plexus

Pubic (obturator anastomotic) vein

Uterovaginal venous plexus

Femoral vein

Great saphenous vein

Vesical venous plexus

External pudendal vein

Anterior abdominal wall (turned down)

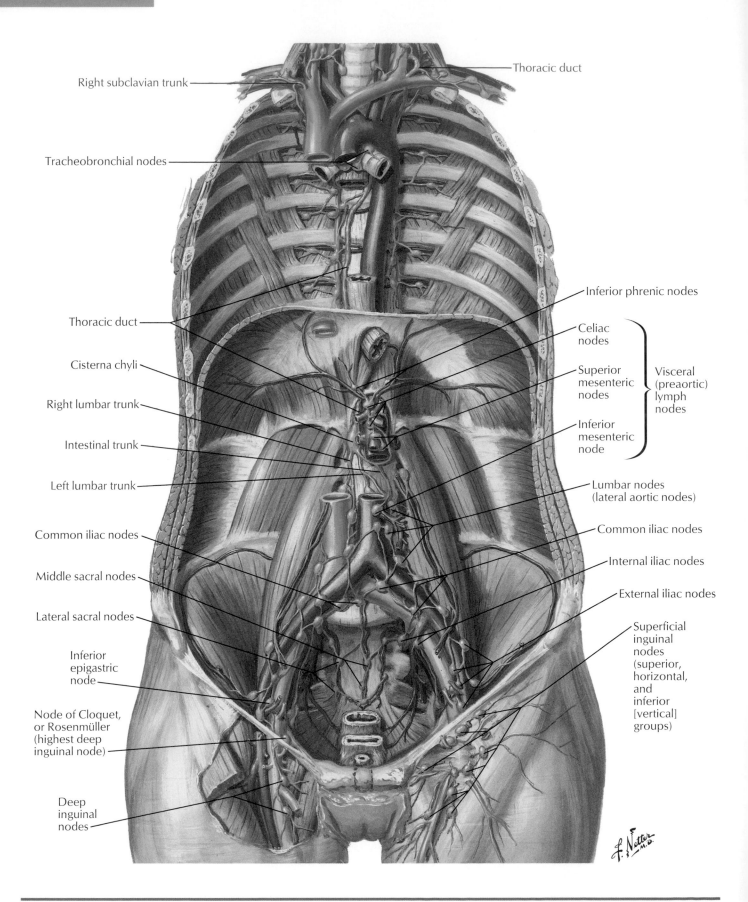

Thoracic duct

Right subclavian trunk

Tracheobronchial nodes

Inferior phrenic nodes

Thoracic duct

Celiac nodes

Cisterna chyli

Superior mesenteric nodes

Visceral (preaortic) lymph nodes

Right lumbar trunk

Intestinal trunk

Inferior mesenteric node

Left lumbar trunk

Lumbar nodes (lateral aortic nodes)

Common iliac nodes

Common iliac nodes

Internal iliac nodes

Middle sacral nodes

External iliac nodes

Lateral sacral nodes

Inferior epigastric node

Superficial inguinal nodes (superior, horizontal, and inferior [vertical] groups)

Node of Cloquet, or Rosenmüller (highest deep inguinal node)

Deep inguinal nodes

Plate 259

Body Wall

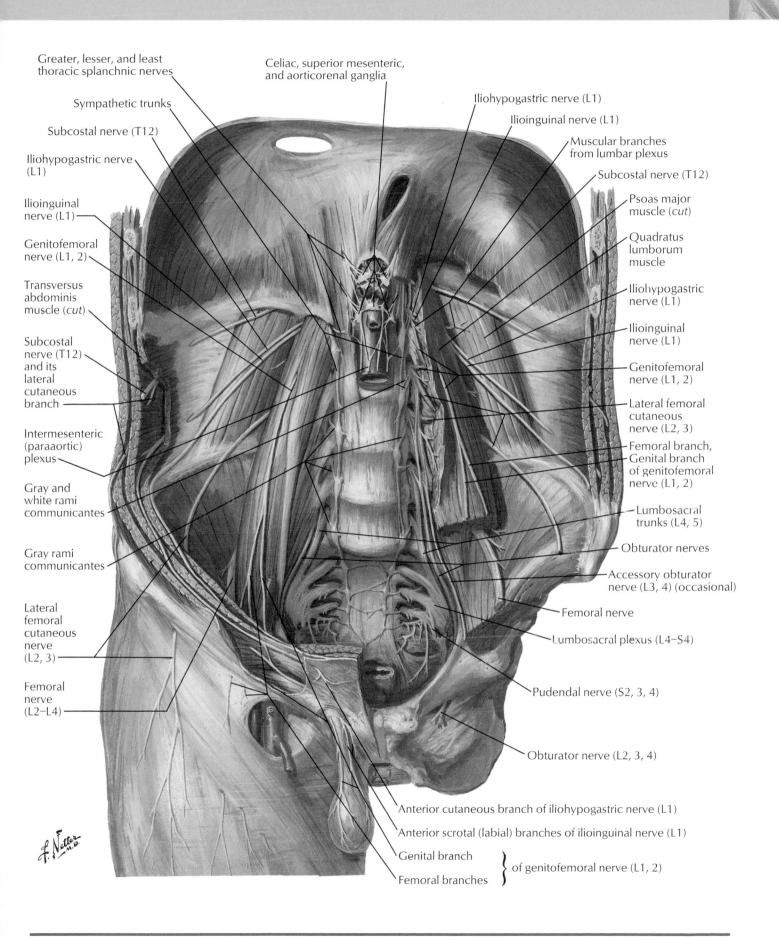

Greater, lesser, and least thoracic splanchnic nerves

Sympathetic trunks

Subcostal nerve (T12)

Iliohypogastric nerve (L1)

Ilioinguinal nerve (L1)

Genitofemoral nerve (L1, 2)

Transversus abdominis muscle (cut)

Subcostal nerve (T12) and its lateral cutaneous branch

Intermesenteric (paraaortic) plexus

Gray and white rami communicantes

Gray rami communicantes

Lateral femoral cutaneous nerve (L2, 3)

Femoral nerve (L2–L4)

Celiac, superior mesenteric, and aorticorenal ganglia

Iliohypogastric nerve (L1)

Ilioinguinal nerve (L1)

Muscular branches from lumbar plexus

Subcostal nerve (T12)

Psoas major muscle (cut)

Quadratus lumborum muscle

Iliohypogastric nerve (L1)

Ilioinguinal nerve (L1)

Genitofemoral nerve (L1, 2)

Lateral femoral cutaneous nerve (L2, 3)

Femoral branch, Genital branch of genitofemoral nerve (L1, 2)

Lumbosacral trunks (L4, 5)

Obturator nerves

Accessory obturator nerve (L3, 4) (occasional)

Femoral nerve

Lumbosacral plexus (L4–S4)

Pudendal nerve (S2, 3, 4)

Obturator nerve (L2, 3, 4)

Anterior cutaneous branch of iliohypogastric nerve (L1)

Anterior scrotal (labial) branches of ilioinguinal nerve (L1)

Genital branch
Femoral branches } of genitofemoral nerve (L1, 2)

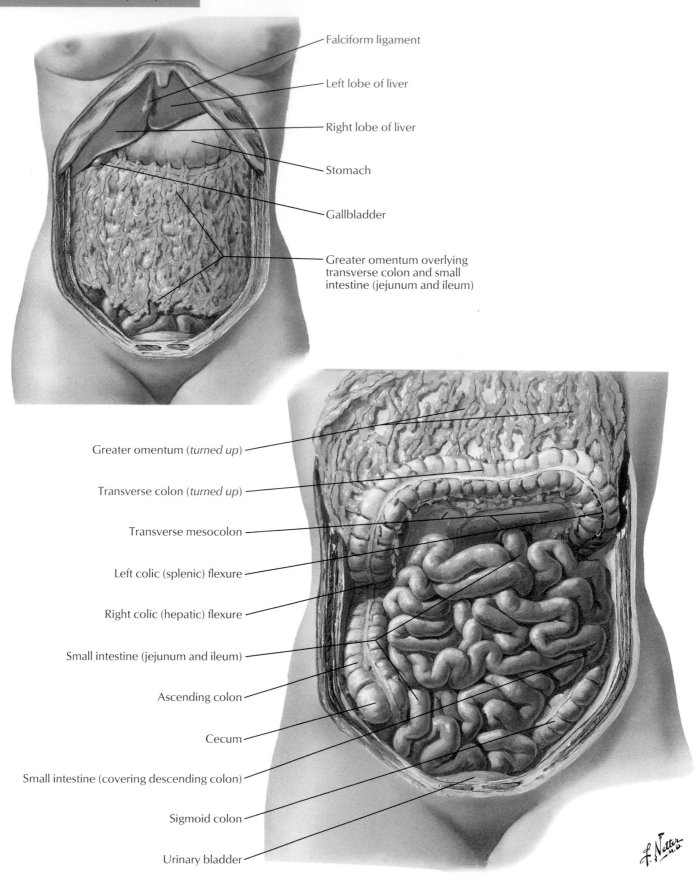

Falciform ligament

Left lobe of liver

Right lobe of liver

Stomach

Gallbladder

Greater omentum overlying transverse colon and small intestine (jejunum and ileum)

Greater omentum (*turned up*)

Transverse colon (*turned up*)

Transverse mesocolon

Left colic (splenic) flexure

Right colic (hepatic) flexure

Small intestine (jejunum and ileum)

Ascending colon

Cecum

Small intestine (covering descending colon)

Sigmoid colon

Urinary bladder

Plate 261

Peritoneal Cavity

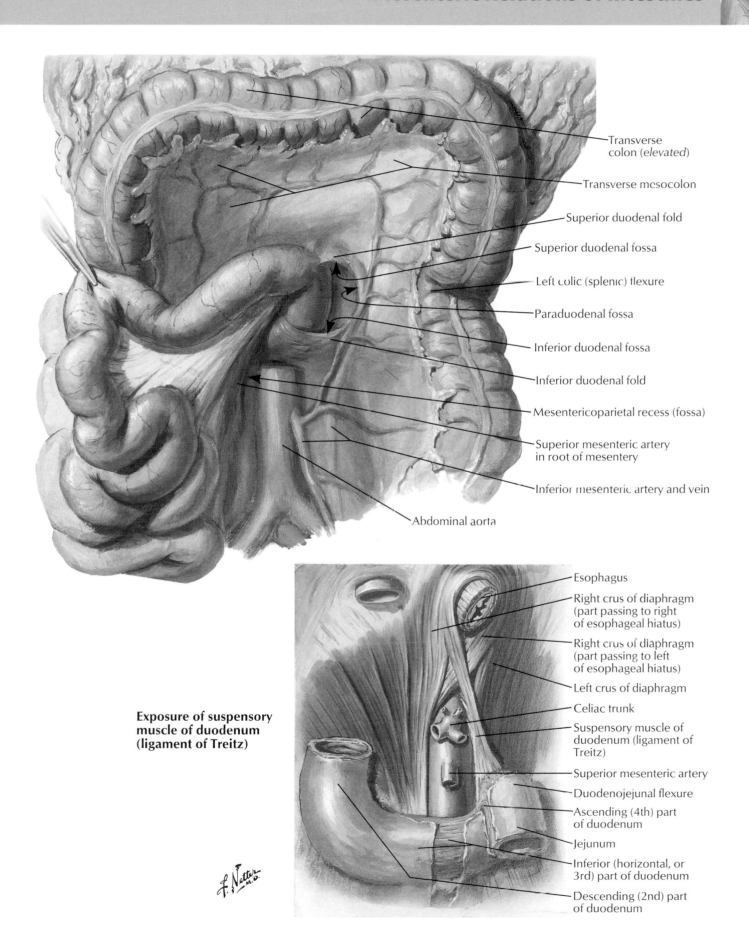

Transverse colon (*elevated*)

Transverse mesocolon

Superior duodenal fold

Superior duodenal fossa

Left colic (splenic) flexure

Paraduodenal fossa

Inferior duodenal fossa

Inferior duodenal fold

Mesentericoparietal recess (fossa)

Superior mesenteric artery in root of mesentery

Inferior mesenteric artery and vein

Abdominal aorta

Exposure of suspensory muscle of duodenum (ligament of Treitz)

Esophagus

Right crus of diaphragm (part passing to right of esophageal hiatus)

Right crus of diaphragm (part passing to left of esophageal hiatus)

Left crus of diaphragm

Celiac trunk

Suspensory muscle of duodenum (ligament of Treitz)

Superior mesenteric artery

Duodenojejunal flexure

Ascending (4th) part of duodenum

Jejunum

Inferior (horizontal, or 3rd) part of duodenum

Descending (2nd) part of duodenum

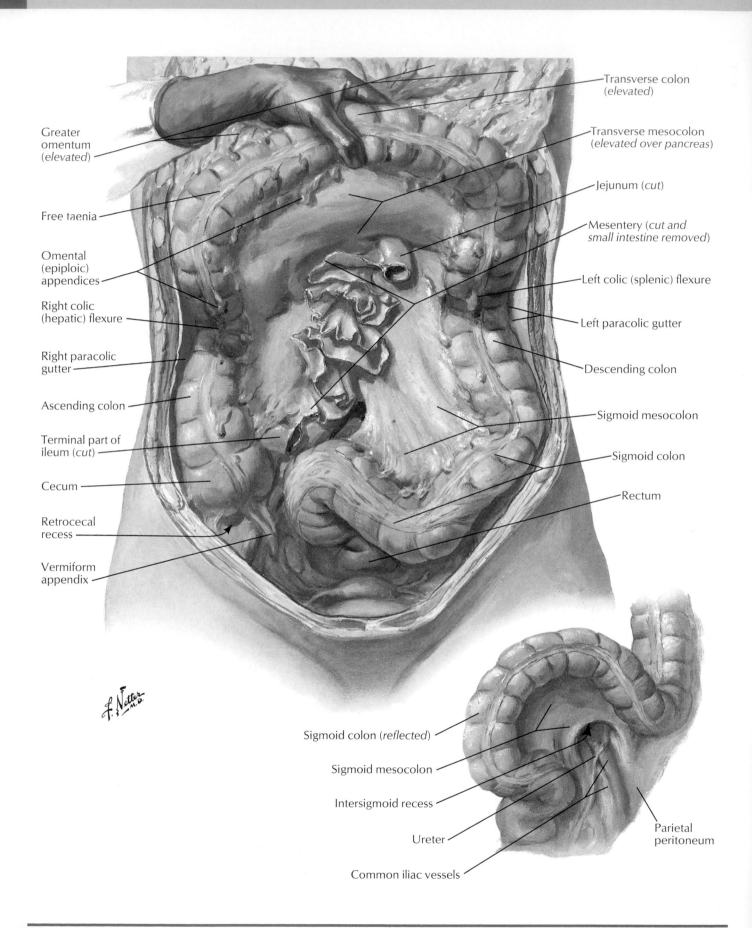

Greater omentum (*elevated*)

Free taenia

Omental (epiploic) appendices

Right colic (hepatic) flexure

Right paracolic gutter

Ascending colon

Terminal part of ileum (*cut*)

Cecum

Retrocecal recess

Vermiform appendix

Transverse colon (*elevated*)

Transverse mesocolon (*elevated over pancreas*)

Jejunum (*cut*)

Mesentery (*cut and small intestine removed*)

Left colic (splenic) flexure

Left paracolic gutter

Descending colon

Sigmoid mesocolon

Sigmoid colon

Rectum

Sigmoid colon (*reflected*)

Sigmoid mesocolon

Intersigmoid recess

Ureter

Common iliac vessels

Parietal peritoneum

Plate 263

Peritoneal Cavity

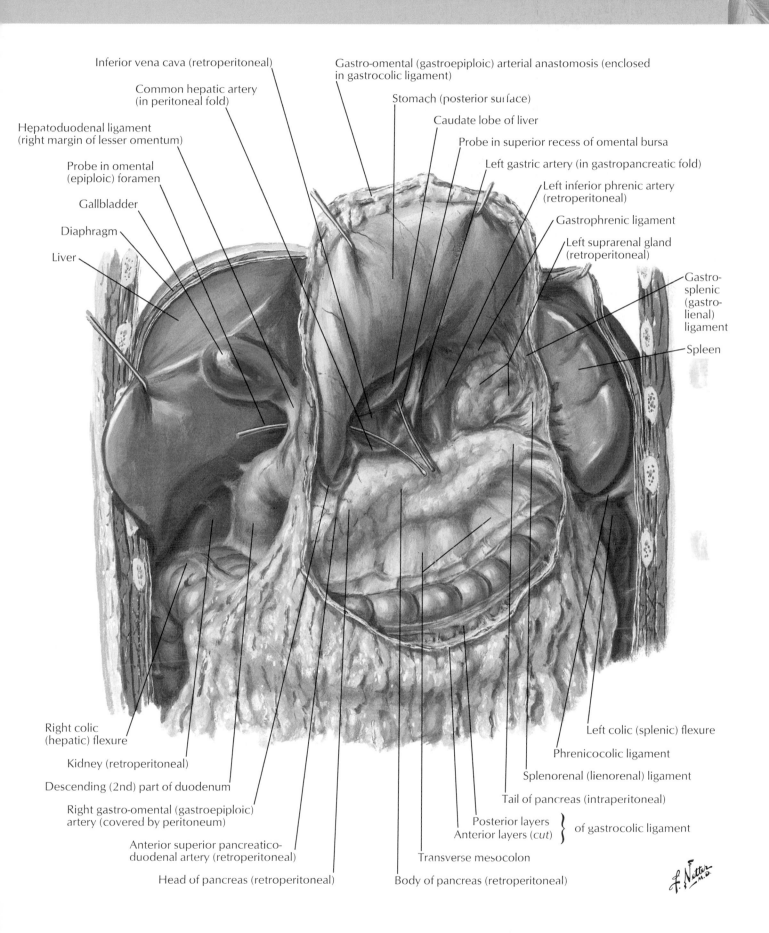

Inferior vena cava (retroperitoneal)

Common hepatic artery (in peritoneal fold)

Hepatoduodenal ligament (right margin of lesser omentum)

Probe in omental (epiploic) foramen

Gallbladder

Diaphragm

Liver

Gastro-omental (gastroepiploic) arterial anastomosis (enclosed in gastrocolic ligament)

Stomach (posterior surface)

Caudate lobe of liver

Probe in superior recess of omental bursa

Left gastric artery (in gastropancreatic fold)

Left inferior phrenic artery (retroperitoneal)

Gastrophrenic ligament

Left suprarenal gland (retroperitoneal)

Gastro-splenic (gastro-lienal) ligament

Spleen

Right colic (hepatic) flexure

Kidney (retroperitoneal)

Descending (2nd) part of duodenum

Right gastro-omental (gastroepiploic) artery (covered by peritoneum)

Anterior superior pancreatico-duodenal artery (retroperitoneal)

Head of pancreas (retroperitoneal)

Left colic (splenic) flexure

Phrenicocolic ligament

Splenorenal (lienorenal) ligament

Tail of pancreas (intraperitoneal)

Posterior layers } of gastrocolic ligament
Anterior layers (cut)

Transverse mesocolon

Body of pancreas (retroperitoneal)

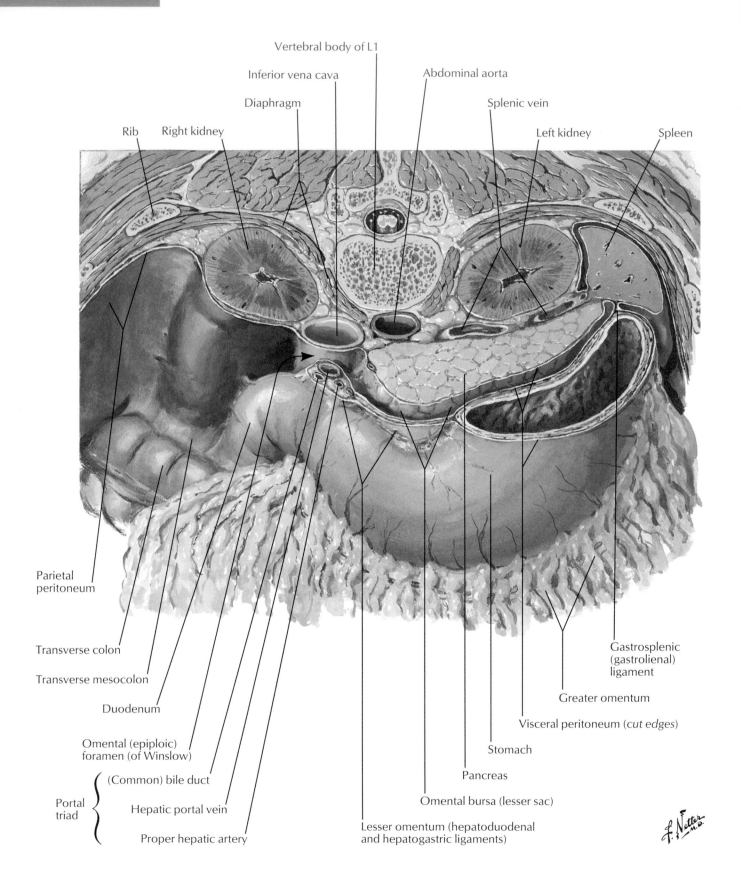

Vertebral body of L1

Inferior vena cava

Abdominal aorta

Diaphragm

Splenic vein

Rib   Right kidney

Left kidney

Spleen

Parietal peritoneum

Transverse colon

Transverse mesocolon

Duodenum

Omental (epiploic) foramen (of Winslow)

Portal triad {
(Common) bile duct

Hepatic portal vein

Proper hepatic artery

Lesser omentum (hepatoduodenal and hepatogastric ligaments)

Omental bursa (lesser sac)

Pancreas

Stomach

Visceral peritoneum (*cut edges*)

Greater omentum

Gastrosplenic (gastrolienal) ligament

Plate 265

Peritoneal Cavity

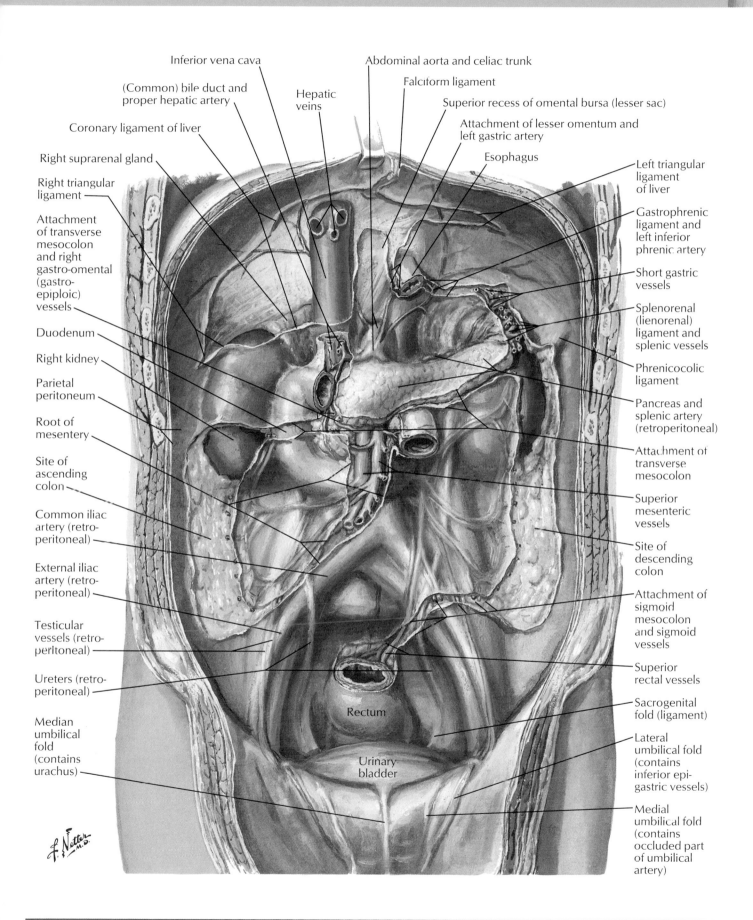

Inferior vena cava

(Common) bile duct and proper hepatic artery

Hepatic veins

Abdominal aorta and celiac trunk

Falciform ligament

Superior recess of omental bursa (lesser sac)

Coronary ligament of liver

Attachment of lesser omentum and left gastric artery

Right suprarenal gland

Esophagus

Right triangular ligament

Attachment of transverse mesocolon and right gastro-omental (gastro-epiploic) vessels

Duodenum

Right kidney

Parietal peritoneum

Root of mesentery

Site of ascending colon

Common iliac artery (retro-peritoneal)

External iliac artery (retro-peritoneal)

Testicular vessels (retro-peritoneal)

Ureters (retro-peritoneal)

Median umbilical fold (contains urachus)

Left triangular ligament of liver

Gastrophrenic ligament and left inferior phrenic artery

Short gastric vessels

Splenorenal (lienorenal) ligament and splenic vessels

Phrenicocolic ligament

Pancreas and splenic artery (retroperitoneal)

Attachment of transverse mesocolon

Superior mesenteric vessels

Site of descending colon

Attachment of sigmoid mesocolon and sigmoid vessels

Superior rectal vessels

Sacrogenital fold (ligament)

Lateral umbilical fold (contains inferior epigastric vessels)

Medial umbilical fold (contains occluded part of umbilical artery)

Rectum

Urinary bladder

f. Netter M.D.

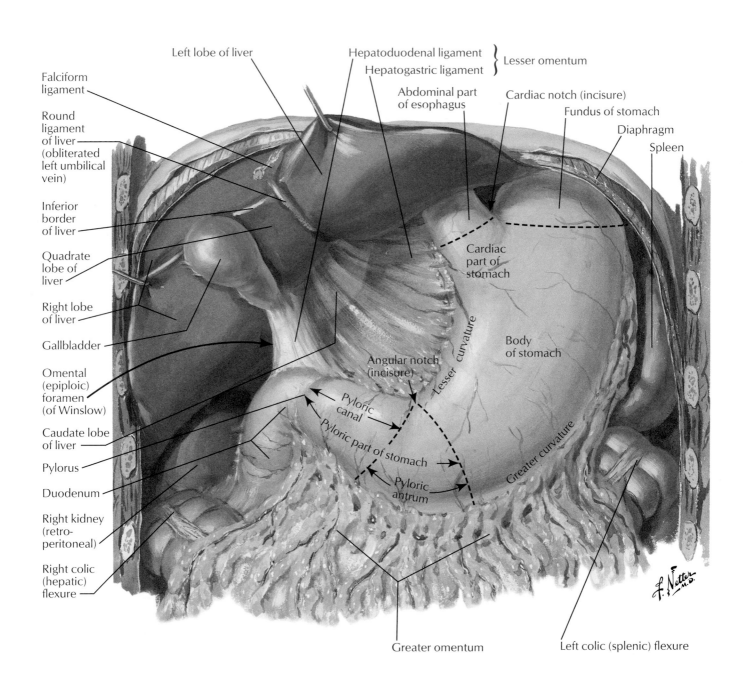

Falciform ligament

Round ligament of liver (obliterated left umbilical vein)

Inferior border of liver

Quadrate lobe of liver

Right lobe of liver

Gallbladder

Omental (epiploic) foramen (of Winslow)

Caudate lobe of liver

Pylorus

Duodenum

Right kidney (retroperitoneal)

Right colic (hepatic) flexure

Left lobe of liver

Hepatoduodenal ligament
Hepatogastric ligament } Lesser omentum

Abdominal part of esophagus

Cardiac notch (incisure)

Fundus of stomach

Diaphragm

Spleen

Cardiac part of stomach

Body of stomach

Lesser curvature

Angular notch (incisure)

Pyloric canal

Pyloric part of stomach

Pyloric antrum

Greater curvature

Greater omentum

Left colic (splenic) flexure

F. Netter

Plate 267   **Viscera (Gut)**

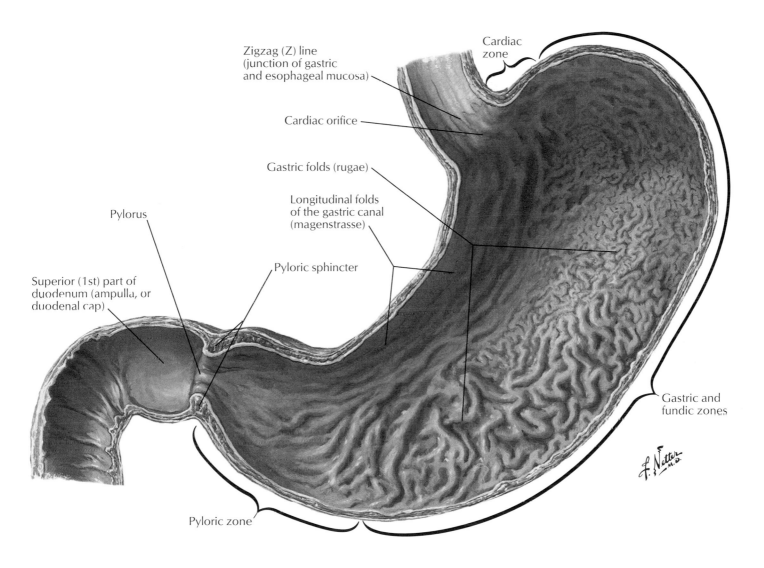

Zigzag (Z) line
(junction of gastric
and esophageal mucosa)

Cardiac
zone

Cardiac orifice

Gastric folds (rugae)

Longitudinal folds
of the gastric canal
(magenstrasse)

Pylorus

Pyloric sphincter

Superior (1st) part of
duodenum (ampulla, or
duodenal cap)

Gastric and
fundic zones

Pyloric zone

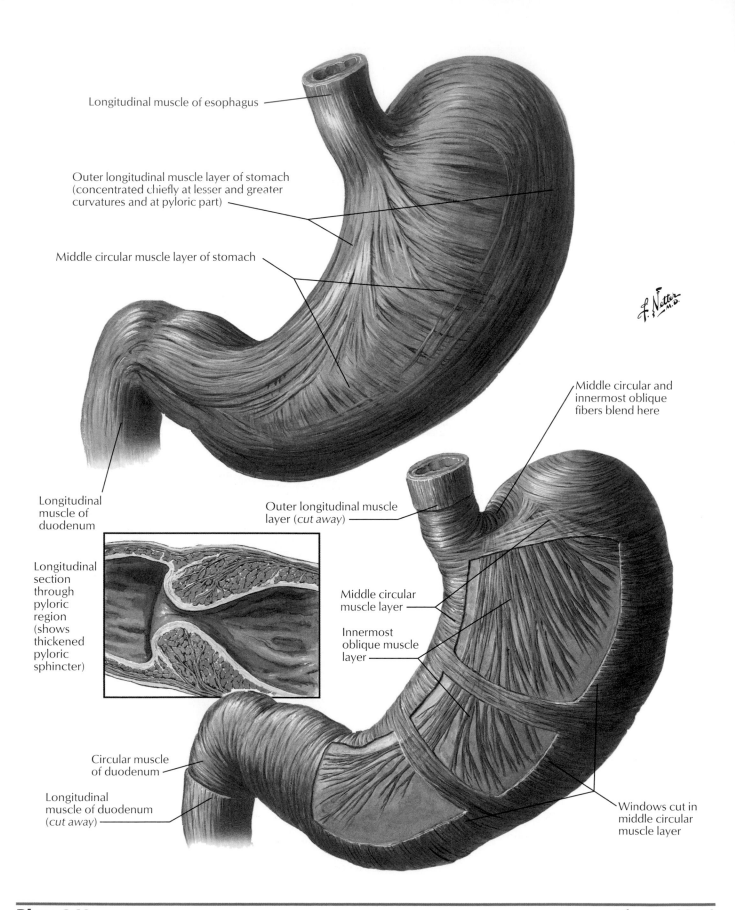

Longitudinal muscle of esophagus

Outer longitudinal muscle layer of stomach
(concentrated chiefly at lesser and greater
curvatures and at pyloric part)

Middle circular muscle layer of stomach

Longitudinal
muscle of
duodenum

Longitudinal
section
through
pyloric
region
(shows
thickened
pyloric
sphincter)

Circular muscle
of duodenum

Longitudinal
muscle of duodenum
(cut away)

Middle circular and
innermost oblique
fibers blend here

Outer longitudinal muscle
layer (cut away)

Middle circular
muscle layer

Innermost
oblique muscle
layer

Windows cut in
middle circular
muscle layer

Plate 269 **Viscera (Gut)**

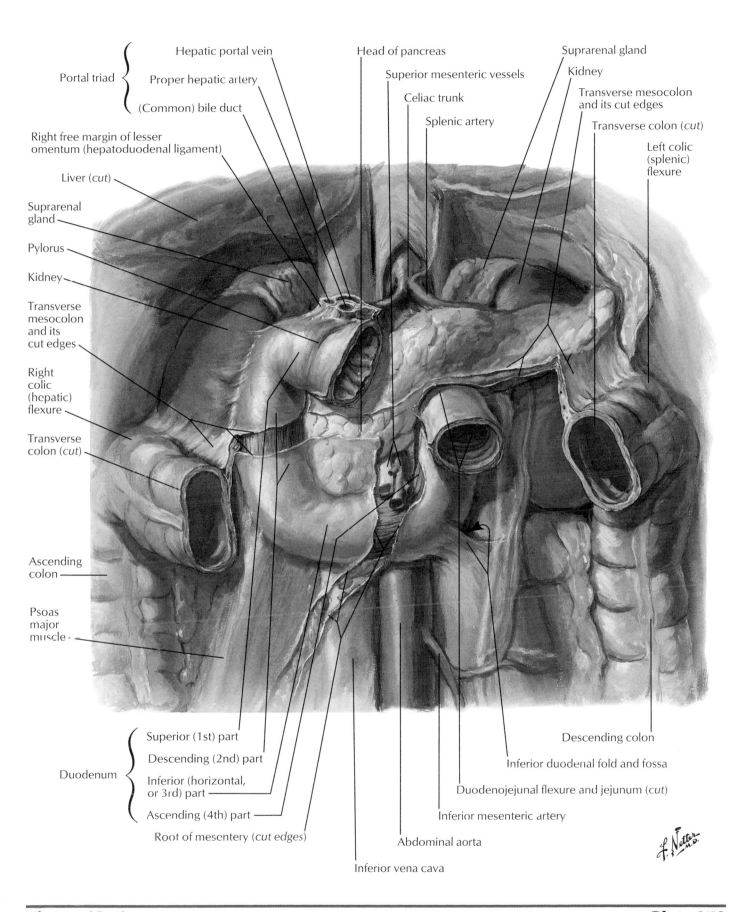

Portal triad
- Hepatic portal vein
- Proper hepatic artery
- (Common) bile duct

Head of pancreas

Superior mesenteric vessels

Celiac trunk

Splenic artery

Suprarenal gland

Kidney

Transverse mesocolon and its cut edges

Transverse colon (cut)

Right free margin of lesser omentum (hepatoduodenal ligament)

Left colic (splenic) flexure

Liver (cut)

Suprarenal gland

Pylorus

Kidney

Transverse mesocolon and its cut edges

Right colic (hepatic) flexure

Transverse colon (cut)

Ascending colon

Psoas major muscle

Duodenum
- Superior (1st) part
- Descending (2nd) part
- Inferior (horizontal, or 3rd) part
- Ascending (4th) part

Root of mesentery (cut edges)

Inferior vena cava

Abdominal aorta

Inferior mesenteric artery

Duodenojejunal flexure and jejunum (cut)

Inferior duodenal fold and fossa

Descending colon

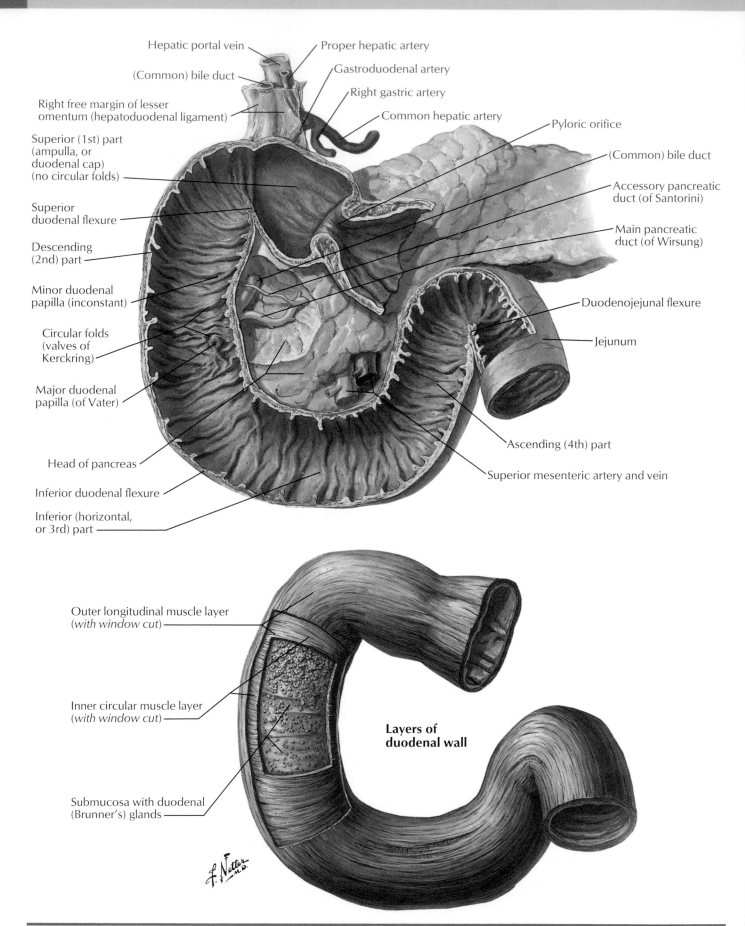

Hepatic portal vein

(Common) bile duct

Right free margin of lesser omentum (hepatoduodenal ligament)

Proper hepatic artery

Gastroduodenal artery

Right gastric artery

Common hepatic artery

Superior (1st) part (ampulla, or duodenal cap) (no circular folds)

Superior duodenal flexure

Descending (2nd) part

Minor duodenal papilla (inconstant)

Circular folds (valves of Kerckring)

Major duodenal papilla (of Vater)

Head of pancreas

Inferior duodenal flexure

Inferior (horizontal, or 3rd) part

Pyloric orifice

(Common) bile duct

Accessory pancreatic duct (of Santorini)

Main pancreatic duct (of Wirsung)

Duodenojejunal flexure

Jejunum

Ascending (4th) part

Superior mesenteric artery and vein

Outer longitudinal muscle layer (*with window cut*)

Inner circular muscle layer (*with window cut*)

Layers of duodenal wall

Submucosa with duodenal (Brunner's) glands

Plate 271

Viscera (Gut)

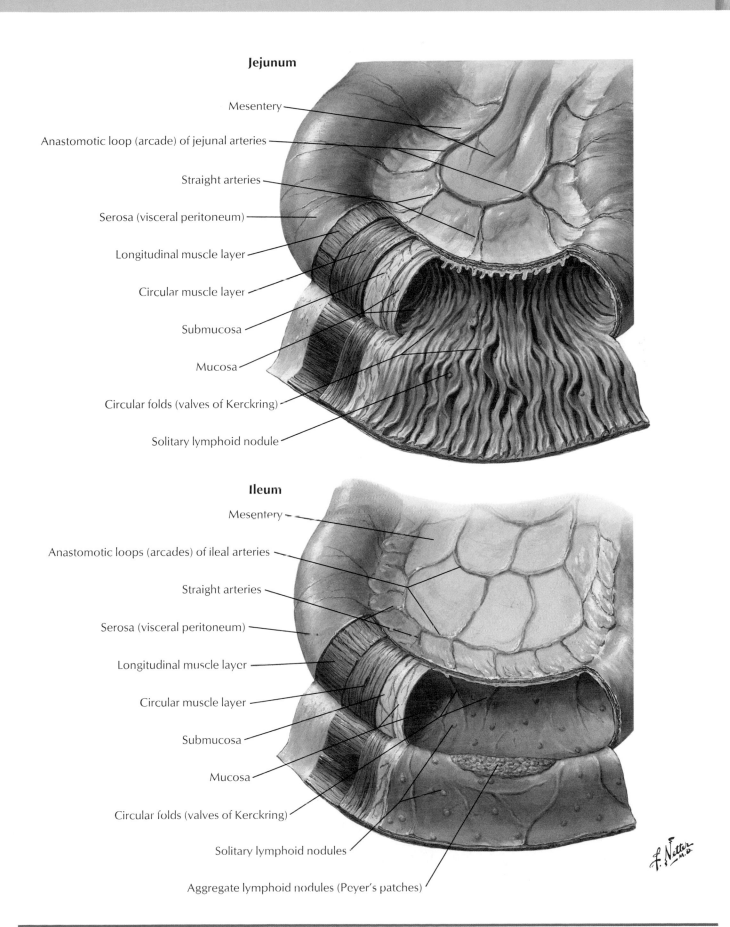

Jejunum

Mesentery

Anastomotic loop (arcade) of jejunal arteries

Straight arteries

Serosa (visceral peritoneum)

Longitudinal muscle layer

Circular muscle layer

Submucosa

Mucosa

Circular folds (valves of Kerckring)

Solitary lymphoid nodule

Ileum

Mesentery

Anastomotic loops (arcades) of ileal arteries

Straight arteries

Serosa (visceral peritoneum)

Longitudinal muscle layer

Circular muscle layer

Submucosa

Mucosa

Circular folds (valves of Kerckring)

Solitary lymphoid nodules

Aggregate lymphoid nodules (Peyer's patches)

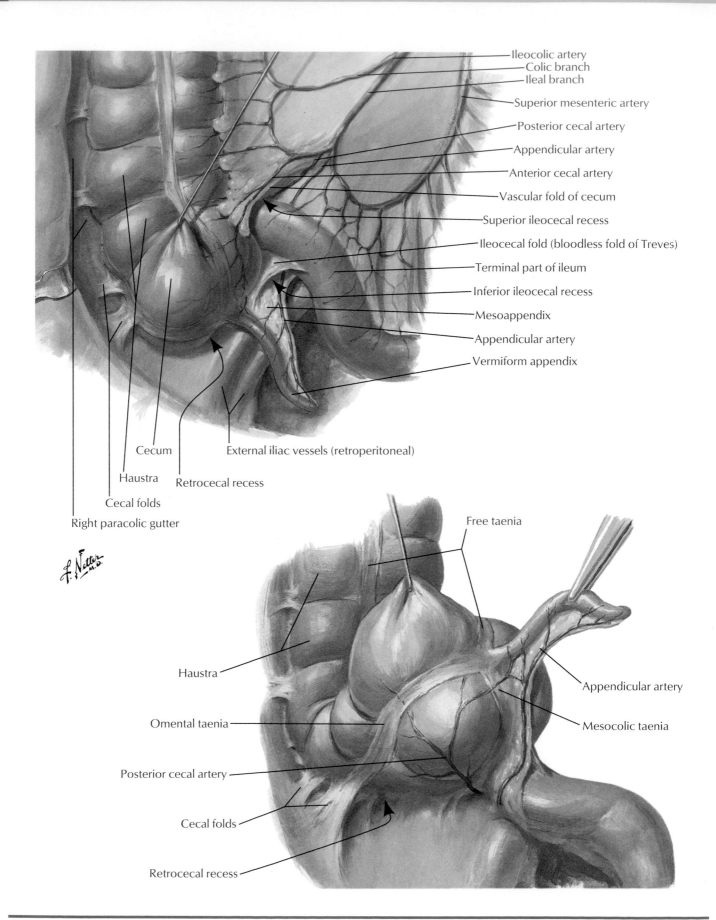

Ileocolic artery
Colic branch
Ileal branch
Superior mesenteric artery
Posterior cecal artery
Appendicular artery
Anterior cecal artery
Vascular fold of cecum
Superior ileocecal recess
Ileocecal fold (bloodless fold of Treves)
Terminal part of ileum
Inferior ileocecal recess
Mesoappendix
Appendicular artery
Vermiform appendix

External iliac vessels (retroperitoneal)

Cecum
Haustra
Retrocecal recess
Cecal folds
Right paracolic gutter

Free taenia

Haustra

Appendicular artery

Omental taenia

Mesocolic taenia

Posterior cecal artery

Cecal folds

Retrocecal recess

Plate 273   **Viscera (Gut)**

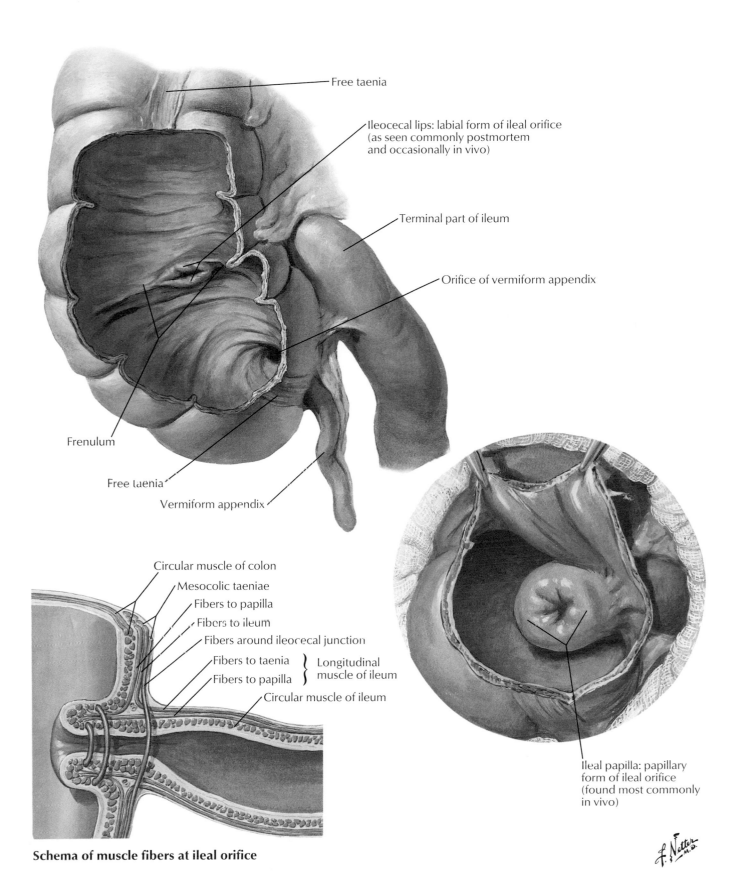

Free taenia

Ileocecal lips: labial form of ileal orifice (as seen commonly postmortem and occasionally in vivo)

Terminal part of ileum

Orifice of vermiform appendix

Frenulum

Free taenia

Vermiform appendix

Circular muscle of colon

Mesocolic taeniae

Fibers to papilla

Fibers to ileum

Fibers around ileocecal junction

Fibers to taenia } Longitudinal muscle of ileum

Fibers to papilla

Circular muscle of ileum

Ileal papilla: papillary form of ileal orifice (found most commonly in vivo)

Schema of muscle fibers at ileal orifice

Barium radiograph of unusually long appendix

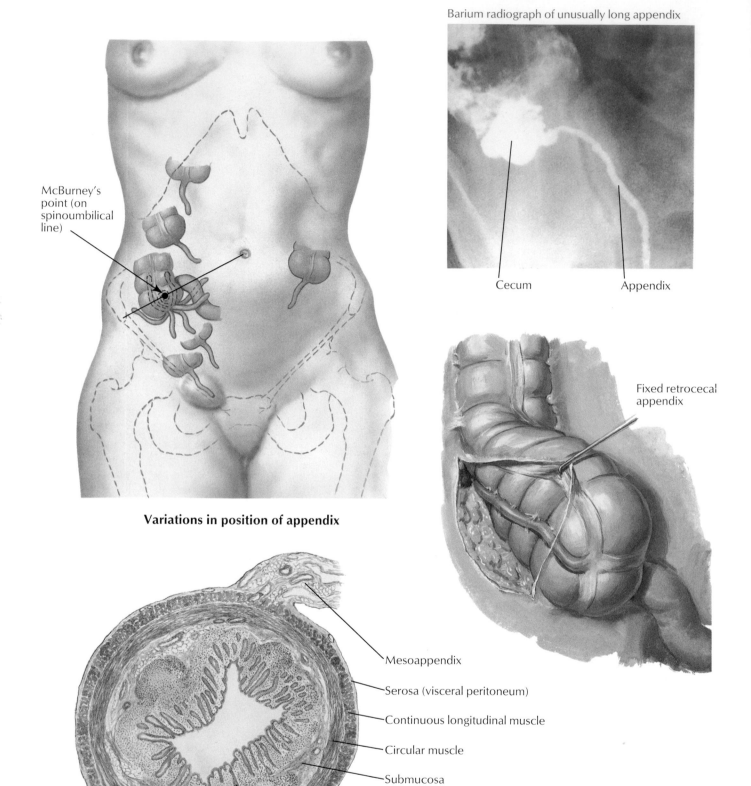

McBurney's point (on spinoumbilical line)

Cecum

Appendix

Variations in position of appendix

Fixed retrocecal appendix

Mesoappendix

Serosa (visceral peritoneum)

Continuous longitudinal muscle

Circular muscle

Submucosa

Aggregate lymphoid nodules

Crypts of Lieberkühn

Plate 275

Viscera (Gut)

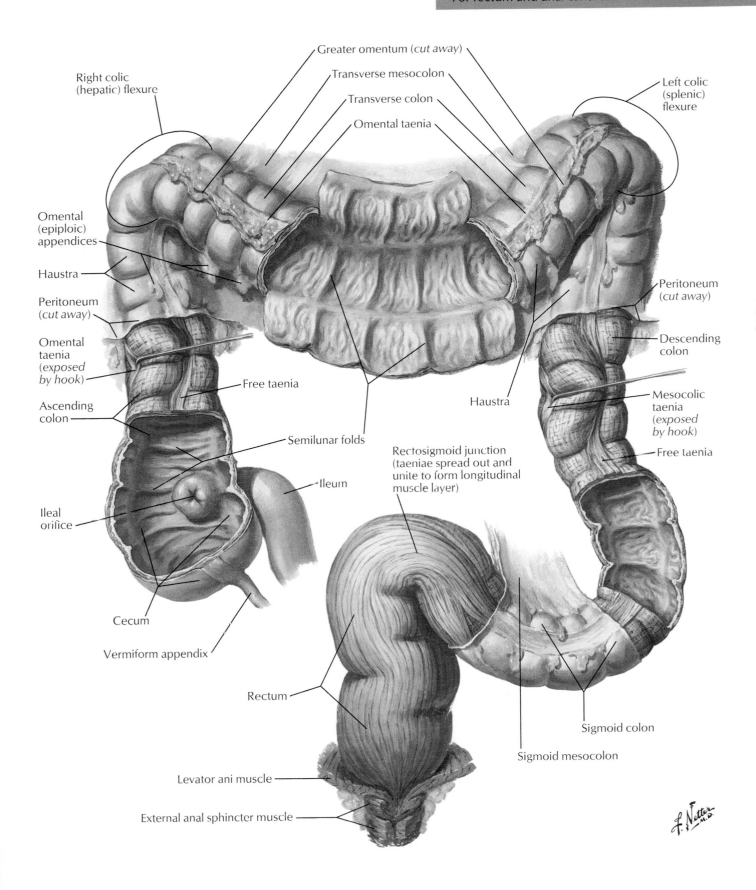

Right colic (hepatic) flexure

Greater omentum (*cut away*)

Transverse mesocolon

Transverse colon

Omental taenia

Left colic (splenic) flexure

Omental (epiploic) appendices

Haustra

Peritoneum (*cut away*)

Omental taenia (*exposed by hook*)

Ascending colon

Free taenia

Semilunar folds

Ileum

Haustra

Peritoneum (*cut away*)

Descending colon

Mesocolic taenia (*exposed by hook*)

Free taenia

Ileal orifice

Rectosigmoid junction (taeniae spread out and unite to form longitudinal muscle layer)

Cecum

Vermiform appendix

Rectum

Sigmoid colon

Sigmoid mesocolon

Levator ani muscle

External anal sphincter muscle

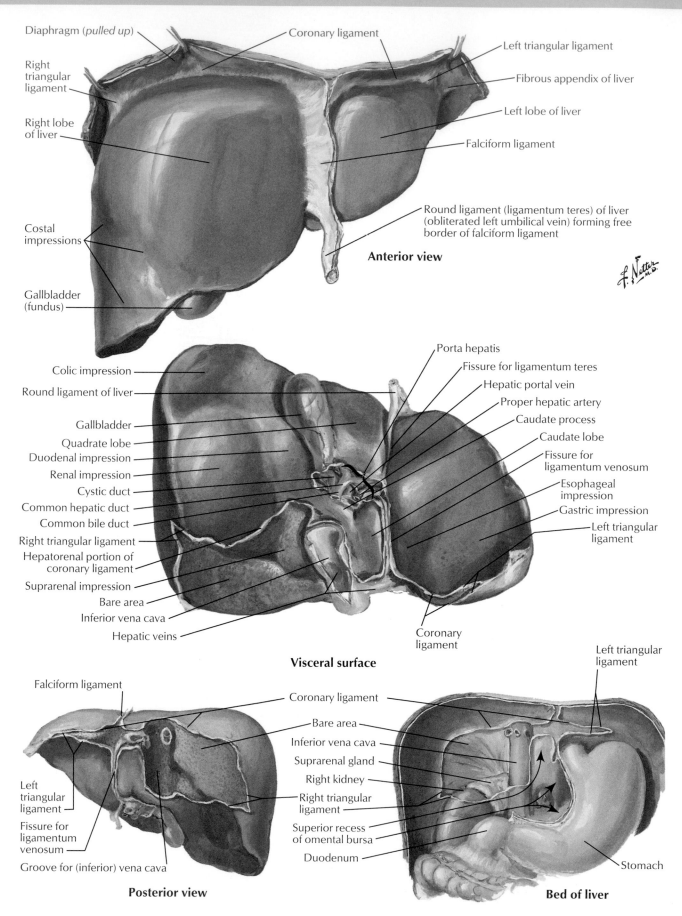

Diaphragm (*pulled up*)

Coronary ligament

Left triangular ligament

Right triangular ligament

Fibrous appendix of liver

Right lobe of liver

Left lobe of liver

Falciform ligament

Costal impressions

Round ligament (ligamentum teres) of liver (obliterated left umbilical vein) forming free border of falciform ligament

Anterior view

Gallbladder (fundus)

Colic impression

Porta hepatis

Fissure for ligamentum teres

Round ligament of liver

Hepatic portal vein

Proper hepatic artery

Gallbladder

Caudate process

Quadrate lobe

Caudate lobe

Duodenal impression

Fissure for ligamentum venosum

Renal impression

Cystic duct

Esophageal impression

Common hepatic duct

Gastric impression

Common bile duct

Left triangular ligament

Right triangular ligament

Hepatorenal portion of coronary ligament

Suprarenal impression

Bare area

Inferior vena cava

Coronary ligament

Hepatic veins

Visceral surface

Falciform ligament

Left triangular ligament

Coronary ligament

Bare area

Inferior vena cava

Suprarenal gland

Right kidney

Left triangular ligament

Right triangular ligament

Fissure for ligamentum venosum

Superior recess of omental bursa

Duodenum

Groove for (inferior) vena cava

Stomach

Posterior view

Bed of liver

Plate 277

Viscera (Accessory Organs)

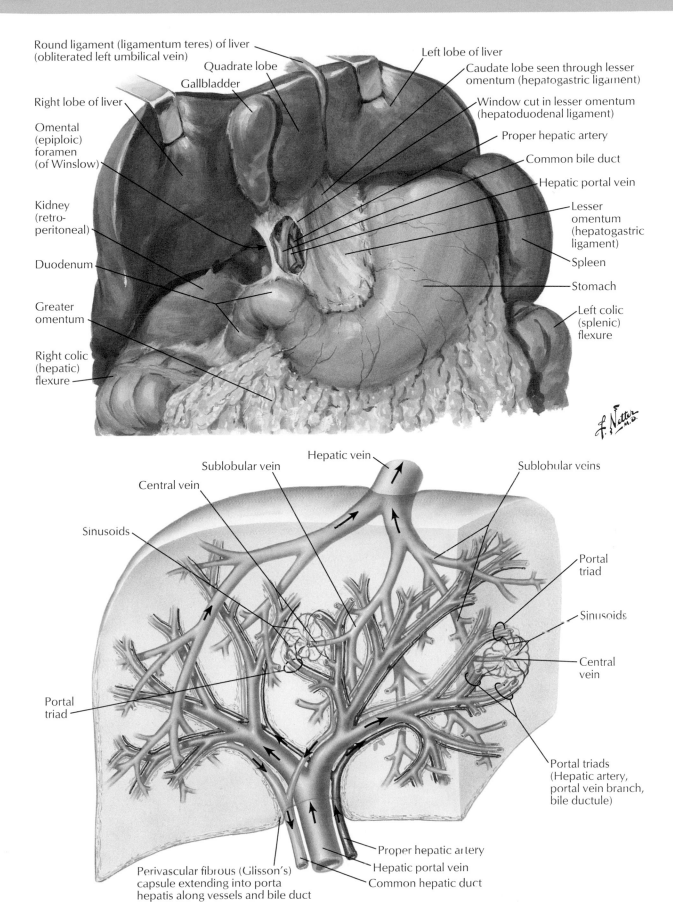

Round ligament (ligamentum teres) of liver
(obliterated left umbilical vein)

Quadrate lobe

Gallbladder

Right lobe of liver

Omental
(epiploic)
foramen
(of Winslow)

Kidney
(retro-
peritoneal)

Duodenum

Greater
omentum

Right colic
(hepatic)
flexure

Left lobe of liver

Caudate lobe seen through lesser
omentum (hepatogastric ligament)

Window cut in lesser omentum
(hepatoduodenal ligament)

Proper hepatic artery

Common bile duct

Hepatic portal vein

Lesser
omentum
(hepatogastric
ligament)

Spleen

Stomach

Left colic
(splenic)
flexure

Hepatic vein

Sublobular vein

Central vein

Sinusoids

Portal
triad

Sublobular veins

Portal
triad

Sinusoids

Central
vein

Portal triads
(Hepatic artery,
portal vein branch,
bile ductule)

Perivascular fibrous (Glisson's)
capsule extending into porta
hepatis along vessels and bile duct

Proper hepatic artery

Hepatic portal vein

Common hepatic duct

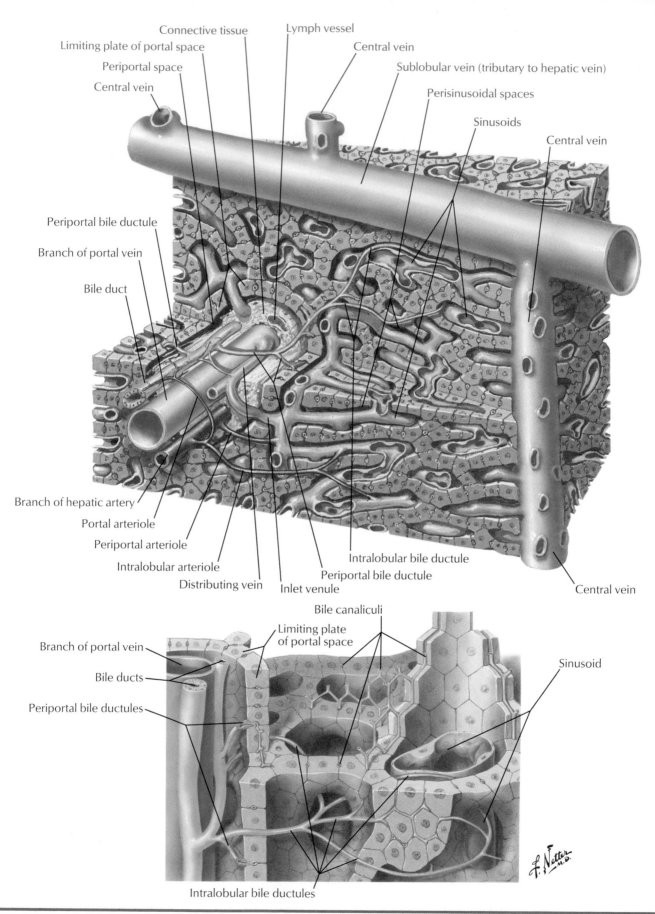

Connective tissue

Lymph vessel

Limiting plate of portal space

Central vein

Periportal space

Sublobular vein (tributary to hepatic vein)

Central vein

Perisinusoidal spaces

Sinusoids

Central vein

Periportal bile ductule

Branch of portal vein

Bile duct

Branch of hepatic artery

Portal arteriole

Periportal arteriole

Intralobular arteriole

Distributing vein

Inlet venule

Intralobular bile ductule

Periportal bile ductule

Central vein

Bile canaliculi

Limiting plate of portal space

Branch of portal vein

Sinusoid

Bile ducts

Periportal bile ductules

Intralobular bile ductules

Plate 279

Viscera (Accessory Organs)

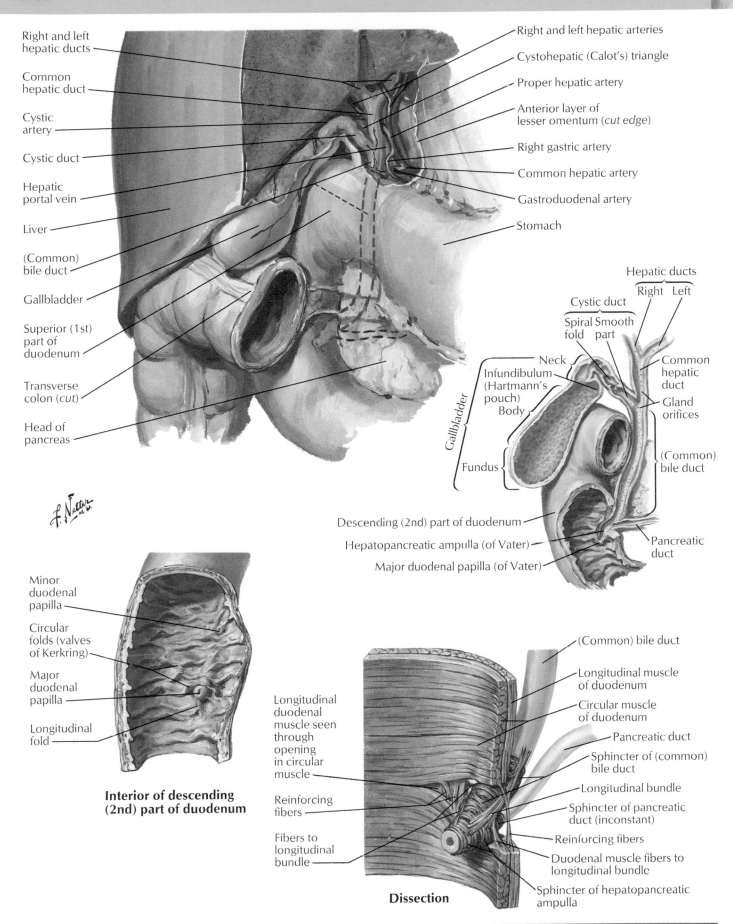

Right and left hepatic ducts

Common hepatic duct

Cystic artery

Cystic duct

Hepatic portal vein

Liver

(Common) bile duct

Gallbladder

Superior (1st) part of duodenum

Transverse colon (cut)

Head of pancreas

Right and left hepatic arteries

Cystohepatic (Calot's) triangle

Proper hepatic artery

Anterior layer of lesser omentum (cut edge)

Right gastric artery

Common hepatic artery

Gastroduodenal artery

Stomach

Hepatic ducts
Right   Left

Cystic duct

Spiral Smooth fold   part

Neck

Infundibulum (Hartmann's pouch)

Body

Gallbladder

Fundus

Common hepatic duct

Gland orifices

(Common) bile duct

Descending (2nd) part of duodenum

Hepatopancreatic ampulla (of Vater)

Major duodenal papilla (of Vater)

Pancreatic duct

Minor duodenal papilla

Circular folds (valves of Kerkring)

Major duodenal papilla

Longitudinal fold

Interior of descending (2nd) part of duodenum

Longitudinal duodenal muscle seen through opening in circular muscle

Reinforcing fibers

Fibers to longitudinal bundle

(Common) bile duct

Longitudinal muscle of duodenum

Circular muscle of duodenum

Pancreatic duct

Sphincter of (common) bile duct

Longitudinal bundle

Sphincter of pancreatic duct (inconstant)

Reinforcing fibers

Duodenal muscle fibers to longitudinal bundle

Sphincter of hepatopancreatic ampulla

Dissection

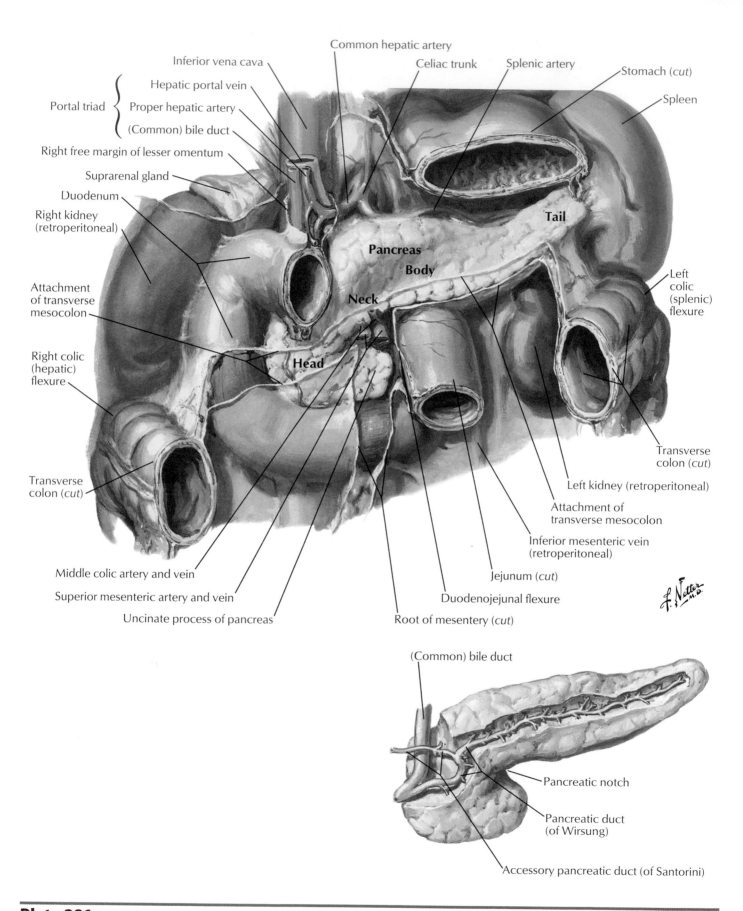

Common hepatic artery

Inferior vena cava

Celiac trunk

Splenic artery

Stomach (*cut*)

Hepatic portal vein

Portal triad

Proper hepatic artery

Spleen

(Common) bile duct

Right free margin of lesser omentum

Suprarenal gland

Duodenum

Right kidney (retroperitoneal)

Tail

Pancreas Body

Left colic (splenic) flexure

Attachment of transverse mesocolon

Neck

Right colic (hepatic) flexure

Head

Transverse colon (*cut*)

Transverse colon (*cut*)

Left kidney (retroperitoneal)

Attachment of transverse mesocolon

Inferior mesenteric vein (retroperitoneal)

Middle colic artery and vein

Jejunum (*cut*)

Superior mesenteric artery and vein

Duodenojejunal flexure

Uncinate process of pancreas

Root of mesentery (*cut*)

(Common) bile duct

Pancreatic notch

Pancreatic duct (of Wirsung)

Accessory pancreatic duct (of Santorini)

Plate 281

Viscera (Accessory Organs)

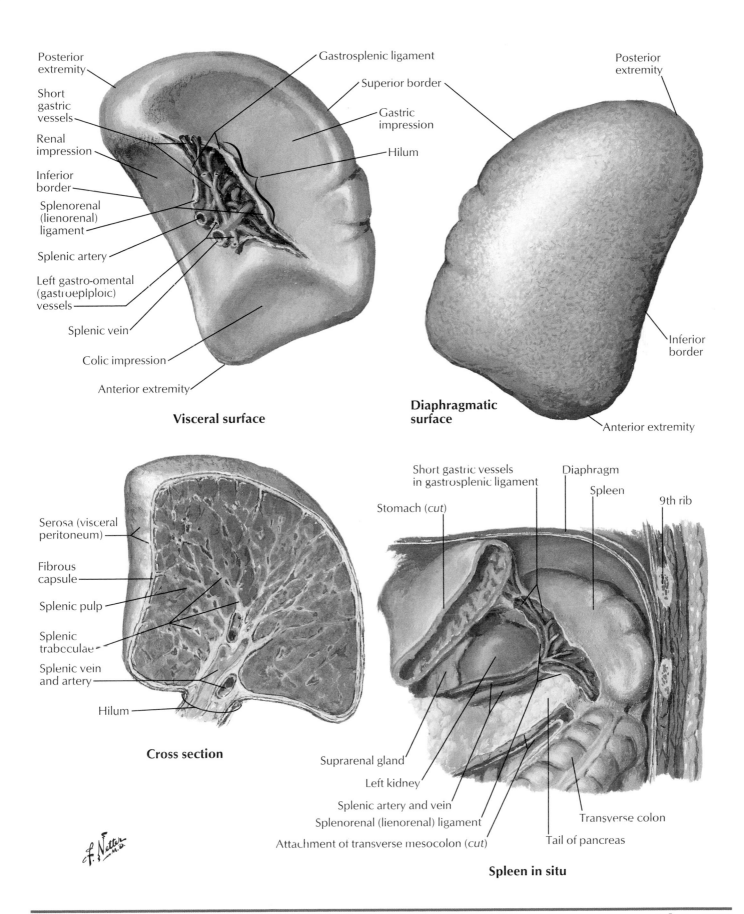

Visceral surface

Posterior extremity
Short gastric vessels
Renal impression
Inferior border
Splenorenal (lienorenal) ligament
Splenic artery
Left gastro-omental (gastroepiploic) vessels
Splenic vein
Colic impression
Anterior extremity

Gastrosplenic ligament
Superior border
Gastric impression
Hilum

Diaphragmatic surface

Posterior extremity
Inferior border
Anterior extremity

Cross section

Serosa (visceral peritoneum)
Fibrous capsule
Splenic pulp
Splenic trabeculae
Splenic vein and artery
Hilum

Spleen in situ

Short gastric vessels in gastrosplenic ligament
Diaphragm
Spleen
9th rib
Stomach (cut)
Suprarenal gland
Left kidney
Splenic artery and vein
Splenorenal (lienorenal) ligament
Attachment of transverse mesocolon (cut)
Tail of pancreas
Transverse colon

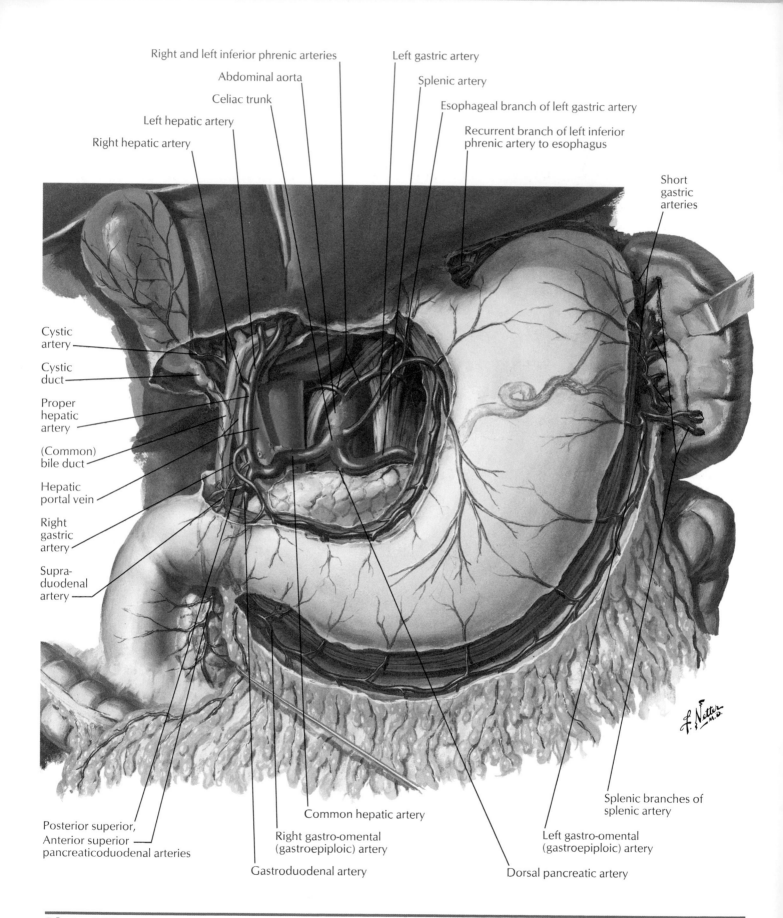

Right and left inferior phrenic arteries

Abdominal aorta

Celiac trunk

Left hepatic artery

Right hepatic artery

Left gastric artery

Splenic artery

Esophageal branch of left gastric artery

Recurrent branch of left inferior phrenic artery to esophagus

Short gastric arteries

Cystic artery

Cystic duct

Proper hepatic artery

(Common) bile duct

Hepatic portal vein

Right gastric artery

Supra-duodenal artery

Splenic branches of splenic artery

Posterior superior, Anterior superior pancreaticoduodenal arteries

Common hepatic artery

Right gastro-omental (gastroepiploic) artery

Gastroduodenal artery

Left gastro-omental (gastroepiploic) artery

Dorsal pancreatic artery

f. Netter M.D.

Plate 283

Visceral Vasculature

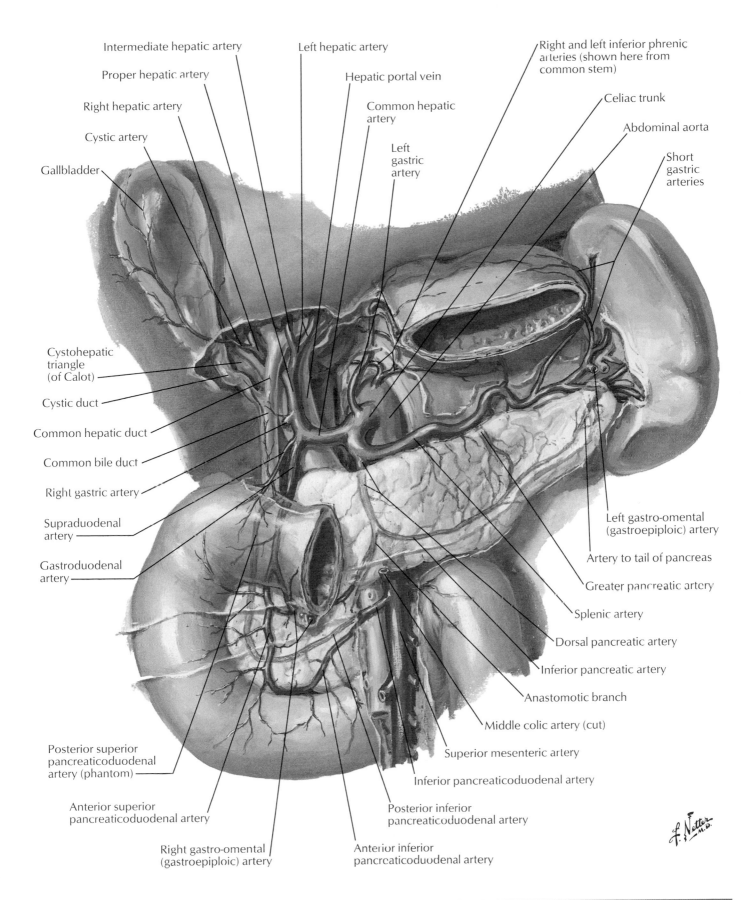

Intermediate hepatic artery

Proper hepatic artery

Right hepatic artery

Cystic artery

Gallbladder

Left hepatic artery

Hepatic portal vein

Common hepatic artery

Left gastric artery

Right and left inferior phrenic arteries (shown here from common stem)

Celiac trunk

Abdominal aorta

Short gastric arteries

Cystohepatic triangle (of Calot)

Cystic duct

Common hepatic duct

Common bile duct

Right gastric artery

Supraduodenal artery

Gastroduodenal artery

Left gastro-omental (gastroepiploic) artery

Artery to tail of pancreas

Greater pancreatic artery

Splenic artery

Dorsal pancreatic artery

Inferior pancreatic artery

Anastomotic branch

Middle colic artery (cut)

Superior mesenteric artery

Inferior pancreaticoduodenal artery

Posterior superior pancreaticoduodenal artery (phantom)

Anterior superior pancreaticoduodenal artery

Right gastro-omental (gastroepiploic) artery

Posterior inferior pancreaticoduodenal artery

Anterior inferior pancreaticoduodenal artery

f. Netter M.D.

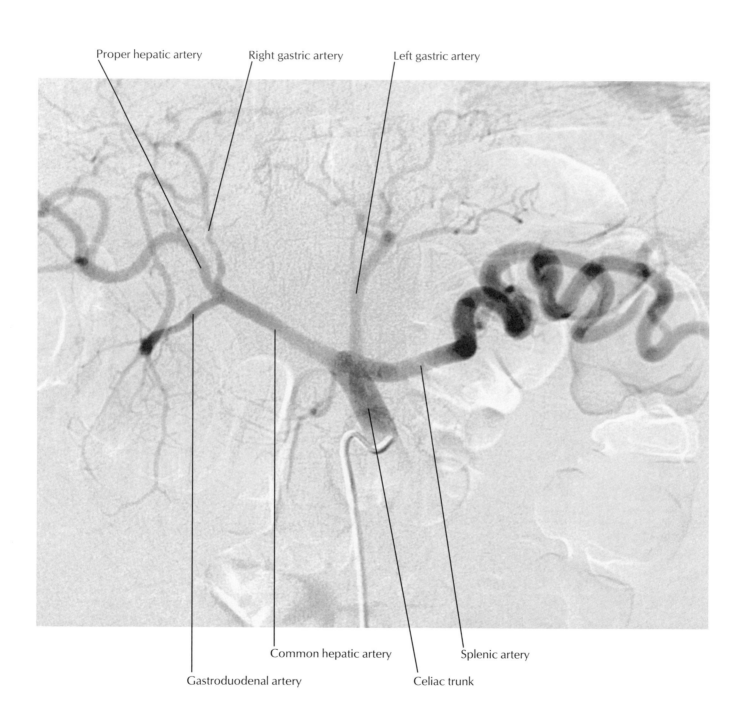

Proper hepatic artery   Right gastric artery   Left gastric artery

Common hepatic artery   Splenic artery

Gastroduodenal artery   Celiac trunk

Plate 285   **Visceral Vasculature**

Duodenum and head of pancreas reflected to left

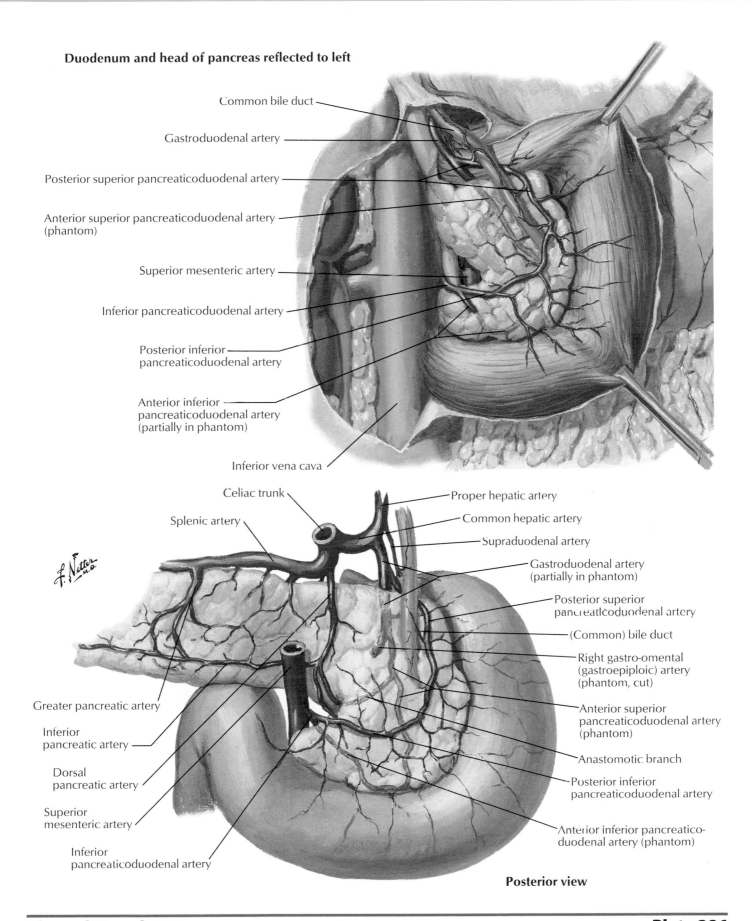

Common bile duct

Gastroduodenal artery

Posterior superior pancreaticoduodenal artery

Anterior superior pancreaticoduodenal artery (phantom)

Superior mesenteric artery

Inferior pancreaticoduodenal artery

Posterior inferior pancreaticoduodenal artery

Anterior inferior pancreaticoduodenal artery (partially in phantom)

Inferior vena cava

Celiac trunk

Splenic artery

Proper hepatic artery

Common hepatic artery

Supraduodenal artery

Gastroduodenal artery (partially in phantom)

Posterior superior pancreaticoduodenal artery

(Common) bile duct

Right gastro-omental (gastroepiploic) artery (phantom, cut)

Anterior superior pancreaticoduodenal artery (phantom)

Anastomotic branch

Posterior inferior pancreaticoduodenal artery

Greater pancreatic artery

Inferior pancreatic artery

Dorsal pancreatic artery

Superior mesenteric artery

Inferior pancreaticoduodenal artery

Anterior inferior pancreatico-duodenal artery (phantom)

Posterior view

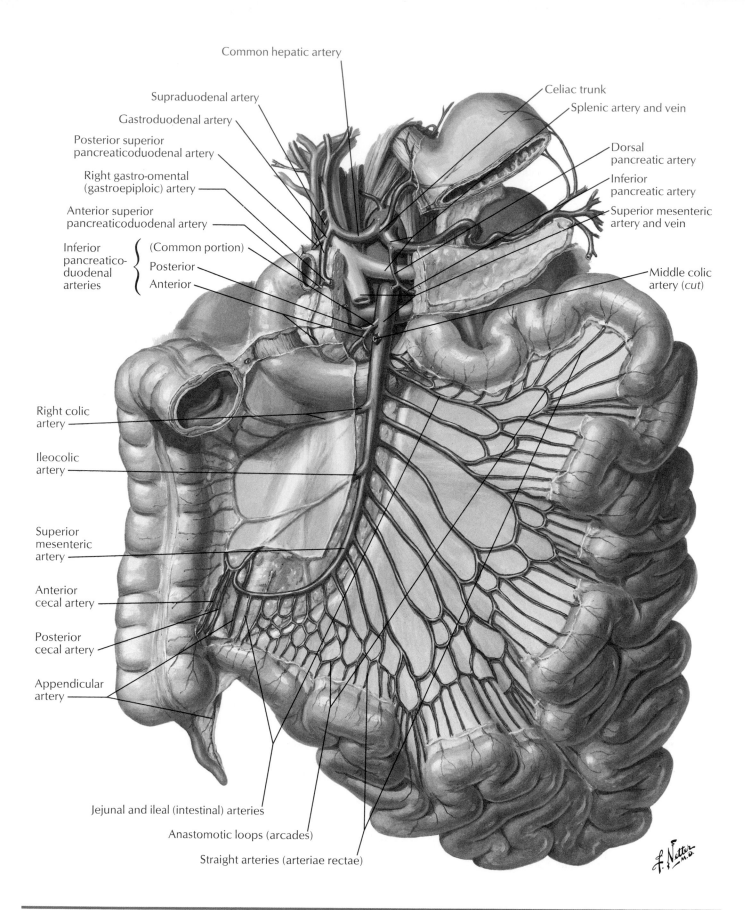

Common hepatic artery

Celiac trunk

Splenic artery and vein

Supraduodenal artery

Gastroduodenal artery

Dorsal pancreatic artery

Posterior superior pancreaticoduodenal artery

Inferior pancreatic artery

Right gastro-omental (gastroepiploic) artery

Superior mesenteric artery and vein

Anterior superior pancreaticoduodenal artery

Inferior pancreatico-duodenal arteries
- (Common portion)
- Posterior
- Anterior

Middle colic artery (*cut*)

Right colic artery

Ileocolic artery

Superior mesenteric artery

Anterior cecal artery

Posterior cecal artery

Appendicular artery

Jejunal and ileal (intestinal) arteries

Anastomotic loops (arcades)

Straight arteries (arteriae rectae)

Plate 287

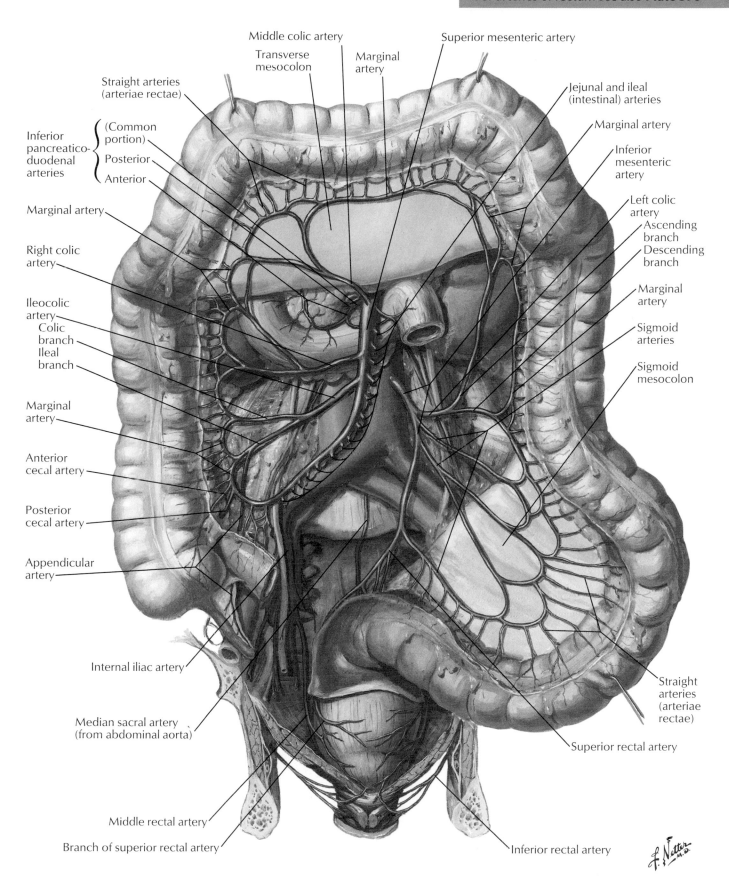

Middle colic artery

Superior mesenteric artery

Transverse mesocolon

Marginal artery

Straight arteries (arteriae rectae)

Jejunal and ileal (intestinal) arteries

Inferior pancreatico-duodenal arteries

(Common portion)

Posterior

Anterior

Marginal artery

Inferior mesenteric artery

Left colic artery

Ascending branch

Descending branch

Marginal artery

Marginal artery

Right colic artery

Ileocolic artery

Colic branch

Ileal branch

Sigmoid arteries

Sigmoid mesocolon

Marginal artery

Anterior cecal artery

Posterior cecal artery

Appendicular artery

Internal iliac artery

Straight arteries (arteriae rectae)

Median sacral artery (from abdominal aorta)

Superior rectal artery

Middle rectal artery

Branch of superior rectal artery

Inferior rectal artery

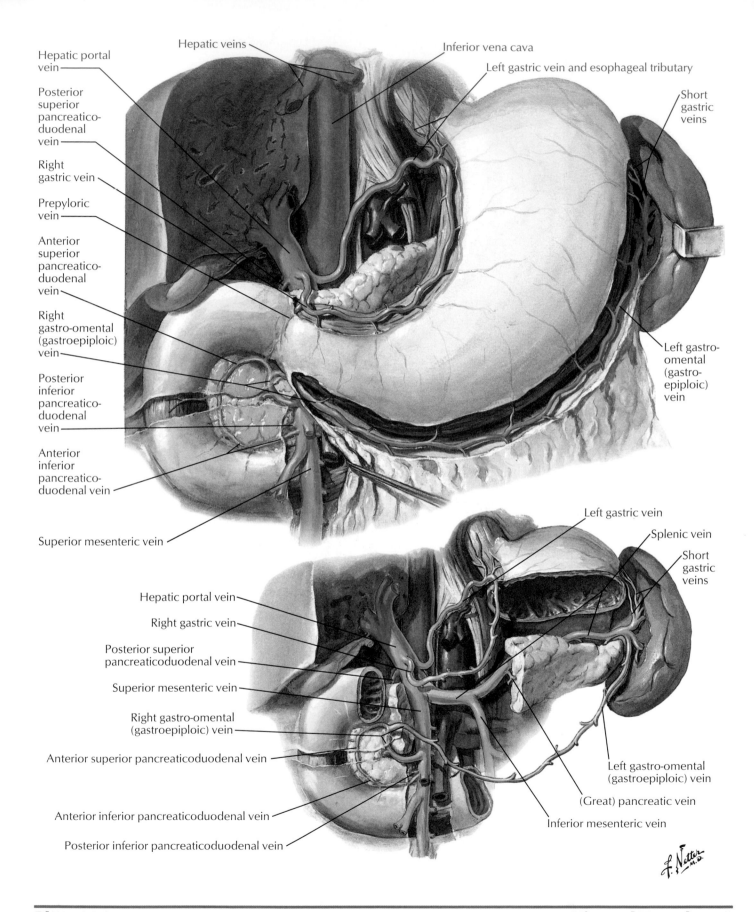

Hepatic veins

Inferior vena cava

Hepatic portal vein

Left gastric vein and esophageal tributary

Posterior superior pancreaticoduodenal vein

Short gastric veins

Right gastric vein

Prepyloric vein

Anterior superior pancreaticoduodenal vein

Right gastro-omental (gastroepiploic) vein

Left gastro-omental (gastroepiploic) vein

Posterior inferior pancreaticoduodenal vein

Anterior inferior pancreaticoduodenal vein

Superior mesenteric vein

Left gastric vein

Splenic vein

Hepatic portal vein

Short gastric veins

Right gastric vein

Posterior superior pancreaticoduodenal vein

Superior mesenteric vein

Right gastro-omental (gastroepiploic) vein

Anterior superior pancreaticoduodenal vein

Left gastro-omental (gastroepiploic) vein

Anterior inferior pancreaticoduodenal vein

(Great) pancreatic vein

Posterior inferior pancreaticoduodenal vein

Inferior mesenteric vein

Plate 289

Visceral Vasculature

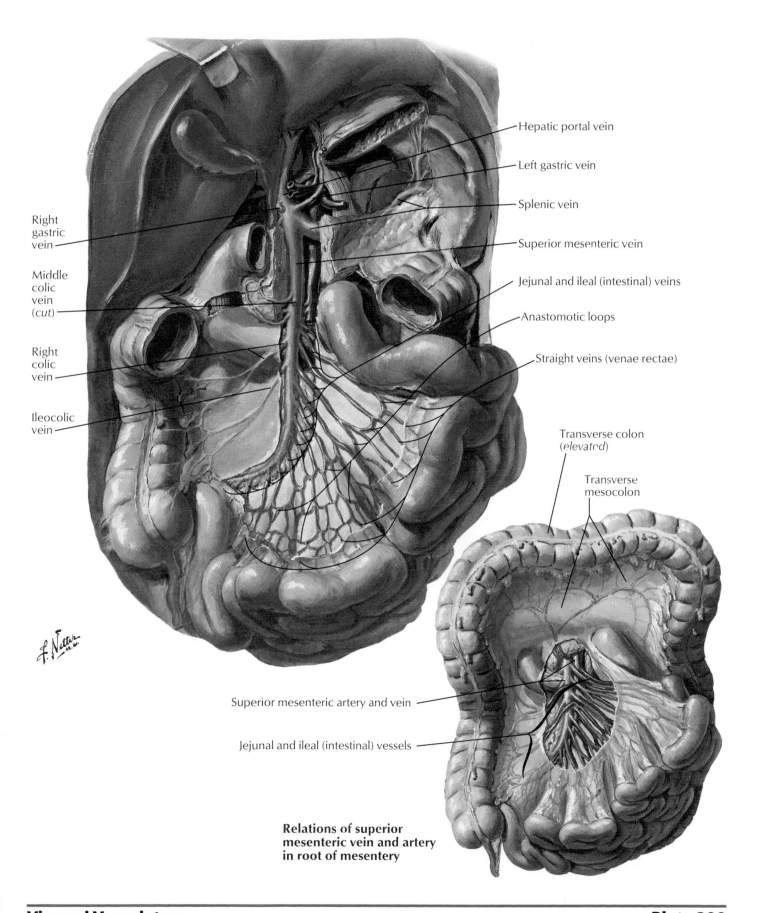

Hepatic portal vein

Left gastric vein

Splenic vein

Superior mesenteric vein

Jejunal and ileal (intestinal) veins

Anastomotic loops

Straight veins (venae rectae)

Right gastric vein

Middle colic vein (*cut*)

Right colic vein

Ileocolic vein

Transverse colon (*elevated*)

Transverse mesocolon

Superior mesenteric artery and vein

Jejunal and ileal (intestinal) vessels

Relations of superior mesenteric vein and artery in root of mesentery

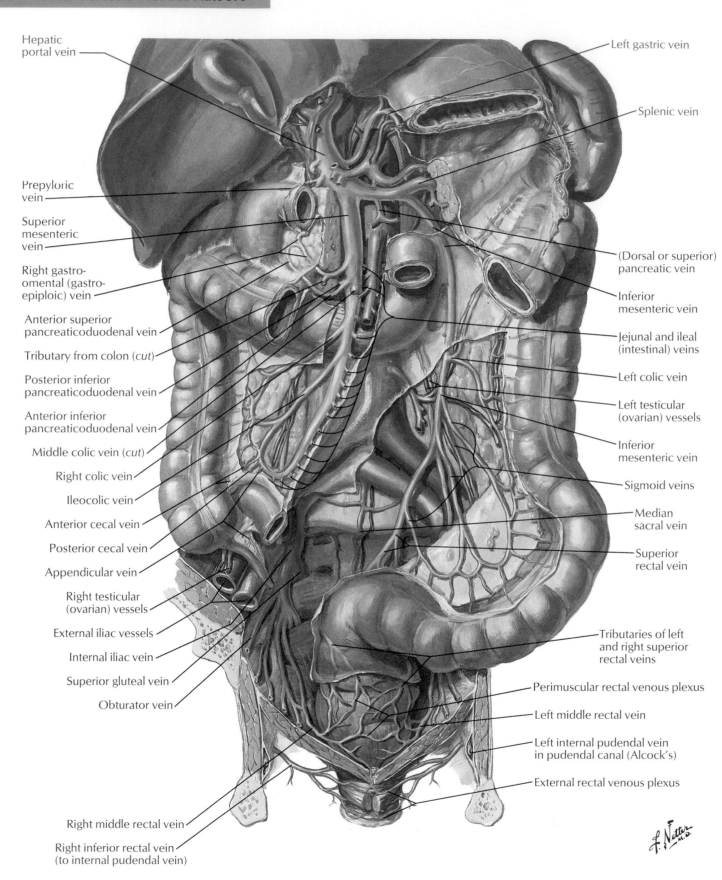

Hepatic portal vein

Left gastric vein

Prepyloric vein

Splenic vein

Superior mesenteric vein

(Dorsal or superior) pancreatic vein

Right gastro-omental (gastro-epiploic) vein

Inferior mesenteric vein

Anterior superior pancreaticoduodenal vein

Jejunal and ileal (intestinal) veins

Tributary from colon (cut)

Left colic vein

Posterior inferior pancreaticoduodenal vein

Left testicular (ovarian) vessels

Anterior inferior pancreaticoduodenal vein

Inferior mesenteric vein

Middle colic vein (cut)

Sigmoid veins

Right colic vein

Median sacral vein

Ileocolic vein

Anterior cecal vein

Superior rectal vein

Posterior cecal vein

Appendicular vein

Tributaries of left and right superior rectal veins

Right testicular (ovarian) vessels

External iliac vessels

Perimuscular rectal venous plexus

Internal iliac vein

Left middle rectal vein

Superior gluteal vein

Left internal pudendal vein in pudendal canal (Alcock's)

Obturator vein

External rectal venous plexus

Right middle rectal vein

Right inferior rectal vein (to internal pudendal vein)

Plate 291

Visceral Vasculature

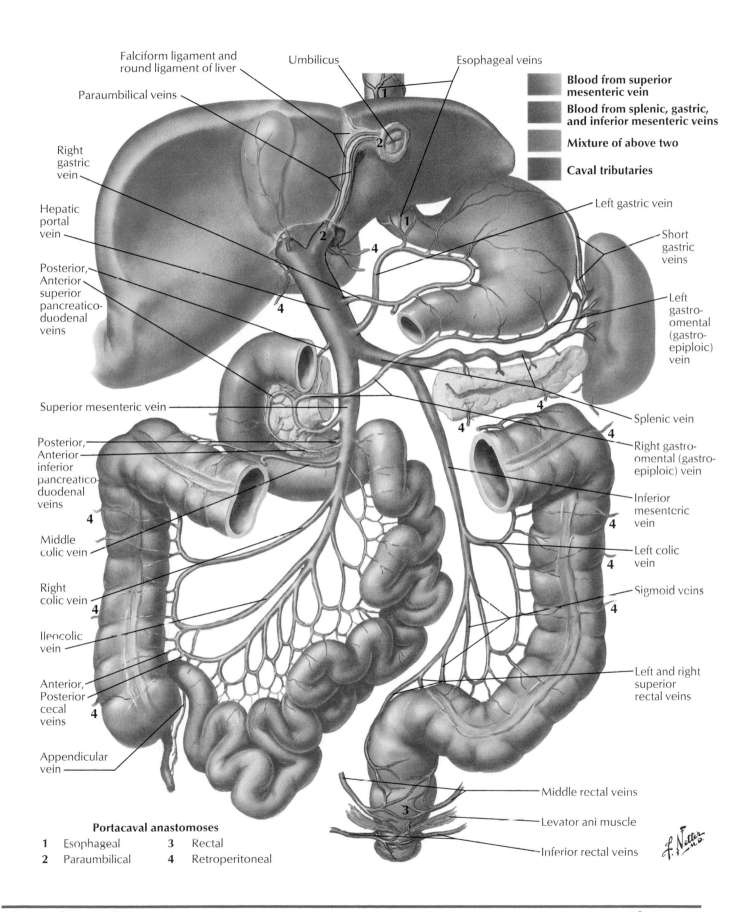

Falciform ligament and round ligament of liver

Umbilicus

Esophageal veins

Paraumbilical veins

Blood from superior mesenteric vein

Blood from splenic, gastric, and inferior mesenteric veins

Mixture of above two

Caval tributaries

Right gastric vein

Left gastric vein

Hepatic portal vein

Short gastric veins

Posterior, Anterior superior pancreatico-duodenal veins

Left gastro-omental (gastro-epiploic) vein

Superior mesenteric vein

Splenic vein

Posterior, Anterior inferior pancreatico-duodenal veins

Right gastro-omental (gastro-epiploic) vein

Middle colic vein

Inferior mesenteric vein

Right colic vein

Left colic vein

Ileocolic vein

Sigmoid veins

Anterior, Posterior cecal veins

Left and right superior rectal veins

Appendicular vein

Middle rectal veins

Levator ani muscle

Inferior rectal veins

Portacaval anastomoses

1	Esophageal	3	Rectal
2	Paraumbilical	4	Retroperitoneal

f. Netter M.D.

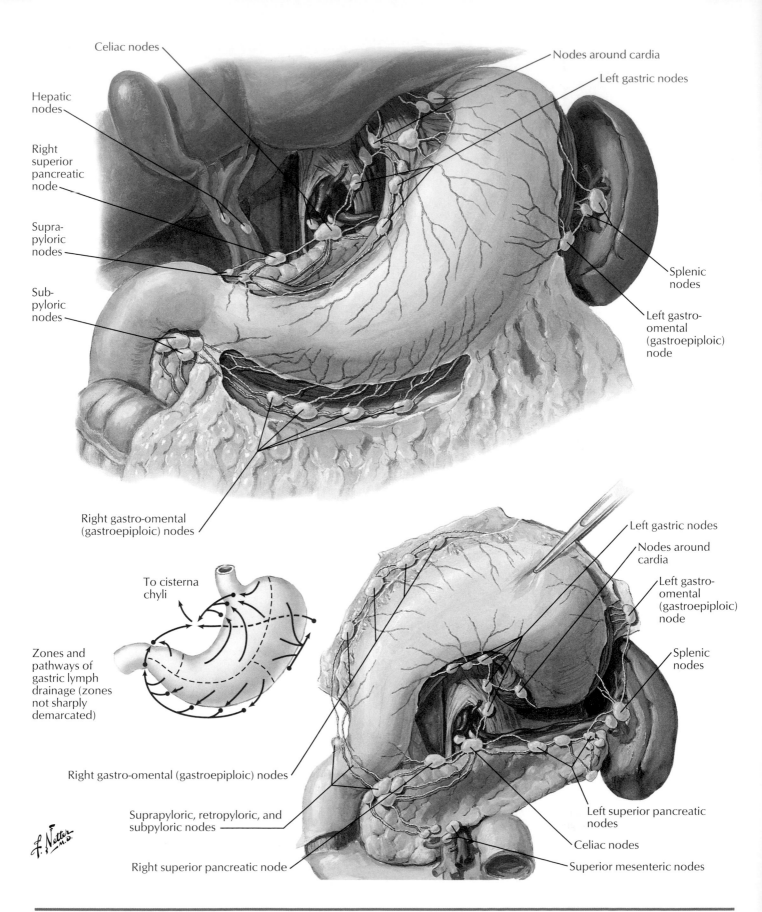

Celiac nodes

Nodes around cardia

Left gastric nodes

Hepatic nodes

Right superior pancreatic node

Supra-pyloric nodes

Sub-pyloric nodes

Splenic nodes

Left gastro-omental (gastroepiploic) node

Right gastro-omental (gastroepiploic) nodes

To cisterna chyli

Zones and pathways of gastric lymph drainage (zones not sharply demarcated)

Left gastric nodes

Nodes around cardia

Left gastro-omental (gastroepiploic) node

Splenic nodes

Right gastro-omental (gastroepiploic) nodes

Suprapyloric, retropyloric, and subpyloric nodes

Left superior pancreatic nodes

Right superior pancreatic node

Celiac nodes

Superior mesenteric nodes

Plate 293

Visceral Vasculature

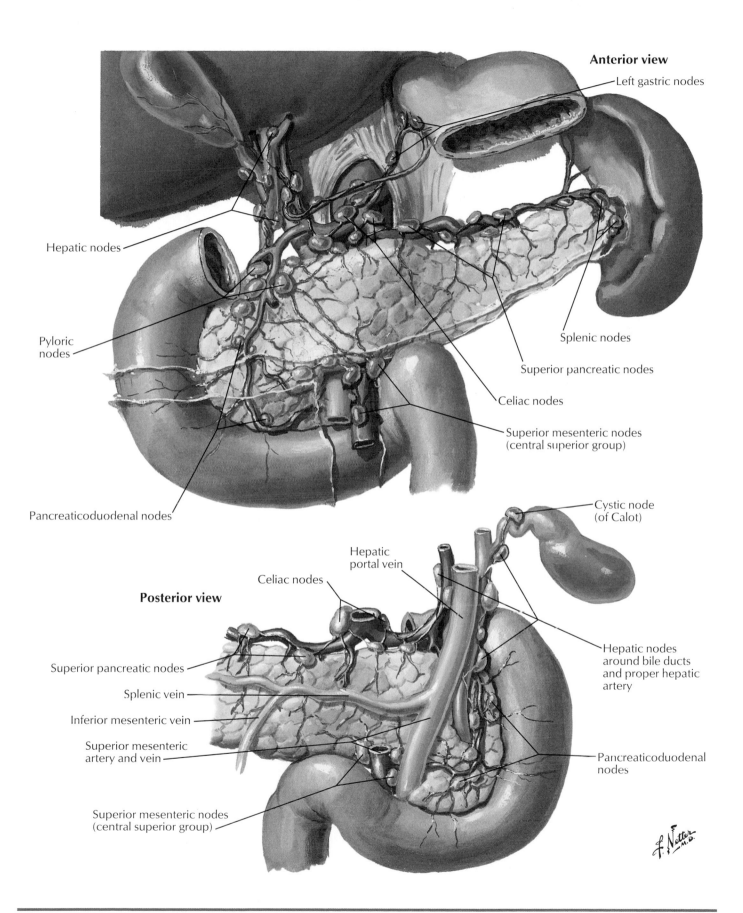

Anterior view

Left gastric nodes

Hepatic nodes

Pyloric nodes

Splenic nodes

Superior pancreatic nodes

Celiac nodes

Superior mesenteric nodes (central superior group)

Pancreaticoduodenal nodes

Cystic node (of Calot)

Hepatic portal vein

Celiac nodes

Posterior view

Superior pancreatic nodes

Splenic vein

Inferior mesenteric vein

Superior mesenteric artery and vein

Superior mesenteric nodes (central superior group)

Hepatic nodes around bile ducts and proper hepatic artery

Pancreaticoduodenal nodes

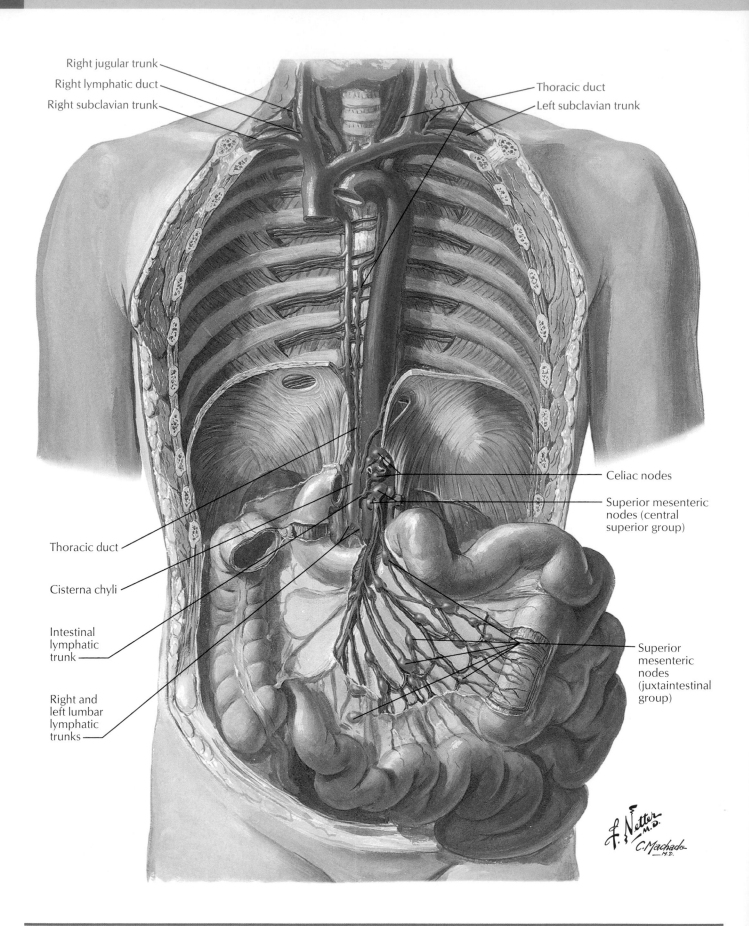

Right jugular trunk

Right lymphatic duct

Right subclavian trunk

Thoracic duct

Left subclavian trunk

Celiac nodes

Superior mesenteric nodes (central superior group)

Thoracic duct

Cisterna chyli

Intestinal lymphatic trunk

Right and left lumbar lymphatic trunks

Superior mesenteric nodes (juxtaintestinal group)

Plate 295 **Visceral Vasculature**

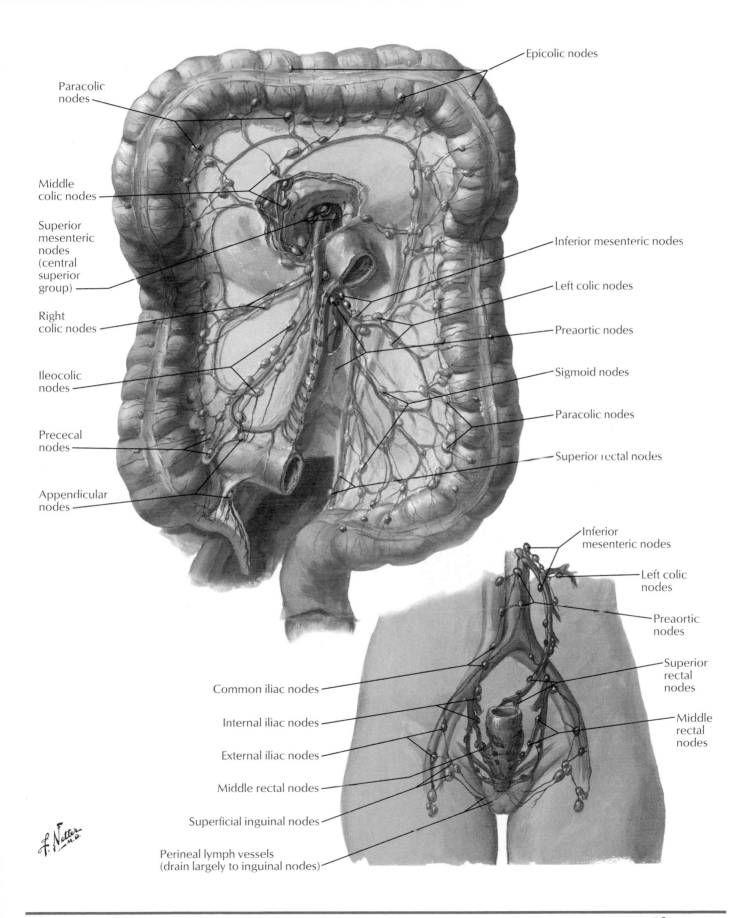

Epicolic nodes

Paracolic nodes

Middle colic nodes

Superior mesenteric nodes (central superior group)

Right colic nodes

Ileocolic nodes

Prececal nodes

Appendicular nodes

Inferior mesenteric nodes

Left colic nodes

Preaortic nodes

Sigmoid nodes

Paracolic nodes

Superior rectal nodes

Inferior mesenteric nodes

Left colic nodes

Preaortic nodes

Superior rectal nodes

Middle rectal nodes

Common iliac nodes

Internal iliac nodes

External iliac nodes

Middle rectal nodes

Superficial inguinal nodes

Perineal lymph vessels (drain largely to inguinal nodes)

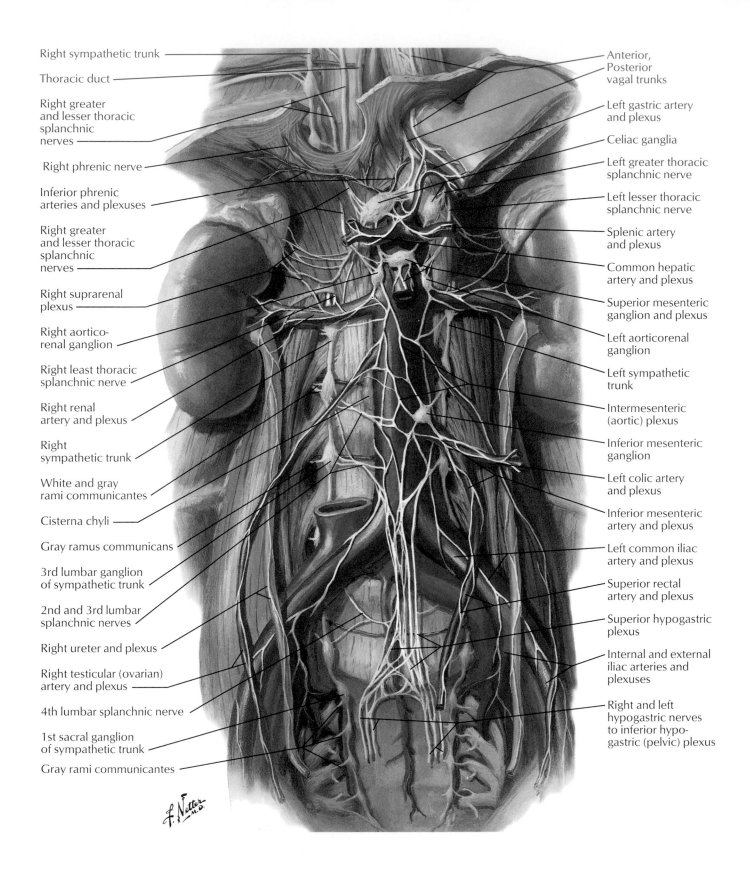

Right sympathetic trunk

Thoracic duct

Right greater and lesser thoracic splanchnic nerves

Right phrenic nerve

Inferior phrenic arteries and plexuses

Right greater and lesser thoracic splanchnic nerves

Right suprarenal plexus

Right aortico-renal ganglion

Right least thoracic splanchnic nerve

Right renal artery and plexus

Right sympathetic trunk

White and gray rami communicantes

Cisterna chyli

Gray ramus communicans

3rd lumbar ganglion of sympathetic trunk

2nd and 3rd lumbar splanchnic nerves

Right ureter and plexus

Right testicular (ovarian) artery and plexus

4th lumbar splanchnic nerve

1st sacral ganglion of sympathetic trunk

Gray rami communicantes

Anterior, Posterior vagal trunks

Left gastric artery and plexus

Celiac ganglia

Left greater thoracic splanchnic nerve

Left lesser thoracic splanchnic nerve

Splenic artery and plexus

Common hepatic artery and plexus

Superior mesenteric ganglion and plexus

Left aorticorenal ganglion

Left sympathetic trunk

Intermesenteric (aortic) plexus

Inferior mesenteric ganglion

Left colic artery and plexus

Inferior mesenteric artery and plexus

Left common iliac artery and plexus

Superior rectal artery and plexus

Superior hypogastric plexus

Internal and external iliac arteries and plexuses

Right and left hypogastric nerves to inferior hypo-gastric (pelvic) plexus

Plate 297   **Innervation**

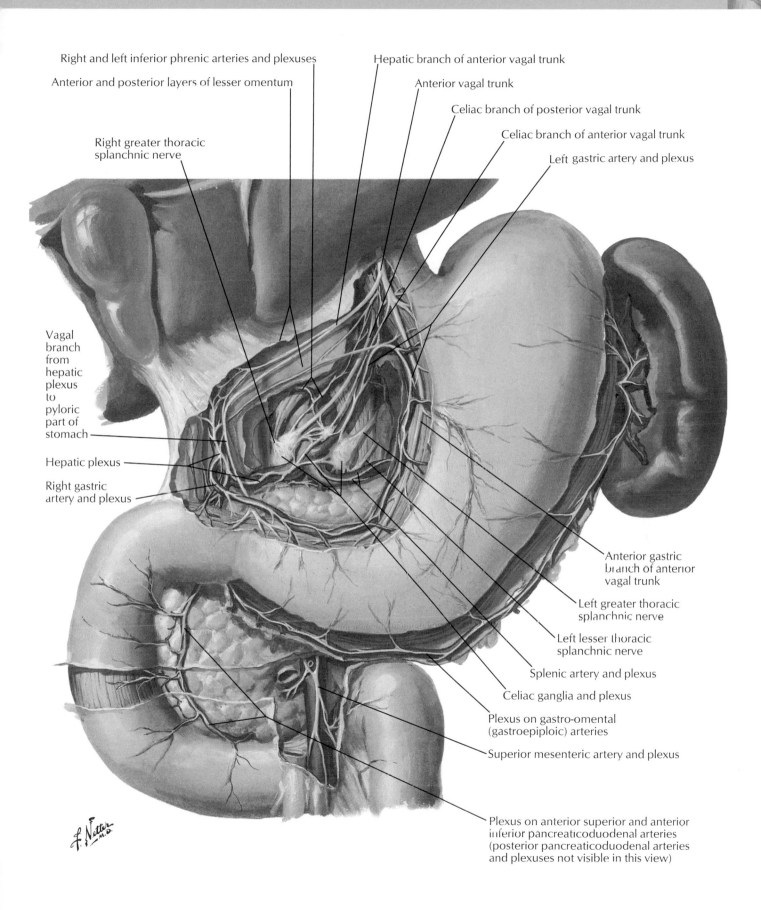

Right and left inferior phrenic arteries and plexuses

Anterior and posterior layers of lesser omentum

Hepatic branch of anterior vagal trunk

Anterior vagal trunk

Celiac branch of posterior vagal trunk

Celiac branch of anterior vagal trunk

Left gastric artery and plexus

Right greater thoracic splanchnic nerve

Vagal branch from hepatic plexus to pyloric part of stomach

Hepatic plexus

Right gastric artery and plexus

Anterior gastric branch of anterior vagal trunk

Left greater thoracic splanchnic nerve

Left lesser thoracic splanchnic nerve

Splenic artery and plexus

Celiac ganglia and plexus

Plexus on gastro-omental (gastroepiploic) arteries

Superior mesenteric artery and plexus

Plexus on anterior superior and anterior inferior pancreaticoduodenal arteries (posterior pancreaticoduodenal arteries and plexuses not visible in this view)

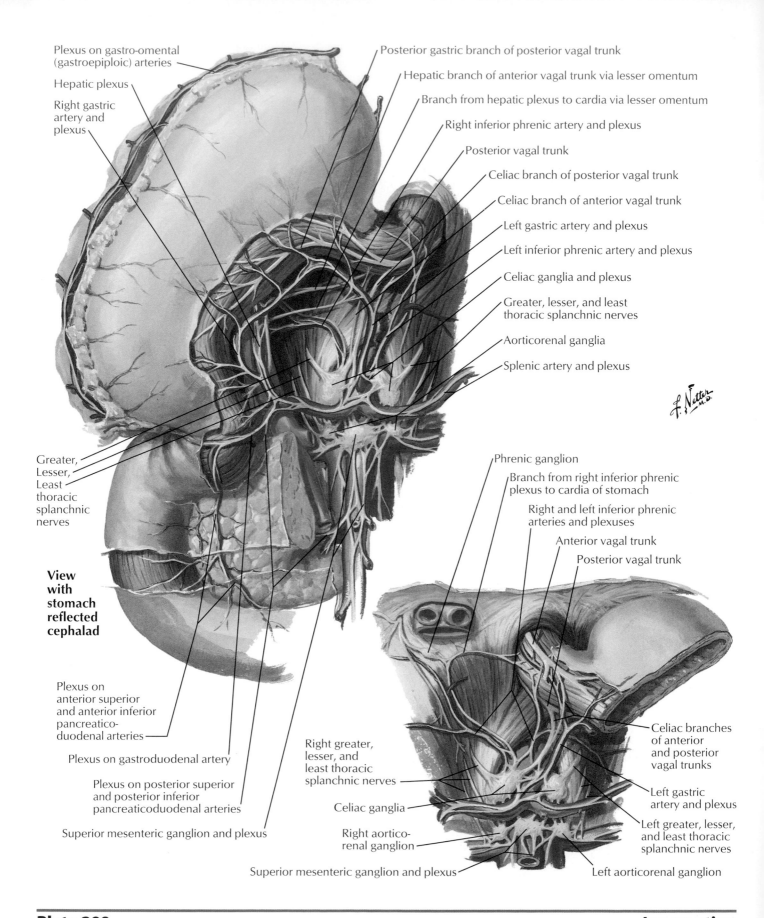

Plexus on gastro-omental (gastroepiploic) arteries

Hepatic plexus

Right gastric artery and plexus

Posterior gastric branch of posterior vagal trunk

Hepatic branch of anterior vagal trunk via lesser omentum

Branch from hepatic plexus to cardia via lesser omentum

Right inferior phrenic artery and plexus

Posterior vagal trunk

Celiac branch of posterior vagal trunk

Celiac branch of anterior vagal trunk

Left gastric artery and plexus

Left inferior phrenic artery and plexus

Celiac ganglia and plexus

Greater, lesser, and least thoracic splanchnic nerves

Aorticorenal ganglia

Splenic artery and plexus

Greater, Lesser, Least thoracic splanchnic nerves

View with stomach reflected cephalad

Plexus on anterior superior and anterior inferior pancreatico-duodenal arteries

Plexus on gastroduodenal artery

Plexus on posterior superior and posterior inferior pancreaticoduodenal arteries

Superior mesenteric ganglion and plexus

Right greater, lesser, and least thoracic splanchnic nerves

Celiac ganglia

Right aortico-renal ganglion

Superior mesenteric ganglion and plexus

Phrenic ganglion

Branch from right inferior phrenic plexus to cardia of stomach

Right and left inferior phrenic arteries and plexuses

Anterior vagal trunk

Posterior vagal trunk

Celiac branches of anterior and posterior vagal trunks

Left gastric artery and plexus

Left greater, lesser, and least thoracic splanchnic nerves

Left aorticorenal ganglion

Plate 299 **Innervation**

Autonomic Innervation of Stomach and Duodenum: Schema

Right 6th thoracic ganglion of sympathetic trunk

Gray, White rami communicantes

Spinal sensory (dorsal root) ganglion

Anterior (ventral) root of spinal nerve

Right greater thoracic splanchnic nerve

Right lesser thoracic splanchnic nerve

Celiac ganglia

Least thoracic splanchnic nerve

Common hepatic artery

Proper hepatic artery

Superior mesenteric ganglion

Aorticorenal ganglia

Right gastric artery

Right renal artery

Gastroduodenal artery

Posterior and anterior superior pancreatico-duodenal arteries

Superior mesenteric artery

Posterior and anterior inferior pancreatico-duodenal arteries

Esophageal plexus

Left greater thoracic splanchnic nerve

Aortic plexus

Left 9th thoracic ganglion of sympathetic trunk

Posterior vagal trunk and celiac branch

Anterior vagal trunk and celiac branch of vagus nerve (X)

Left gastric artery

Celiac trunk

Splenic artery

Short gastric arteries

Left, Right gastro-omental (gastroepiploic) arteries

Sympathetic fibers

Preganglionic ——————

Postganglionic - - - - - - -

Parasympathetic fibers

Preganglionic ——————

Postganglionic - - - - - - -

Afferent fibers ——————

f. Netter
m.d.

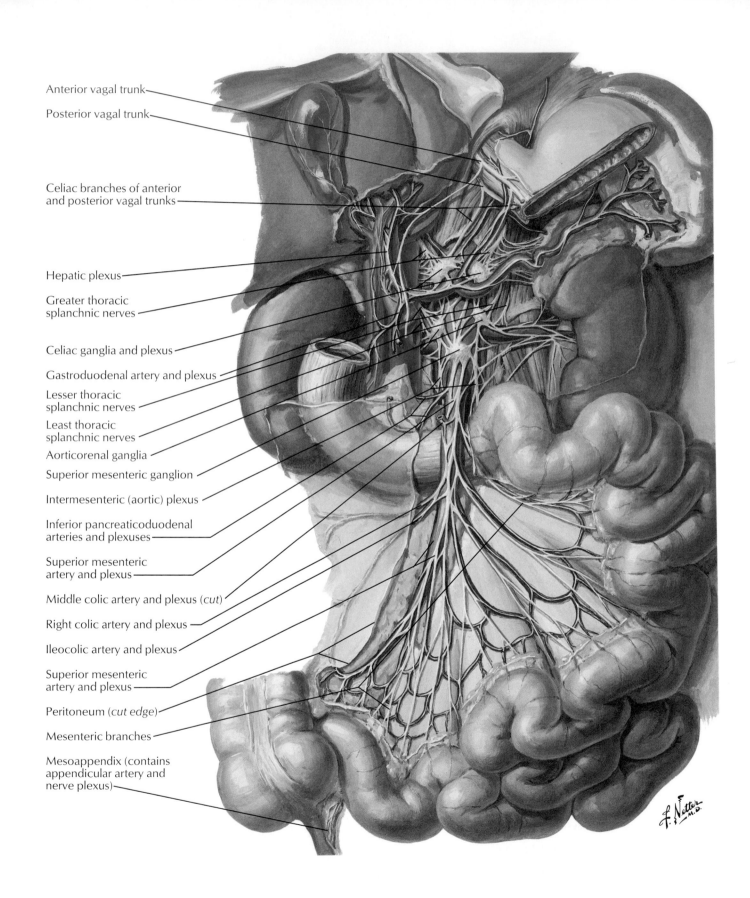

Anterior vagal trunk

Posterior vagal trunk

Celiac branches of anterior
and posterior vagal trunks

Hepatic plexus

Greater thoracic
splanchnic nerves

Celiac ganglia and plexus

Gastroduodenal artery and plexus

Lesser thoracic
splanchnic nerves

Least thoracic
splanchnic nerves

Aorticorenal ganglia

Superior mesenteric ganglion

Intermesenteric (aortic) plexus

Inferior pancreaticoduodenal
arteries and plexuses

Superior mesenteric
artery and plexus

Middle colic artery and plexus (*cut*)

Right colic artery and plexus

Ileocolic artery and plexus

Superior mesenteric
artery and plexus

Peritoneum (*cut edge*)

Mesenteric branches

Mesoappendix (contains
appendicular artery and
nerve plexus)

Plate 301

Innervation

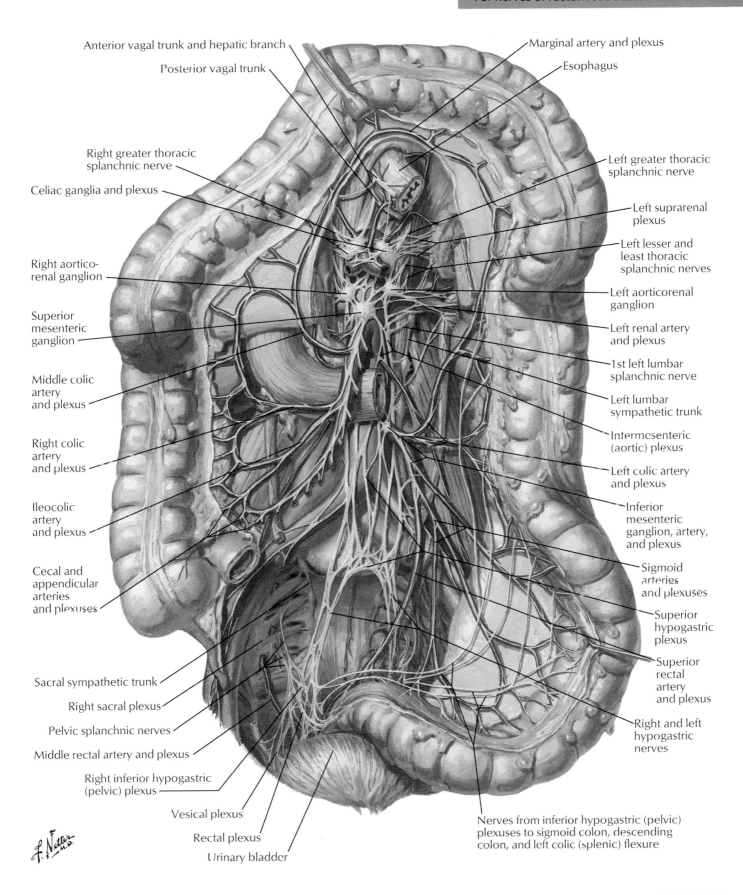

Anterior vagal trunk and hepatic branch

Posterior vagal trunk

Right greater thoracic splanchnic nerve

Celiac ganglia and plexus

Right aortico-renal ganglion

Superior mesenteric ganglion

Middle colic artery and plexus

Right colic artery and plexus

Ileocolic artery and plexus

Cecal and appendicular arteries and plexuses

Sacral sympathetic trunk

Right sacral plexus

Pelvic splanchnic nerves

Middle rectal artery and plexus

Right inferior hypogastric (pelvic) plexus

Vesical plexus

Rectal plexus

Urinary bladder

Marginal artery and plexus

Esophagus

Left greater thoracic splanchnic nerve

Left suprarenal plexus

Left lesser and least thoracic splanchnic nerves

Left aorticorenal ganglion

Left renal artery and plexus

1st left lumbar splanchnic nerve

Left lumbar sympathetic trunk

Intermesenteric (aortic) plexus

Left colic artery and plexus

Inferior mesenteric ganglion, artery, and plexus

Sigmoid arteries and plexuses

Superior hypogastric plexus

Superior rectal artery and plexus

Right and left hypogastric nerves

Nerves from inferior hypogastric (pelvic) plexuses to sigmoid colon, descending colon, and left colic (splenic) flexure

Innervation

Plate 302

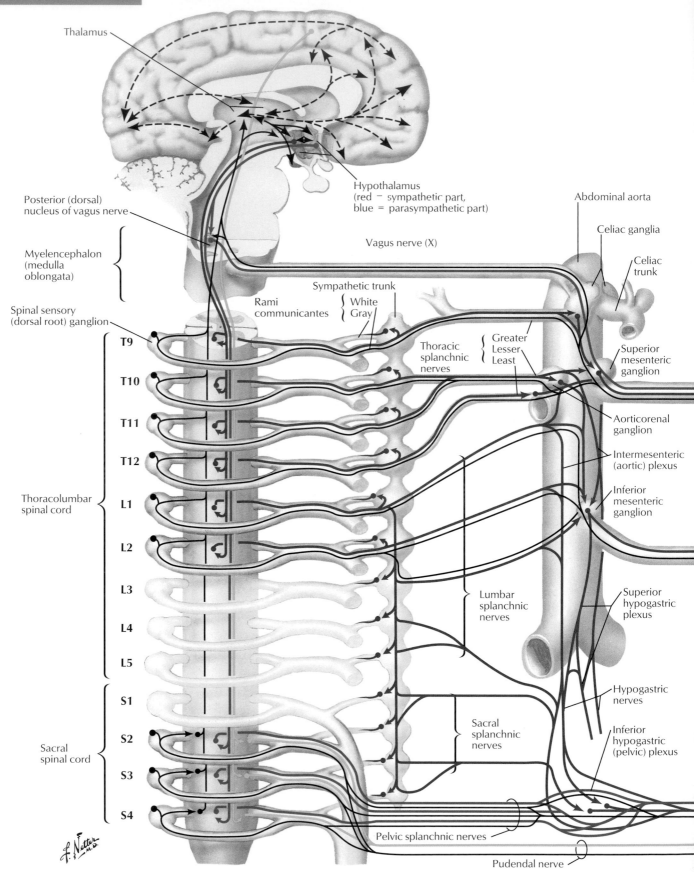

Thalamus

Hypothalamus
(red = sympathetic part,
blue = parasympathetic part)

Abdominal aorta

Celiac ganglia

Celiac trunk

Posterior (dorsal)
nucleus of vagus nerve

Myelencephalon
(medulla
oblongata)

Vagus nerve (X)

Spinal sensory
(dorsal root) ganglion

Sympathetic trunk
White
Gray

Rami
communicantes

Thoracic
splanchnic
nerves

Greater
Lesser
Least

Superior
mesenteric
ganglion

T9

T10

T11

T12

Aorticorenal
ganglion

Intermesenteric
(aortic) plexus

L1

Inferior
mesenteric
ganglion

L2

Thoracolumbar
spinal cord

L3

L4

Lumbar
splanchnic
nerves

Superior
hypogastric
plexus

L5

S1

Hypogastric
nerves

Sacral
splanchnic
nerves

Sacral
spinal cord

S2

S3

Inferior
hypogastric
(pelvic) plexus

S4

Pelvic splanchnic nerves

Pudendal nerve

Plate 303

Innervation

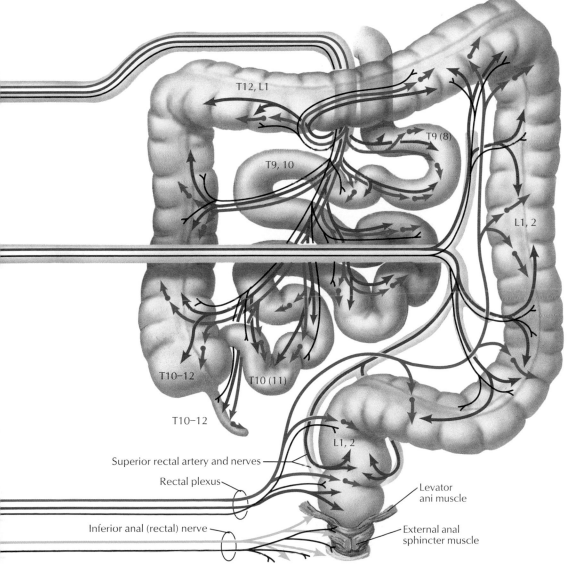

Sympathetic efferents
Parasympathetic efferents
Somatic efferents
Afferents and CNS connections
Indefinite paths

T12, L1

T9 (8)

T9, 10

L1, 2

T10–12

T10 (11)

T10–12

L1, 2

Superior rectal artery and nerves

Rectal plexus

Levator
ani muscle

Inferior anal (rectal) nerve

External anal
sphincter muscle

Chief segmental sources
of sympathetic fibers
innervating different
regions of intestinal
tract are indicated.
Numerous afferent fibers
are carried centripetally
through approximately
the same sympathetic
splanchnic nerves
that transmit
preganglionic fibers.

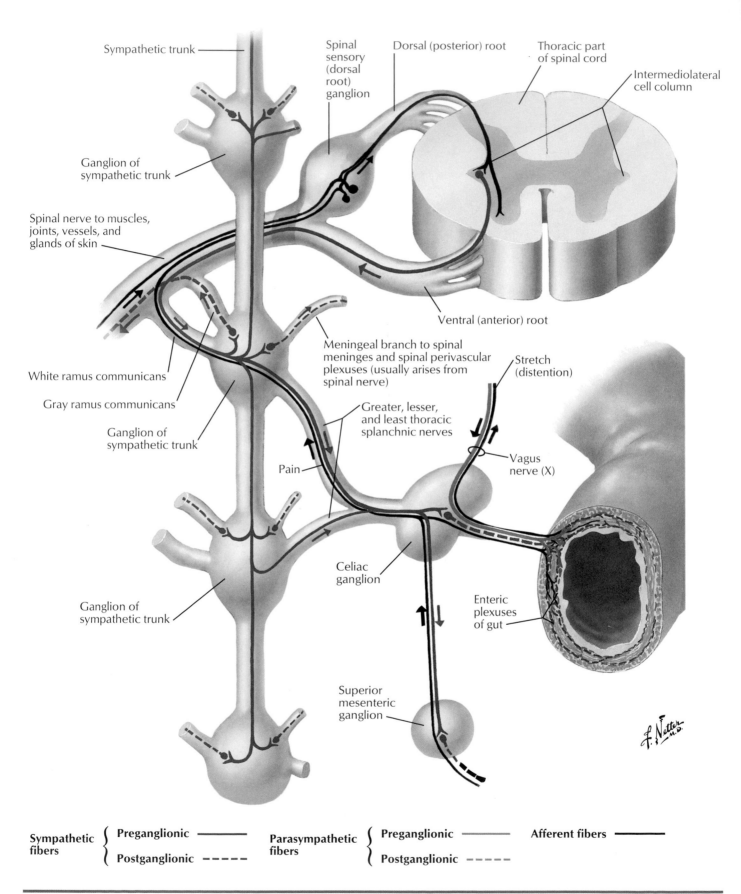

Sympathetic trunk

Spinal sensory (dorsal root) ganglion

Dorsal (posterior) root

Thoracic part of spinal cord

Intermediolateral cell column

Ganglion of sympathetic trunk

Spinal nerve to muscles, joints, vessels, and glands of skin

Ventral (anterior) root

White ramus communicans

Gray ramus communicans

Meningeal branch to spinal meninges and spinal perivascular plexuses (usually arises from spinal nerve)

Stretch (distention)

Ganglion of sympathetic trunk

Greater, lesser, and least thoracic splanchnic nerves

Pain

Vagus nerve (X)

Celiac ganglion

Enteric plexuses of gut

Ganglion of sympathetic trunk

Superior mesenteric ganglion

Sympathetic fibers	Preganglionic ———	Parasympathetic fibers	Preganglionic ———	Afferent fibers ———
	Postganglionic - - - -		Postganglionic - - - -	

Plate 304   **Innervation**

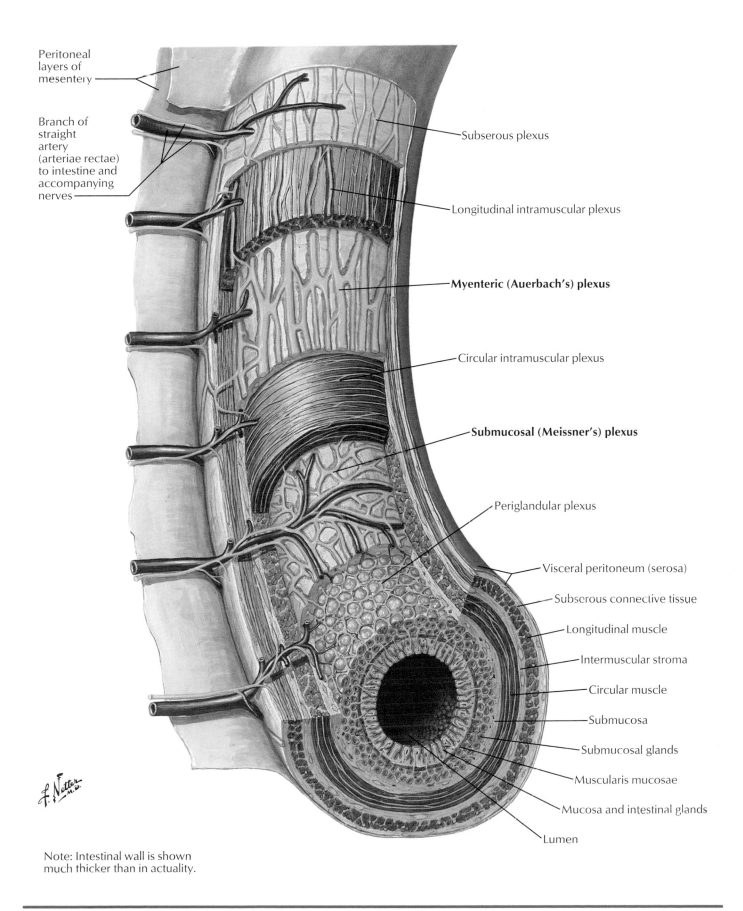

Peritoneal layers of mesentery

Branch of straight artery (arteriae rectae) to intestine and accompanying nerves

Subserous plexus

Longitudinal intramuscular plexus

Myenteric (Auerbach's) plexus

Circular intramuscular plexus

Submucosal (Meissner's) plexus

Periglandular plexus

Visceral peritoneum (serosa)

Subserous connective tissue

Longitudinal muscle

Intermuscular stroma

Circular muscle

Submucosa

Submucosal glands

Muscularis mucosae

Mucosa and intestinal glands

Lumen

Note: Intestinal wall is shown much thicker than in actuality.

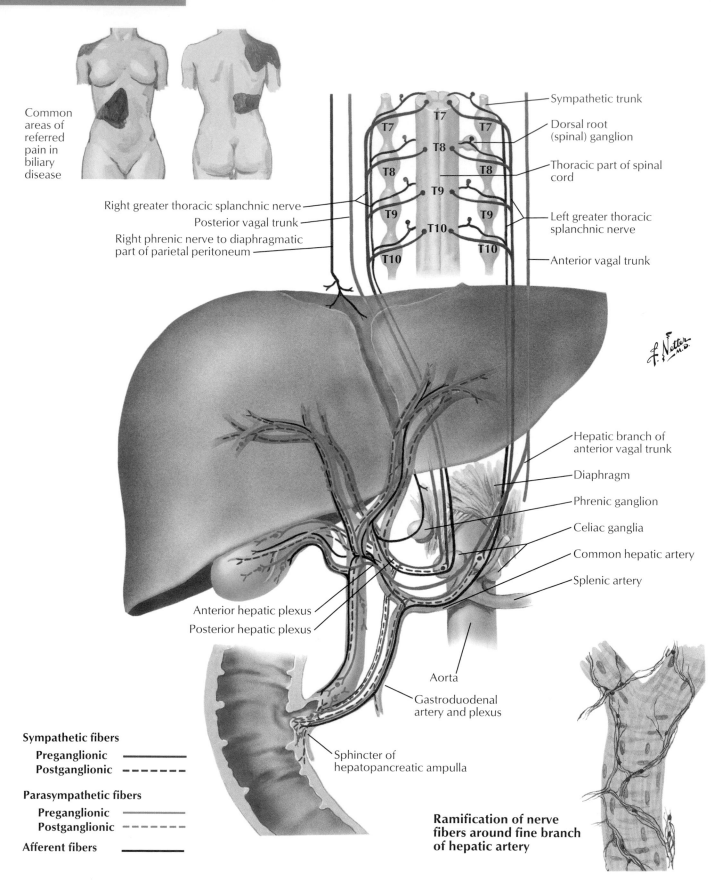

Common areas of referred pain in biliary disease

Sympathetic trunk

Dorsal root (spinal) ganglion

Thoracic part of spinal cord

Left greater thoracic splanchnic nerve

Anterior vagal trunk

Right greater thoracic splanchnic nerve

Posterior vagal trunk

Right phrenic nerve to diaphragmatic part of parietal peritoneum

Hepatic branch of anterior vagal trunk

Diaphragm

Phrenic ganglion

Celiac ganglia

Common hepatic artery

Splenic artery

Anterior hepatic plexus

Posterior hepatic plexus

Aorta

Gastroduodenal artery and plexus

Sphincter of hepatopancreatic ampulla

Sympathetic fibers

Preganglionic ———

Postganglionic − − − −

Parasympathetic fibers

Preganglionic ———

Postganglionic − − − −

Afferent fibers ———

Ramification of nerve fibers around fine branch of hepatic artery

Plate 306

Innervation

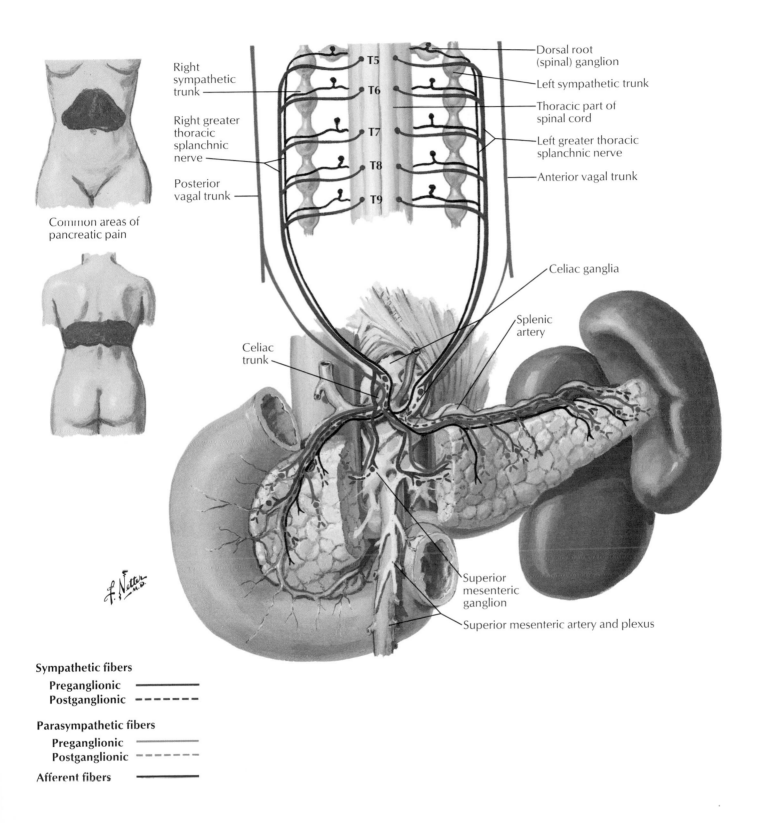

Common areas of pancreatic pain

Right sympathetic trunk

Right greater thoracic splanchnic nerve

Posterior vagal trunk

T5
T6
T7
T8
T9

Dorsal root (spinal) ganglion

Left sympathetic trunk

Thoracic part of spinal cord

Left greater thoracic splanchnic nerve

Anterior vagal trunk

Celiac ganglia

Splenic artery

Celiac trunk

Superior mesenteric ganglion

Superior mesenteric artery and plexus

Sympathetic fibers
  Preganglionic ————
  Postganglionic – – – –

Parasympathetic fibers
  Preganglionic ————
  Postganglionic – – – –

Afferent fibers ————

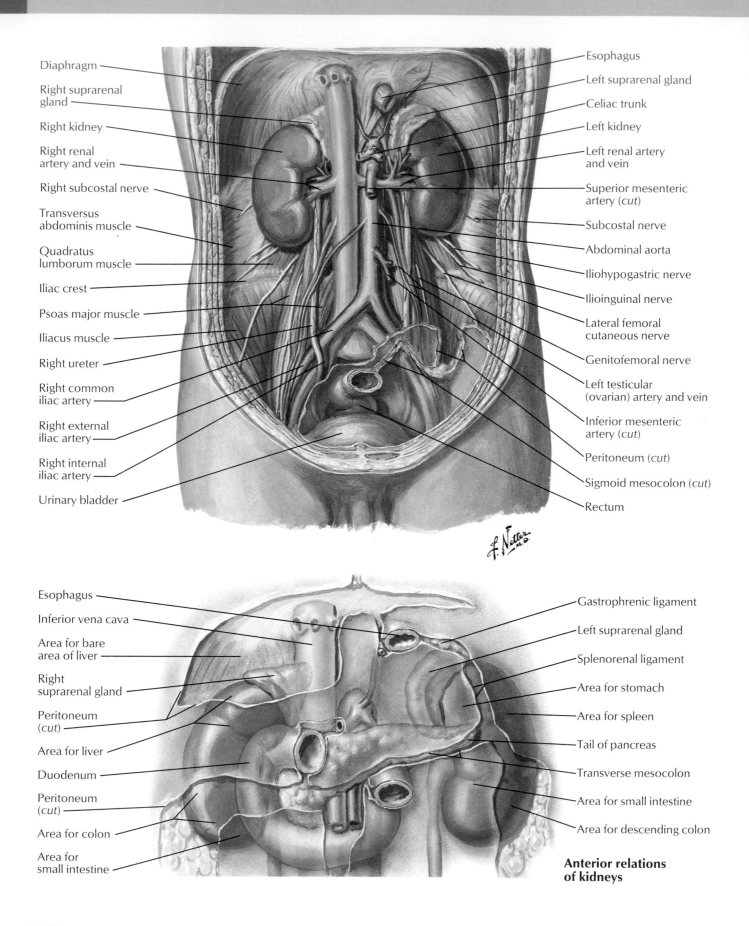

Diaphragm

Right suprarenal gland

Right kidney

Right renal artery and vein

Right subcostal nerve

Transversus abdominis muscle

Quadratus lumborum muscle

Iliac crest

Psoas major muscle

Iliacus muscle

Right ureter

Right common iliac artery

Right external iliac artery

Right internal iliac artery

Urinary bladder

Esophagus

Left suprarenal gland

Celiac trunk

Left kidney

Left renal artery and vein

Superior mesenteric artery (cut)

Subcostal nerve

Abdominal aorta

Iliohypogastric nerve

Ilioinguinal nerve

Lateral femoral cutaneous nerve

Genitofemoral nerve

Left testicular (ovarian) artery and vein

Inferior mesenteric artery (cut)

Peritoneum (cut)

Sigmoid mesocolon (cut)

Rectum

Esophagus

Inferior vena cava

Area for bare area of liver

Right suprarenal gland

Peritoneum (cut)

Area for liver

Duodenum

Peritoneum (cut)

Area for colon

Area for small intestine

Gastrophrenic ligament

Left suprarenal gland

Splenorenal ligament

Area for stomach

Area for spleen

Tail of pancreas

Transverse mesocolon

Area for small intestine

Area for descending colon

Anterior relations of kidneys

Plate 308

Kidneys and Suprarenal Glands

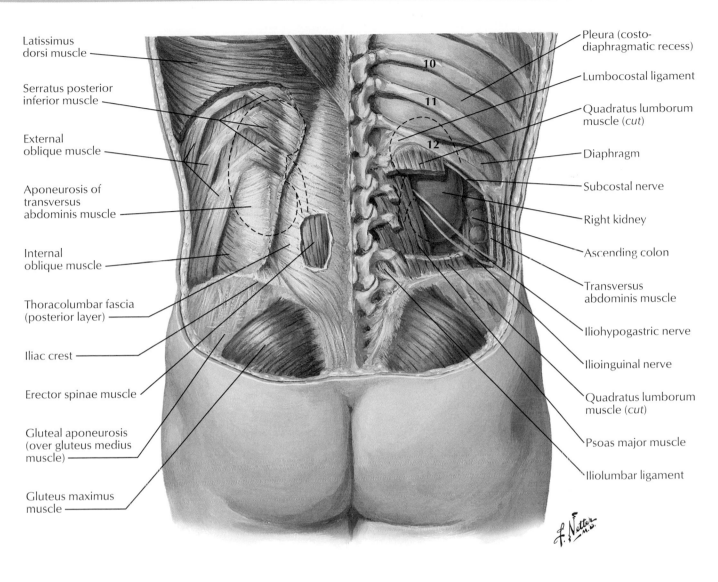

Latissimus dorsi muscle

Serratus posterior inferior muscle

External oblique muscle

Aponeurosis of transversus abdominis muscle

Internal oblique muscle

Thoracolumbar fascia (posterior layer)

Iliac crest

Erector spinae muscle

Gluteal aponeurosis (over gluteus medius muscle)

Gluteus maximus muscle

Pleura (costo-diaphragmatic recess)

Lumbocostal ligament

Quadratus lumborum muscle (cut)

Diaphragm

Subcostal nerve

Right kidney

Ascending colon

Transversus abdominis muscle

Iliohypogastric nerve

Ilioinguinal nerve

Quadratus lumborum muscle (cut)

Psoas major muscle

Iliolumbar ligament

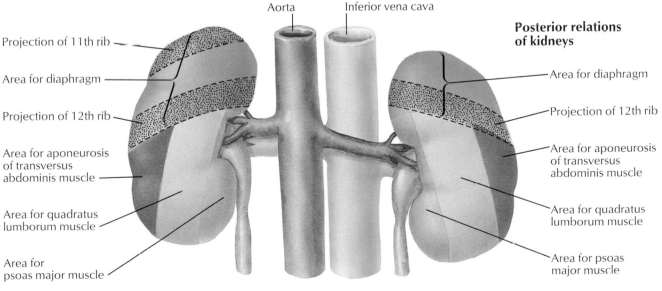

Aorta

Inferior vena cava

Posterior relations of kidneys

Projection of 11th rib

Area for diaphragm

Projection of 12th rib

Area for aponeurosis of transversus abdominis muscle

Area for quadratus lumborum muscle

Area for psoas major muscle

Area for diaphragm

Projection of 12th rib

Area for aponeurosis of transversus abdominis muscle

Area for quadratus lumborum muscle

Area for psoas major muscle

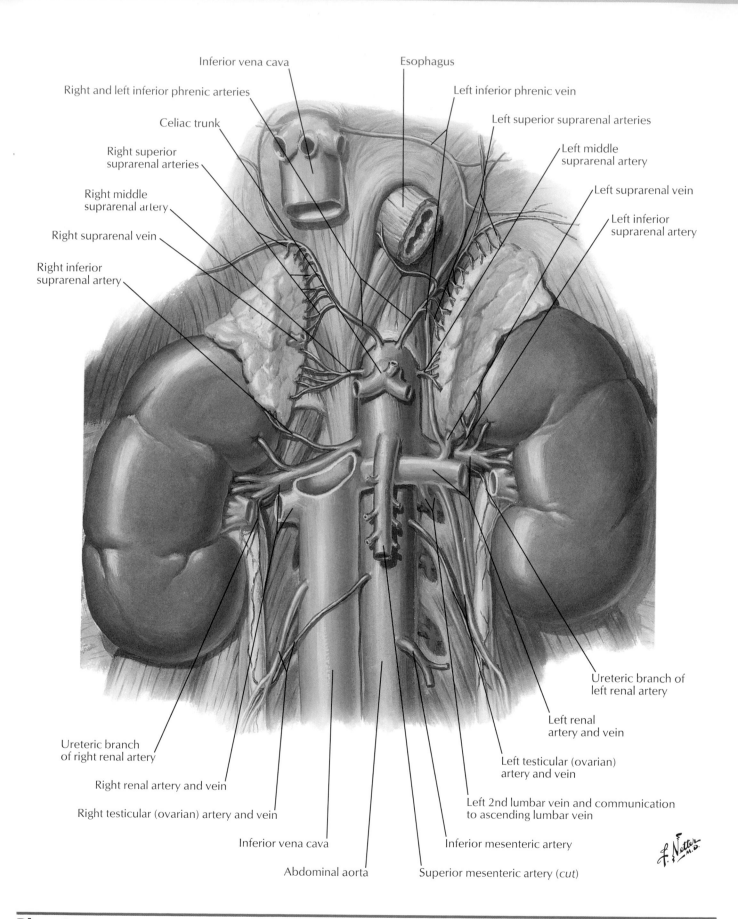

Inferior vena cava

Right and left inferior phrenic arteries

Celiac trunk

Right superior suprarenal arteries

Right middle suprarenal artery

Right suprarenal vein

Right inferior suprarenal artery

Esophagus

Left inferior phrenic vein

Left superior suprarenal arteries

Left middle suprarenal artery

Left suprarenal vein

Left inferior suprarenal artery

Ureteric branch of left renal artery

Left renal artery and vein

Left testicular (ovarian) artery and vein

Left 2nd lumbar vein and communication to ascending lumbar vein

Inferior mesenteric artery

Superior mesenteric artery (cut)

Ureteric branch of right renal artery

Right renal artery and vein

Right testicular (ovarian) artery and vein

Inferior vena cava

Abdominal aorta

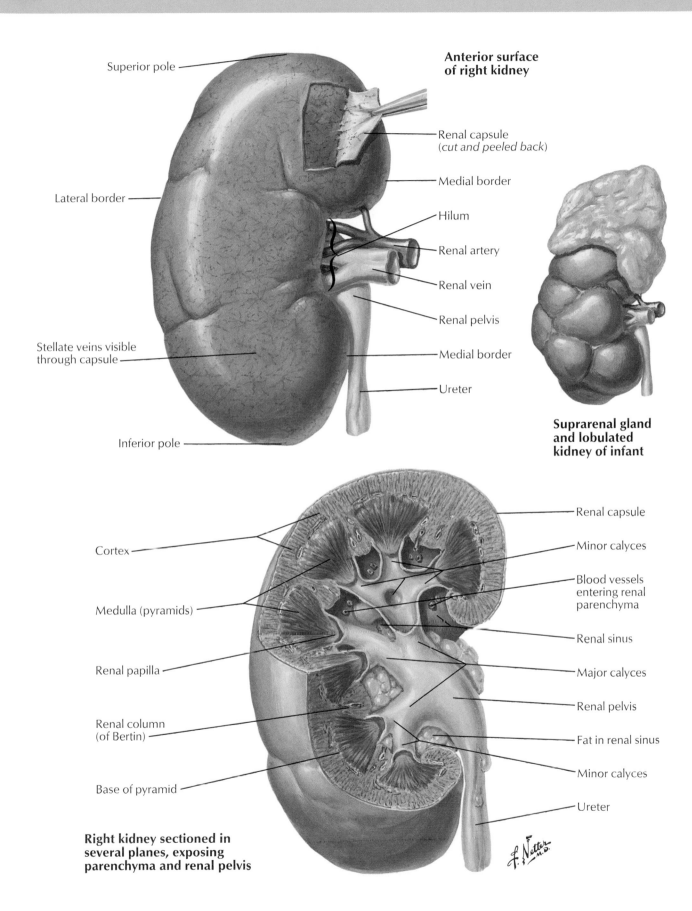

Superior pole

Anterior surface of right kidney

Renal capsule (*cut and peeled back*)

Medial border

Lateral border

Hilum

Renal artery

Renal vein

Renal pelvis

Stellate veins visible through capsule

Medial border

Ureter

Inferior pole

Suprarenal gland and lobulated kidney of infant

Renal capsule

Cortex

Minor calyces

Blood vessels entering renal parenchyma

Medulla (pyramids)

Renal sinus

Renal papilla

Major calyces

Renal column (of Bertin)

Renal pelvis

Fat in renal sinus

Minor calyces

Base of pyramid

Ureter

Right kidney sectioned in several planes, exposing parenchyma and renal pelvis

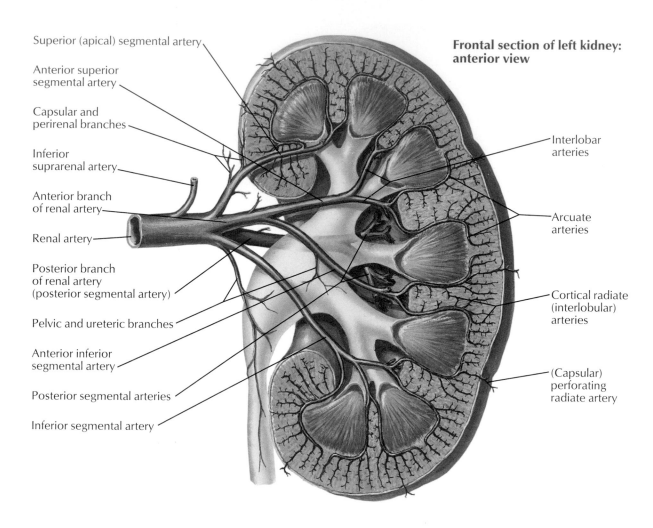

Superior (apical) segmental artery

Anterior superior segmental artery

Capsular and perirenal branches

Inferior suprarenal artery

Anterior branch of renal artery

Renal artery

Posterior branch of renal artery (posterior segmental artery)

Pelvic and ureteric branches

Anterior inferior segmental artery

Posterior segmental arteries

Inferior segmental artery

Frontal section of left kidney: anterior view

Interlobar arteries

Arcuate arteries

Cortical radiate (interlobular) arteries

(Capsular) perforating radiate artery

Vascular renal segments

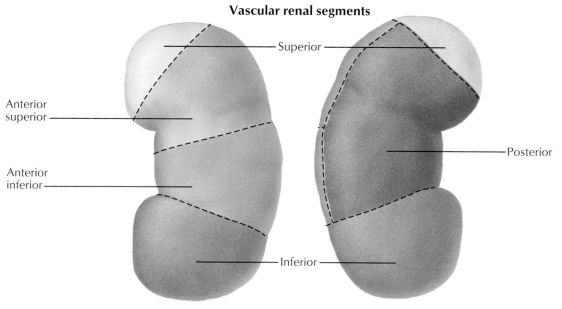

Superior

Anterior superior

Anterior inferior

Posterior

Inferior

Anterior surface of left kidney

Posterior surface of left kidney

Plate 312

Kidneys and Suprarenal Glands

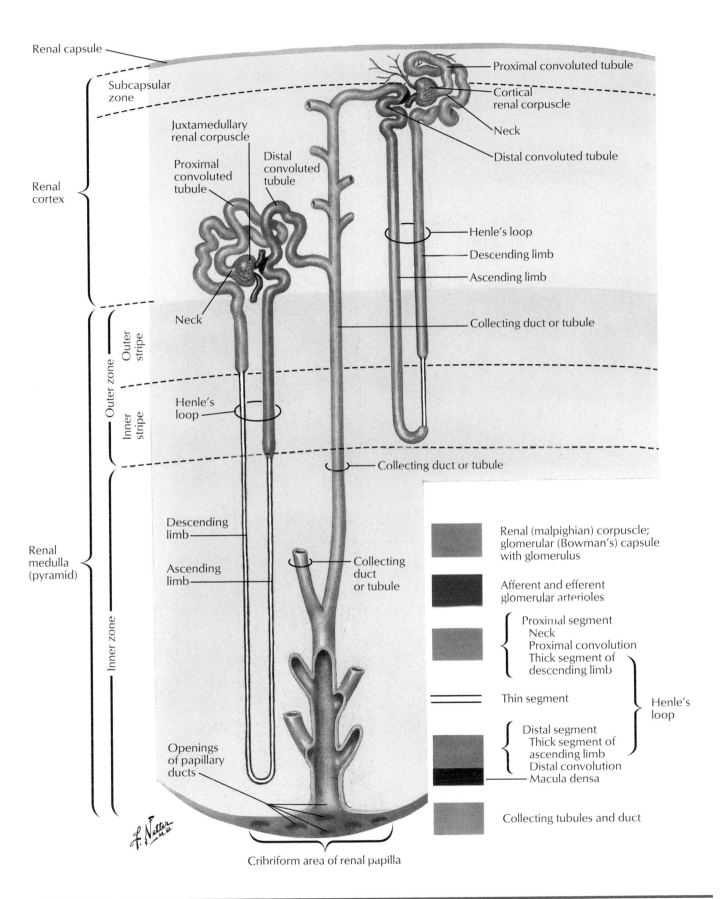

Renal capsule

Subcapsular zone

Renal cortex

Juxtamedullary renal corpuscle

Proximal convoluted tubule

Distal convoluted tubule

Neck

Outer zone — Outer stripe

Inner stripe

Henle's loop

Renal medulla (pyramid)

Descending limb

Ascending limb

Inner zone

Openings of papillary ducts

Proximal convoluted tubule

Cortical renal corpuscle

Neck

Distal convoluted tubule

Henle's loop

Descending limb

Ascending limb

Collecting duct or tubule

Collecting duct or tubule

Collecting duct or tubule

Renal (malpighian) corpuscle; glomerular (Bowman's) capsule with glomerulus

Afferent and efferent glomerular arterioles

Proximal segment
Neck
Proximal convolution
Thick segment of descending limb

Thin segment

Henle's loop

Distal segment
Thick segment of ascending limb
Distal convolution
Macula densa

Collecting tubules and duct

Cribriform area of renal papilla

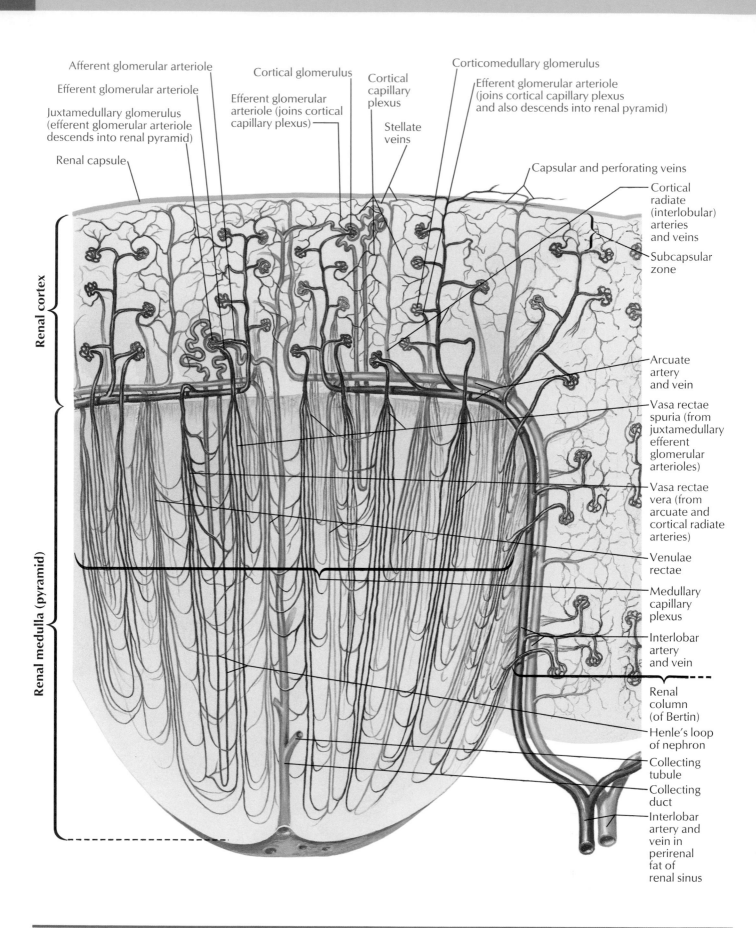

Afferent glomerular arteriole

Efferent glomerular arteriole

Juxtamedullary glomerulus (efferent glomerular arteriole descends into renal pyramid)

Renal capsule

Cortical glomerulus

Efferent glomerular arteriole (joins cortical capillary plexus)

Cortical capillary plexus

Stellate veins

Corticomedullary glomerulus

Efferent glomerular arteriole (joins cortical capillary plexus and also descends into renal pyramid)

Capsular and perforating veins

Cortical radiate (interlobular) arteries and veins

Subcapsular zone

Arcuate artery and vein

Vasa rectae spuria (from juxtamedullary efferent glomerular arterioles)

Vasa rectae vera (from arcuate and cortical radiate arteries)

Venulae rectae

Medullary capillary plexus

Interlobar artery and vein

Renal column (of Bertin)

Henle's loop of nephron

Collecting tubule

Collecting duct

Interlobar artery and vein in perirenal fat of renal sinus

Renal cortex

Renal medulla (pyramid)

Plate 314   **Kidneys and Suprarenal Glands**

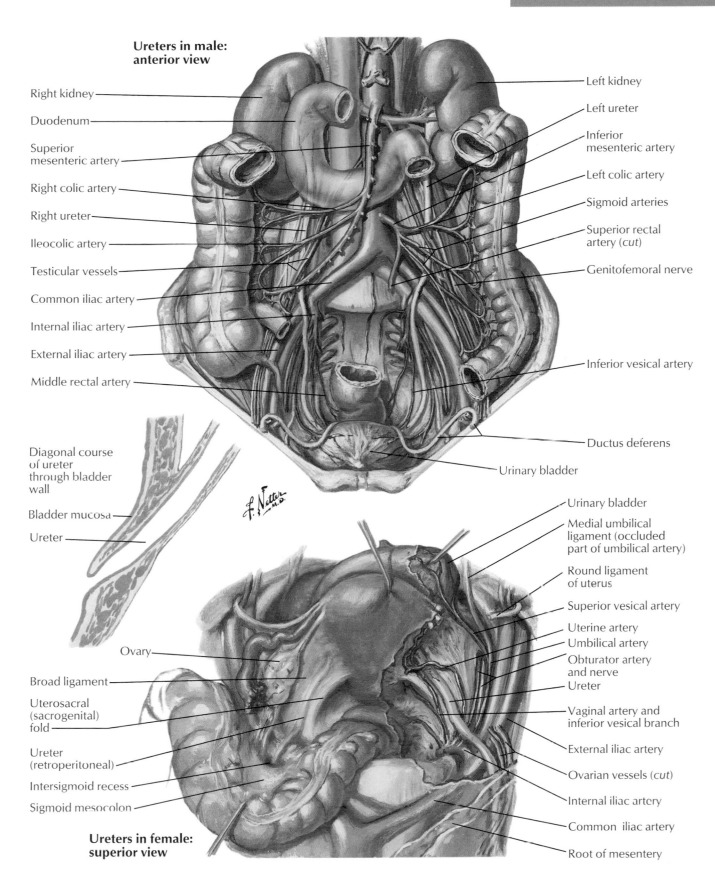

Ureters in male: anterior view

Right kidney

Duodenum

Superior mesenteric artery

Right colic artery

Right ureter

Ileocolic artery

Testicular vessels

Common iliac artery

Internal iliac artery

External iliac artery

Middle rectal artery

Left kidney

Left ureter

Inferior mesenteric artery

Left colic artery

Sigmoid arteries

Superior rectal artery (*cut*)

Genitofemoral nerve

Inferior vesical artery

Ductus deferens

Urinary bladder

Diagonal course of ureter through bladder wall

Bladder mucosa

Ureter

Urinary bladder

Medial umbilical ligament (occluded part of umbilical artery)

Round ligament of uterus

Superior vesical artery

Uterine artery

Umbilical artery

Obturator artery and nerve

Ureter

Vaginal artery and inferior vesical branch

External iliac artery

Ovarian vessels (*cut*)

Internal iliac artery

Common iliac artery

Root of mesentery

Ovary

Broad ligament

Uterosacral (sacrogenital) fold

Ureter (retroperitoneal)

Intersigmoid recess

Sigmoid mesocolon

Ureters in female: superior view

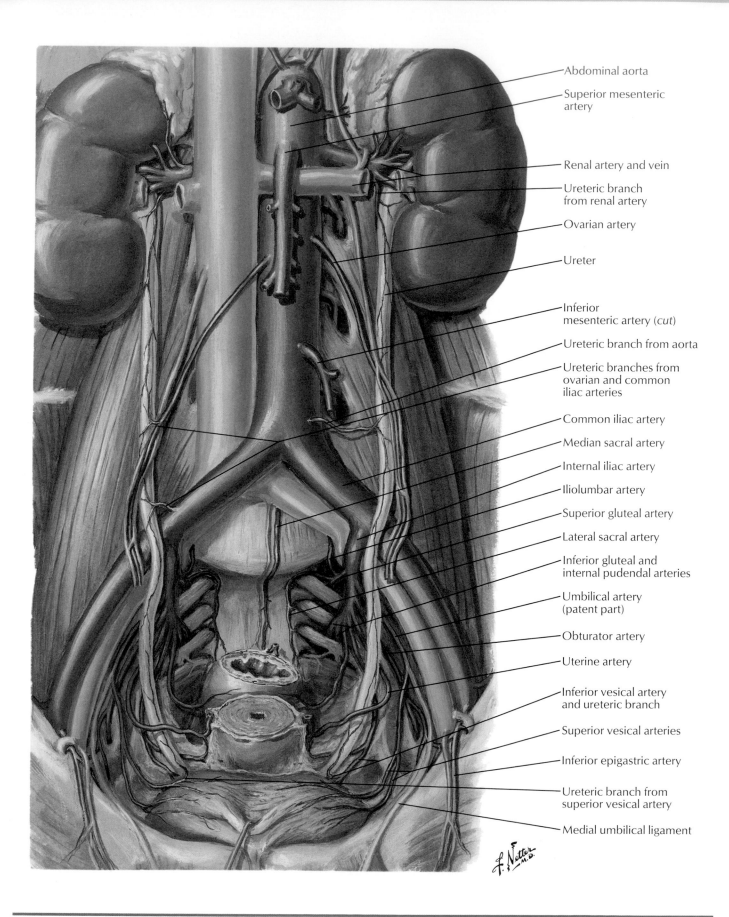

Abdominal aorta

Superior mesenteric artery

Renal artery and vein

Ureteric branch from renal artery

Ovarian artery

Ureter

Inferior mesenteric artery (*cut*)

Ureteric branch from aorta

Ureteric branches from ovarian and common iliac arteries

Common iliac artery

Median sacral artery

Internal iliac artery

Iliolumbar artery

Superior gluteal artery

Lateral sacral artery

Inferior gluteal and internal pudendal arteries

Umbilical artery (patent part)

Obturator artery

Uterine artery

Inferior vesical artery and ureteric branch

Superior vesical arteries

Inferior epigastric artery

Ureteric branch from superior vesical artery

Medial umbilical ligament

Plate 316   **Kidneys and Suprarenal Glands**

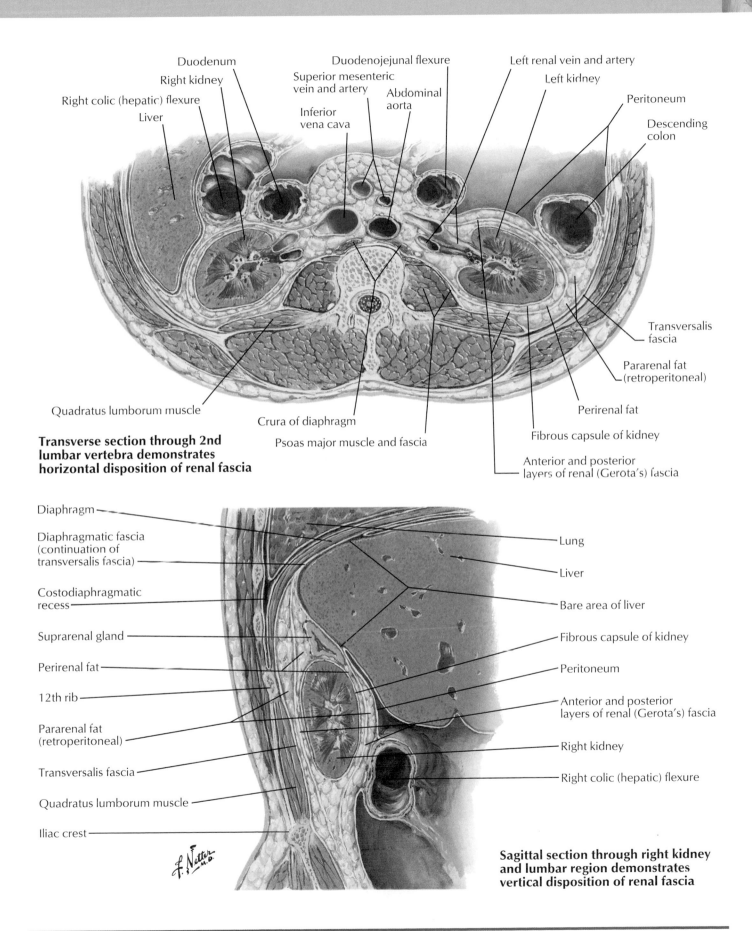

Duodenum
Right kidney
Right colic (hepatic) flexure
Liver
Duodenojejunal flexure
Superior mesenteric vein and artery
Inferior vena cava
Abdominal aorta
Left renal vein and artery
Left kidney
Peritoneum
Descending colon
Transversalis fascia
Pararenal fat (retroperitoneal)
Perirenal fat
Fibrous capsule of kidney
Anterior and posterior layers of renal (Gerota's) fascia
Quadratus lumborum muscle
Crura of diaphragm
Psoas major muscle and fascia

Transverse section through 2nd lumbar vertebra demonstrates horizontal disposition of renal fascia

Diaphragm
Diaphragmatic fascia (continuation of transversalis fascia)
Costodiaphragmatic recess
Suprarenal gland
Perirenal fat
12th rib
Pararenal fat (retroperitoneal)
Transversalis fascia
Quadratus lumborum muscle
Iliac crest
Lung
Liver
Bare area of liver
Fibrous capsule of kidney
Peritoneum
Anterior and posterior layers of renal (Gerota's) fascia
Right kidney
Right colic (hepatic) flexure

Sagittal section through right kidney and lumbar region demonstrates vertical disposition of renal fascia

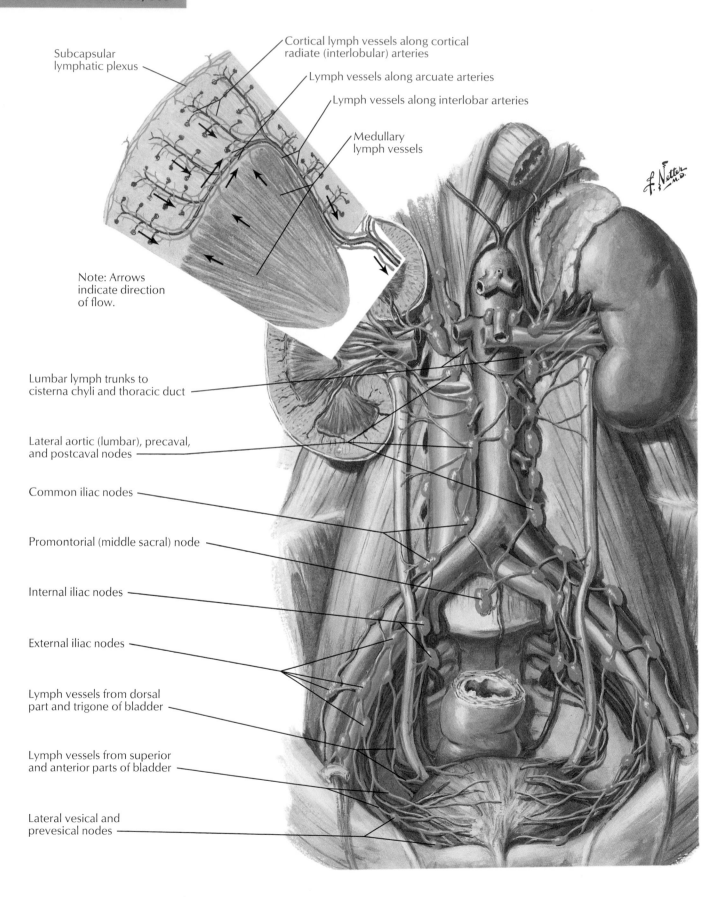

Subcapsular lymphatic plexus

Cortical lymph vessels along cortical radiate (interlobular) arteries

Lymph vessels along arcuate arteries

Lymph vessels along interlobar arteries

Medullary lymph vessels

Note: Arrows indicate direction of flow.

Lumbar lymph trunks to cisterna chyli and thoracic duct

Lateral aortic (lumbar), precaval, and postcaval nodes

Common iliac nodes

Promontorial (middle sacral) node

Internal iliac nodes

External iliac nodes

Lymph vessels from dorsal part and trigone of bladder

Lymph vessels from superior and anterior parts of bladder

Lateral vesical and prevesical nodes

Plate 318

Kidneys and Suprarenal Glands

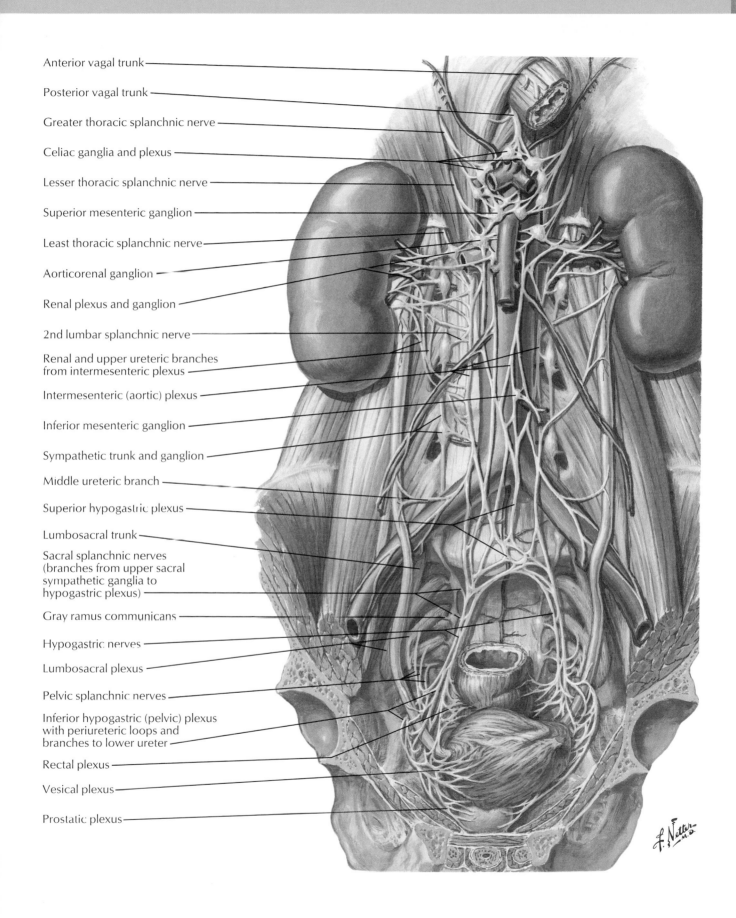

Anterior vagal trunk

Posterior vagal trunk

Greater thoracic splanchnic nerve

Celiac ganglia and plexus

Lesser thoracic splanchnic nerve

Superior mesenteric ganglion

Least thoracic splanchnic nerve

Aorticorenal ganglion

Renal plexus and ganglion

2nd lumbar splanchnic nerve

Renal and upper ureteric branches from intermesenteric plexus

Intermesenteric (aortic) plexus

Inferior mesenteric ganglion

Sympathetic trunk and ganglion

Middle ureteric branch

Superior hypogastric plexus

Lumbosacral trunk

Sacral splanchnic nerves (branches from upper sacral sympathetic ganglia to hypogastric plexus)

Gray ramus communicans

Hypogastric nerves

Lumbosacral plexus

Pelvic splanchnic nerves

Inferior hypogastric (pelvic) plexus with periureteric loops and branches to lower ureter

Rectal plexus

Vesical plexus

Prostatic plexus

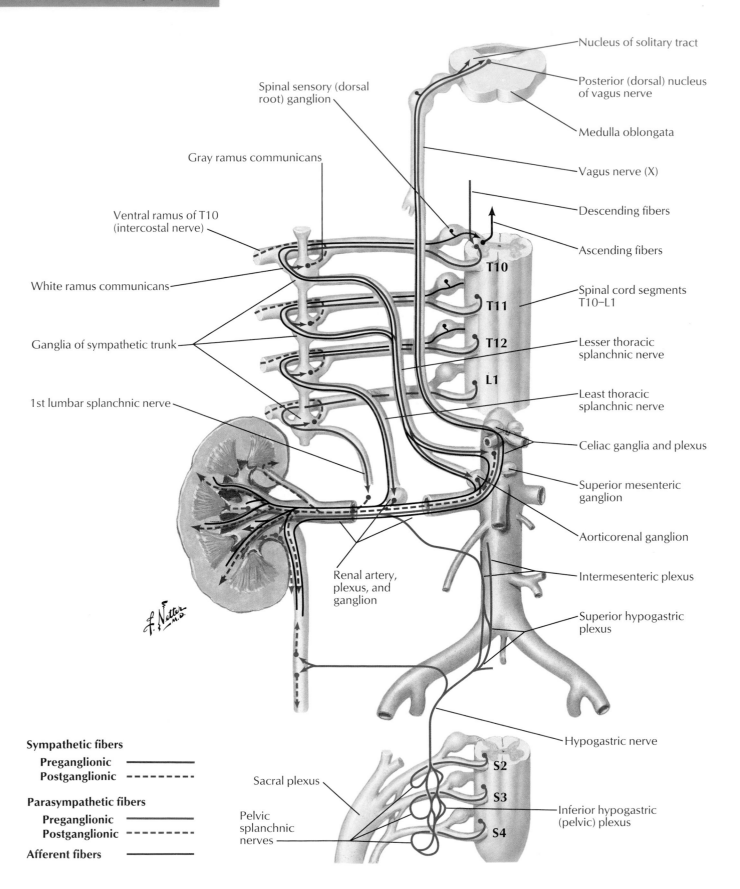

Nucleus of solitary tract

Posterior (dorsal) nucleus of vagus nerve

Medulla oblongata

Spinal sensory (dorsal root) ganglion

Vagus nerve (X)

Gray ramus communicans

Descending fibers

Ventral ramus of T10 (intercostal nerve)

Ascending fibers

T10

White ramus communicans

Spinal cord segments T10–L1

T11

Ganglia of sympathetic trunk

T12

Lesser thoracic splanchnic nerve

L1

1st lumbar splanchnic nerve

Least thoracic splanchnic nerve

Celiac ganglia and plexus

Superior mesenteric ganglion

Aorticorenal ganglion

Renal artery, plexus, and ganglion

Intermesenteric plexus

Superior hypogastric plexus

Hypogastric nerve

Sympathetic fibers
Preganglionic ——
Postganglionic - - - -

Parasympathetic fibers
Preganglionic ——
Postganglionic - - - -

Afferent fibers ——

Sacral plexus

Pelvic splanchnic nerves

S2

S3

S4

Inferior hypogastric (pelvic) plexus

Plate 320

Kidneys and Suprarenal Glands

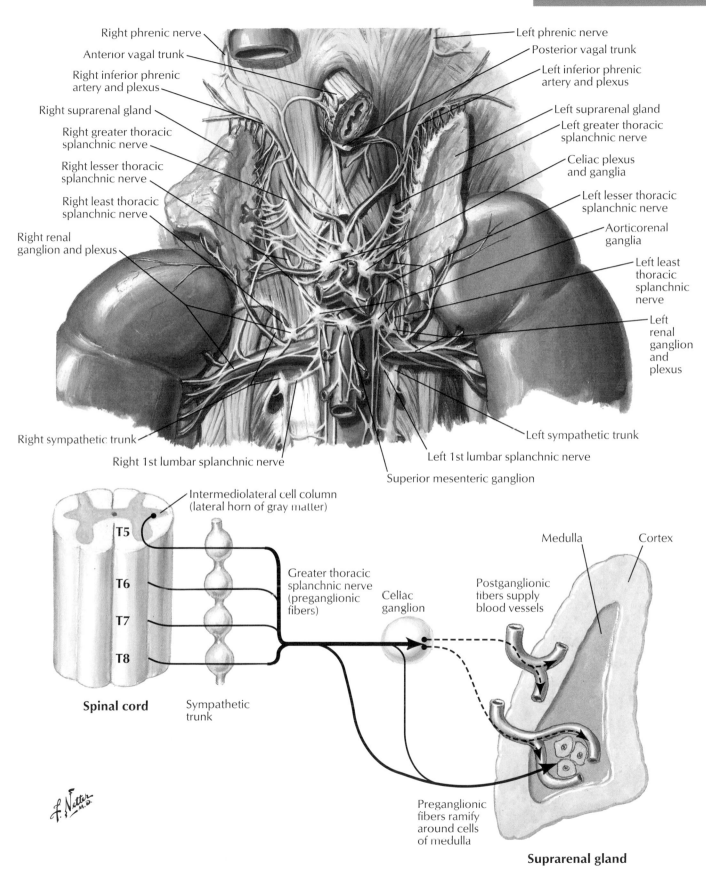

Right phrenic nerve
Anterior vagal trunk
Right inferior phrenic artery and plexus
Right suprarenal gland
Right greater thoracic splanchnic nerve
Right lesser thoracic splanchnic nerve
Right least thoracic splanchnic nerve
Right renal ganglion and plexus
Right sympathetic trunk
Right 1st lumbar splanchnic nerve

Left phrenic nerve
Posterior vagal trunk
Left inferior phrenic artery and plexus
Left suprarenal gland
Left greater thoracic splanchnic nerve
Celiac plexus and ganglia
Left lesser thoracic splanchnic nerve
Aorticorenal ganglia
Left least thoracic splanchnic nerve
Left renal ganglion and plexus
Left sympathetic trunk
Left 1st lumbar splanchnic nerve
Superior mesenteric ganglion

Intermediolateral cell column (lateral horn of gray matter)

T5
T6
T7
T8

Spinal cord

Sympathetic trunk

Greater thoracic splanchnic nerve (preganglionic fibers)

Celiac ganglion

Medulla   Cortex

Postganglionic fibers supply blood vessels

Preganglionic fibers ramify around cells of medulla

Suprarenal gland

f. Netter
M.D.

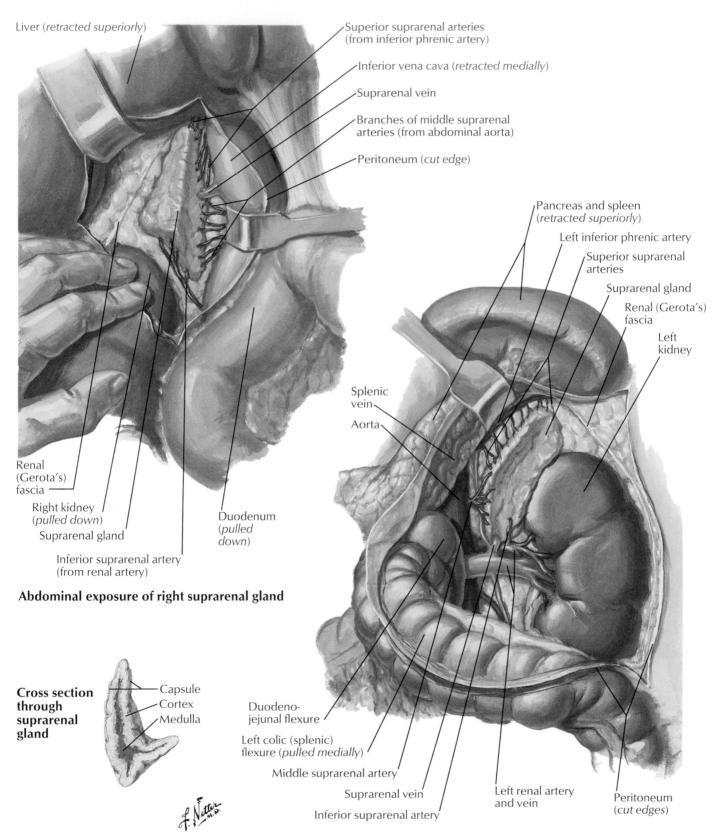

Liver (*retracted superiorly*)

Superior suprarenal arteries
(from inferior phrenic artery)

Inferior vena cava (*retracted medially*)

Suprarenal vein

Branches of middle suprarenal
arteries (from abdominal aorta)

Peritoneum (*cut edge*)

Pancreas and spleen
(*retracted superiorly*)

Left inferior phrenic artery

Superior suprarenal
arteries

Suprarenal gland

Renal (Gerota's)
fascia

Left
kidney

Splenic
vein

Aorta

Renal
(Gerota's)
fascia

Right kidney
(*pulled down*)

Suprarenal gland

Inferior suprarenal artery
(from renal artery)

Duodenum
(*pulled
down*)

Abdominal exposure of right suprarenal gland

**Cross section
through
suprarenal
gland**

Capsule

Cortex

Medulla

Duodeno-
jejunal flexure

Left colic (splenic)
flexure (*pulled medially*)

Middle suprarenal artery

Suprarenal vein

Inferior suprarenal artery

Left renal artery
and vein

Peritoneum
(*cut edges*)

Abdominal exposure of left suprarenal gland

Plate 322   **Kidneys and Suprarenal Glands**

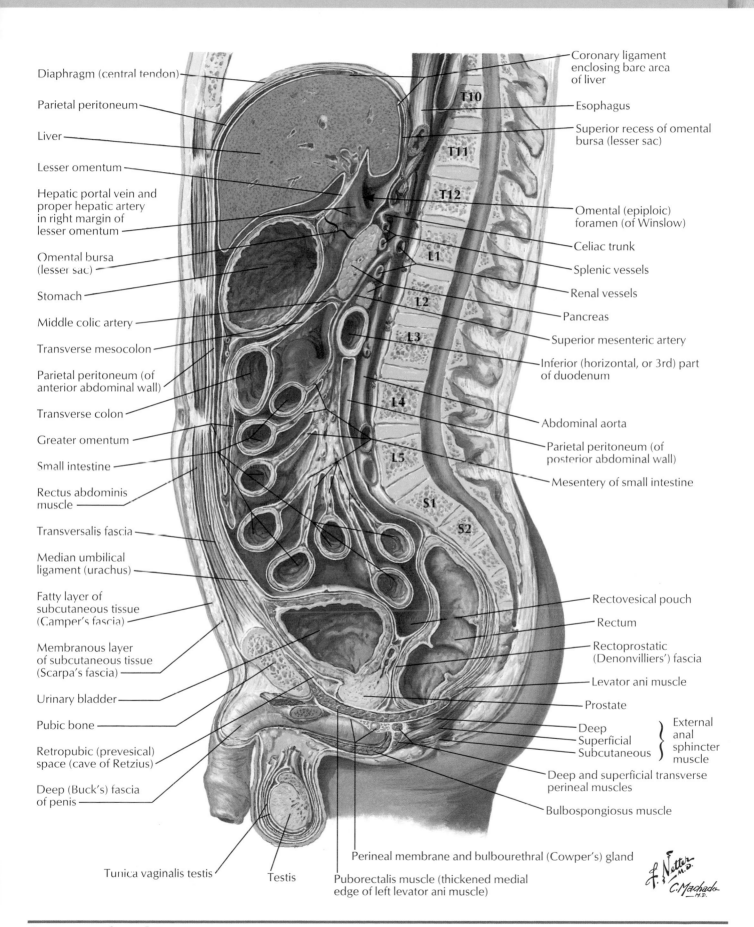

Diaphragm (central tendon)

Parietal peritoneum

Liver

Lesser omentum

Hepatic portal vein and proper hepatic artery in right margin of lesser omentum

Omental bursa (lesser sac)

Stomach

Middle colic artery

Transverse mesocolon

Parietal peritoneum (of anterior abdominal wall)

Transverse colon

Greater omentum

Small intestine

Rectus abdominis muscle

Transversalis fascia

Median umbilical ligament (urachus)

Fatty layer of subcutaneous tissue (Camper's fascia)

Membranous layer of subcutaneous tissue (Scarpa's fascia)

Urinary bladder

Pubic bone

Retropubic (prevesical) space (cave of Retzius)

Deep (Buck's) fascia of penis

Tunica vaginalis testis

Testis

Coronary ligament enclosing bare area of liver

T10

Esophagus

Superior recess of omental bursa (lesser sac)

T11

T12

Omental (epiploic) foramen (of Winslow)

Celiac trunk

L1

Splenic vessels

Renal vessels

L2

Pancreas

Superior mesenteric artery

L3

Inferior (horizontal, or 3rd) part of duodenum

L4

Abdominal aorta

Parietal peritoneum (of posterior abdominal wall)

L5

Mesentery of small intestine

S1

S2

Rectovesical pouch

Rectum

Rectoprostatic (Denonvilliers') fascia

Levator ani muscle

Prostate

Deep

Superficial   External anal sphincter muscle

Subcutaneous

Deep and superficial transverse perineal muscles

Bulbospongiosus muscle

Perineal membrane and bulbourethral (Cowper's) gland

Puborectalis muscle (thickened medial edge of left levator ani muscle)

f. Netter, M.D.
C. Machado, M.D.

Series of abdominal axial CT images from superior (A) to inferior (D)

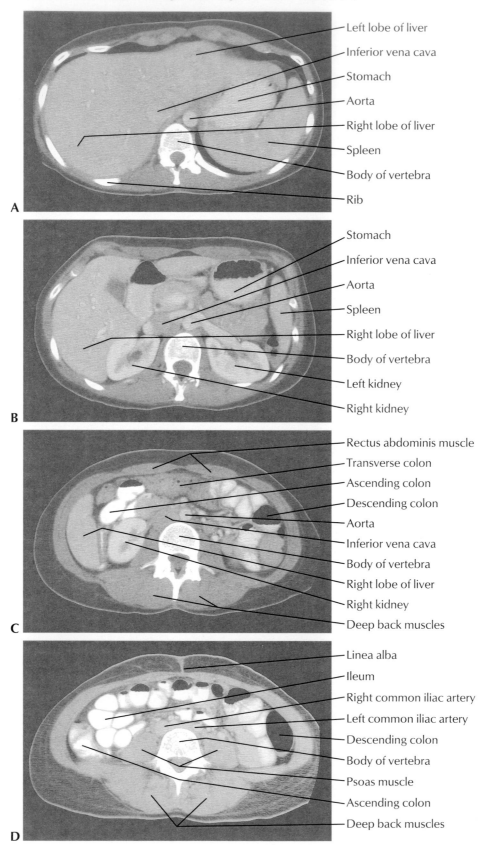

Left lobe of liver
Inferior vena cava
Stomach
Aorta
Right lobe of liver
Spleen
Body of vertebra
Rib

A

Stomach
Inferior vena cava
Aorta
Spleen
Right lobe of liver
Body of vertebra
Left kidney
Right kidney

B

Rectus abdominis muscle
Transverse colon
Ascending colon
Descending colon
Aorta
Inferior vena cava
Body of vertebra
Right lobe of liver
Right kidney
Deep back muscles

C

Linea alba
Ileum
Right common iliac artery
Left common iliac artery
Descending colon
Body of vertebra
Psoas muscle
Ascending colon
Deep back muscles

D

Plate 324   **Cross-sectional Anatomy**

Transverse Section: Level of T10, Esophagogastric Junction

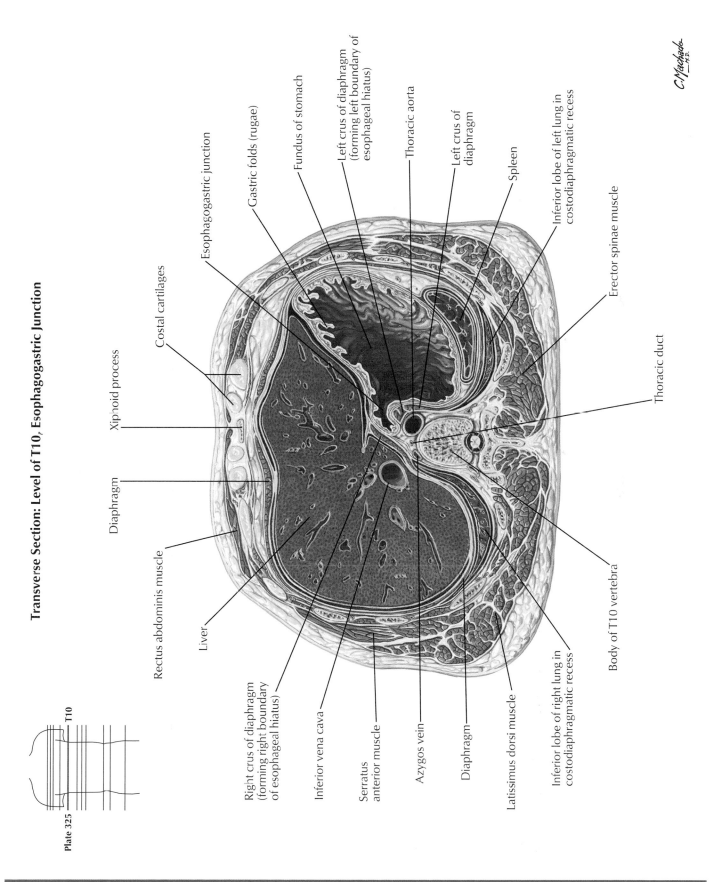

T10

Plate 325

Left crus of diaphragm (forming left boundary of esophageal hiatus)

Thoracic aorta

Left crus of diaphragm

Spleen

Inferior lobe of left lung in costodiaphragmatic recess

Erector spinae muscle

Fundus of stomach

Gastric folds (rugae)

Esophagogastric junction

Costal cartilages

Xiphoid process

Diaphragm

Rectus abdominis muscle

Liver

Thoracic duct

Right crus of diaphragm (forming right boundary of esophageal hiatus)

Inferior vena cava

Serratus anterior muscle

Azygos vein

Diaphragm

Latissimus dorsi muscle

Inferior lobe of right lung in costodiaphragmatic recess

Body of T10 vertebra

Transverse Section: Level of T12, Inferior to Xiphoid

Transverse colon
(ascending to left colic flexure)

Bifurcation of
celiac trunk

Descending colon
(descending from left
colic flexure)

Spleen

Splenic artery and vein

Left suprarenal gland

Superior pole of
left kidney

Left crus of diaphragm

Thoracic aorta

Jejunum

Stomach

Pancreas

Pyloric canal

Pylorus

Right colic (hepatic) flexure of colon

Gallbladder

Superior (1st) part
of duodenum

Hepatoduodenal
ligament

Liver

Common
bile duct

Proper
hepatic
artery

Portal vein

Portal triad

Inferior vena cava

Right suprarenal gland

Right crus of diaphragm

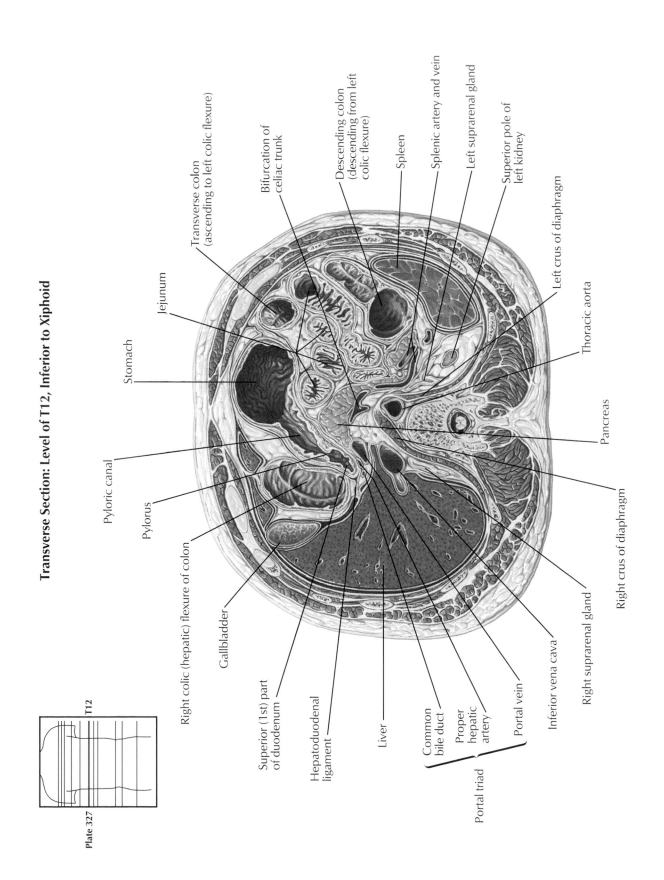

T12

Plate 327

Plate 326

Cross-sectional Anatomy

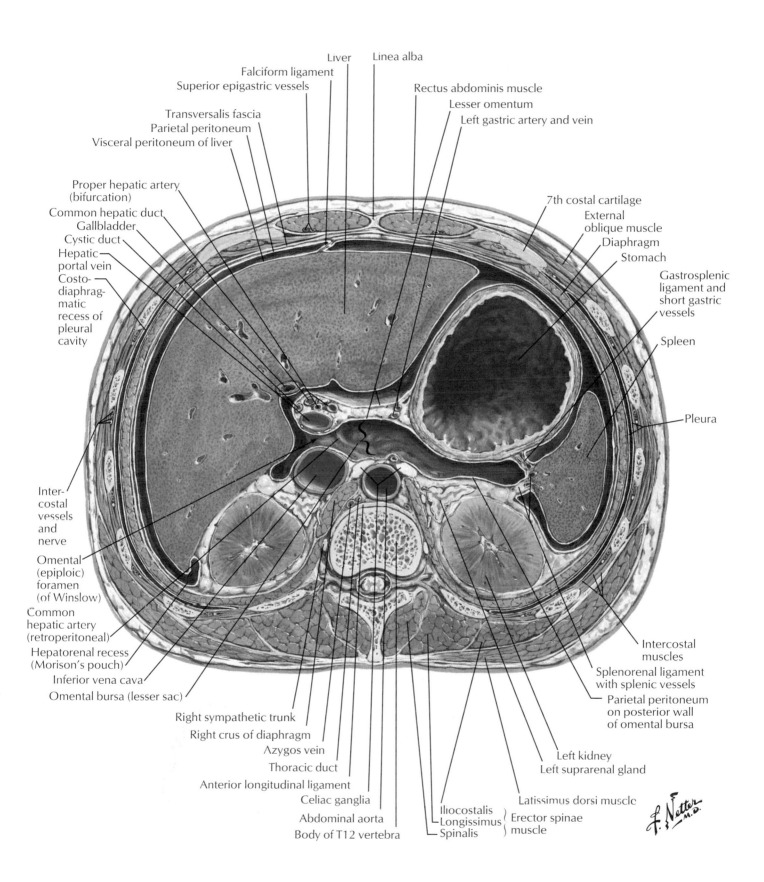

Liver

Falciform ligament

Superior epigastric vessels

Transversalis fascia

Parietal peritoneum

Visceral peritoneum of liver

Proper hepatic artery (bifurcation)

Common hepatic duct

Gallbladder

Cystic duct

Hepatic portal vein

Costo-diaphrag-matic recess of pleural cavity

Inter-costal vessels and nerve

Omental (epiploic) foramen (of Winslow)

Common hepatic artery (retroperitoneal)

Hepatorenal recess (Morison's pouch)

Inferior vena cava

Omental bursa (lesser sac)

Right sympathetic trunk

Right crus of diaphragm

Azygos vein

Thoracic duct

Anterior longitudinal ligament

Celiac ganglia

Abdominal aorta

Body of T12 vertebra

Linea alba

Rectus abdominis muscle

Lesser omentum

Left gastric artery and vein

7th costal cartilage

External oblique muscle

Diaphragm

Stomach

Gastrosplenic ligament and short gastric vessels

Spleen

Pleura

Intercostal muscles

Splenorenal ligament with splenic vessels

Parietal peritoneum on posterior wall of omental bursa

Left kidney

Left suprarenal gland

Latissimus dorsi muscle

Iliocostalis
Longissimus } Erector spinae
Spinalis   } muscle

Transverse Section: Level of T12–L1 Intervertebral Disc

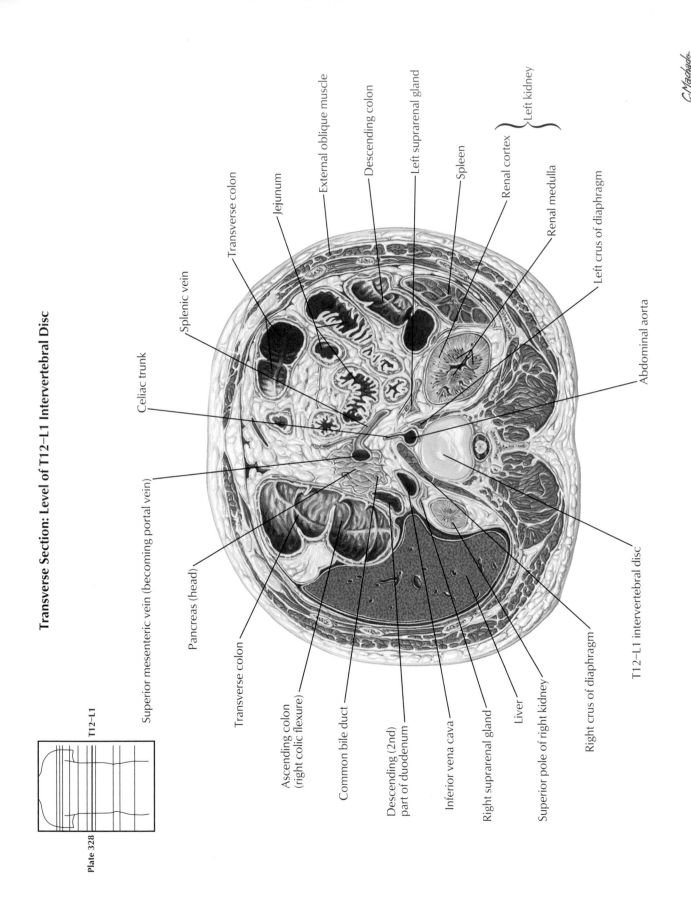

Transverse colon

Jejunum

External oblique muscle

Descending colon

Left suprarenal gland

Spleen

Renal cortex

Renal medulla

Left kidney

Left crus of diaphragm

Splenic vein

Celiac trunk

Abdominal aorta

Superior mesenteric vein (becoming portal vein)

Pancreas (head)

Transverse colon

Ascending colon (right colic flexure)

Common bile duct

Descending (2nd) part of duodenum

Inferior vena cava

Right suprarenal gland

Liver

Superior pole of right kidney

Right crus of diaphragm

T12–L1 intervertebral disc

T12–L1

Plate 328

Plate 328   **Cross-sectional Anatomy**

Transverse Section: Level of L1–2 Intervertebral Disc

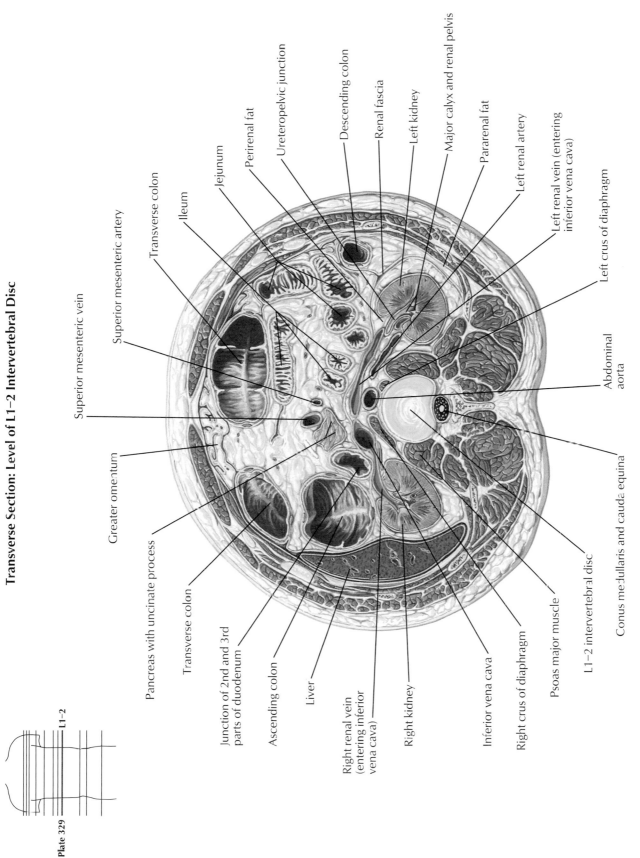

Superior mesenteric vein

Superior mesenteric artery

Transverse colon

Ileum

Jejunum

Perirenal fat

Ureteropelvic junction

Descending colon

Renal fascia

Left kidney

Major calyx and renal pelvis

Pararenal fat

Left renal artery

Left renal vein (entering inferior vena cava)

Left crus of diaphragm

Abdominal aorta

Conus medullaris and cauda equina

Greater omentum

Pancreas with uncinate process

Transverse colon

Junction of 2nd and 3rd parts of duodenum

Ascending colon

Liver

Right renal vein (entering inferior vena cava)

Right kidney

Inferior vena cava

Right crus of diaphragm

Psoas major muscle

L1–2 intervertebral disc

L1–2

Plate 329

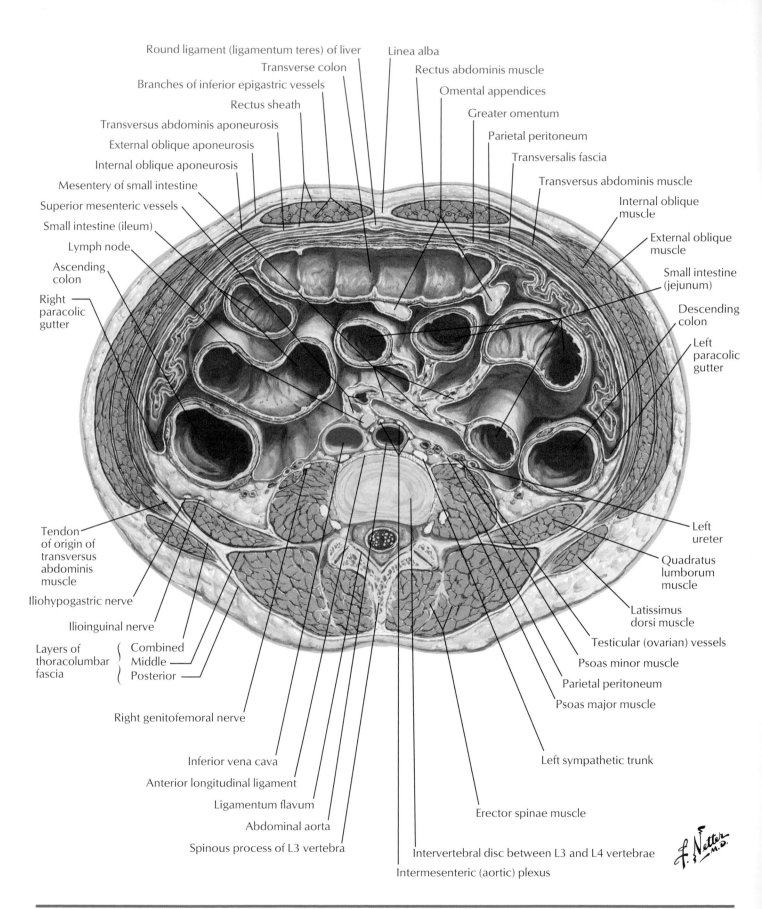

Round ligament (ligamentum teres) of liver

Transverse colon

Branches of inferior epigastric vessels

Rectus sheath

Transversus abdominis aponeurosis

External oblique aponeurosis

Internal oblique aponeurosis

Mesentery of small intestine

Superior mesenteric vessels

Small intestine (ileum)

Lymph node

Ascending colon

Right paracolic gutter

Tendon of origin of transversus abdominis muscle

Iliohypogastric nerve

Ilioinguinal nerve

Layers of thoracolumbar fascia

Combined

Middle

Posterior

Right genitofemoral nerve

Inferior vena cava

Anterior longitudinal ligament

Ligamentum flavum

Abdominal aorta

Spinous process of L3 vertebra

Linea alba

Rectus abdominis muscle

Omental appendices

Greater omentum

Parietal peritoneum

Transversalis fascia

Transversus abdominis muscle

Internal oblique muscle

External oblique muscle

Small intestine (jejunum)

Descending colon

Left paracolic gutter

Left ureter

Quadratus lumborum muscle

Latissimus dorsi muscle

Testicular (ovarian) vessels

Psoas minor muscle

Parietal peritoneum

Psoas major muscle

Left sympathetic trunk

Erector spinae muscle

Intervertebral disc between L3 and L4 vertebrae

Intermesenteric (aortic) plexus

Plate 330 **Cross-sectional Anatomy**

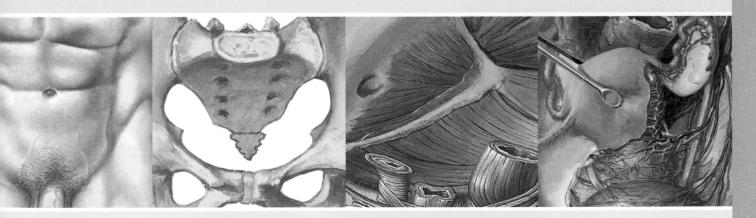

Section 5 PELVIS AND PERINEUM

Innervation
Plates 389-397

Cross-sectional Anatomy
Plates 398-399

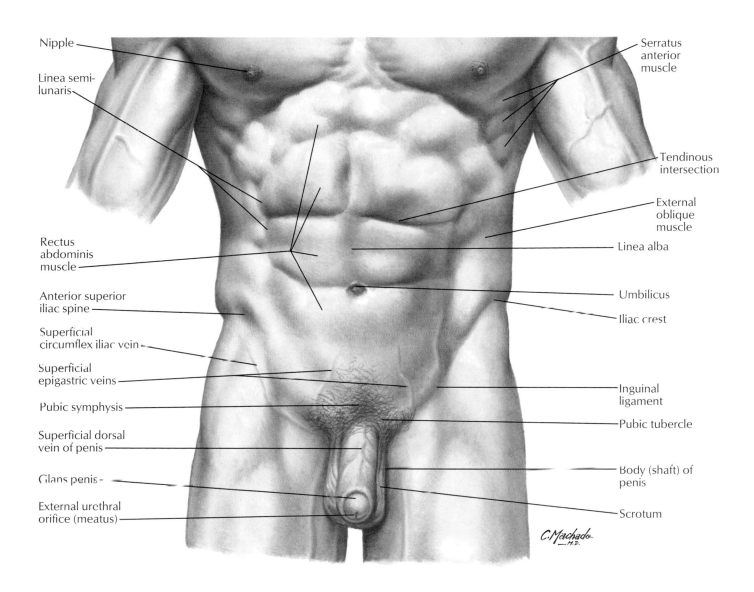

Nipple

Linea semi-lunaris

Rectus abdominis muscle

Anterior superior iliac spine

Superficial circumflex iliac vein

Superficial epigastric veins

Pubic symphysis

Superficial dorsal vein of penis

Glans penis

External urethral orifice (meatus)

Serratus anterior muscle

Tendinous intersection

External oblique muscle

Linea alba

Umbilicus

Iliac crest

Inguinal ligament

Pubic tubercle

Body (shaft) of penis

Scrotum

C. Machado
M.D.

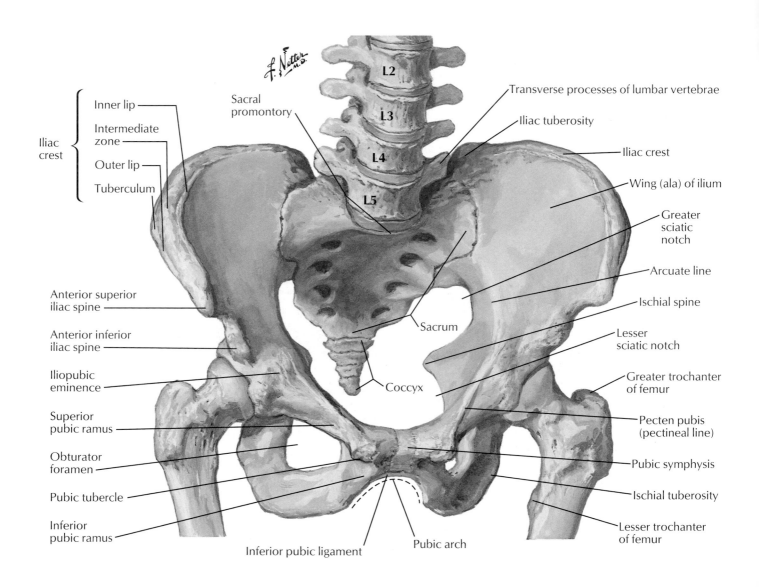

Inner lip

Intermediate zone

Outer lip

Tuberculum

Iliac crest

Sacral promontory

L2

L3

L4

L5

Transverse processes of lumbar vertebrae

Iliac tuberosity

Iliac crest

Wing (ala) of ilium

Greater sciatic notch

Arcuate line

Ischial spine

Lesser sciatic notch

Greater trochanter of femur

Sacrum

Anterior superior iliac spine

Anterior inferior iliac spine

Iliopubic eminence

Superior pubic ramus

Obturator foramen

Pubic tubercle

Inferior pubic ramus

Coccyx

Pecten pubis (pectineal line)

Pubic symphysis

Ischial tuberosity

Lesser trochanter of femur

Inferior pubic ligament

Pubic arch

Plate 332 **Bones and Ligaments**

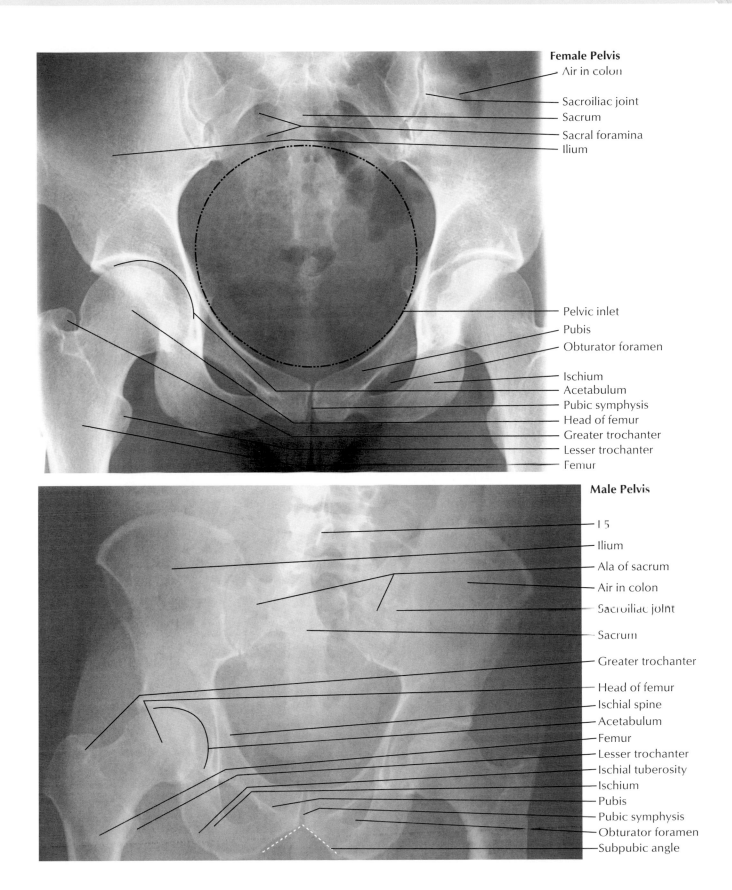

Female Pelvis
- Air in colon
- Sacroiliac joint
- Sacrum
- Sacral foramina
- Ilium

- Pelvic inlet
- Pubis
- Obturator foramen
- Ischium
- Acetabulum
- Pubic symphysis
- Head of femur
- Greater trochanter
- Lesser trochanter
- Femur

Male Pelvis
- L 5
- Ilium
- Ala of sacrum
- Air in colon
- Sacroiliac joint
- Sacrum
- Greater trochanter
- Head of femur
- Ischial spine
- Acetabulum
- Femur
- Lesser trochanter
- Ischial tuberosity
- Ischium
- Pubis
- Pubic symphysis
- Obturator foramen
- Subpubic angle

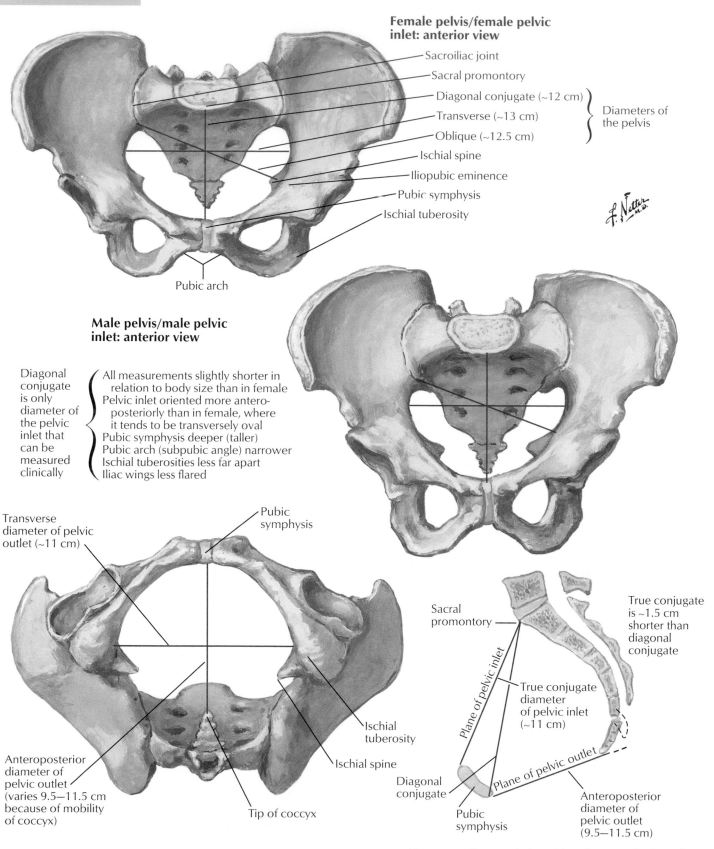

Female pelvis/female pelvic inlet: anterior view

- Sacroiliac joint
- Sacral promontory
- Diagonal conjugate (~12 cm)
- Transverse (~13 cm)
- Oblique (~12.5 cm)
- Ischial spine
- Iliopubic eminence
- Pubic symphysis
- Ischial tuberosity

Diameters of the pelvis

f. Netter M.D.

Pubic arch

Male pelvis/male pelvic inlet: anterior view

Diagonal conjugate is only diameter of the pelvic inlet that can be measured clinically

- All measurements slightly shorter in relation to body size than in female
- Pelvic inlet oriented more antero-posteriorly than in female, where it tends to be transversely oval
- Pubic symphysis deeper (taller)
- Pubic arch (subpubic angle) narrower
- Ischial tuberosities less far apart
- Iliac wings less flared

Transverse diameter of pelvic outlet (~11 cm)

Pubic symphysis

Ischial tuberosity

Ischial spine

Anteroposterior diameter of pelvic outlet (varies 9.5–11.5 cm because of mobility of coccyx)

Tip of coccyx

Female pelvis/female pelvic outlet: inferior view

Sacral promontory

True conjugate is ~1.5 cm shorter than diagonal conjugate

Plane of pelvic inlet

True conjugate diameter of pelvic inlet (~11 cm)

Diagonal conjugate

Plane of pelvic outlet

Pubic symphysis

Anteroposterior diameter of pelvic outlet (9.5–11.5 cm)

Transverse diameter is the widest distance of pelvic inlet

Female: sagittal section

Plate 334

Bones and Ligaments

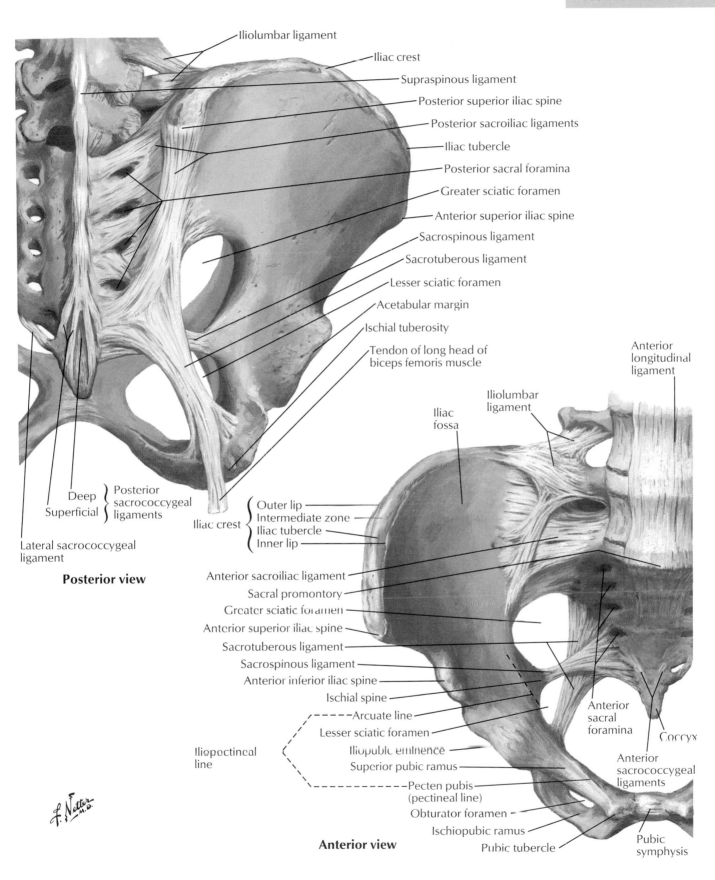

Iliolumbar ligament

Iliac crest

Supraspinous ligament

Posterior superior iliac spine

Posterior sacroiliac ligaments

Iliac tubercle

Posterior sacral foramina

Greater sciatic foramen

Anterior superior iliac spine

Sacrospinous ligament

Sacrotuberous ligament

Lesser sciatic foramen

Acetabular margin

Ischial tuberosity

Tendon of long head of biceps femoris muscle

Deep

Superficial

} Posterior sacrococcygeal ligaments

Lateral sacrococcygeal ligament

Posterior view

Iliac crest {
Outer lip
Intermediate zone
Iliac tubercle
Inner lip
}

Anterior sacroiliac ligament

Sacral promontory

Greater sciatic foramen

Anterior superior iliac spine

Sacrotuberous ligament

Sacrospinous ligament

Anterior inferior iliac spine

Ischial spine

Arcuate line

Lesser sciatic foramen

Iliopectineal line {

Iliopubic eminence

Superior pubic ramus

Pecten pubis (pectineal line)

Obturator foramen

Ischiopubic ramus

Pubic tubercle

Iliac fossa

Iliolumbar ligament

Anterior longitudinal ligament

Anterior sacral foramina

Coccyx

Anterior sacrococcygeal ligaments

Pubic symphysis

Anterior view

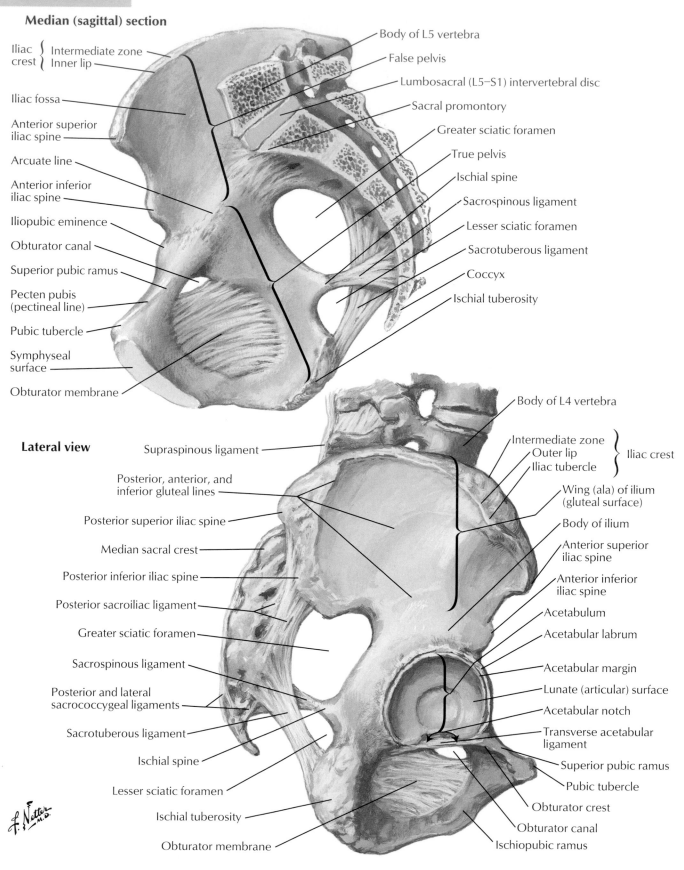

Median (sagittal) section

Iliac crest { Intermediate zone / Inner lip

Iliac fossa

Anterior superior iliac spine

Arcuate line

Anterior inferior iliac spine

Iliopubic eminence

Obturator canal

Superior pubic ramus

Pecten pubis (pectineal line)

Pubic tubercle

Symphyseal surface

Obturator membrane

Body of L5 vertebra

False pelvis

Lumbosacral (L5–S1) intervertebral disc

Sacral promontory

Greater sciatic foramen

True pelvis

Ischial spine

Sacrospinous ligament

Lesser sciatic foramen

Sacrotuberous ligament

Coccyx

Ischial tuberosity

Lateral view

Supraspinous ligament

Posterior, anterior, and inferior gluteal lines

Posterior superior iliac spine

Median sacral crest

Posterior inferior iliac spine

Posterior sacroiliac ligament

Greater sciatic foramen

Sacrospinous ligament

Posterior and lateral sacrococcygeal ligaments

Sacrotuberous ligament

Ischial spine

Lesser sciatic foramen

Ischial tuberosity

Obturator membrane

Body of L4 vertebra

Intermediate zone / Outer lip / Iliac tubercle } Iliac crest

Wing (ala) of ilium (gluteal surface)

Body of ilium

Anterior superior iliac spine

Anterior inferior iliac spine

Acetabulum

Acetabular labrum

Acetabular margin

Lunate (articular) surface

Acetabular notch

Transverse acetabular ligament

Superior pubic ramus

Pubic tubercle

Obturator crest

Obturator canal

Ischiopubic ramus

Plate 336

Bones and Ligaments

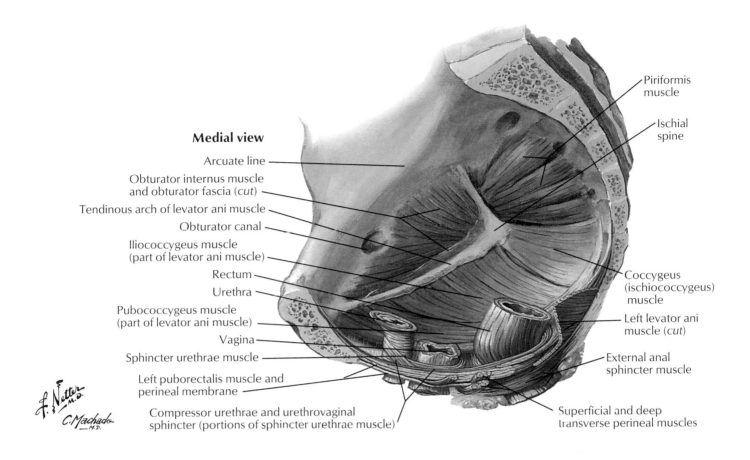

Medial view

Arcuate line

Obturator internus muscle
and obturator fascia (*cut*)

Tendinous arch of levator ani muscle

Obturator canal

Iliococcygeus muscle
(part of levator ani muscle)

Rectum

Urethra

Pubococcygeus muscle
(part of levator ani muscle)

Vagina

Sphincter urethrae muscle

Left puborectalis muscle and
perineal membrane

Compressor urethrae and urethrovaginal
sphincter (portions of sphincter urethrae muscle)

Piriformis
muscle

Ischial
spine

Coccygeus
(ischiococcygeus)
muscle

Left levator ani
muscle (*cut*)

External anal
sphincter muscle

Superficial and deep
transverse perineal muscles

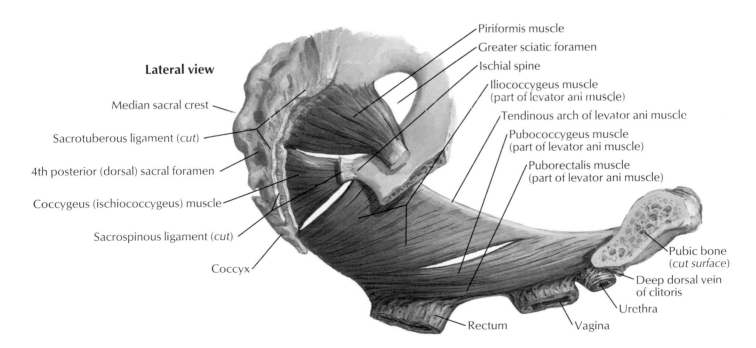

Lateral view

Median sacral crest

Sacrotuberous ligament (*cut*)

4th posterior (dorsal) sacral foramen

Coccygeus (ischiococcygeus) muscle

Sacrospinous ligament (*cut*)

Coccyx

Rectum

Piriformis muscle

Greater sciatic foramen

Ischial spine

Iliococcygeus muscle
(part of levator ani muscle)

Tendinous arch of levator ani muscle

Pubococcygeus muscle
(part of levator ani muscle)

Puborectalis muscle
(part of levator ani muscle)

Pubic bone
(*cut surface*)

Deep dorsal vein
of clitoris

Urethra

Vagina

For urogenital diaphragm see **Plate 358**

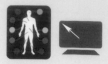

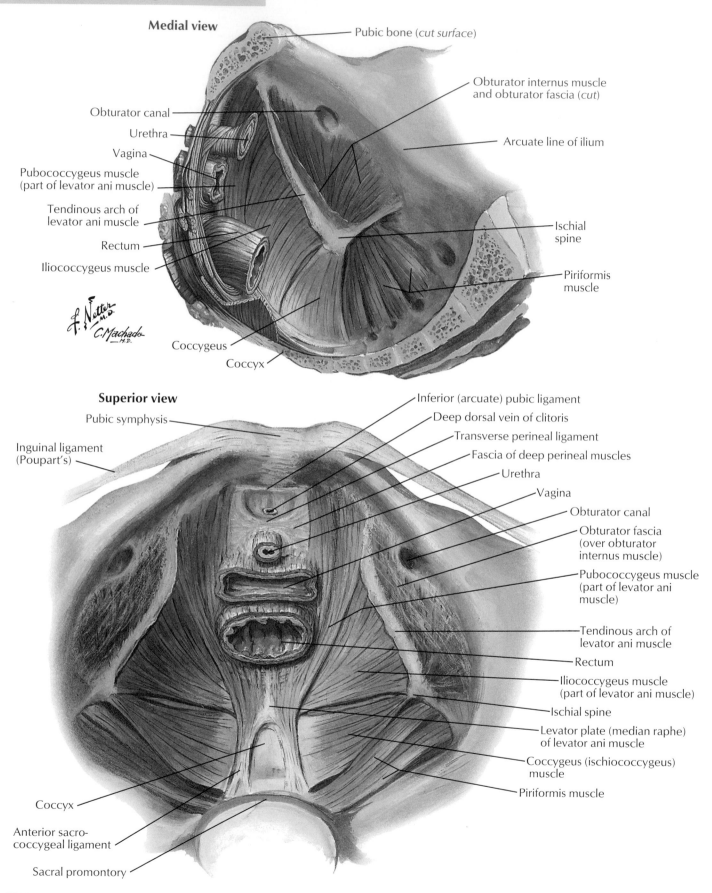

Medial view

Pubic bone (*cut surface*)

Obturator internus muscle
and obturator fascia (*cut*)

Obturator canal

Urethra

Vagina

Pubococcygeus muscle
(part of levator ani muscle)

Tendinous arch of
levator ani muscle

Rectum

Iliococcygeus muscle

Arcuate line of ilium

Ischial
spine

Piriformis
muscle

Coccygeus

Coccyx

Superior view

Pubic symphysis

Inguinal ligament
(Poupart's)

Inferior (arcuate) pubic ligament

Deep dorsal vein of clitoris

Transverse perineal ligament

Fascia of deep perineal muscles

Urethra

Vagina

Obturator canal

Obturator fascia
(over obturator
internus muscle)

Pubococcygeus muscle
(part of levator ani
muscle)

Tendinous arch of
levator ani muscle

Rectum

Iliococcygeus muscle
(part of levator ani muscle)

Ischial spine

Levator plate (median raphe)
of levator ani muscle

Coccygeus (ischiococcygeus)
muscle

Piriformis muscle

Coccyx

Anterior sacro-
coccygeal ligament

Sacral promontory

Plate 338

Pelvic Floor and Contents

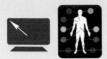

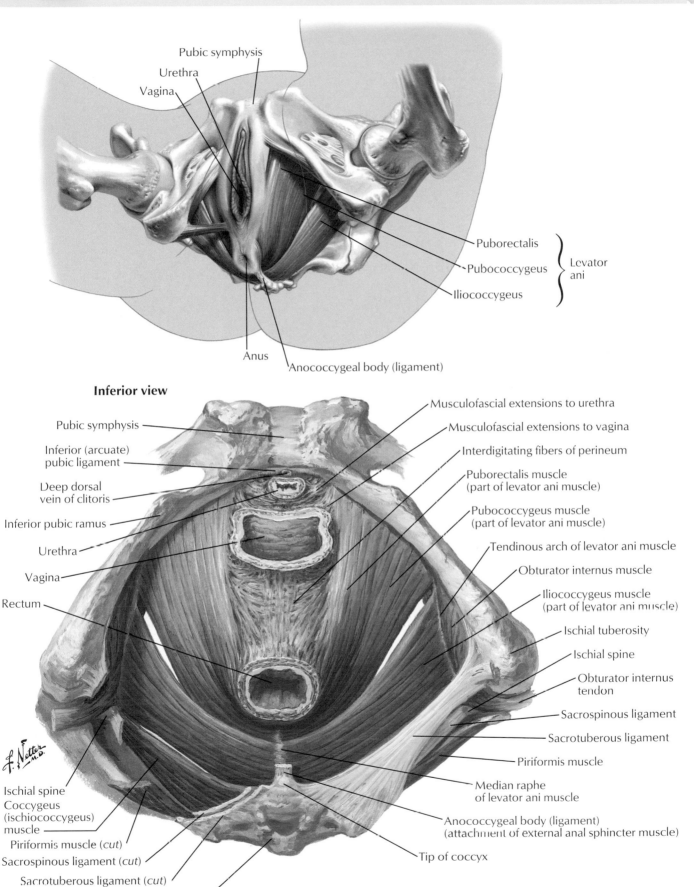

Pubic symphysis

Urethra

Vagina

Puborectalis

Pubococcygeus ⎫
⎬ Levator
Iliococcygeus ⎭ ani

Anus

Anococcygeal body (ligament)

Inferior view

Pubic symphysis

Inferior (arcuate) pubic ligament

Deep dorsal vein of clitoris

Inferior pubic ramus

Urethra

Vagina

Rectum

Ischial spine
Coccygeus (ischiococcygeus) muscle

Piriformis muscle (*cut*)

Sacrospinous ligament (*cut*)

Sacrotuberous ligament (*cut*)

Sacrum

Musculofascial extensions to urethra

Musculofascial extensions to vagina

Interdigitating fibers of perineum

Puborectalis muscle (part of levator ani muscle)

Pubococcygeus muscle (part of levator ani muscle)

Tendinous arch of levator ani muscle

Obturator internus muscle

Iliococcygeus muscle (part of levator ani muscle)

Ischial tuberosity

Ischial spine

Obturator internus tendon

Sacrospinous ligament

Sacrotuberous ligament

Piriformis muscle

Median raphe of levator ani muscle

Anococcygeal body (ligament) (attachment of external anal sphincter muscle)

Tip of coccyx

Pelvic Diaphragm: Male

See also **Plates 256, 259, 372**

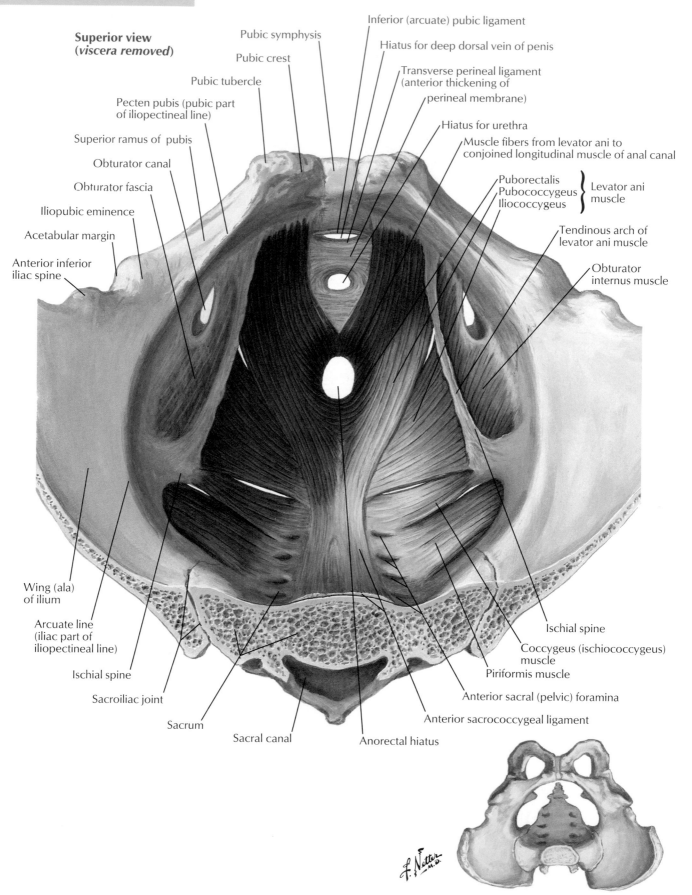

Superior view
(*viscera removed*)

Pubic symphysis

Pubic crest

Pubic tubercle

Pecten pubis (pubic part of iliopectineal line)

Superior ramus of pubis

Obturator canal

Obturator fascia

Iliopubic eminence

Acetabular margin

Anterior inferior iliac spine

Inferior (arcuate) pubic ligament

Hiatus for deep dorsal vein of penis

Transverse perineal ligament (anterior thickening of perineal membrane)

Hiatus for urethra

Muscle fibers from levator ani to conjoined longitudinal muscle of anal canal

Puborectalis
Pubococcygeus } Levator ani
Iliococcygeus } muscle

Tendinous arch of levator ani muscle

Obturator internus muscle

Wing (ala) of ilium

Arcuate line (iliac part of iliopectineal line)

Ischial spine

Sacroiliac joint

Sacrum

Sacral canal

Anorectal hiatus

Ischial spine

Coccygeus (ischiococcygeus) muscle

Piriformis muscle

Anterior sacral (pelvic) foramina

Anterior sacrococcygeal ligament

Plate 340

Pelvic Floor and Contents

Inferior view

Deep dorsal veins of penis

Fat in retropubic (prevesical) space

Sphincter urethrae muscle ascending
anterior aspect of prostate

Urethra

Rectoprostatic (Denonvilliers') fascia

Medial border (pillar)
of levator ani muscle

Perineal membrane (*cut away*)

Ischiopubic
ramus

Pubic symphysis

Inferior pubic (arcuate) ligament

Perineal body

Fibromuscular extensions of levator
ani muscle to prostate

Pubic tubercle

Rectourethralis superior muscle

Prerectal muscle fibers (of Luschka)
from levator ani muscle

Muscle fibers from levator
ani to conjoined longitudinal
muscle of anal canal

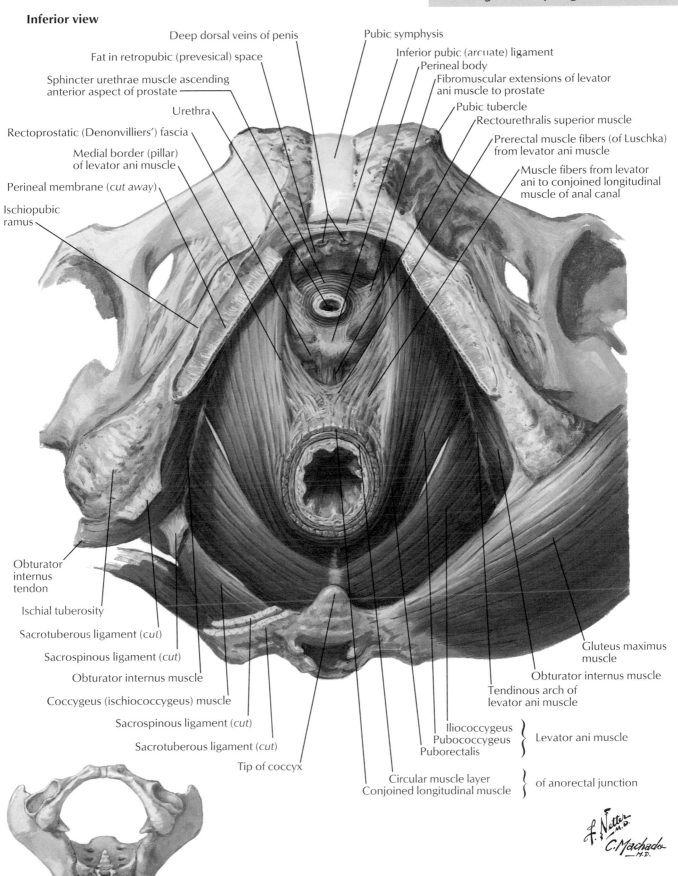

Obturator
internus
tendon

Ischial tuberosity

Sacrotuberous ligament (*cut*)

Sacrospinous ligament (*cut*)

Obturator internus muscle

Coccygeus (ischiococcygeus) muscle

Sacrospinous ligament (*cut*)

Sacrotuberous ligament (*cut*)

Tip of coccyx

Gluteus maximus
muscle

Obturator internus muscle

Tendinous arch of
levator ani muscle

Iliococcygeus
Pubococcygeus   } Levator ani muscle
Puborectalis

Circular muscle layer   } of anorectal junction
Conjoined longitudinal muscle

Pelvic Floor and Contents

Plate 341

Paramedian (sagittal) dissection

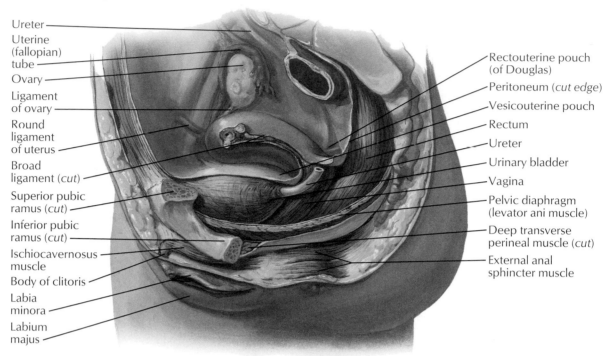

Ureter

Uterine (fallopian) tube

Ovary

Ligament of ovary

Round ligament of uterus

Broad ligament (*cut*)

Superior pubic ramus (*cut*)

Inferior pubic ramus (*cut*)

Ischiocavernosus muscle

Body of clitoris

Labia minora

Labium majus

Rectouterine pouch (of Douglas)

Peritoneum (*cut edge*)

Vesicouterine pouch

Rectum

Ureter

Urinary bladder

Vagina

Pelvic diaphragm (levator ani muscle)

Deep transverse perineal muscle (*cut*)

External anal sphincter muscle

Median (sagittal) section

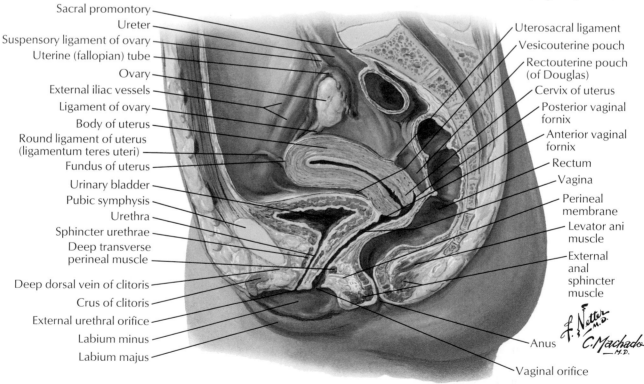

Sacral promontory

Ureter

Suspensory ligament of ovary

Uterine (fallopian) tube

Ovary

External iliac vessels

Ligament of ovary

Body of uterus

Round ligament of uterus (ligamentum teres uteri)

Fundus of uterus

Urinary bladder

Pubic symphysis

Urethra

Sphincter urethrae

Deep transverse perineal muscle

Deep dorsal vein of clitoris

Crus of clitoris

External urethral orifice

Labium minus

Labium majus

Uterosacral ligament

Vesicouterine pouch

Rectouterine pouch (of Douglas)

Cervix of uterus

Posterior vaginal fornix

Anterior vaginal fornix

Rectum

Vagina

Perineal membrane

Levator ani muscle

External anal sphincter muscle

Anus

Vaginal orifice

F. Netter M.D.

C. Machado M.D.

Plate 342   **Pelvic Floor and Contents**

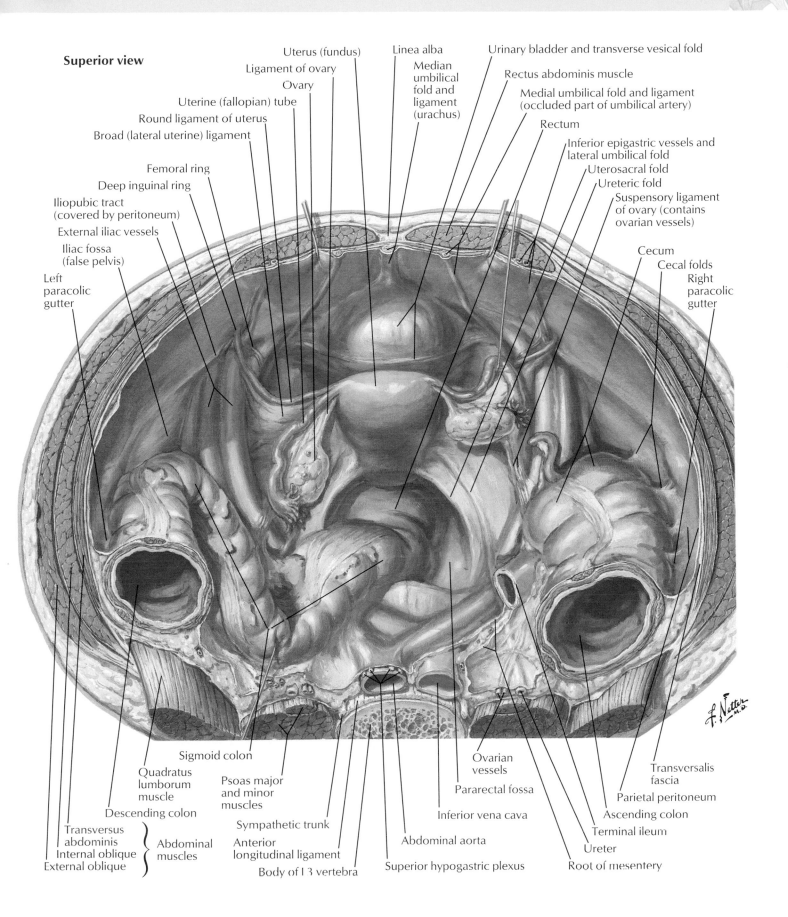

Superior view

Uterus (fundus)
Ligament of ovary
Ovary
Uterine (fallopian) tube
Round ligament of uterus
Broad (lateral uterine) ligament
Femoral ring
Deep inguinal ring
Iliopubic tract (covered by peritoneum)
External iliac vessels
Iliac fossa (false pelvis)
Left paracolic gutter

Linea alba
Median umbilical fold and ligament (urachus)

Urinary bladder and transverse vesical fold
Rectus abdominis muscle
Medial umbilical fold and ligament (occluded part of umbilical artery)
Rectum
Inferior epigastric vessels and lateral umbilical fold
Uterosacral fold
Ureteric fold
Suspensory ligament of ovary (contains ovarian vessels)
Cecum
Cecal folds
Right paracolic gutter

Sigmoid colon
Quadratus lumborum muscle
Descending colon
Transversus abdominis
Internal oblique
External oblique
} Abdominal muscles
Psoas major and minor muscles
Anterior longitudinal ligament
Body of L3 vertebra
Sympathetic trunk
Superior hypogastric plexus
Abdominal aorta
Inferior vena cava
Pararectal fossa
Ovarian vessels
Terminal ileum
Ureter
Root of mesentery
Ascending colon
Parietal peritoneum
Transversalis fascia

f. Netter M.D.

Pelvic Floor and Contents

Plate 343

Superior view with peritoneum intact

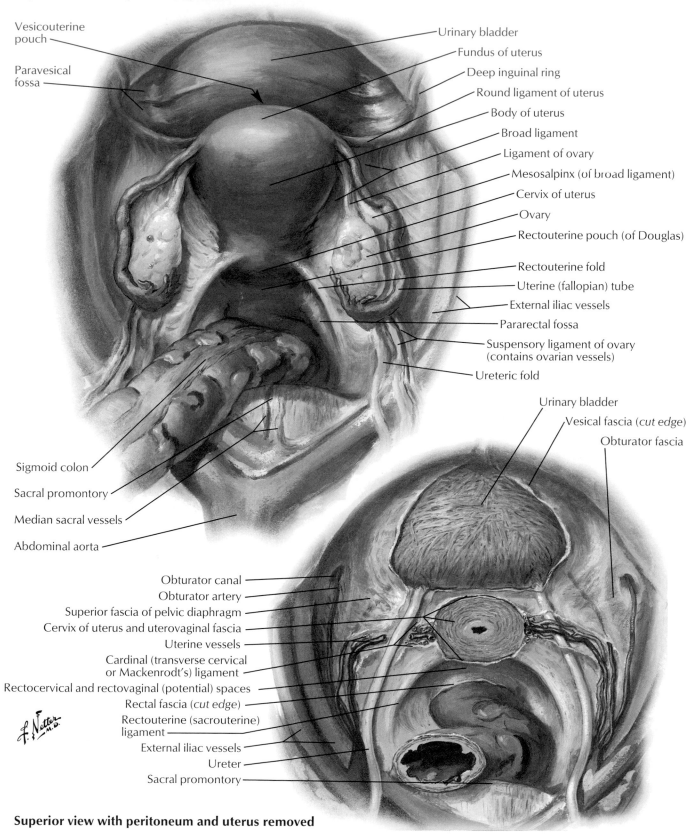

Vesicouterine pouch

Paravesical fossa

Urinary bladder

Fundus of uterus

Deep inguinal ring

Round ligament of uterus

Body of uterus

Broad ligament

Ligament of ovary

Mesosalpinx (of broad ligament)

Cervix of uterus

Ovary

Rectouterine pouch (of Douglas)

Rectouterine fold

Uterine (fallopian) tube

External iliac vessels

Pararectal fossa

Suspensory ligament of ovary (contains ovarian vessels)

Ureteric fold

Sigmoid colon

Sacral promontory

Median sacral vessels

Abdominal aorta

Urinary bladder

Vesical fascia (*cut edge*)

Obturator fascia

Obturator canal

Obturator artery

Superior fascia of pelvic diaphragm

Cervix of uterus and uterovaginal fascia

Uterine vessels

Cardinal (transverse cervical or Mackenrodt's) ligament

Rectocervical and rectovaginal (potential) spaces

Rectal fascia (*cut edge*)

Rectouterine (sacrouterine) ligament

External iliac vessels

Ureter

Sacral promontory

Superior view with peritoneum and uterus removed

Plate 344 **Pelvic Floor and Contents**

Female: superior view (peritoneum and loose areolar tissue removed)

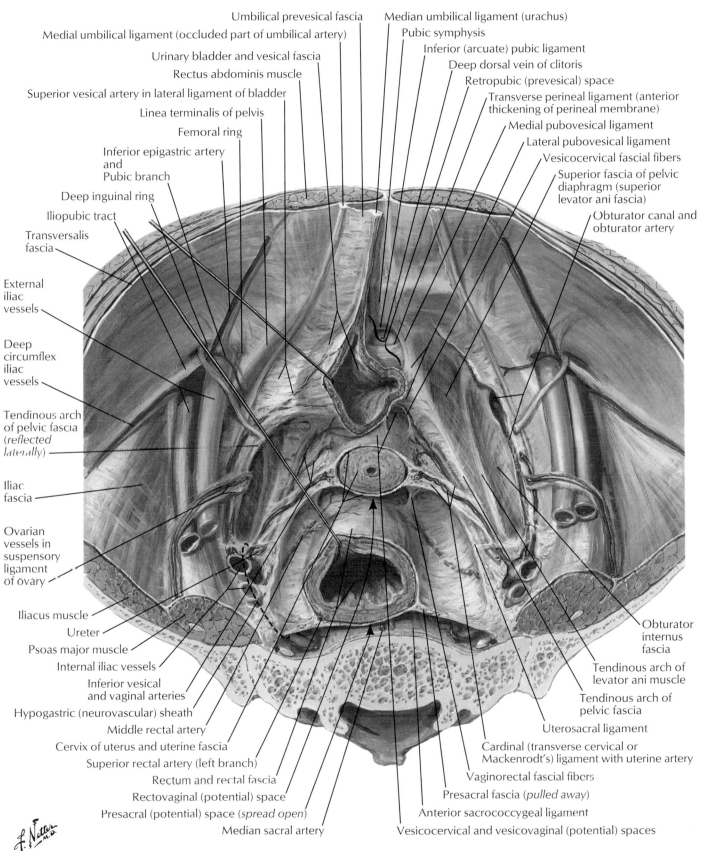

Umbilical prevesical fascia

Medial umbilical ligament (occluded part of umbilical artery)

Urinary bladder and vesical fascia

Rectus abdominis muscle

Superior vesical artery in lateral ligament of bladder

Linea terminalis of pelvis

Femoral ring

Inferior epigastric artery and Pubic branch

Deep inguinal ring

Iliopubic tract

Transversalis fascia

External iliac vessels

Deep circumflex iliac vessels

Tendinous arch of pelvic fascia (*reflected laterally*)

Iliac fascia

Ovarian vessels in suspensory ligament of ovary

Iliacus muscle

Ureter

Psoas major muscle

Internal iliac vessels

Inferior vesical and vaginal arteries

Hypogastric (neurovascular) sheath

Middle rectal artery

Cervix of uterus and uterine fascia

Superior rectal artery (left branch)

Rectum and rectal fascia

Rectovaginal (potential) space

Presacral (potential) space (*spread open*)

Median sacral artery

Median umbilical ligament (urachus)

Pubic symphysis

Inferior (arcuate) pubic ligament

Deep dorsal vein of clitoris

Retropubic (prevesical) space

Transverse perineal ligament (anterior thickening of perineal membrane)

Medial pubovesical ligament

Lateral pubovesical ligament

Vesicocervical fascial fibers

Superior fascia of pelvic diaphragm (superior levator ani fascia)

Obturator canal and obturator artery

Obturator internus fascia

Tendinous arch of levator ani muscle

Tendinous arch of pelvic fascia

Uterosacral ligament

Cardinal (transverse cervical or Mackenrodt's) ligament with uterine artery

Vaginorectal fascial fibers

Presacral fascia (*pulled away*)

Anterior sacrococcygeal ligament

Vesicocervical and vesicovaginal (potential) spaces

Paramedian (sagittal) dissection

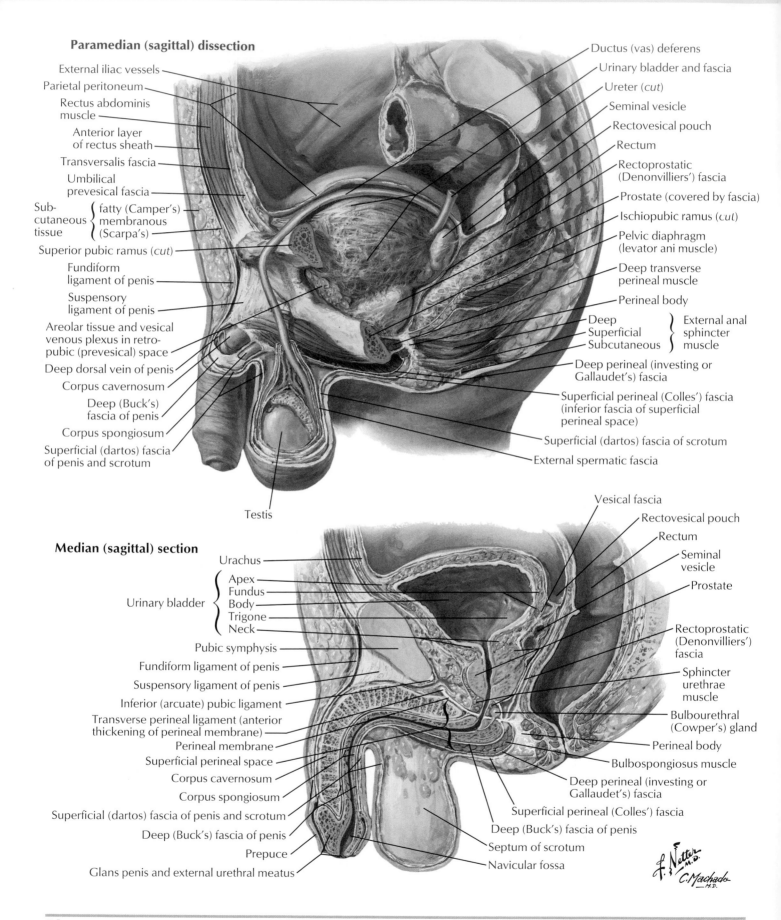

External iliac vessels

Parietal peritoneum

Rectus abdominis muscle

Anterior layer of rectus sheath

Transversalis fascia

Umbilical prevesical fascia

Sub-cutaneous tissue { fatty (Camper's) / membranous (Scarpa's)

Superior pubic ramus (cut)

Fundiform ligament of penis

Suspensory ligament of penis

Areolar tissue and vesical venous plexus in retro-pubic (prevesical) space

Deep dorsal vein of penis

Corpus cavernosum

Deep (Buck's) fascia of penis

Corpus spongiosum

Superficial (dartos) fascia of penis and scrotum

Testis

Ductus (vas) deferens

Urinary bladder and fascia

Ureter (cut)

Seminal vesicle

Rectovesical pouch

Rectum

Rectoprostatic (Denonvilliers') fascia

Prostate (covered by fascia)

Ischiopubic ramus (cut)

Pelvic diaphragm (levator ani muscle)

Deep transverse perineal muscle

Perineal body

Deep / Superficial / Subcutaneous } External anal sphincter muscle

Deep perineal (investing or Gallaudet's) fascia

Superficial perineal (Colles') fascia (inferior fascia of superficial perineal space)

Superficial (dartos) fascia of scrotum

External spermatic fascia

Median (sagittal) section

Urachus

Urinary bladder { Apex / Fundus / Body / Trigone / Neck

Pubic symphysis

Fundiform ligament of penis

Suspensory ligament of penis

Inferior (arcuate) pubic ligament

Transverse perineal ligament (anterior thickening of perineal membrane)

Perineal membrane

Superficial perineal space

Corpus cavernosum

Corpus spongiosum

Superficial (dartos) fascia of penis and scrotum

Deep (Buck's) fascia of penis

Prepuce

Glans penis and external urethral meatus

Vesical fascia

Rectovesical pouch

Rectum

Seminal vesicle

Prostate

Rectoprostatic (Denonvilliers') fascia

Sphincter urethrae muscle

Bulbourethral (Cowper's) gland

Perineal body

Bulbospongiosus muscle

Deep perineal (investing or Gallaudet's) fascia

Superficial perineal (Colles') fascia

Deep (Buck's) fascia of penis

Septum of scrotum

Navicular fossa

Plate 346 **Pelvic Floor and Contents**

Superior view

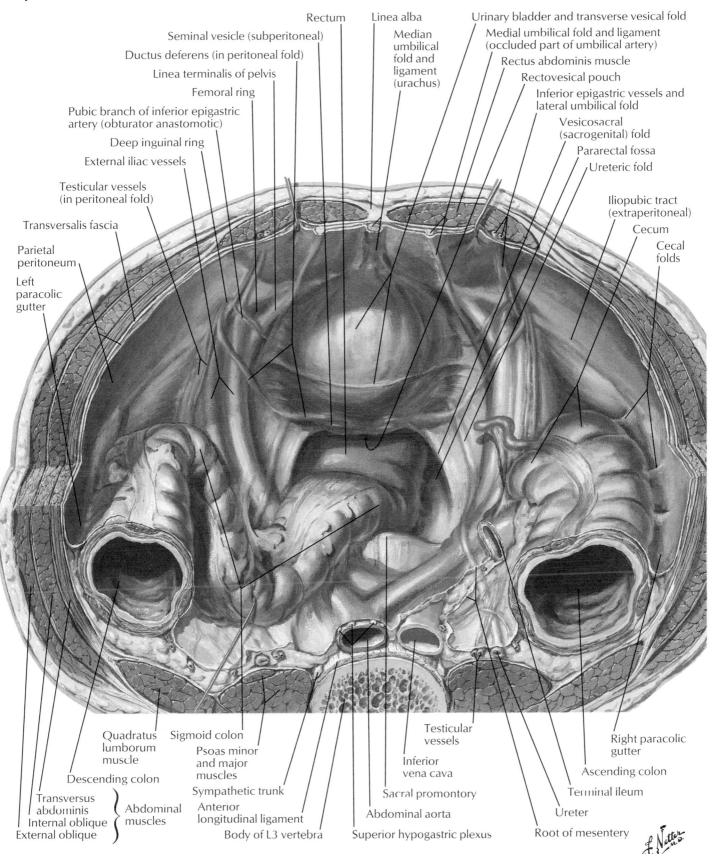

Rectum

Linea alba

Urinary bladder and transverse vesical fold

Seminal vesicle (subperitoneal)

Ductus deferens (in peritoneal fold)

Linea terminalis of pelvis

Femoral ring

Median umbilical fold and ligament (urachus)

Medial umbilical fold and ligament (occluded part of umbilical artery)

Rectus abdominis muscle

Rectovesical pouch

Pubic branch of inferior epigastric artery (obturator anastomotic)

Deep inguinal ring

External iliac vessels

Testicular vessels (in peritoneal fold)

Transversalis fascia

Parietal peritoneum

Left paracolic gutter

Inferior epigastric vessels and lateral umbilical fold

Vesicosacral (sacrogenital) fold

Pararectal fossa

Ureteric fold

Iliopubic tract (extraperitoneal)

Cecum

Cecal folds

Quadratus lumborum muscle

Sigmoid colon

Descending colon

Psoas minor and major muscles

Sympathetic trunk

Transversus abdominis

Internal oblique

External oblique

} Abdominal muscles

Anterior longitudinal ligament

Body of L3 vertebra

Testicular vessels

Inferior vena cava

Sacral promontory

Abdominal aorta

Superior hypogastric plexus

Right paracolic gutter

Ascending colon

Terminal ileum

Ureter

Root of mesentery

f. Netter m.d.

Pelvic Floor and Contents

Plate 347

Female: midsagittal section

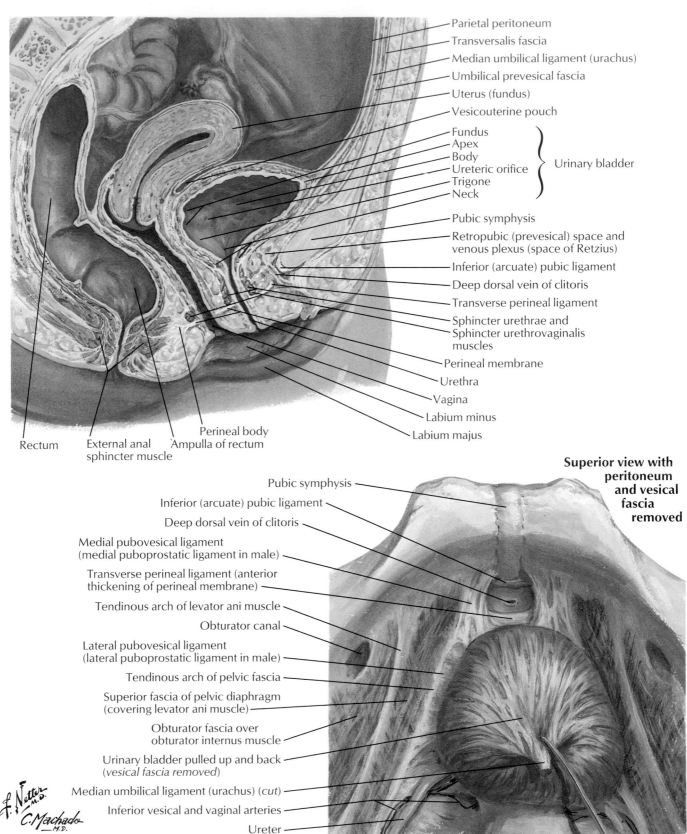

Parietal peritoneum

Transversalis fascia

Median umbilical ligament (urachus)

Umbilical prevesical fascia

Uterus (fundus)

Vesicouterine pouch

Fundus
Apex
Body
Ureteric orifice } Urinary bladder
Trigone
Neck

Pubic symphysis

Retropubic (prevesical) space and venous plexus (space of Retzius)

Inferior (arcuate) pubic ligament

Deep dorsal vein of clitoris

Transverse perineal ligament

Sphincter urethrae and Sphincter urethrovaginalis muscles

Perineal membrane

Urethra

Vagina

Labium minus

Labium majus

Rectum

External anal sphincter muscle

Ampulla of rectum

Perineal body

Superior view with peritoneum and vesical fascia removed

Pubic symphysis

Inferior (arcuate) pubic ligament

Deep dorsal vein of clitoris

Medial pubovesical ligament (medial puboprostatic ligament in male)

Transverse perineal ligament (anterior thickening of perineal membrane)

Tendinous arch of levator ani muscle

Obturator canal

Lateral pubovesical ligament (lateral puboprostatic ligament in male)

Tendinous arch of pelvic fascia

Superior fascia of pelvic diaphragm (covering levator ani muscle)

Obturator fascia over obturator internus muscle

Urinary bladder pulled up and back (vesical fascia removed)

Median umbilical ligament (urachus) (cut)

Inferior vesical and vaginal arteries

Ureter

Plate 348

Urinary Bladder

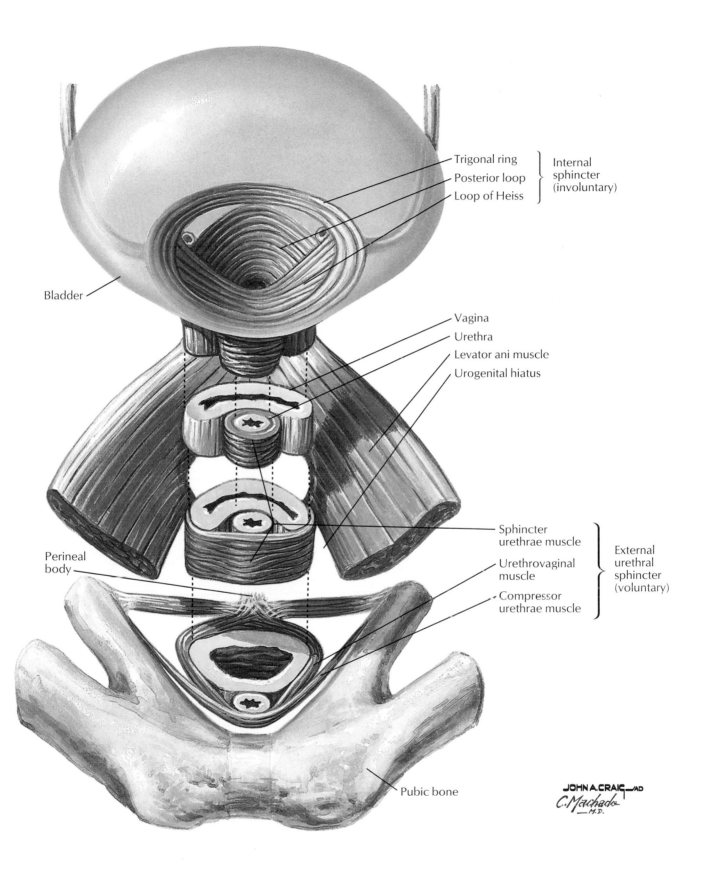

Bladder

Trigonal ring
Posterior loop
Loop of Heiss

Internal
sphincter
(involuntary)

Vagina
Urethra
Levator ani muscle
Urogenital hiatus

Perineal
body

Sphincter
urethrae muscle

Urethrovaginal
muscle

Compressor
urethrae muscle

External
urethral
sphincter
(voluntary)

Pubic bone

JOHN A. CRAIG—MD
C. Machado
—M.D.

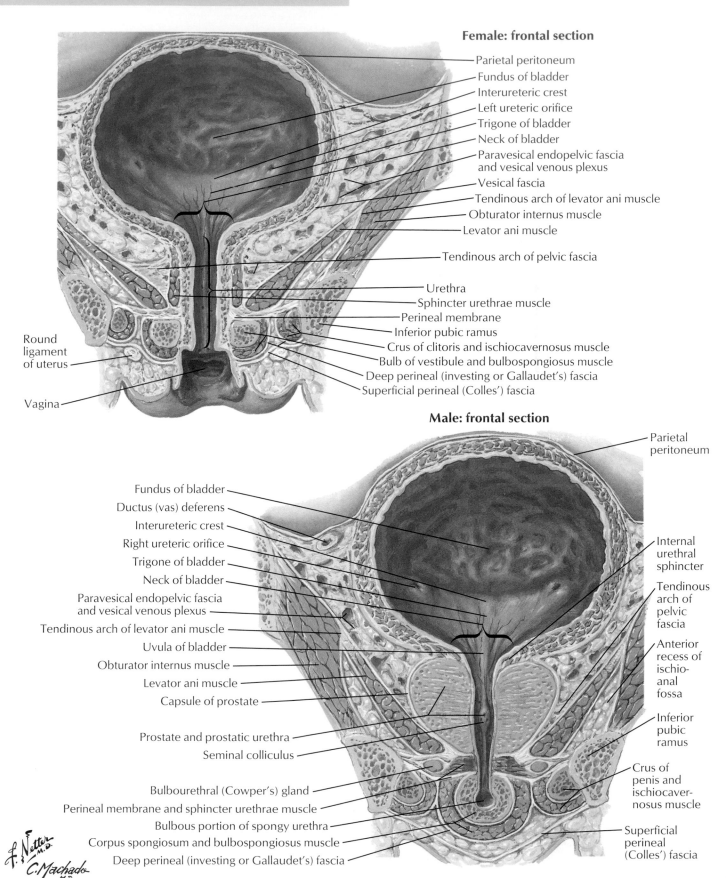

Female: frontal section

Parietal peritoneum
Fundus of bladder
Interureteric crest
Left ureteric orifice
Trigone of bladder
Neck of bladder
Paravesical endopelvic fascia and vesical venous plexus
Vesical fascia
Tendinous arch of levator ani muscle
Obturator internus muscle
Levator ani muscle

Tendinous arch of pelvic fascia

Urethra
Sphincter urethrae muscle
Perineal membrane
Inferior pubic ramus
Crus of clitoris and ischiocavernosus muscle
Bulb of vestibule and bulbospongiosus muscle
Deep perineal (investing or Gallaudet's) fascia
Superficial perineal (Colles') fascia

Round ligament of uterus

Vagina

Male: frontal section

Parietal peritoneum

Fundus of bladder
Ductus (vas) deferens
Interureteric crest
Right ureteric orifice
Trigone of bladder
Neck of bladder
Paravesical endopelvic fascia and vesical venous plexus
Tendinous arch of levator ani muscle
Uvula of bladder
Obturator internus muscle
Levator ani muscle
Capsule of prostate

Prostate and prostatic urethra
Seminal colliculus

Bulbourethral (Cowper's) gland
Perineal membrane and sphincter urethrae muscle
Bulbous portion of spongy urethra
Corpus spongiosum and bulbospongiosus muscle
Deep perineal (investing or Gallaudet's) fascia

Internal urethral sphincter

Tendinous arch of pelvic fascia

Anterior recess of ischio-anal fossa

Inferior pubic ramus

Crus of penis and ischiocaver-nosus muscle

Superficial perineal (Colles') fascia

Plate 350

Urinary Bladder

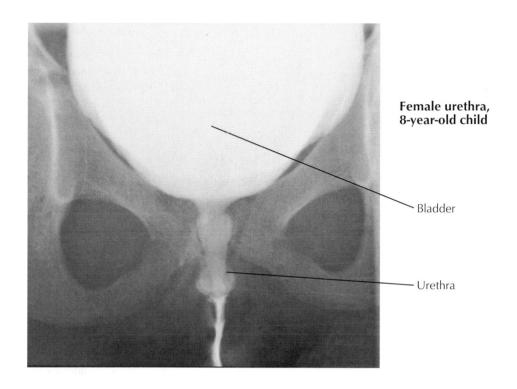

Female urethra,
8-year-old child

Bladder

Urethra

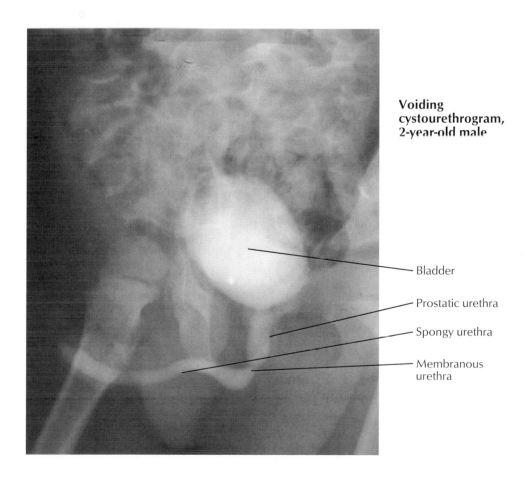

Voiding
cystourethrogram,
2-year-old male

Bladder

Prostatic urethra

Spongy urethra

Membranous
urethra

See also **Plates 380, 382, 384, 386, 392, 394, 395**

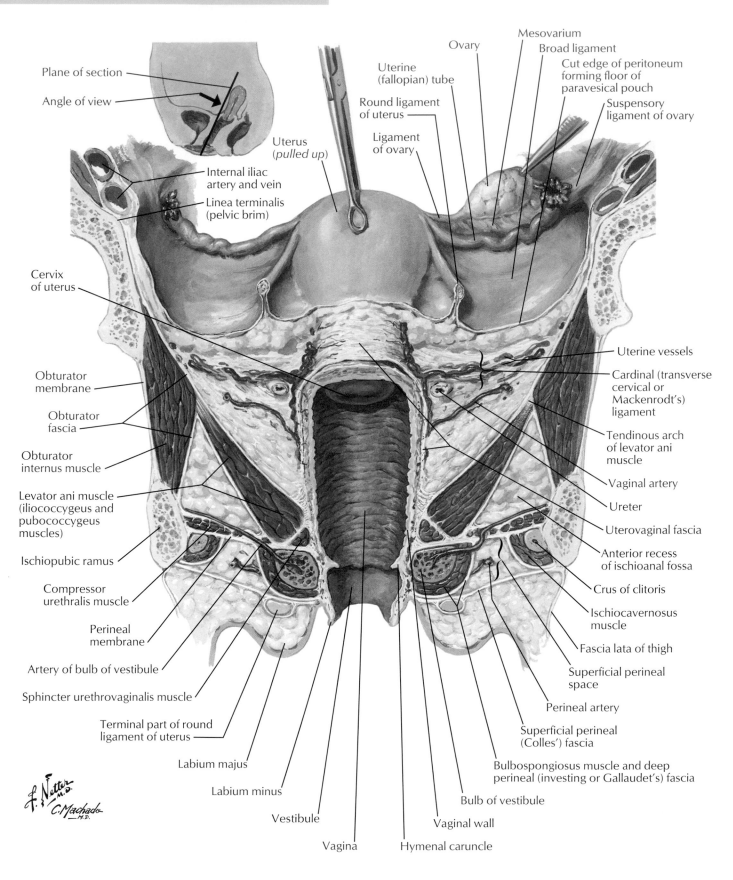

Plane of section

Angle of view

Uterus
(*pulled up*)

Round ligament
of uterus

Uterine
(fallopian) tube

Ligament
of ovary

Ovary

Mesovarium

Broad ligament

Cut edge of peritoneum
forming floor of
paravesical pouch

Suspensory
ligament of ovary

Internal iliac
artery and vein

Linea terminalis
(pelvic brim)

Cervix
of uterus

Uterine vessels

Cardinal (transverse
cervical or
Mackenrodt's)
ligament

Obturator
membrane

Obturator
fascia

Tendinous arch
of levator ani
muscle

Vaginal artery

Obturator
internus muscle

Ureter

Uterovaginal fascia

Levator ani muscle
(iliococcygeus and
pubococcygeus
muscles)

Anterior recess
of ischioanal fossa

Ischiopubic ramus

Crus of clitoris

Compressor
urethralis muscle

Ischiocavernosus
muscle

Perineal
membrane

Fascia lata of thigh

Artery of bulb of vestibule

Superficial perineal
space

Sphincter urethrovaginalis muscle

Perineal artery

Terminal part of round
ligament of uterus

Superficial perineal
(Colles') fascia

Labium majus

Bulbospongiosus muscle and deep
perineal (investing or Gallaudet's) fascia

Labium minus

Bulb of vestibule

Vestibule

Vaginal wall

Vagina

Hymenal caruncle

Plate 352

Uterus, Vagina, and Supporting Structures

Fascial ligaments of the uterus

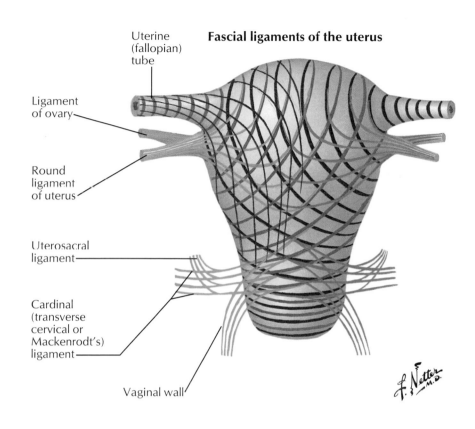

Uterine (fallopian) tube

Ligament of ovary

Round ligament of uterus

Uterosacral ligament

Cardinal (transverse cervical or Mackenrodt's) ligament

Vaginal wall

Pelvic fascia and ligaments

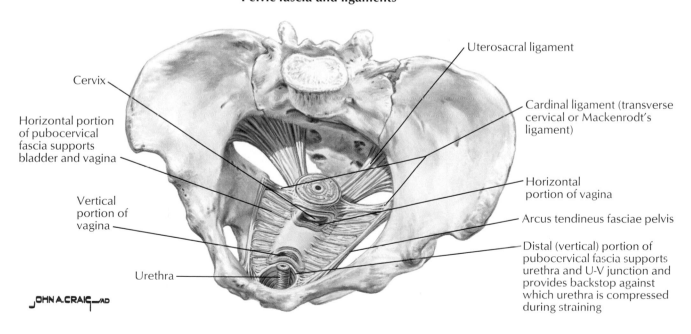

Cervix

Horizontal portion of pubocervical fascia supports bladder and vagina

Vertical portion of vagina

Urethra

Uterosacral ligament

Cardinal ligament (transverse cervical or Mackenrodt's ligament)

Horizontal portion of vagina

Arcus tendineus fasciae pelvis

Distal (vertical) portion of pubocervical fascia supports urethra and U-V junction and provides backstop against which urethra is compressed during straining

JOHN A.CRAIG—AD

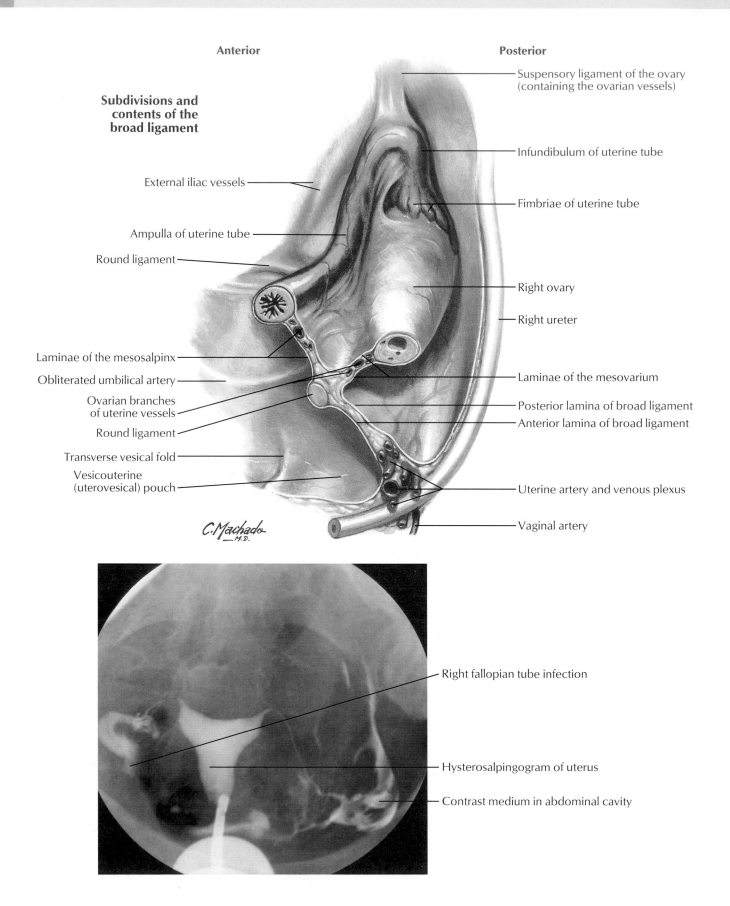

Anterior

Posterior

Suspensory ligament of the ovary
(containing the ovarian vessels)

**Subdivisions and
contents of the
broad ligament**

Infundibulum of uterine tube

External iliac vessels

Fimbriae of uterine tube

Ampulla of uterine tube

Round ligament

Right ovary

Right ureter

Laminae of the mesosalpinx

Obliterated umbilical artery

Laminae of the mesovarium

Ovarian branches
of uterine vessels

Posterior lamina of broad ligament

Round ligament

Anterior lamina of broad ligament

Transverse vesical fold

Vesicouterine
(uterovesical) pouch

Uterine artery and venous plexus

Vaginal artery

C.Machado
_M.D._

Right fallopian tube infection

Hysterosalpingogram of uterus

Contrast medium in abdominal cavity

Plate 354

Uterus, Vagina, and Supporting Structures

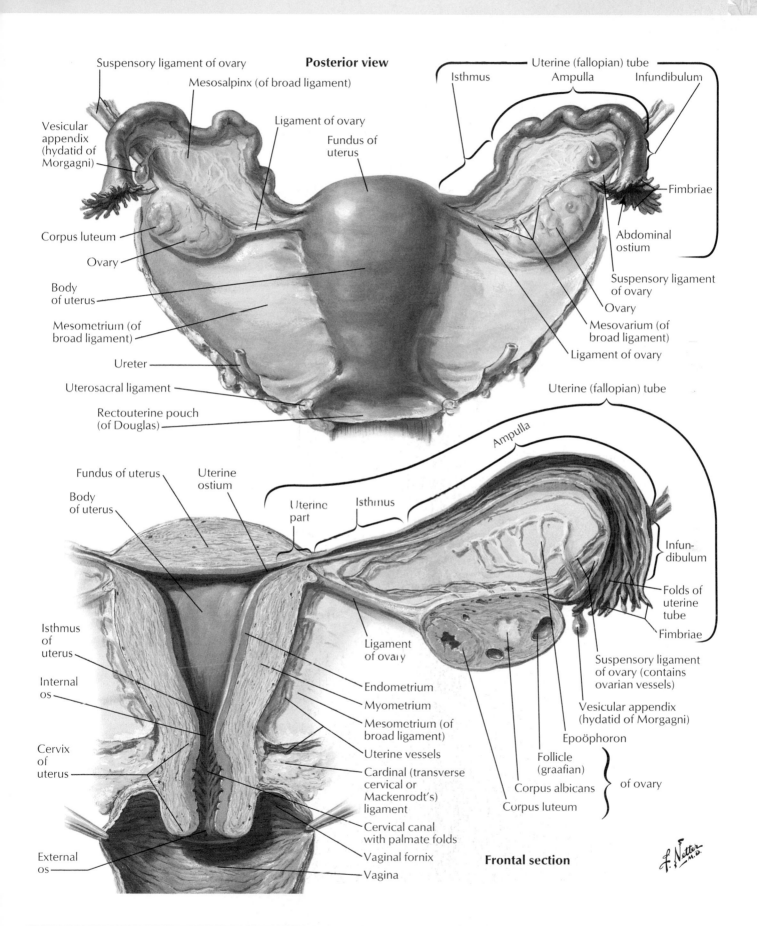

Posterior view

Suspensory ligament of ovary

Mesosalpinx (of broad ligament)

Uterine (fallopian) tube

Isthmus

Ampulla

Infundibulum

Vesicular appendix (hydatid of Morgagni)

Ligament of ovary

Fundus of uterus

Fimbriae

Corpus luteum

Abdominal ostium

Ovary

Body of uterus

Suspensory ligament of ovary

Mesometrium (of broad ligament)

Ovary

Ureter

Mesovarium (of broad ligament)

Uterosacral ligament

Ligament of ovary

Rectouterine pouch (of Douglas)

Uterine (fallopian) tube

Ampulla

Fundus of uterus

Uterine ostium

Body of uterus

Uterine part

Isthmus

Infundibulum

Isthmus of uterus

Folds of uterine tube

Internal os

Fimbriae

Ligament of ovary

Cervix of uterus

Suspensory ligament of ovary (contains ovarian vessels)

Endometrium

Myometrium

Vesicular appendix (hydatid of Morgagni)

Mesometrium (of broad ligament)

Epoöphoron

Uterine vessels

Cardinal (transverse cervical or Mackenrodt's) ligament

Follicle (graafian)

Corpus albicans

of ovary

Corpus luteum

Cervical canal with palmate folds

External os

Vaginal fornix

Frontal section

Vagina

Uterus, Vagina, and Supporting Structures

Plate 355

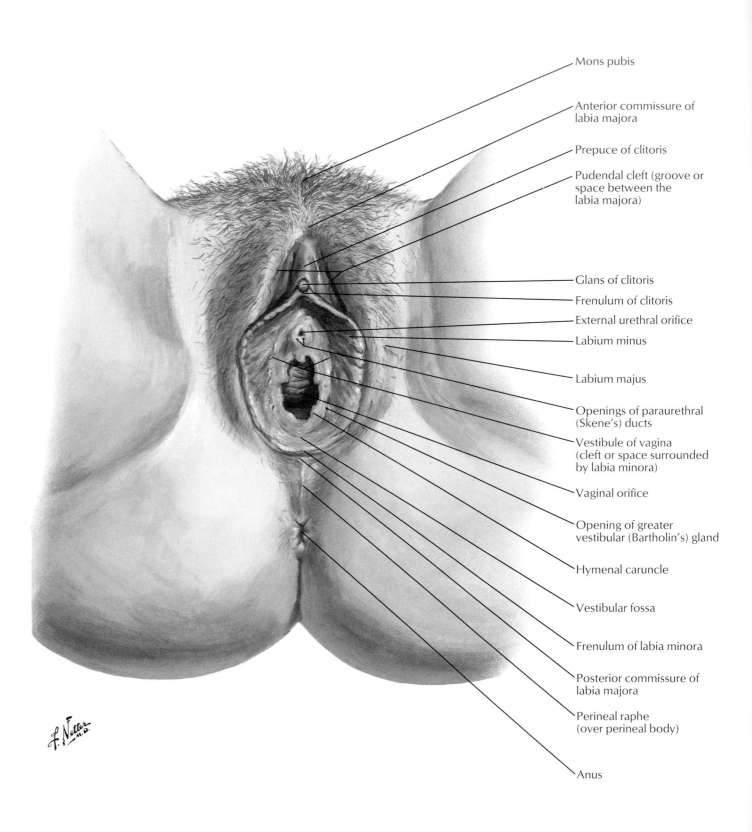

Mons pubis

Anterior commissure of labia majora

Prepuce of clitoris

Pudendal cleft (groove or space between the labia majora)

Glans of clitoris

Frenulum of clitoris

External urethral orifice

Labium minus

Labium majus

Openings of paraurethral (Skene's) ducts

Vestibule of vagina (cleft or space surrounded by labia minora)

Vaginal orifice

Opening of greater vestibular (Bartholin's) gland

Hymenal caruncle

Vestibular fossa

Frenulum of labia minora

Posterior commissure of labia majora

Perineal raphe (over perineal body)

Anus

Plate 356

Perineum and External Genitalia: Female

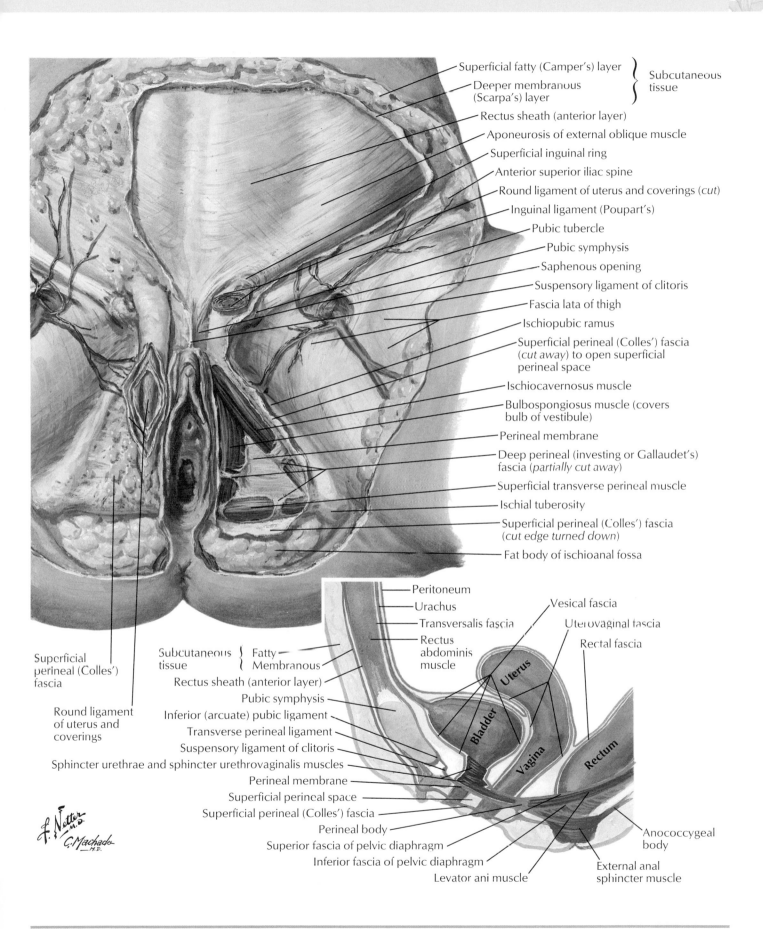

Superficial fatty (Camper's) layer
Deeper membranous (Scarpa's) layer
⎱ Subcutaneous tissue

Rectus sheath (anterior layer)

Aponeurosis of external oblique muscle

Superficial inguinal ring

Anterior superior iliac spine

Round ligament of uterus and coverings (cut)

Inguinal ligament (Poupart's)

Pubic tubercle

Pubic symphysis

Saphenous opening

Suspensory ligament of clitoris

Fascia lata of thigh

Ischiopubic ramus

Superficial perineal (Colles') fascia (cut away) to open superficial perineal space

Ischiocavernosus muscle

Bulbospongiosus muscle (covers bulb of vestibule)

Perineal membrane

Deep perineal (investing or Gallaudet's) fascia (partially cut away)

Superficial transverse perineal muscle

Ischial tuberosity

Superficial perineal (Colles') fascia (cut edge turned down)

Fat body of ischioanal fossa

Superficial perineal (Colles') fascia

Round ligament of uterus and coverings

Subcutaneous tissue ⎱ Fatty / Membranous

Rectus sheath (anterior layer)

Pubic symphysis

Inferior (arcuate) pubic ligament

Transverse perineal ligament

Suspensory ligament of clitoris

Sphincter urethrae and sphincter urethrovaginalis muscles

Perineal membrane

Superficial perineal space

Superficial perineal (Colles') fascia

Perineal body

Superior fascia of pelvic diaphragm

Inferior fascia of pelvic diaphragm

Levator ani muscle

Peritoneum
Urachus
Transversalis fascia
Rectus abdominis muscle

Vesical fascia
Uterovaginal fascia
Rectal fascia

Uterus
Bladder
Vagina
Rectum

Anococcygeal body

External anal sphincter muscle

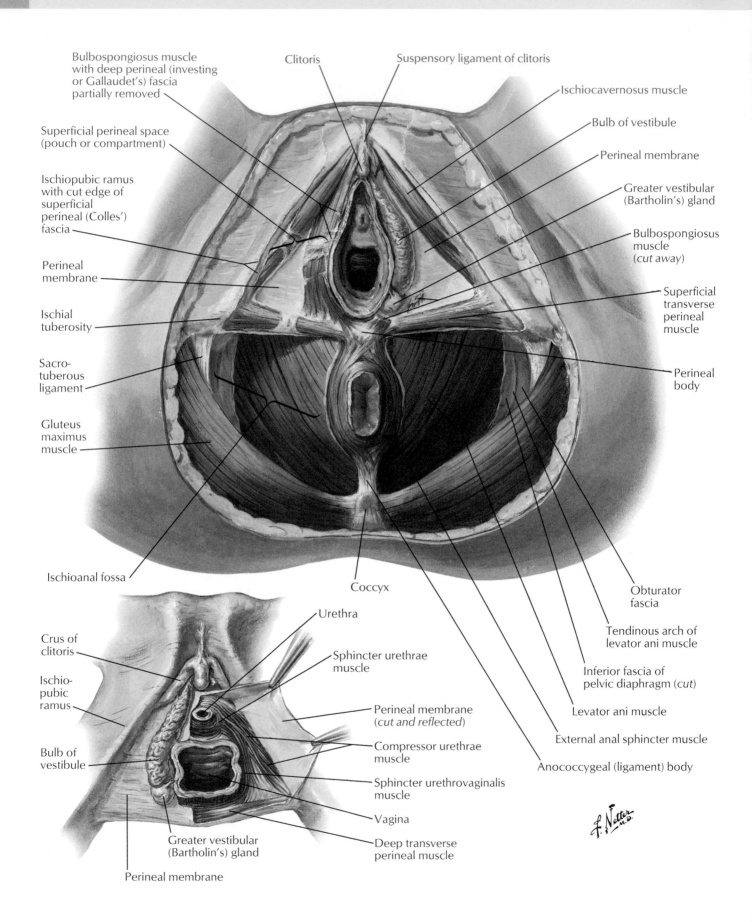

Bulbospongiosus muscle with deep perineal (investing or Gallaudet's) fascia partially removed

Clitoris

Suspensory ligament of clitoris

Ischiocavernosus muscle

Bulb of vestibule

Perineal membrane

Superficial perineal space (pouch or compartment)

Greater vestibular (Bartholin's) gland

Ischiopubic ramus with cut edge of superficial perineal (Colles') fascia

Bulbospongiosus muscle (cut away)

Perineal membrane

Superficial transverse perineal muscle

Ischial tuberosity

Sacro-tuberous ligament

Perineal body

Gluteus maximus muscle

Ischioanal fossa

Coccyx

Obturator fascia

Tendinous arch of levator ani muscle

Inferior fascia of pelvic diaphragm (cut)

Levator ani muscle

External anal sphincter muscle

Anococcygeal (ligament) body

Crus of clitoris

Urethra

Sphincter urethrae muscle

Ischio-pubic ramus

Perineal membrane (cut and reflected)

Compressor urethrae muscle

Bulb of vestibule

Sphincter urethrovaginalis muscle

Vagina

Greater vestibular (Bartholin's) gland

Deep transverse perineal muscle

Perineal membrane

f. Netter M.D.

Plate 358

Perineum and External Genitalia: Female

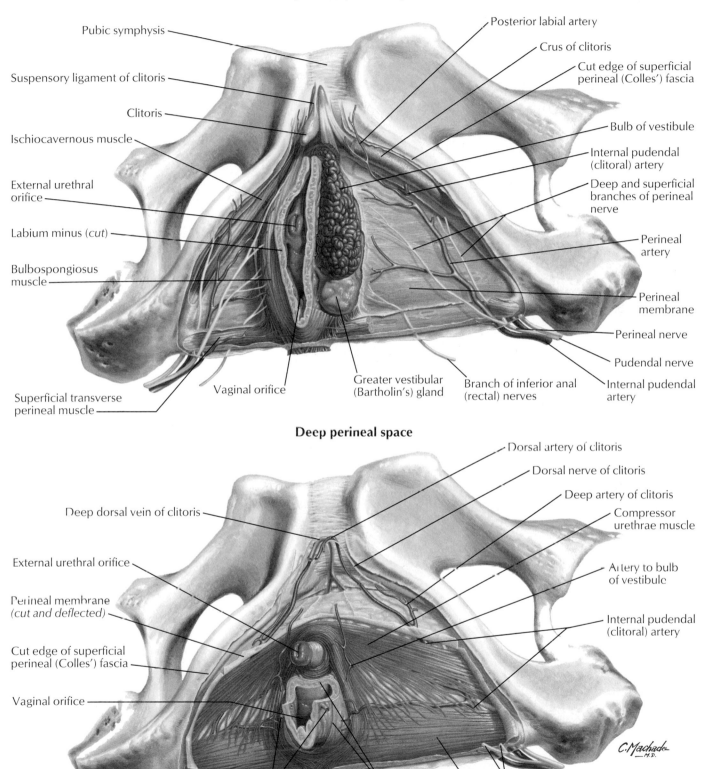

Superficial perineal space

Pubic symphysis

Suspensory ligament of clitoris

Clitoris

Ischiocavernous muscle

External urethral orifice

Labium minus (cut)

Bulbospongiosus muscle

Superficial transverse perineal muscle

Vaginal orifice

Greater vestibular (Bartholin's) gland

Branch of inferior anal (rectal) nerves

Posterior labial artery

Crus of clitoris

Cut edge of superficial perineal (Colles') fascia

Bulb of vestibule

Internal pudendal (clitoral) artery

Deep and superficial branches of perineal nerve

Perineal artery

Perineal membrane

Perineal nerve

Pudendal nerve

Internal pudendal artery

Deep perineal space

Deep dorsal vein of clitoris

External urethral orifice

Perineal membrane (cut and deflected)

Cut edge of superficial perineal (Colles') fascia

Vaginal orifice

Greater vestibular (Bartholin's) glands

Vaginal wall

Deep transverse perineal muscle

Dorsal artery of clitoris

Dorsal nerve of clitoris

Deep artery of clitoris

Compressor urethrae muscle

Artery to bulb of vestibule

Internal pudendal (clitoral) artery

Deep and superficial branches of perineal nerve (cut)

C. Machado M.D.

Perineum and External Genitalia: Female

Plate 359

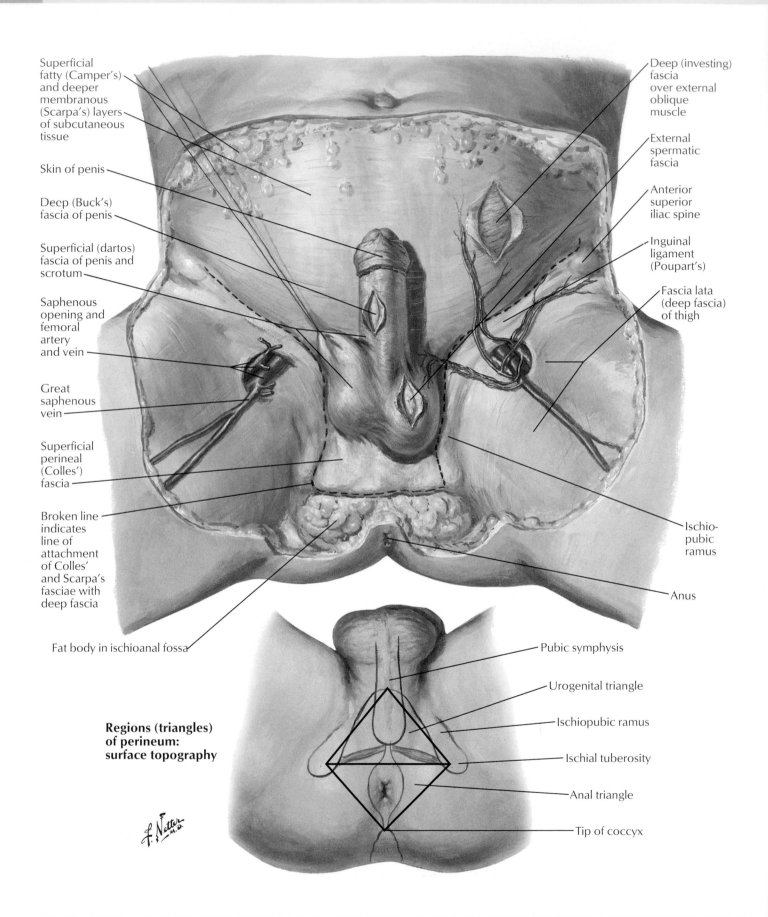

Superficial fatty (Camper's) and deeper membranous (Scarpa's) layers of subcutaneous tissue

Skin of penis

Deep (Buck's) fascia of penis

Superficial (dartos) fascia of penis and scrotum

Saphenous opening and femoral artery and vein

Great saphenous vein

Superficial perineal (Colles') fascia

Broken line indicates line of attachment of Colles' and Scarpa's fasciae with deep fascia

Fat body in ischioanal fossa

Deep (investing) fascia over external oblique muscle

External spermatic fascia

Anterior superior iliac spine

Inguinal ligament (Poupart's)

Fascia lata (deep fascia) of thigh

Ischio-pubic ramus

Anus

Regions (triangles) of perineum: surface topography

Pubic symphysis

Urogenital triangle

Ischiopubic ramus

Ischial tuberosity

Anal triangle

Tip of coccyx

f. Netter

Plate 360

Perineum and External Genitalia: Male

See also **Plates 383, 385, 388-391, 396**

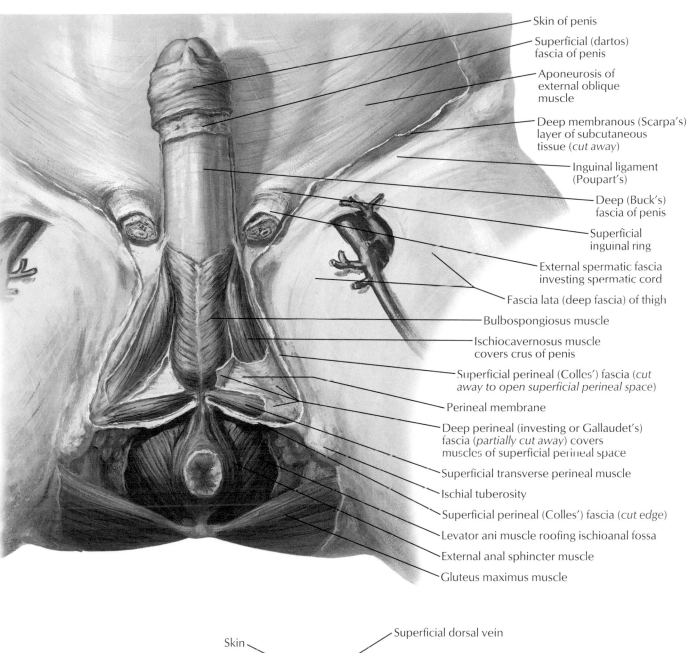

Skin of penis

Superficial (dartos) fascia of penis

Aponeurosis of external oblique muscle

Deep membranous (Scarpa's) layer of subcutaneous tissue (*cut away*)

Inguinal ligament (Poupart's)

Deep (Buck's) fascia of penis

Superficial inguinal ring

External spermatic fascia investing spermatic cord

Fascia lata (deep fascia) of thigh

Bulbospongiosus muscle

Ischiocavernosus muscle covers crus of penis

Superficial perineal (Colles') fascia (*cut away to open superficial perineal space*)

Perineal membrane

Deep perineal (investing or Gallaudet's) fascia (*partially cut away*) covers muscles of superficial perineal space

Superficial transverse perineal muscle

Ischial tuberosity

Superficial perineal (Colles') fascia (*cut edge*)

Levator ani muscle roofing ischioanal fossa

External anal sphincter muscle

Gluteus maximus muscle

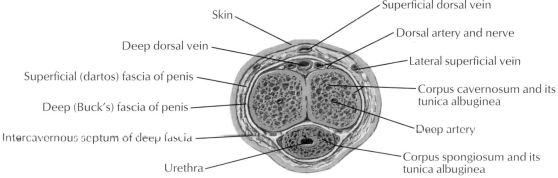

Skin

Superficial dorsal vein

Deep dorsal vein

Dorsal artery and nerve

Superficial (dartos) fascia of penis

Lateral superficial vein

Deep (Buck's) fascia of penis

Corpus cavernosum and its tunica albuginea

Intercavernous septum of deep fascia

Deep artery

Urethra

Corpus spongiosum and its tunica albuginea

Transverse section through body of penis

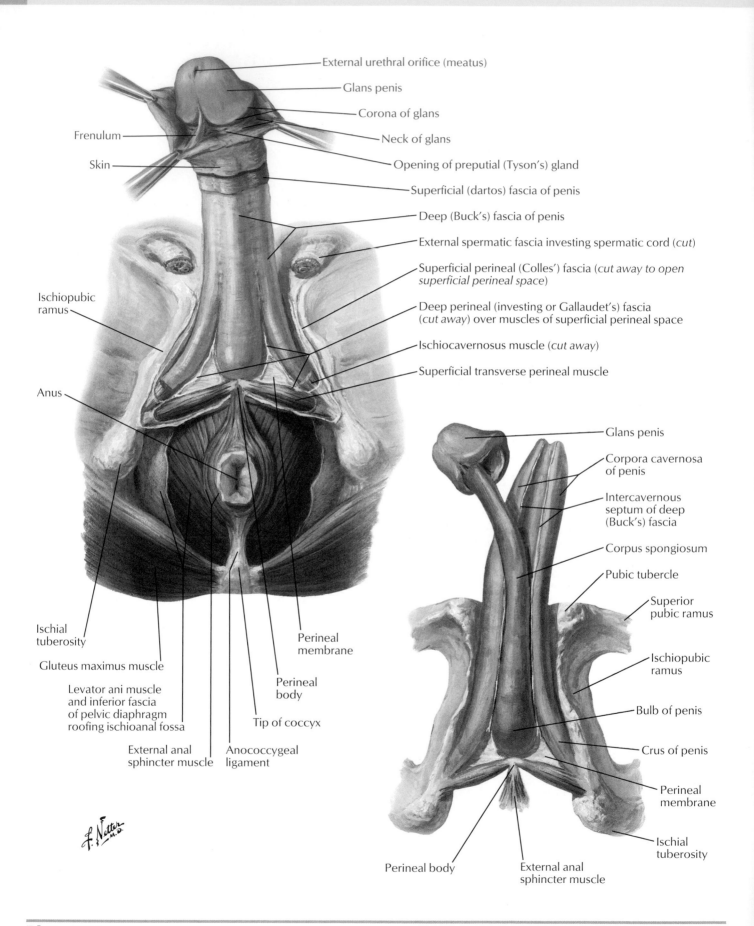

External urethral orifice (meatus)

Glans penis

Corona of glans

Neck of glans

Frenulum

Opening of preputial (Tyson's) gland

Skin

Superficial (dartos) fascia of penis

Deep (Buck's) fascia of penis

External spermatic fascia investing spermatic cord (*cut*)

Superficial perineal (Colles') fascia (*cut away to open superficial perineal space*)

Ischiopubic ramus

Deep perineal (investing or Gallaudet's) fascia (*cut away*) over muscles of superficial perineal space

Ischiocavernosus muscle (*cut away*)

Superficial transverse perineal muscle

Anus

Ischial tuberosity

Gluteus maximus muscle

Levator ani muscle and inferior fascia of pelvic diaphragm roofing ischioanal fossa

Perineal membrane

Perineal body

External anal sphincter muscle

Anococcygeal ligament

Tip of coccyx

Glans penis

Corpora cavernosa of penis

Intercavernous septum of deep (Buck's) fascia

Corpus spongiosum

Pubic tubercle

Superior pubic ramus

Ischiopubic ramus

Bulb of penis

Crus of penis

Perineal membrane

Ischial tuberosity

Perineal body

External anal sphincter muscle

Plate 362

Perineum and External Genitalia: Male

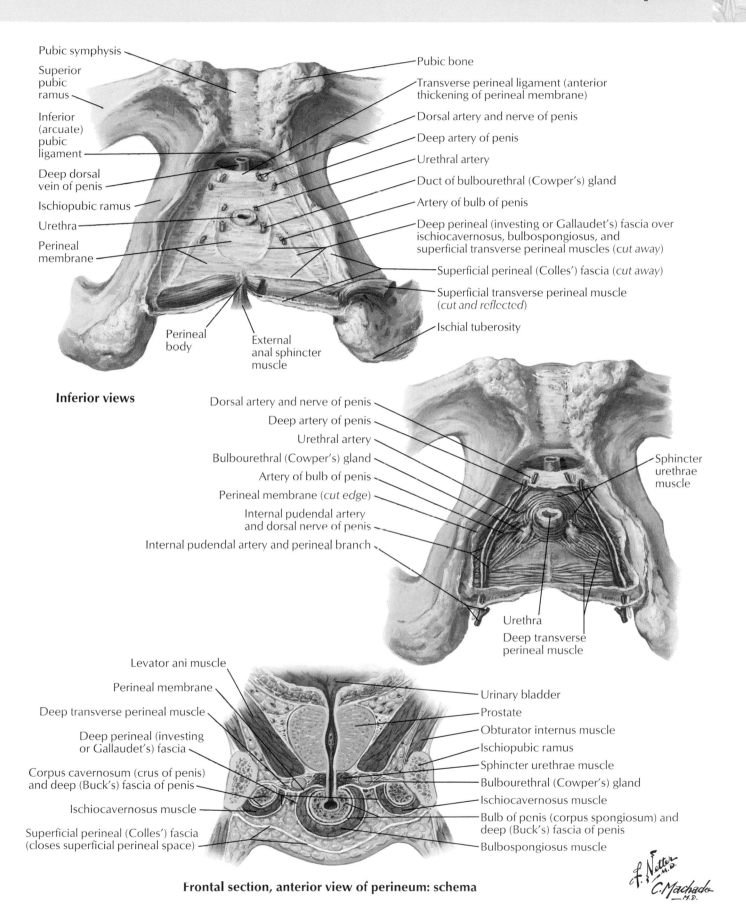

Inferior views

Pubic symphysis

Superior pubic ramus

Inferior (arcuate) pubic ligament

Deep dorsal vein of penis

Ischiopubic ramus

Urethra

Perineal membrane

Perineal body

External anal sphincter muscle

Pubic bone

Transverse perineal ligament (anterior thickening of perineal membrane)

Dorsal artery and nerve of penis

Deep artery of penis

Urethral artery

Duct of bulbourethral (Cowper's) gland

Artery of bulb of penis

Deep perineal (investing or Gallaudet's) fascia over ischiocavernosus, bulbospongiosus, and superficial transverse perineal muscles (*cut away*)

Superficial perineal (Colles') fascia (*cut away*)

Superficial transverse perineal muscle (*cut and reflected*)

Ischial tuberosity

Dorsal artery and nerve of penis

Deep artery of penis

Urethral artery

Bulbourethral (Cowper's) gland

Artery of bulb of penis

Perineal membrane (*cut edge*)

Internal pudendal artery and dorsal nerve of penis

Internal pudendal artery and perineal branch

Sphincter urethrae muscle

Urethra

Deep transverse perineal muscle

Levator ani muscle

Perineal membrane

Deep transverse perineal muscle

Deep perineal (investing or Gallaudet's) fascia

Corpus cavernosum (crus of penis) and deep (Buck's) fascia of penis

Ischiocavernosus muscle

Superficial perineal (Colles') fascia (closes superficial perineal space)

Urinary bladder

Prostate

Obturator internus muscle

Ischiopubic ramus

Sphincter urethrae muscle

Bulbourethral (Cowper's) gland

Ischiocavernosus muscle

Bulb of penis (corpus spongiosum) and deep (Buck's) fascia of penis

Bulbospongiosus muscle

Frontal section, anterior view of perineum: schema

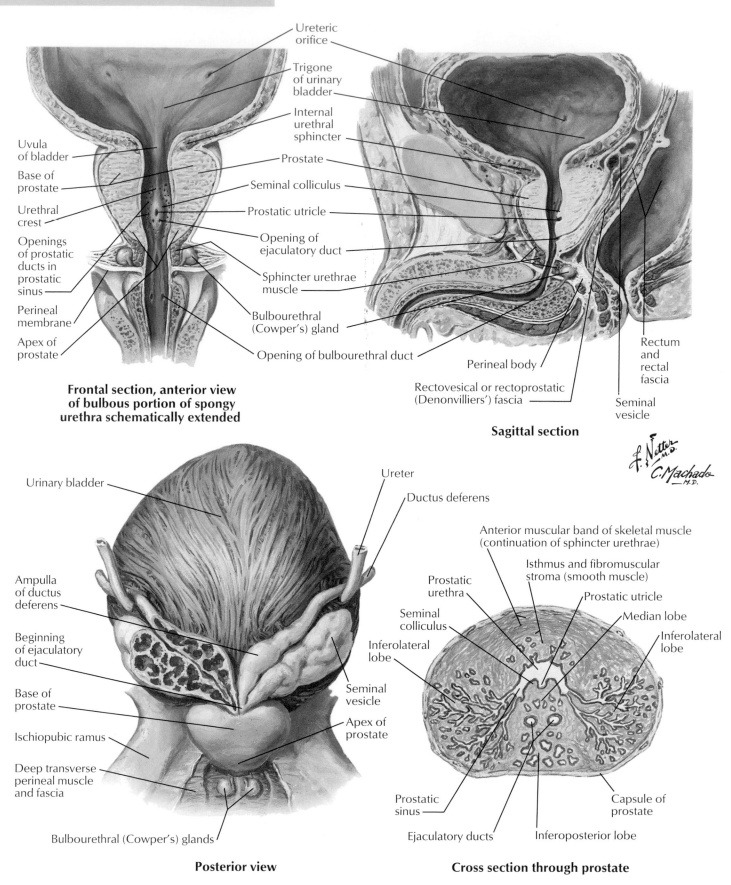

Ureteric orifice

Trigone of urinary bladder

Internal urethral sphincter

Uvula of bladder

Base of prostate

Urethral crest

Openings of prostatic ducts in prostatic sinus

Perineal membrane

Apex of prostate

Prostate

Seminal colliculus

Prostatic utricle

Opening of ejaculatory duct

Sphincter urethrae muscle

Bulbourethral (Cowper's) gland

Opening of bulbourethral duct

Rectum and rectal fascia

Seminal vesicle

Perineal body

Rectovesical or rectoprostatic (Denonvilliers') fascia

Frontal section, anterior view of bulbous portion of spongy urethra schematically extended

Sagittal section

Urinary bladder

Ureter

Ductus deferens

Ampulla of ductus deferens

Beginning of ejaculatory duct

Base of prostate

Ischiopubic ramus

Deep transverse perineal muscle and fascia

Bulbourethral (Cowper's) glands

Seminal vesicle

Apex of prostate

Posterior view

Anterior muscular band of skeletal muscle (continuation of sphincter urethrae)

Isthmus and fibromuscular stroma (smooth muscle)

Prostatic urethra

Prostatic utricle

Seminal colliculus

Median lobe

Inferolateral lobe

Inferolateral lobe

Prostatic sinus

Capsule of prostate

Ejaculatory ducts

Inferoposterior lobe

Cross section through prostate

Plate 364

Perineum and External Genitalia: Male

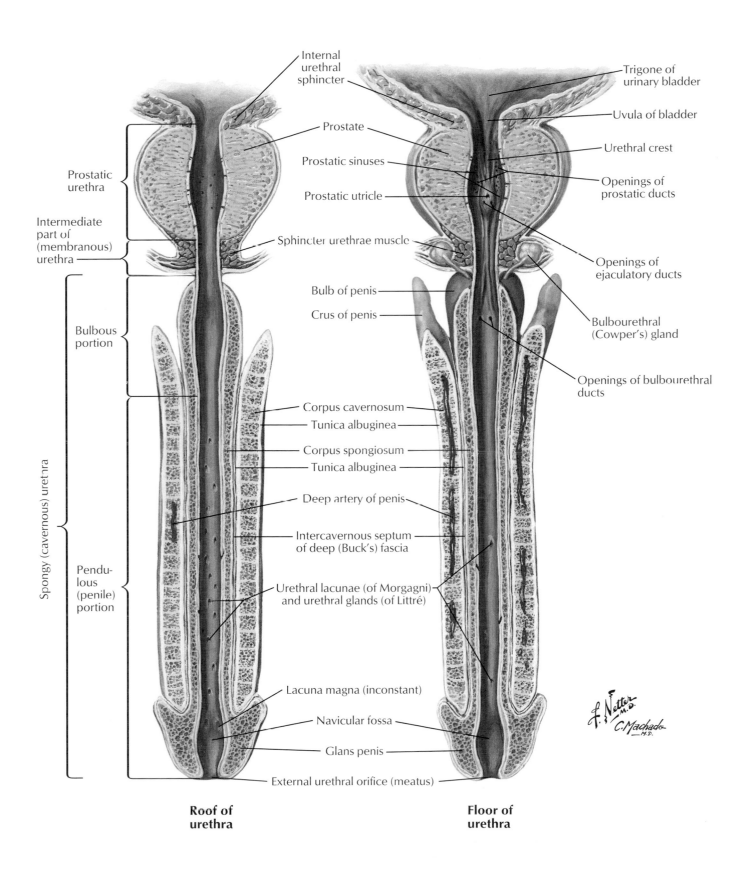

Internal urethral sphincter

Trigone of urinary bladder

Prostate

Uvula of bladder

Prostatic sinuses

Urethral crest

Prostatic urtricle

Openings of prostatic ducts

Prostatic urethra

Sphincter urethrae muscle

Intermediate part of (membranous) urethra

Openings of ejaculatory ducts

Bulb of penis

Crus of penis

Bulbourethral (Cowper's) gland

Bulbous portion

Openings of bulbourethral ducts

Corpus cavernosum

Tunica albuginea

Corpus spongiosum

Spongy (cavernous) urethra

Tunica albuginea

Deep artery of penis

Intercavernous septum of deep (Buck's) fascia

Pendulous (penile) portion

Urethral lacunae (of Morgagni) and urethral glands (of Littré)

Lacuna magna (inconstant)

Navicular fossa

Glans penis

External urethral orifice (meatus)

Roof of urethra

Floor of urethra

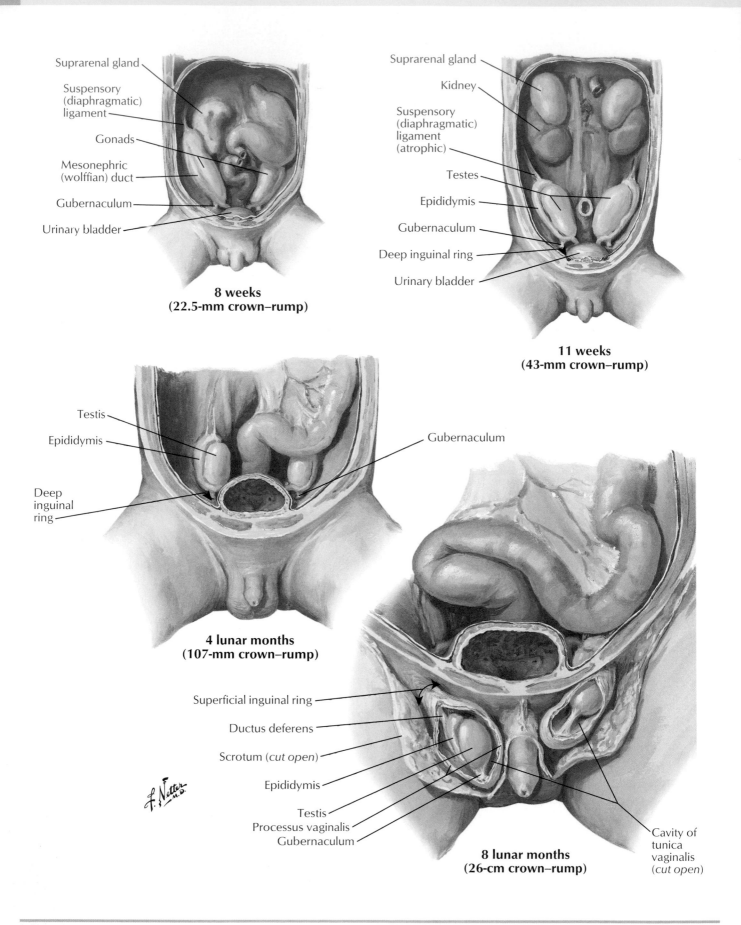

Suprarenal gland
Suspensory (diaphragmatic) ligament
Gonads
Mesonephric (wolffian) duct
Gubernaculum
Urinary bladder

**8 weeks
(22.5-mm crown–rump)**

Suprarenal gland
Kidney
Suspensory (diaphragmatic) ligament (atrophic)
Testes
Epididymis
Gubernaculum
Deep inguinal ring
Urinary bladder

**11 weeks
(43-mm crown–rump)**

Testis
Epididymis
Deep inguinal ring

Gubernaculum

**4 lunar months
(107-mm crown–rump)**

Superficial inguinal ring
Ductus deferens
Scrotum (*cut open*)
Epididymis
Testis
Processus vaginalis
Gubernaculum

Cavity of tunica vaginalis (*cut open*)

**8 lunar months
(26-cm crown–rump)**

Plate 366

Perineum and External Genitalia: Male

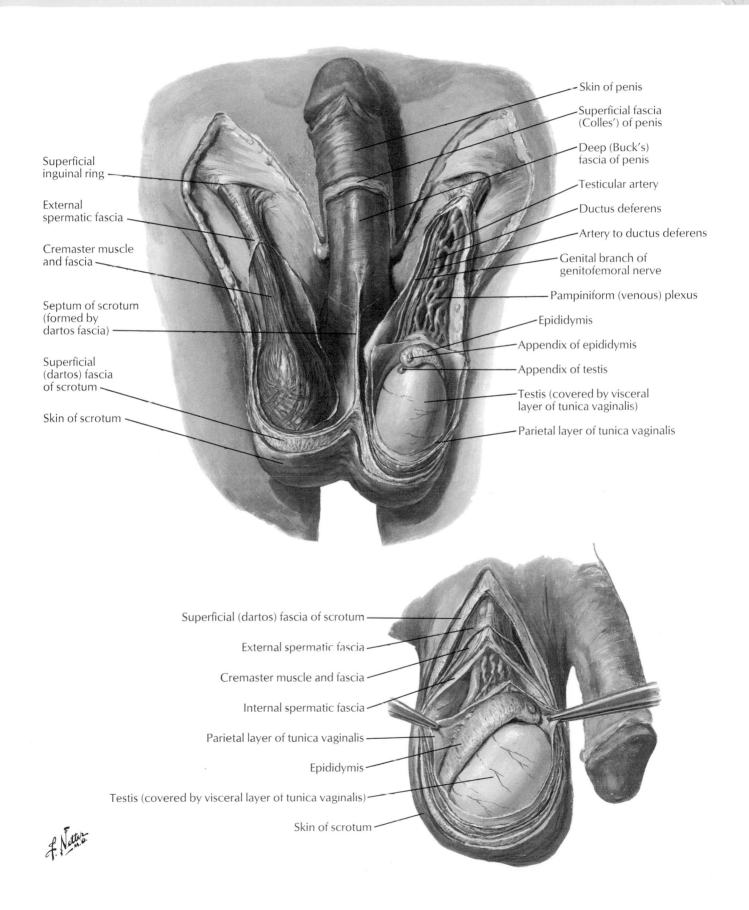

Skin of penis

Superficial fascia (Colles') of penis

Deep (Buck's) fascia of penis

Testicular artery

Ductus deferens

Artery to ductus deferens

Genital branch of genitofemoral nerve

Pampiniform (venous) plexus

Epididymis

Appendix of epididymis

Appendix of testis

Testis (covered by visceral layer of tunica vaginalis)

Parietal layer of tunica vaginalis

Superficial inguinal ring

External spermatic fascia

Cremaster muscle and fascia

Septum of scrotum (formed by dartos fascia)

Superficial (dartos) fascia of scrotum

Skin of scrotum

Superficial (dartos) fascia of scrotum

External spermatic fascia

Cremaster muscle and fascia

Internal spermatic fascia

Parietal layer of tunica vaginalis

Epididymis

Testis (covered by visceral layer of tunica vaginalis)

Skin of scrotum

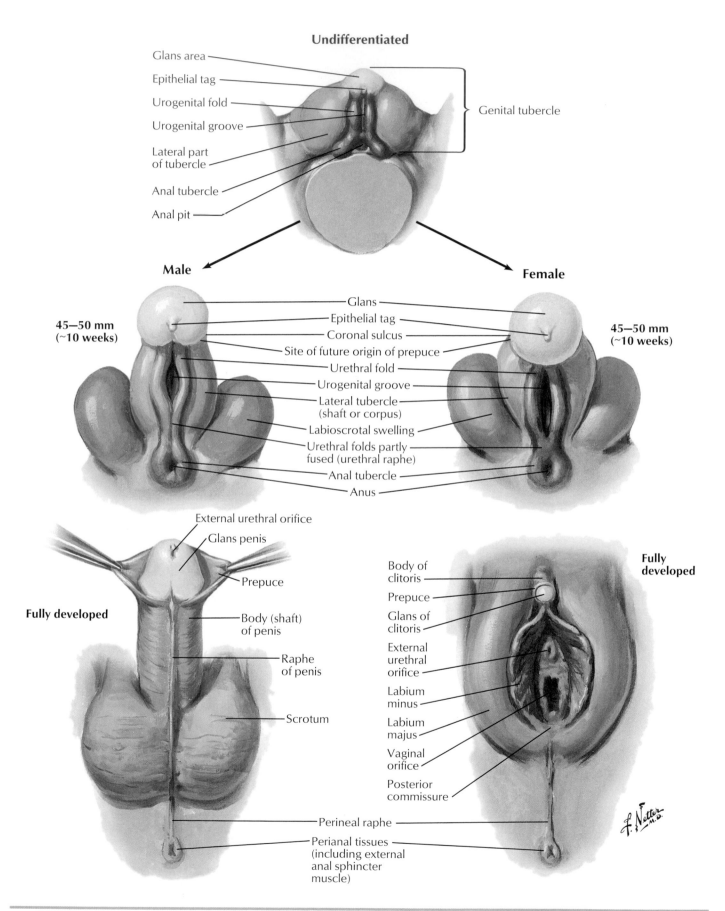

Undifferentiated

- Glans area
- Epithelial tag
- Urogenital fold
- Urogenital groove
- Lateral part of tubercle
- Anal tubercle
- Anal pit
- Genital tubercle

Male

Female

45–50 mm (~10 weeks)

45–50 mm (~10 weeks)

- Glans
- Epithelial tag
- Coronal sulcus
- Site of future origin of prepuce
- Urethral fold
- Urogenital groove
- Lateral tubercle (shaft or corpus)
- Labioscrotal swelling
- Urethral folds partly fused (urethral raphe)
- Anal tubercle
- Anus

Fully developed

- External urethral orifice
- Glans penis
- Prepuce
- Body (shaft) of penis
- Raphe of penis
- Scrotum

Fully developed

- Body of clitoris
- Prepuce
- Glans of clitoris
- External urethral orifice
- Labium minus
- Labium majus
- Vaginal orifice
- Posterior commissure

- Perineal raphe
- Perianal tissues (including external anal sphincter muscle)

Plate 368 **Homologues of Genitalia**

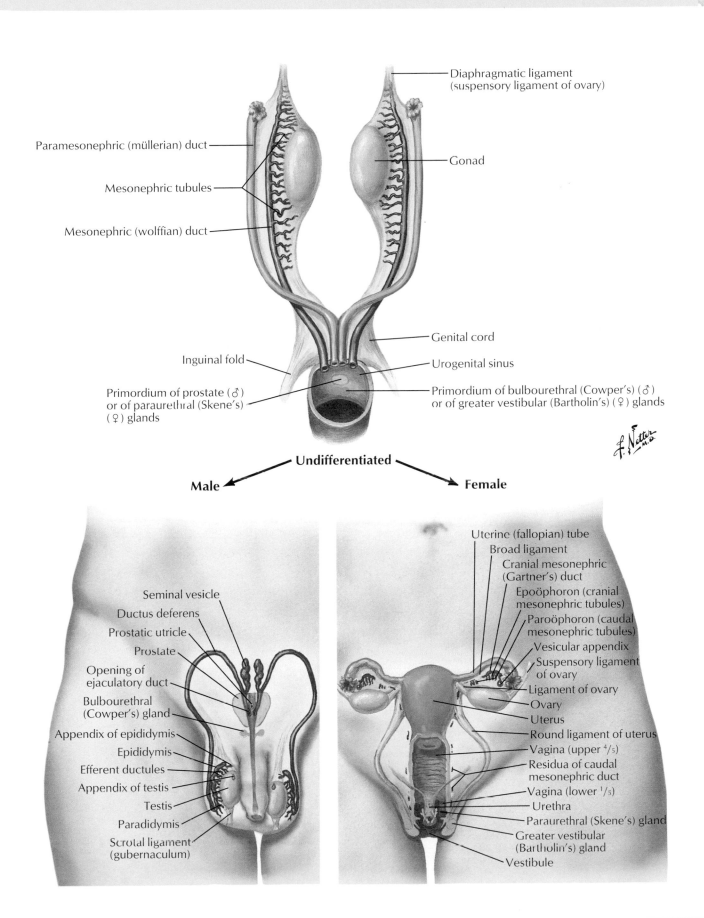

Diaphragmatic ligament
(suspensory ligament of ovary)

Paramesonephric (müllerian) duct

Mesonephric tubules

Mesonephric (wolffian) duct

Gonad

Genital cord

Inguinal fold

Urogenital sinus

Primordium of prostate (♂)
or of paraurethral (Skene's)
(♀) glands

Primordium of bulbourethral (Cowper's) (♂)
or of greater vestibular (Bartholin's) (♀) glands

Undifferentiated

Male

Female

Seminal vesicle

Ductus deferens

Prostatic utricle

Prostate

Opening of
ejaculatory duct

Bulbourethral
(Cowper's) gland

Appendix of epididymis

Epididymis

Efferent ductules

Appendix of testis

Testis

Paradidymis

Scrotal ligament
(gubernaculum)

Uterine (fallopian) tube

Broad ligament

Cranial mesonephric
(Gartner's) duct

Epoöphoron (cranial
mesonephric tubules)

Paroöphoron (caudal
mesonephric tubules)

Vesicular appendix

Suspensory ligament
of ovary

Ligament of ovary

Ovary

Uterus

Round ligament of uterus

Vagina (upper $^4/_5$)

Residua of caudal
mesonephric duct

Vagina (lower $^1/_5$)

Urethra

Paraurethral (Skene's) gland

Greater vestibular
(Bartholin's) gland

Vestibule

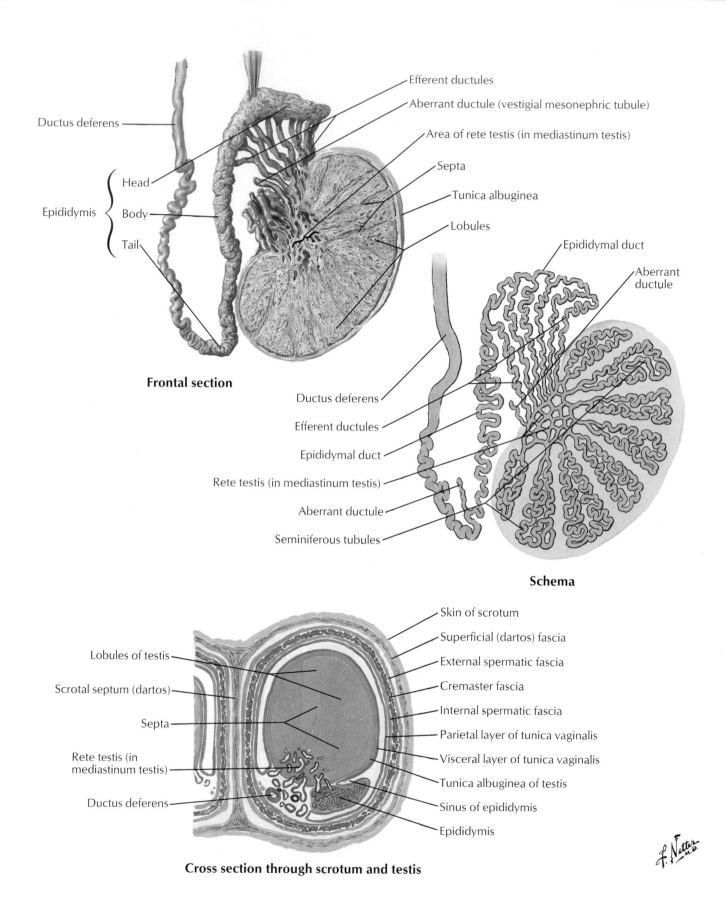

Efferent ductules

Aberrant ductule (vestigial mesonephric tubule)

Area of rete testis (in mediastinum testis)

Septa

Tunica albuginea

Lobules

Ductus deferens

Head

Epididymis { Body

Tail

Frontal section

Epididymal duct

Aberrant ductule

Ductus deferens

Efferent ductules

Epididymal duct

Rete testis (in mediastinum testis)

Aberrant ductule

Seminiferous tubules

Schema

Lobules of testis

Scrotal septum (dartos)

Septa

Rete testis (in mediastinum testis)

Ductus deferens

Skin of scrotum

Superficial (dartos) fascia

External spermatic fascia

Cremaster fascia

Internal spermatic fascia

Parietal layer of tunica vaginalis

Visceral layer of tunica vaginalis

Tunica albuginea of testis

Sinus of epididymis

Epididymis

Cross section through scrotum and testis

Plate 370

Testis, Epididymis, and Ductus Deferens

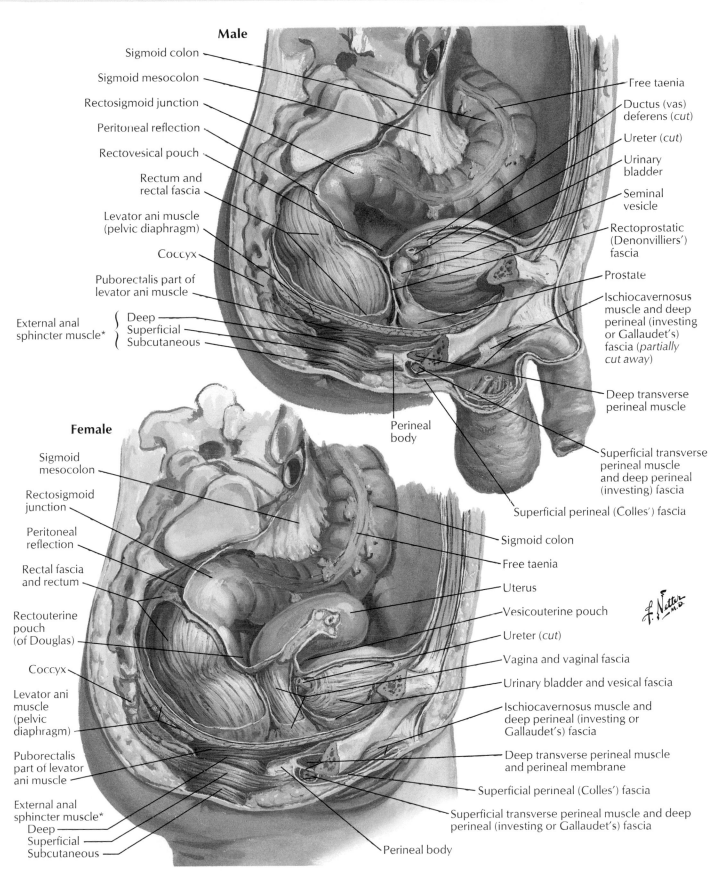

Male

Sigmoid colon

Sigmoid mesocolon

Rectosigmoid junction

Peritoneal reflection

Rectovesical pouch

Rectum and rectal fascia

Levator ani muscle (pelvic diaphragm)

Coccyx

Puborectalis part of levator ani muscle

External anal sphincter muscle* { Deep / Superficial / Subcutaneous

Free taenia

Ductus (vas) deferens (cut)

Ureter (cut)

Urinary bladder

Seminal vesicle

Rectoprostatic (Denonvilliers') fascia

Prostate

Ischiocavernosus muscle and deep perineal (investing or Gallaudet's) fascia (partially cut away)

Deep transverse perineal muscle

Superficial transverse perineal muscle and deep perineal (investing) fascia

Superficial perineal (Colles') fascia

Perineal body

Female

Sigmoid mesocolon

Rectosigmoid junction

Peritoneal reflection

Rectal fascia and rectum

Rectouterine pouch (of Douglas)

Coccyx

Levator ani muscle (pelvic diaphragm)

Puborectalis part of levator ani muscle

External anal sphincter muscle* Deep / Superficial / Subcutaneous

Sigmoid colon

Free taenia

Uterus

Vesicouterine pouch

Ureter (cut)

Vagina and vaginal fascia

Urinary bladder and vesical fascia

Ischiocavernosus muscle and deep perineal (investing or Gallaudet's) fascia

Deep transverse perineal muscle and perineal membrane

Superficial perineal (Colles') fascia

Superficial transverse perineal muscle and deep perineal (investing or Gallaudet's) fascia

Perineal body

*Parts variable and often indistinct

Rectum

Plate 371

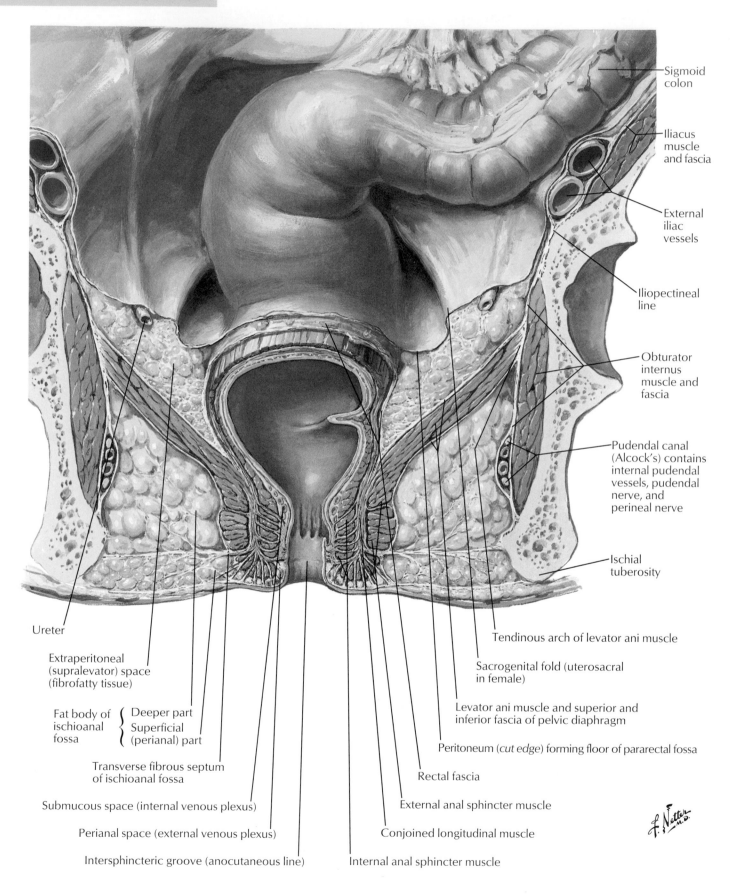

Sigmoid colon

Iliacus muscle and fascia

External iliac vessels

Iliopectineal line

Obturator internus muscle and fascia

Pudendal canal (Alcock's) contains internal pudendal vessels, pudendal nerve, and perineal nerve

Ischial tuberosity

Tendinous arch of levator ani muscle

Sacrogenital fold (uterosacral in female)

Levator ani muscle and superior and inferior fascia of pelvic diaphragm

Peritoneum (*cut edge*) forming floor of pararectal fossa

Rectal fascia

External anal sphincter muscle

Conjoined longitudinal muscle

Internal anal sphincter muscle

Ureter

Extraperitoneal (supralevator) space (fibrofatty tissue)

Fat body of ischioanal fossa { Deeper part / Superficial (perianal) part

Transverse fibrous septum of ischioanal fossa

Submucous space (internal venous plexus)

Perianal space (external venous plexus)

Intersphincteric groove (anocutaneous line)

f. Netter
M.D.

Plate 372

Rectum

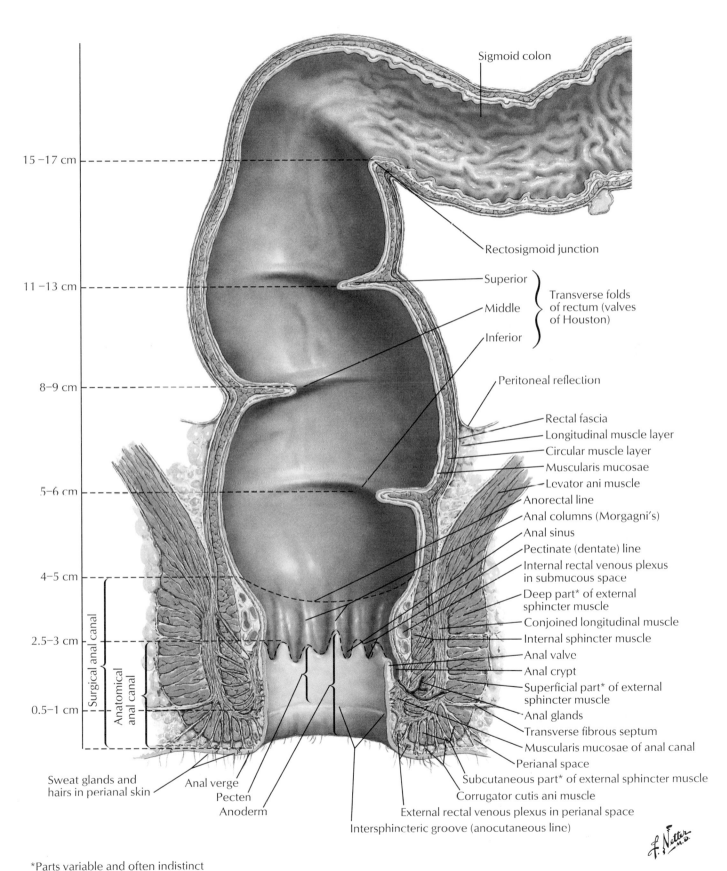

Sigmoid colon

Rectosigmoid junction

Superior

Middle　Transverse folds of rectum (valves of Houston)

Inferior

Peritoneal reflection

Rectal fascia

Longitudinal muscle layer

Circular muscle layer

Muscularis mucosae

Levator ani muscle

Anorectal line

Anal columns (Morgagni's)

Anal sinus

Pectinate (dentate) line

Internal rectal venous plexus in submucous space

Deep part* of external sphincter muscle

Conjoined longitudinal muscle

Internal sphincter muscle

Anal valve

Anal crypt

Superficial part* of external sphincter muscle

Anal glands

Transverse fibrous septum

Muscularis mucosae of anal canal

Perianal space

Subcutaneous part* of external sphincter muscle

Corrugator cutis ani muscle

External rectal venous plexus in perianal space

Intersphincteric groove (anocutaneous line)

15 –17 cm

11 –13 cm

8–9 cm

5–6 cm

4–5 cm

2.5–3 cm

0.5–1 cm

Surgical anal canal

Anatomical anal canal

Sweat glands and hairs in perianal skin

Anal verge

Pecten

Anoderm

*Parts variable and often indistinct

Anorectal Musculature

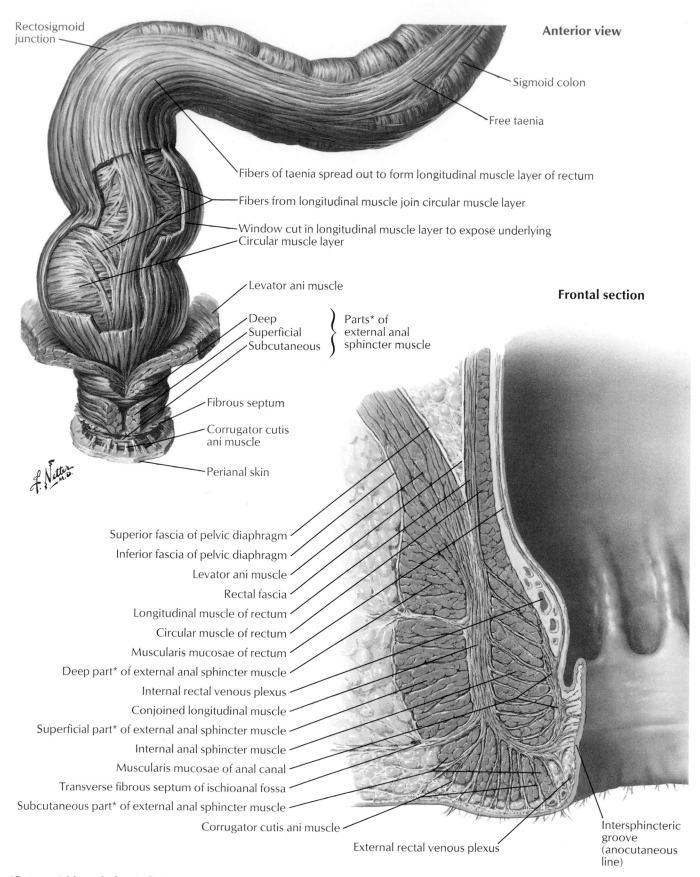

Anterior view

Rectosigmoid junction

Sigmoid colon

Free taenia

Fibers of taenia spread out to form longitudinal muscle layer of rectum

Fibers from longitudinal muscle join circular muscle layer

Window cut in longitudinal muscle layer to expose underlying Circular muscle layer

Levator ani muscle

Deep
Superficial
Subcutaneous
} Parts* of external anal sphincter muscle

Frontal section

Fibrous septum

Corrugator cutis ani muscle

Perianal skin

Superior fascia of pelvic diaphragm

Inferior fascia of pelvic diaphragm

Levator ani muscle

Rectal fascia

Longitudinal muscle of rectum

Circular muscle of rectum

Muscularis mucosae of rectum

Deep part* of external anal sphincter muscle

Internal rectal venous plexus

Conjoined longitudinal muscle

Superficial part* of external anal sphincter muscle

Internal anal sphincter muscle

Muscularis mucosae of anal canal

Transverse fibrous septum of ischioanal fossa

Subcutaneous part* of external anal sphincter muscle

Corrugator cutis ani muscle

External rectal venous plexus

Intersphincteric groove (anocutaneous line)

*Parts variable and often indistinct

Plate 374

Rectum

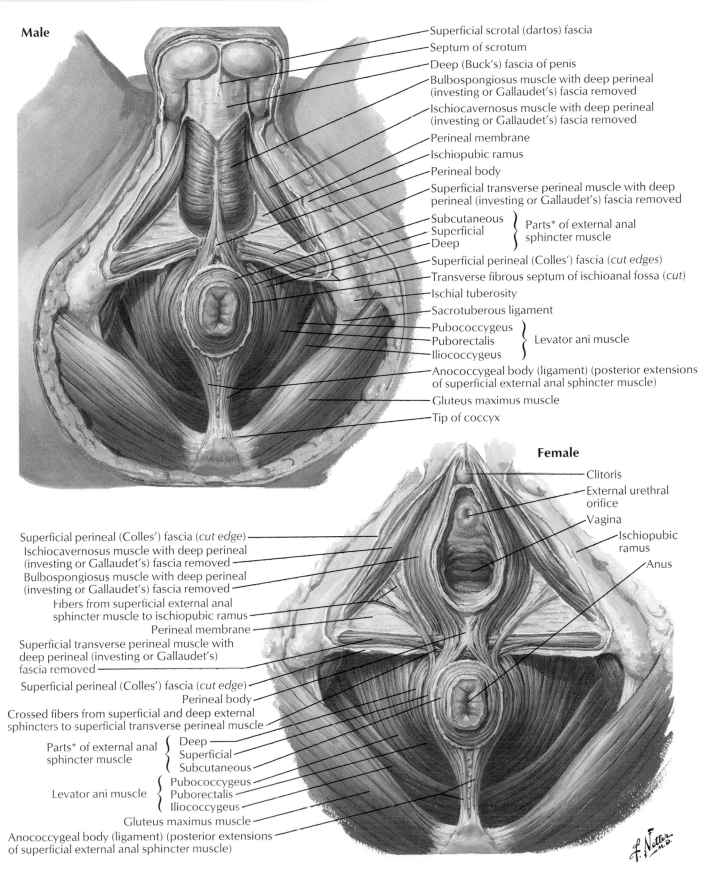

Male

Superficial scrotal (dartos) fascia

Septum of scrotum

Deep (Buck's) fascia of penis

Bulbospongiosus muscle with deep perineal (investing or Gallaudet's) fascia removed

Ischiocavernosus muscle with deep perineal (investing or Gallaudet's) fascia removed

Perineal membrane

Ischiopubic ramus

Perineal body

Superficial transverse perineal muscle with deep perineal (investing or Gallaudet's) fascia removed

Subcutaneous
Superficial } Parts* of external anal
Deep sphincter muscle

Superficial perineal (Colles') fascia (cut edges)

Transverse fibrous septum of ischioanal fossa (cut)

Ischial tuberosity

Sacrotuberous ligament

Pubococcygeus
Puborectalis } Levator ani muscle
Iliococcygeus

Anococcygeal body (ligament) (posterior extensions of superficial external anal sphincter muscle)

Gluteus maximus muscle

Tip of coccyx

Female

Clitoris

External urethral orifice

Vagina

Ischiopubic ramus

Anus

Superficial perineal (Colles') fascia (cut edge)

Ischiocavernosus muscle with deep perineal (investing or Gallaudet's) fascia removed

Bulbospongiosus muscle with deep perineal (investing or Gallaudet's) fascia removed

Fibers from superficial external anal sphincter muscle to ischiopubic ramus

Perineal membrane

Superficial transverse perineal muscle with deep perineal (investing or Gallaudet's) fascia removed

Superficial perineal (Colles') fascia (cut edge)

Perineal body

Crossed fibers from superficial and deep external sphincters to superficial transverse perineal muscle

Parts* of external anal { Deep
sphincter muscle { Superficial
{ Subcutaneous

Levator ani muscle { Pubococcygeus
{ Puborectalis
{ Iliococcygeus

Gluteus maximus muscle

Anococcygeal body (ligament) (posterior extensions of superficial external anal sphincter muscle)

*Parts variable and often indistinct

Rectum

Plate 375

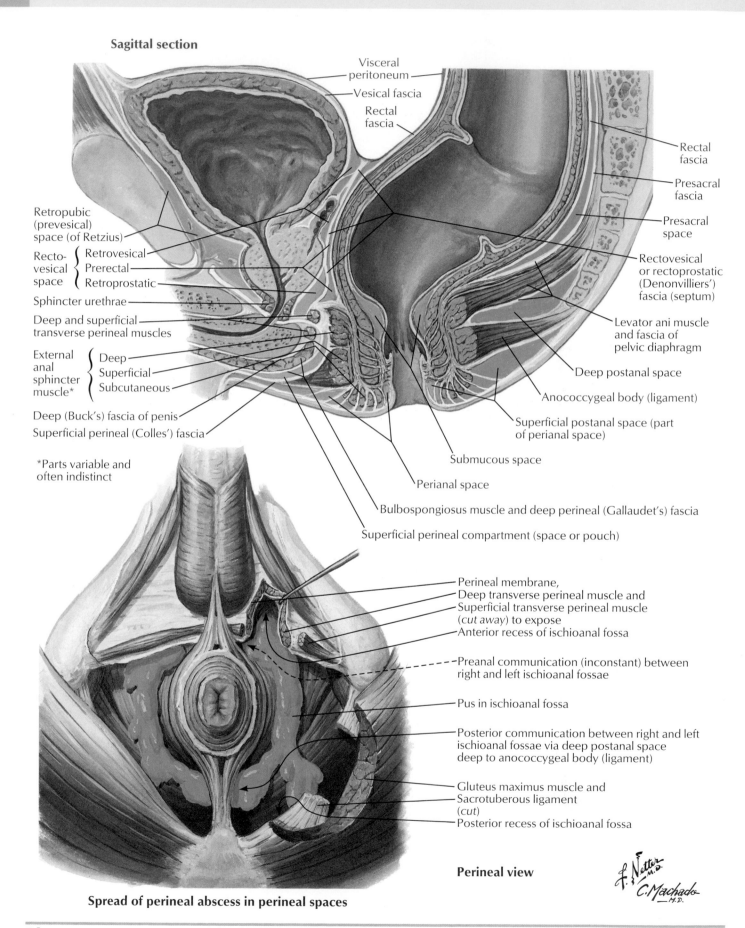

Sagittal section

Visceral peritoneum

Vesical fascia

Rectal fascia

Rectal fascia

Presacral fascia

Presacral space

Retropubic (prevesical) space (of Retzius)

Recto-vesical space { Retrovesical / Prerectal / Retroprostatic

Rectovesical or rectoprostatic (Denonvilliers') fascia (septum)

Sphincter urethrae

Deep and superficial transverse perineal muscles

Levator ani muscle and fascia of pelvic diaphragm

External anal sphincter muscle* { Deep / Superficial / Subcutaneous

Deep postanal space

Anococcygeal body (ligament)

Deep (Buck's) fascia of penis

Superficial perineal (Colles') fascia

Superficial postanal space (part of perianal space)

*Parts variable and often indistinct

Submucous space

Perianal space

Bulbospongiosus muscle and deep perineal (Gallaudet's) fascia

Superficial perineal compartment (space or pouch)

Perineal membrane,
Deep transverse perineal muscle and
Superficial transverse perineal muscle
(*cut away*) to expose
Anterior recess of ischioanal fossa

Preanal communication (inconstant) between right and left ischioanal fossae

Pus in ischioanal fossa

Posterior communication between right and left ischioanal fossae via deep postanal space deep to anococcygeal body (ligament)

Gluteus maximus muscle and
Sacrotuberous ligament
(*cut*)
Posterior recess of ischioanal fossa

Perineal view

Spread of perineal abscess in perineal spaces

Plate 376

Rectum

Median (A) and paramedian (B) sagittal MR images of female pelvis

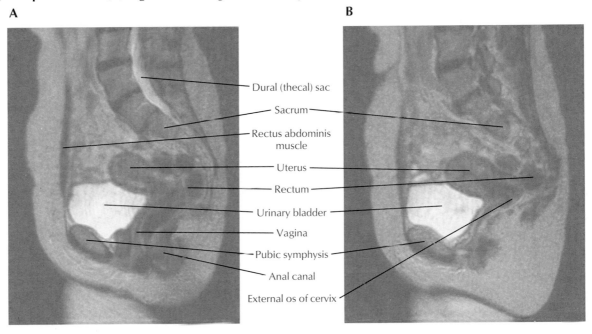

A B

Dural (thecal) sac

Sacrum

Rectus abdominis muscle

Uterus

Rectum

Urinary bladder

Vagina

Pubic symphysis

Anal canal

External os of cervix

Median (C) and paramedian (D) sagittal MR images of male pelvis

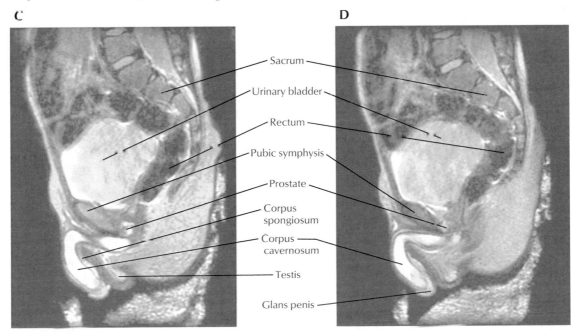

C D

Sacrum

Urinary bladder

Rectum

Pubic symphysis

Prostate

Corpus spongiosum

Corpus cavernosum

Testis

Glans penis

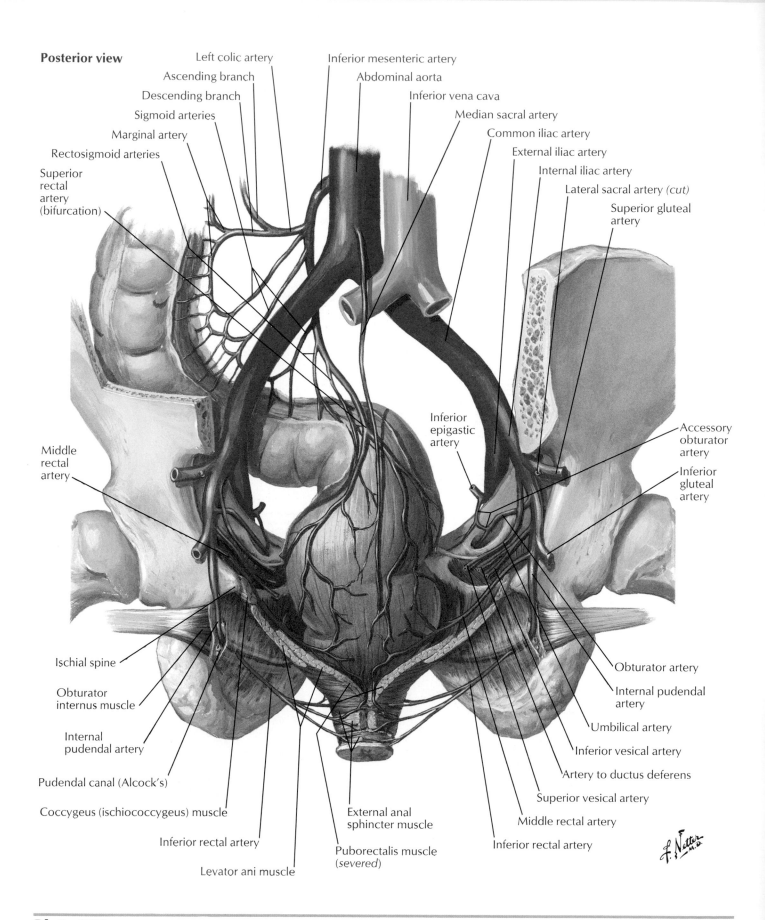

Posterior view

Left colic artery
Ascending branch
Descending branch
Sigmoid arteries
Marginal artery
Rectosigmoid arteries
Superior rectal artery (bifurcation)
Middle rectal artery
Ischial spine
Obturator internus muscle
Internal pudendal artery
Pudendal canal (Alcock's)
Coccygeus (ischiococcygeus) muscle
Inferior rectal artery
Levator ani muscle
External anal sphincter muscle
Puborectalis muscle (severed)
Inferior mesenteric artery
Abdominal aorta
Inferior vena cava
Median sacral artery
Common iliac artery
External iliac artery
Internal iliac artery
Lateral sacral artery (cut)
Superior gluteal artery
Inferior epigastric artery
Accessory obturator artery
Inferior gluteal artery
Obturator artery
Internal pudendal artery
Umbilical artery
Inferior vesical artery
Artery to ductus deferens
Superior vesical artery
Middle rectal artery
Inferior rectal artery

Plate 378   **Vasculature**

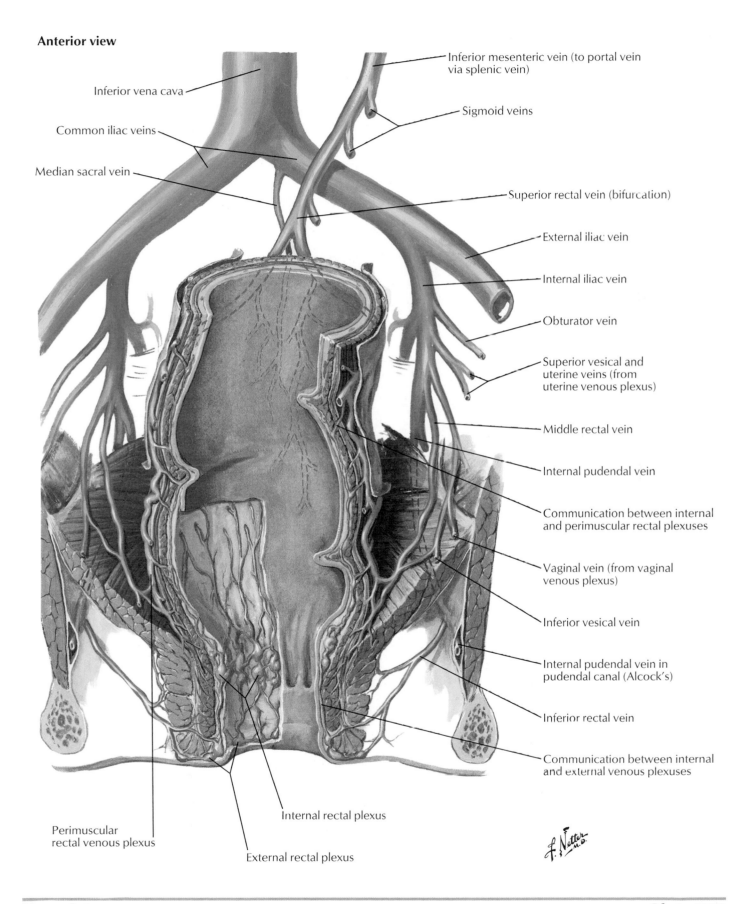

Anterior view

Inferior vena cava

Common iliac veins

Median sacral vein

Inferior mesenteric vein (to portal vein via splenic vein)

Sigmoid veins

Superior rectal vein (bifurcation)

External iliac vein

Internal iliac vein

Obturator vein

Superior vesical and uterine veins (from uterine venous plexus)

Middle rectal vein

Internal pudendal vein

Communication between internal and perimuscular rectal plexuses

Vaginal vein (from vaginal venous plexus)

Inferior vesical vein

Internal pudendal vein in pudendal canal (Alcock's)

Inferior rectal vein

Communication between internal and external venous plexuses

Internal rectal plexus

Perimuscular rectal venous plexus

External rectal plexus

Anterior view

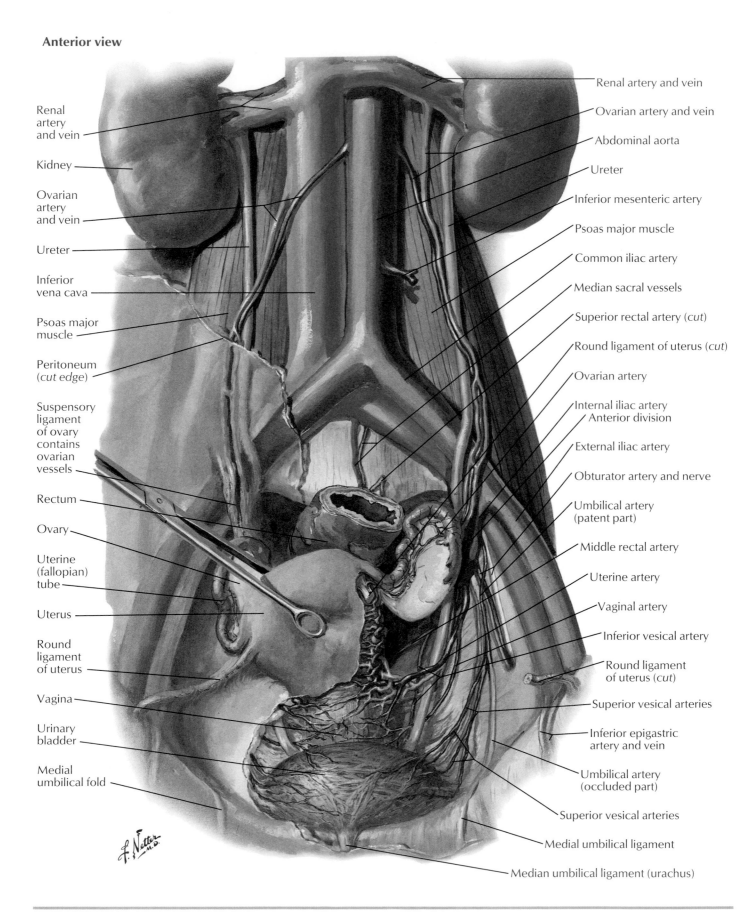

Renal artery and vein

Ovarian artery and vein

Abdominal aorta

Ureter

Inferior mesenteric artery

Psoas major muscle

Common iliac artery

Median sacral vessels

Superior rectal artery (*cut*)

Round ligament of uterus (*cut*)

Ovarian artery

Internal iliac artery
Anterior division

External iliac artery

Obturator artery and nerve

Umbilical artery
(patent part)

Middle rectal artery

Uterine artery

Vaginal artery

Inferior vesical artery

Round ligament
of uterus (*cut*)

Superior vesical arteries

Inferior epigastric
artery and vein

Umbilical artery
(occluded part)

Superior vesical arteries

Medial umbilical ligament

Median umbilical ligament (urachus)

Renal
artery
and vein

Kidney

Ovarian
artery
and vein

Ureter

Inferior
vena cava

Psoas major
muscle

Peritoneum
(*cut edge*)

Suspensory
ligament
of ovary
contains
ovarian
vessels

Rectum

Ovary

Uterine
(fallopian)
tube

Uterus

Round
ligament
of uterus

Vagina

Urinary
bladder

Medial
umbilical fold

F. Netter M.D.

Plate 380 | **Vasculature**

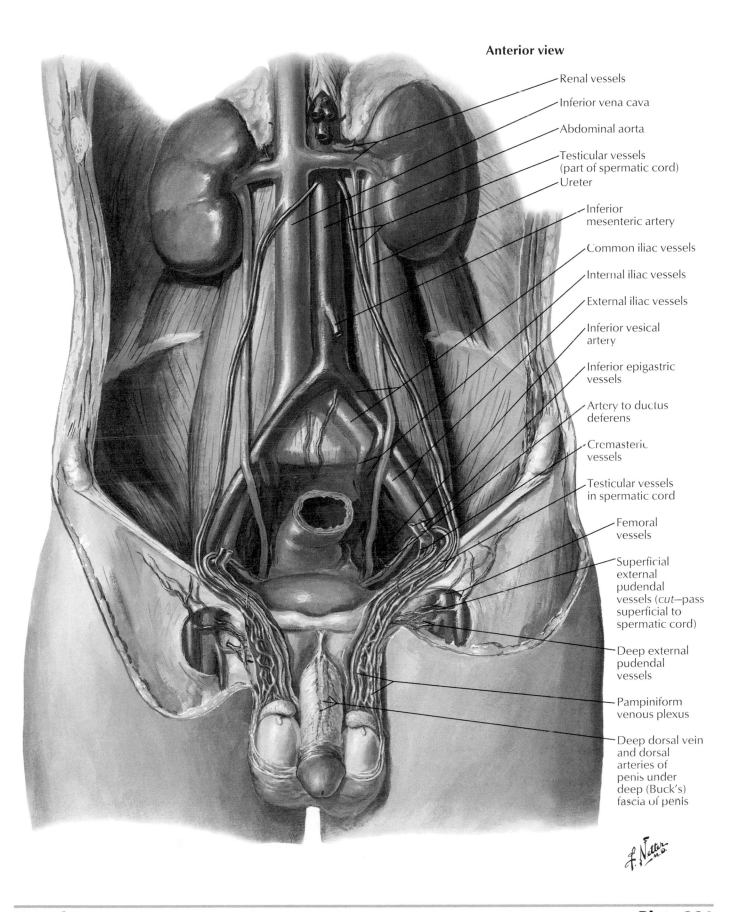

Anterior view

Renal vessels

Inferior vena cava

Abdominal aorta

Testicular vessels (part of spermatic cord)

Ureter

Inferior mesenteric artery

Common iliac vessels

Internal iliac vessels

External iliac vessels

Inferior vesical artery

Inferior epigastric vessels

Artery to ductus deferens

Cremasteric vessels

Testicular vessels in spermatic cord

Femoral vessels

Superficial external pudendal vessels (cut–pass superficial to spermatic cord)

Deep external pudendal vessels

Pampiniform venous plexus

Deep dorsal vein and dorsal arteries of penis under deep (Buck's) fascia of penis

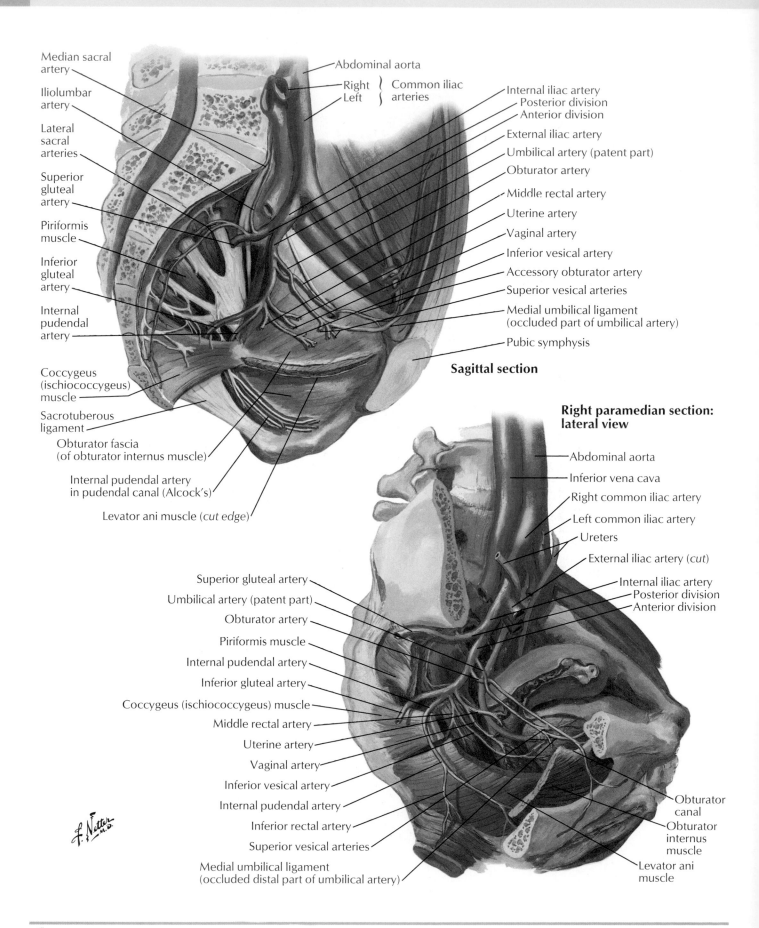

Median sacral artery

Iliolumbar artery

Lateral sacral arteries

Superior gluteal artery

Piriformis muscle

Inferior gluteal artery

Internal pudendal artery

Coccygeus (ischiococcygeus) muscle

Sacrotuberous ligament

Obturator fascia (of obturator internus muscle)

Internal pudendal artery in pudendal canal (Alcock's)

Levator ani muscle (*cut edge*)

Abdominal aorta

Right } Common iliac
Left } arteries

Internal iliac artery
Posterior division
Anterior division

External iliac artery

Umbilical artery (patent part)

Obturator artery

Middle rectal artery

Uterine artery

Vaginal artery

Inferior vesical artery

Accessory obturator artery

Superior vesical arteries

Medial umbilical ligament (occluded part of umbilical artery)

Pubic symphysis

Sagittal section

Right paramedian section: lateral view

Abdominal aorta

Inferior vena cava

Right common iliac artery

Left common iliac artery

Ureters

External iliac artery (*cut*)

Internal iliac artery
Posterior division
Anterior division

Superior gluteal artery

Umbilical artery (patent part)

Obturator artery

Piriformis muscle

Internal pudendal artery

Inferior gluteal artery

Coccygeus (ischiococcygeus) muscle

Middle rectal artery

Uterine artery

Vaginal artery

Inferior vesical artery

Internal pudendal artery

Inferior rectal artery

Superior vesical arteries

Medial umbilical ligament (occluded distal part of umbilical artery)

Obturator canal

Obturator internus muscle

Levator ani muscle

Plate 382

Vasculature

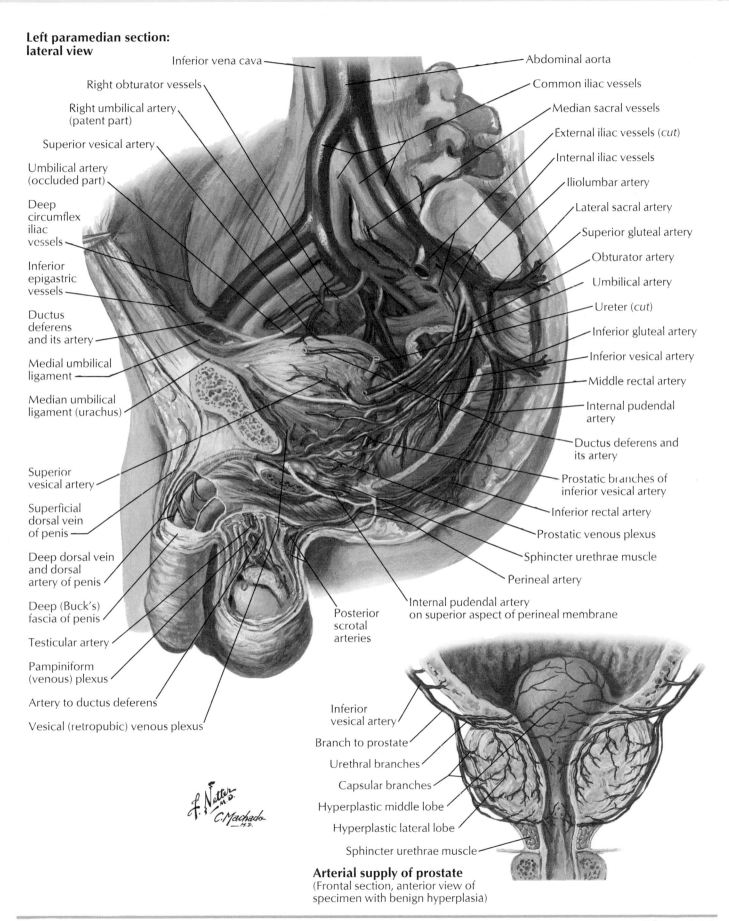

Left paramedian section: lateral view

Inferior vena cava

Right obturator vessels

Right umbilical artery (patent part)

Superior vesical artery

Umbilical artery (occluded part)

Deep circumflex iliac vessels

Inferior epigastric vessels

Ductus deferens and its artery

Medial umbilical ligament

Median umbilical ligament (urachus)

Superior vesical artery

Superficial dorsal vein of penis

Deep dorsal vein and dorsal artery of penis

Deep (Buck's) fascia of penis

Testicular artery

Pampiniform (venous) plexus

Artery to ductus deferens

Vesical (retropubic) venous plexus

Abdominal aorta

Common iliac vessels

Median sacral vessels

External iliac vessels (cut)

Internal iliac vessels

Iliolumbar artery

Lateral sacral artery

Superior gluteal artery

Obturator artery

Umbilical artery

Ureter (cut)

Inferior gluteal artery

Inferior vesical artery

Middle rectal artery

Internal pudendal artery

Ductus deferens and its artery

Prostatic branches of inferior vesical artery

Inferior rectal artery

Prostatic venous plexus

Sphincter urethrae muscle

Perineal artery

Posterior scrotal arteries

Internal pudendal artery on superior aspect of perineal membrane

Inferior vesical artery

Branch to prostate

Urethral branches

Capsular branches

Hyperplastic middle lobe

Hyperplastic lateral lobe

Sphincter urethrae muscle

Arterial supply of prostate
(Frontal section, anterior view of specimen with benign hyperplasia)

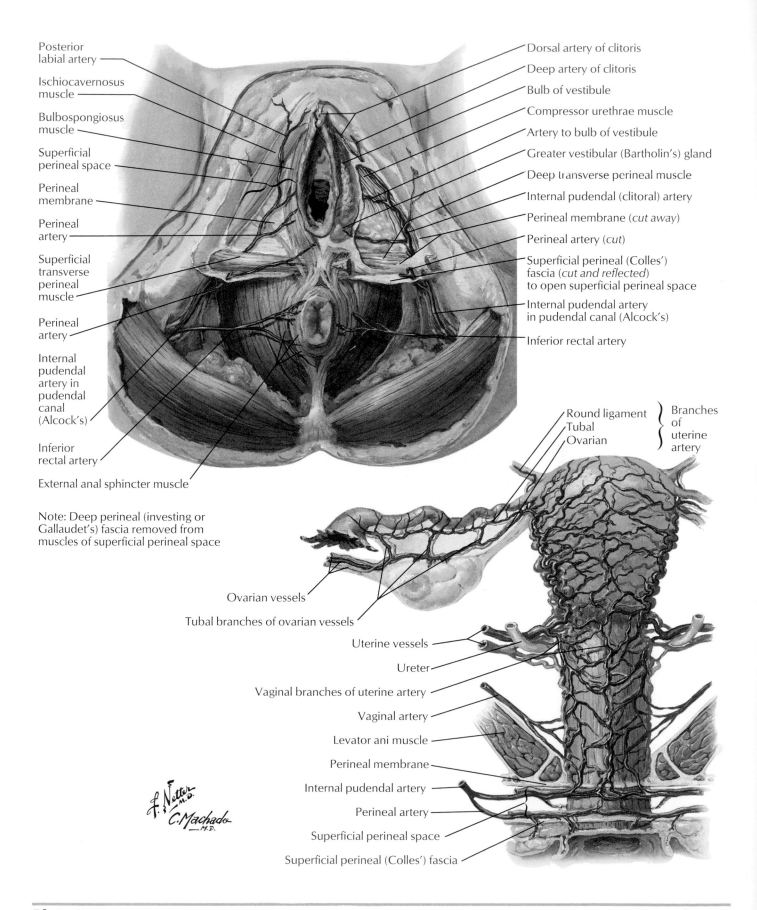

Posterior labial artery

Ischiocavernosus muscle

Bulbospongiosus muscle

Superficial perineal space

Perineal membrane

Perineal artery

Superficial transverse perineal muscle

Perineal artery

Internal pudendal artery in pudendal canal (Alcock's)

Inferior rectal artery

External anal sphincter muscle

Note: Deep perineal (investing or Gallaudet's) fascia removed from muscles of superficial perineal space

Dorsal artery of clitoris

Deep artery of clitoris

Bulb of vestibule

Compressor urethrae muscle

Artery to bulb of vestibule

Greater vestibular (Bartholin's) gland

Deep transverse perineal muscle

Internal pudendal (clitoral) artery

Perineal membrane (*cut away*)

Perineal artery (*cut*)

Superficial perineal (Colles') fascia (*cut and reflected*) to open superficial perineal space

Internal pudendal artery in pudendal canal (Alcock's)

Inferior rectal artery

Round ligament
Tubal
Ovarian
} Branches of uterine artery

Ovarian vessels

Tubal branches of ovarian vessels

Uterine vessels

Ureter

Vaginal branches of uterine artery

Vaginal artery

Levator ani muscle

Perineal membrane

Internal pudendal artery

Perineal artery

Superficial perineal space

Superficial perineal (Colles') fascia

Plate 384

Vasculature

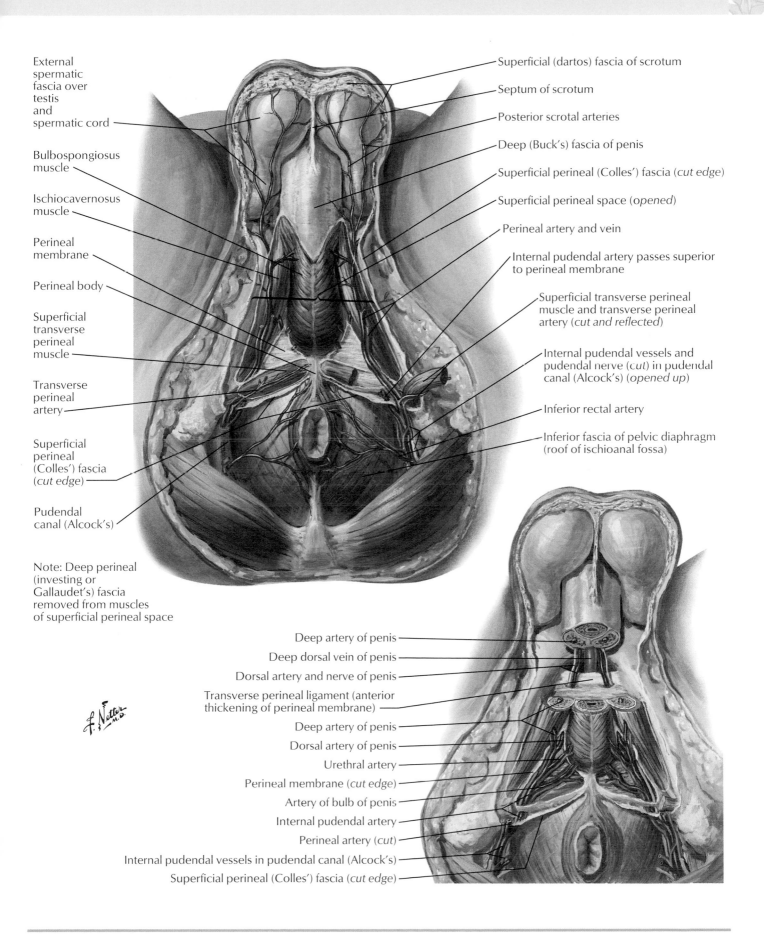

External spermatic fascia over testis and spermatic cord

Bulbospongiosus muscle

Ischiocavernosus muscle

Perineal membrane

Perineal body

Superficial transverse perineal muscle

Transverse perineal artery

Superficial perineal (Colles') fascia (cut edge)

Pudendal canal (Alcock's)

Note: Deep perineal (investing or Gallaudet's) fascia removed from muscles of superficial perineal space

Superficial (dartos) fascia of scrotum

Septum of scrotum

Posterior scrotal arteries

Deep (Buck's) fascia of penis

Superficial perineal (Colles') fascia (cut edge)

Superficial perineal space (opened)

Perineal artery and vein

Internal pudendal artery passes superior to perineal membrane

Superficial transverse perineal muscle and transverse perineal artery (cut and reflected)

Internal pudendal vessels and pudendal nerve (cut) in pudendal canal (Alcock's) (opened up)

Inferior rectal artery

Inferior fascia of pelvic diaphragm (roof of ischioanal fossa)

Deep artery of penis

Deep dorsal vein of penis

Dorsal artery and nerve of penis

Transverse perineal ligament (anterior thickening of perineal membrane)

Deep artery of penis

Dorsal artery of penis

Urethral artery

Perineal membrane (cut edge)

Artery of bulb of penis

Internal pudendal artery

Perineal artery (cut)

Internal pudendal vessels in pudendal canal (Alcock's)

Superficial perineal (Colles') fascia (cut edge)

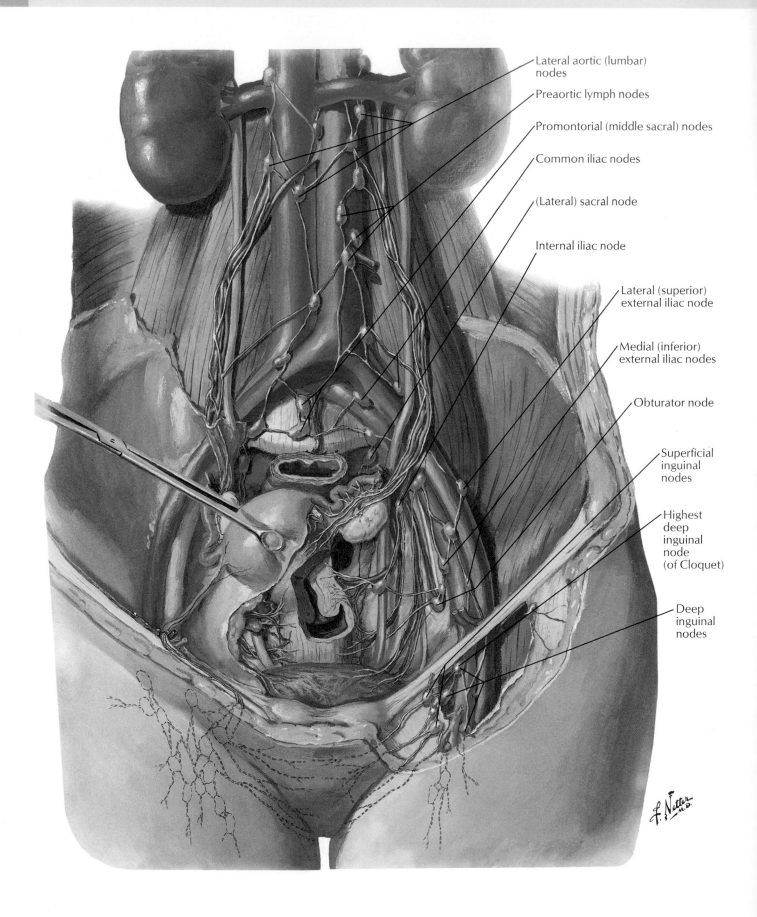

Lateral aortic (lumbar) nodes

Preaortic lymph nodes

Promontorial (middle sacral) nodes

Common iliac nodes

(Lateral) sacral node

Internal iliac node

Lateral (superior) external iliac node

Medial (inferior) external iliac nodes

Obturator node

Superficial inguinal nodes

Highest deep inguinal node (of Cloquet)

Deep inguinal nodes

Plate 386

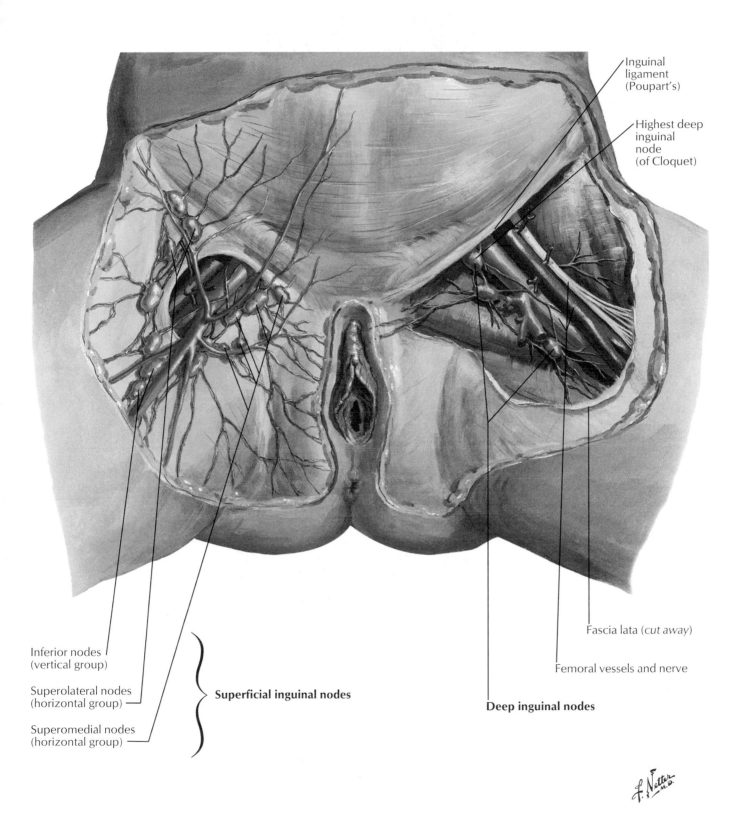

Inguinal ligament (Poupart's)

Highest deep inguinal node (of Cloquet)

Fascia lata (*cut away*)

Femoral vessels and nerve

Deep inguinal nodes

Inferior nodes (vertical group)

Superolateral nodes (horizontal group)

Superomedial nodes (horizontal group)

Superficial inguinal nodes

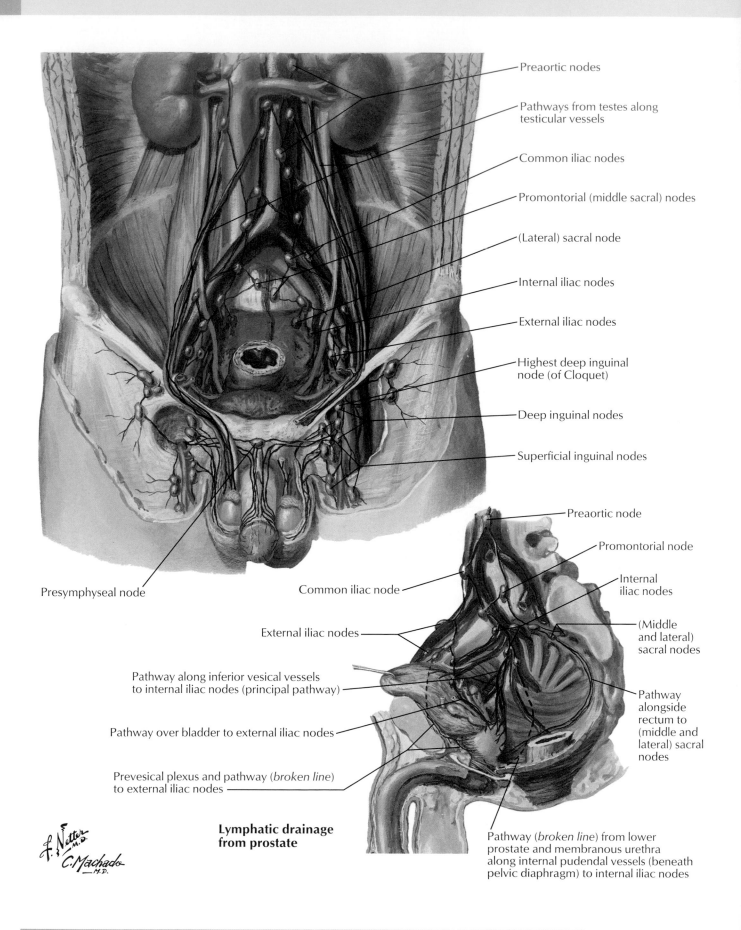

Preaortic nodes

Pathways from testes along testicular vessels

Common iliac nodes

Promontorial (middle sacral) nodes

(Lateral) sacral node

Internal iliac nodes

External iliac nodes

Highest deep inguinal node (of Cloquet)

Deep inguinal nodes

Superficial inguinal nodes

Presymphyseal node

Preaortic node

Promontorial node

Internal iliac nodes

Common iliac node

(Middle and lateral) sacral nodes

External iliac nodes

Pathway alongside rectum to (middle and lateral) sacral nodes

Pathway along inferior vesical vessels to internal iliac nodes (principal pathway)

Pathway over bladder to external iliac nodes

Prevesical plexus and pathway (*broken line*) to external iliac nodes

Lymphatic drainage from prostate

Pathway (*broken line*) from lower prostate and membranous urethra along internal pudendal vessels (beneath pelvic diaphragm) to internal iliac nodes

Plate 388 **Vasculature**

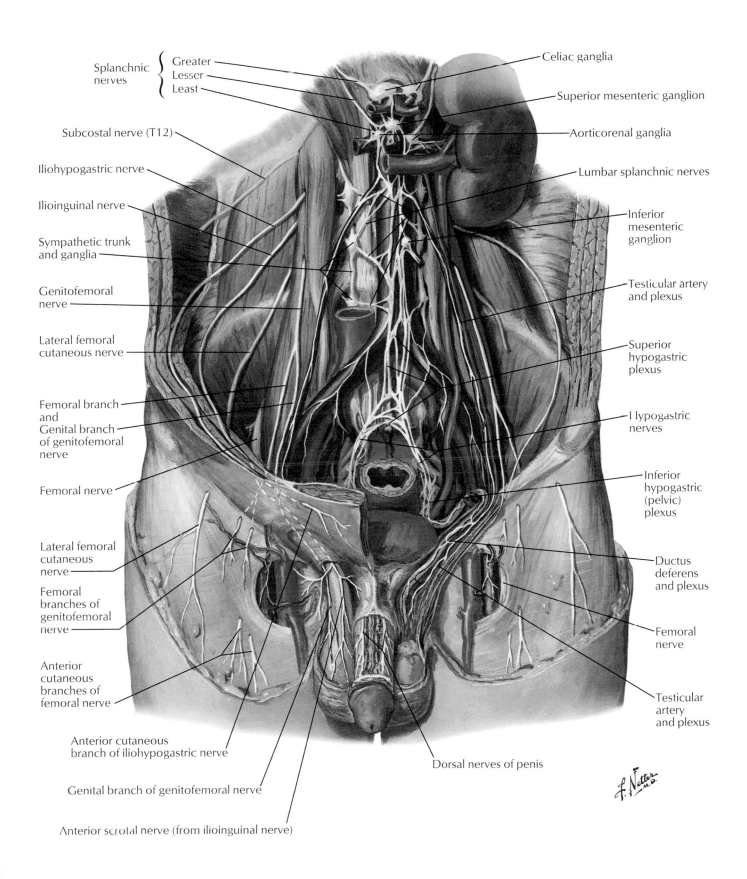

Splanchnic nerves
{ Greater
Lesser
Least }

Celiac ganglia

Superior mesenteric ganglion

Subcostal nerve (T12)

Aorticorenal ganglia

Iliohypogastric nerve

Lumbar splanchnic nerves

Ilioinguinal nerve

Inferior mesenteric ganglion

Sympathetic trunk and ganglia

Testicular artery and plexus

Genitofemoral nerve

Superior hypogastric plexus

Lateral femoral cutaneous nerve

Hypogastric nerves

Femoral branch and Genital branch of genitofemoral nerve

Inferior hypogastric (pelvic) plexus

Femoral nerve

Lateral femoral cutaneous nerve

Ductus deferens and plexus

Femoral branches of genitofemoral nerve

Femoral nerve

Anterior cutaneous branches of femoral nerve

Testicular artery and plexus

Anterior cutaneous branch of iliohypogastric nerve

Dorsal nerves of penis

Genital branch of genitofemoral nerve

Anterior scrotal nerve (from ilioinguinal nerve)

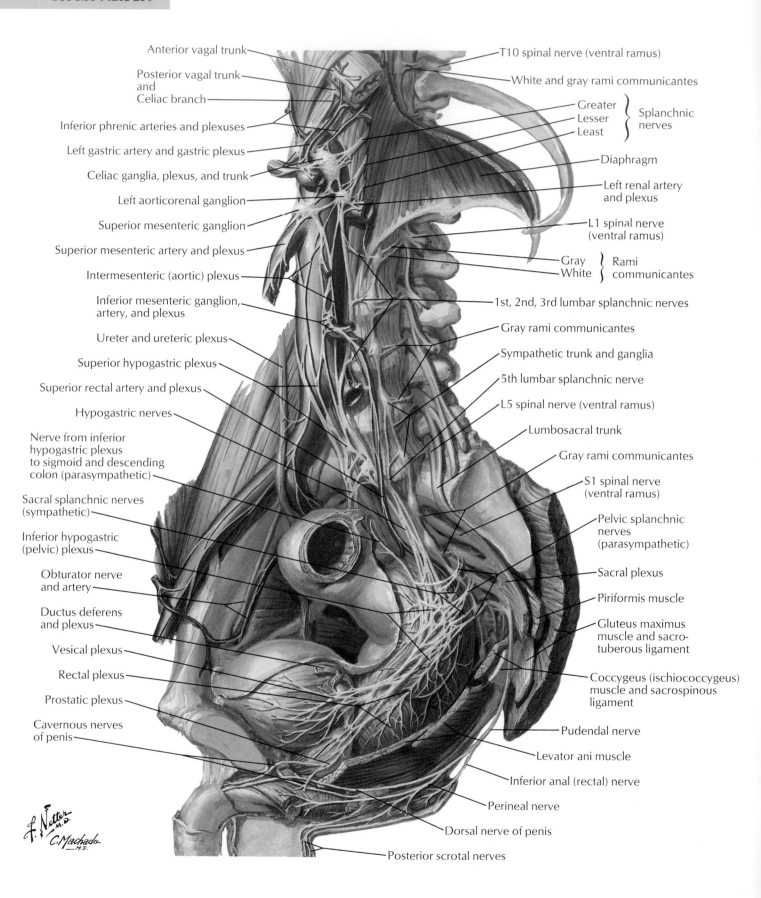

Anterior vagal trunk

Posterior vagal trunk and Celiac branch

Inferior phrenic arteries and plexuses

Left gastric artery and gastric plexus

Celiac ganglia, plexus, and trunk

Left aorticorenal ganglion

Superior mesenteric ganglion

Superior mesenteric artery and plexus

Intermesenteric (aortic) plexus

Inferior mesenteric ganglion, artery, and plexus

Ureter and ureteric plexus

Superior hypogastric plexus

Superior rectal artery and plexus

Hypogastric nerves

Nerve from inferior hypogastric plexus to sigmoid and descending colon (parasympathetic)

Sacral splanchnic nerves (sympathetic)

Inferior hypogastric (pelvic) plexus

Obturator nerve and artery

Ductus deferens and plexus

Vesical plexus

Rectal plexus

Prostatic plexus

Cavernous nerves of penis

T10 spinal nerve (ventral ramus)

White and gray rami communicantes

Greater
Lesser
Least
} Splanchnic nerves

Diaphragm

Left renal artery and plexus

L1 spinal nerve (ventral ramus)

Gray
White
} Rami communicantes

1st, 2nd, 3rd lumbar splanchnic nerves

Gray rami communicantes

Sympathetic trunk and ganglia

5th lumbar splanchnic nerve

L5 spinal nerve (ventral ramus)

Lumbosacral trunk

Gray rami communicantes

S1 spinal nerve (ventral ramus)

Pelvic splanchnic nerves (parasympathetic)

Sacral plexus

Piriformis muscle

Gluteus maximus muscle and sacro-tuberous ligament

Coccygeus (ischiococcygeus) muscle and sacrospinous ligament

Pudendal nerve

Levator ani muscle

Inferior anal (rectal) nerve

Perineal nerve

Dorsal nerve of penis

Posterior scrotal nerves

Plate 390

Innervation

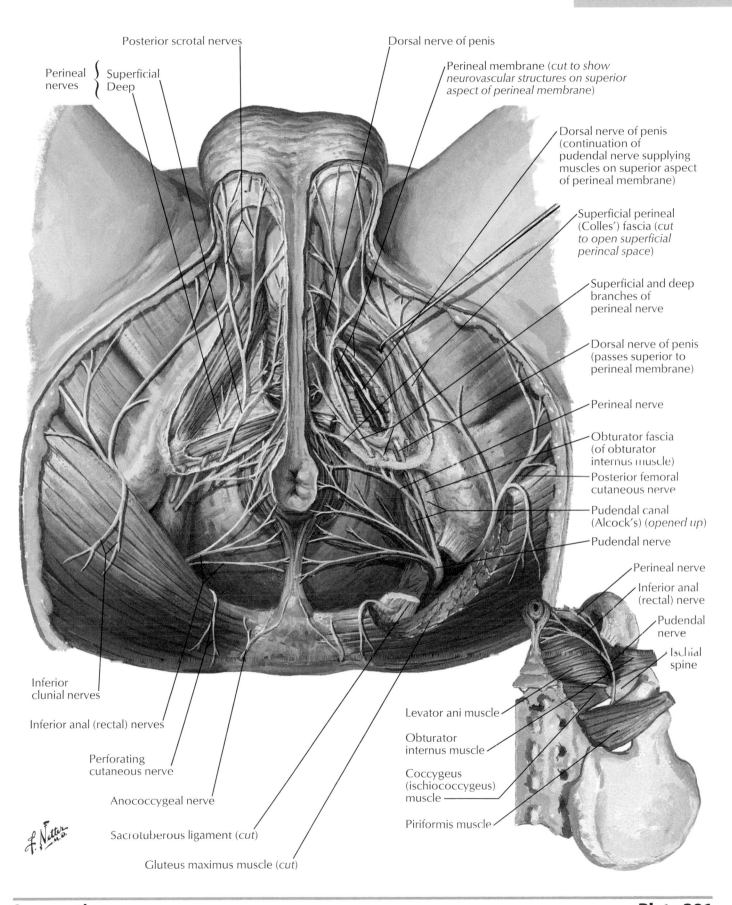

Posterior scrotal nerves

Dorsal nerve of penis

Perineal nerves { Superficial Deep

Perineal membrane (cut to show neurovascular structures on superior aspect of perineal membrane)

Dorsal nerve of penis (continuation of pudendal nerve supplying muscles on superior aspect of perineal membrane)

Superficial perineal (Colles') fascia (cut to open superficial perineal space)

Superficial and deep branches of perineal nerve

Dorsal nerve of penis (passes superior to perineal membrane)

Perineal nerve

Obturator fascia (of obturator internus muscle)

Posterior femoral cutaneous nerve

Pudendal canal (Alcock's) (opened up)

Pudendal nerve

Perineal nerve

Inferior anal (rectal) nerve

Pudendal nerve

Ischial spine

Levator ani muscle

Obturator internus muscle

Coccygeus (ischiococcygeus) muscle

Piriformis muscle

Inferior clunial nerves

Inferior anal (rectal) nerves

Perforating cutaneous nerve

Anococcygeal nerve

Sacrotuberous ligament (cut)

Gluteus maximus muscle (cut)

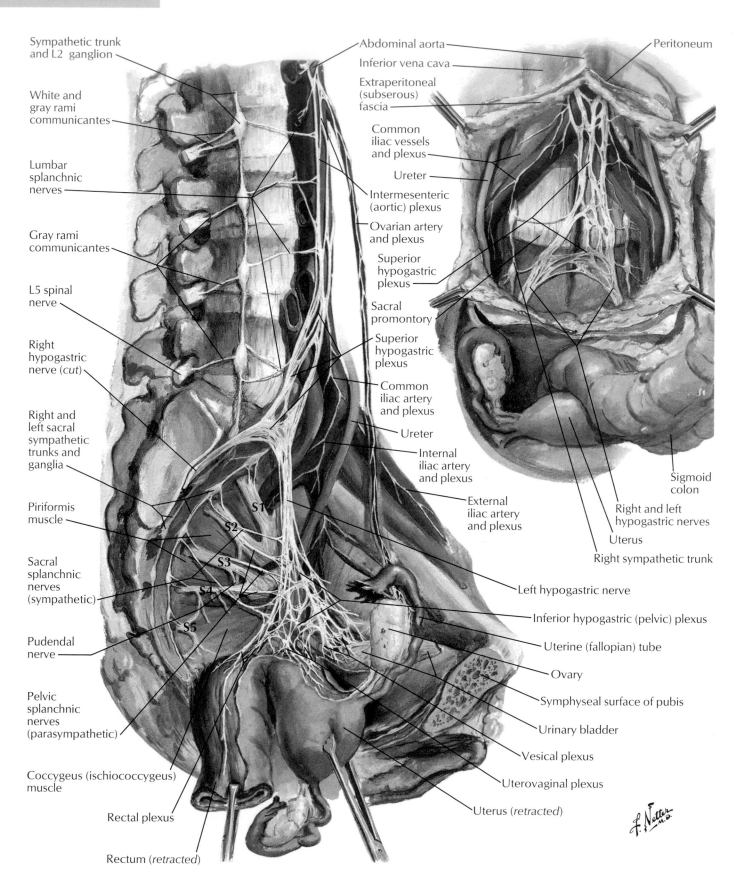

Sympathetic trunk and L2 ganglion

White and gray rami communicantes

Lumbar splanchnic nerves

Gray rami communicantes

L5 spinal nerve

Right hypogastric nerve (*cut*)

Right and left sacral sympathetic trunks and ganglia

Piriformis muscle

Sacral splanchnic nerves (sympathetic)

Pudendal nerve

Pelvic splanchnic nerves (parasympathetic)

Coccygeus (ischiococcygeus) muscle

Rectal plexus

Rectum (*retracted*)

Abdominal aorta

Inferior vena cava

Extraperitoneal (subserous) fascia

Common iliac vessels and plexus

Ureter

Intermesenteric (aortic) plexus

Ovarian artery and plexus

Superior hypogastric plexus

Sacral promontory

Superior hypogastric plexus

Common iliac artery and plexus

Ureter

Internal iliac artery and plexus

External iliac artery and plexus

Peritoneum

Sigmoid colon

Right and left hypogastric nerves

Uterus

Right sympathetic trunk

Left hypogastric nerve

Inferior hypogastric (pelvic) plexus

Uterine (fallopian) tube

Ovary

Symphyseal surface of pubis

Urinary bladder

Vesical plexus

Uterovaginal plexus

Uterus (*retracted*)

S1

S2

S3

S4

S5

Plate 392

Innervation

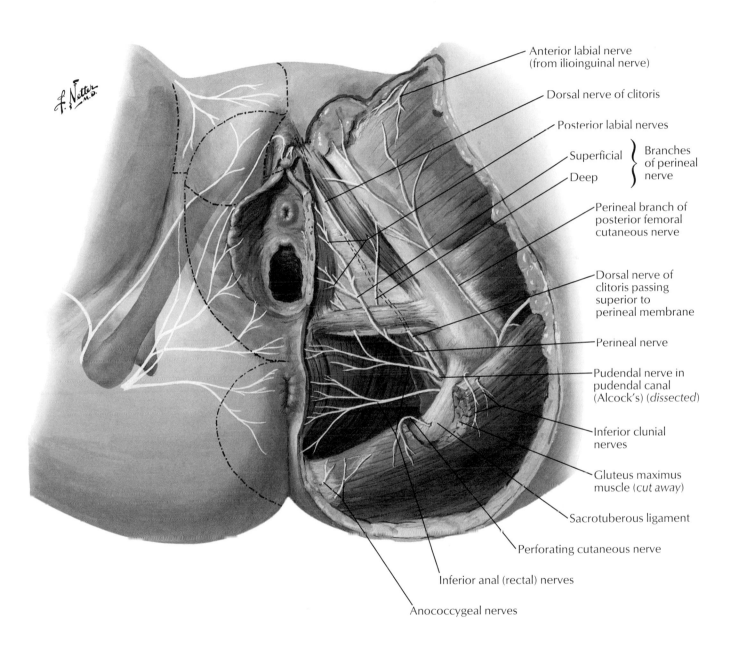

Anterior labial nerve (from ilioinguinal nerve)

Dorsal nerve of clitoris

Posterior labial nerves

Superficial } Branches of perineal nerve

Deep

Perineal branch of posterior femoral cutaneous nerve

Dorsal nerve of clitoris passing superior to perineal membrane

Perineal nerve

Pudendal nerve in pudendal canal (Alcock's) (*dissected*)

Inferior clunial nerves

Gluteus maximus muscle (*cut away*)

Sacrotuberous ligament

Perforating cutaneous nerve

Inferior anal (rectal) nerves

Anococcygeal nerves

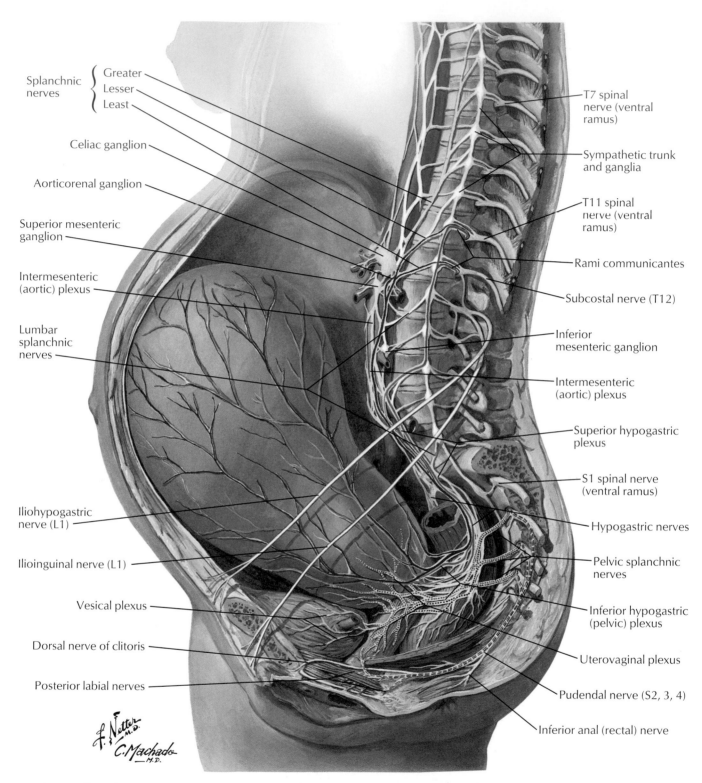

Splanchnic nerves { Greater / Lesser / Least

Celiac ganglion

Aorticorenal ganglion

Superior mesenteric ganglion

Intermesenteric (aortic) plexus

Lumbar splanchnic nerves

Iliohypogastric nerve (L1)

Ilioinguinal nerve (L1)

Vesical plexus

Dorsal nerve of clitoris

Posterior labial nerves

T7 spinal nerve (ventral ramus)

Sympathetic trunk and ganglia

T11 spinal nerve (ventral ramus)

Rami communicantes

Subcostal nerve (T12)

Inferior mesenteric ganglion

Intermesenteric (aortic) plexus

Superior hypogastric plexus

S1 spinal nerve (ventral ramus)

Hypogastric nerves

Pelvic splanchnic nerves

Inferior hypogastric (pelvic) plexus

Uterovaginal plexus

Pudendal nerve (S2, 3, 4)

Inferior anal (rectal) nerve

———— Sensory fibers from uterine body and fundus accompany sympathetic fibers via hypogastric plexuses to T11, 12 (L1?)

———— Motor fibers to uterine body and fundus (sympathetic)

·············· Sensory fibers from cervix and upper vagina accompany pelvic splanchnic nerves (parasympathetic) to S2, 3, 4

············ Motor fibers to lower uterine segment, cervix, and upper vagina (parasympathetic)

– – – – Sensory fibers from lower vagina and perineum accompany somatic fibers via pudendal nerve to S2, 3, 4

– – – – – Motor fibers to lower vagina and perineum via pudendal nerve (somatic)

Plate 394

Innervation

See also **Plates 160, 161**

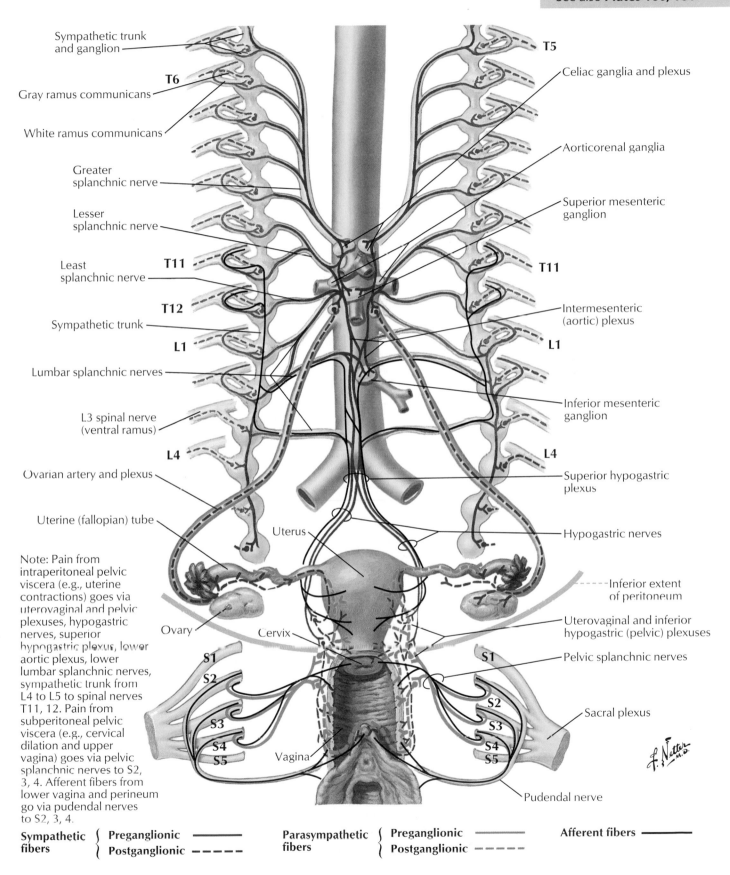

Sympathetic trunk and ganglion

Gray ramus communicans

White ramus communicans

Greater splanchnic nerve

Lesser splanchnic nerve

Least splanchnic nerve

Sympathetic trunk

Lumbar splanchnic nerves

L3 spinal nerve (ventral ramus)

Ovarian artery and plexus

Uterine (fallopian) tube

T6

T11

T12

L1

L4

Celiac ganglia and plexus

Aorticorenal ganglia

Superior mesenteric ganglion

T5

T11

L1

L4

Intermesenteric (aortic) plexus

Inferior mesenteric ganglion

Superior hypogastric plexus

Hypogastric nerves

Inferior extent of peritoneum

Uterovaginal and inferior hypogastric (pelvic) plexuses

Pelvic splanchnic nerves

Sacral plexus

Pudendal nerve

Uterus

Ovary

Cervix

Vagina

S1
S2
S3
S4
S5

S1
S2
S3
S4
S5

Note: Pain from intraperitoneal pelvic viscera (e.g., uterine contractions) goes via uterovaginal and pelvic plexuses, hypogastric nerves, superior hypogastric plexus, lower aortic plexus, lower lumbar splanchnic nerves, sympathetic trunk from L4 to L5 to spinal nerves T11, 12. Pain from subperitoneal pelvic viscera (e.g., cervical dilation and upper vagina) goes via pelvic splanchnic nerves to S2, 3, 4. Afferent fibers from lower vagina and perineum go via pudendal nerves to S2, 3, 4.

| Sympathetic fibers | Preganglionic ——— | Parasympathetic fibers | Preganglionic ——— | Afferent fibers ——— |
| | Postganglionic - - - - | | Postganglionic - - - - | |

Innervation of Male Reproductive Organs: Schema

See also **Plates 160, 161**

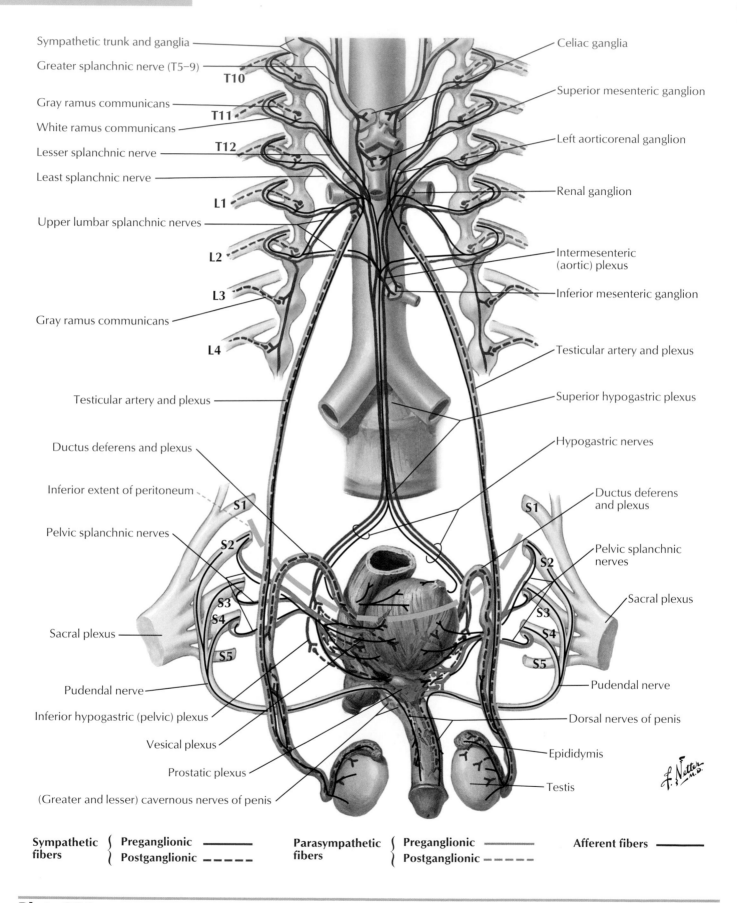

Sympathetic trunk and ganglia

Greater splanchnic nerve (T5–9)

T10

Gray ramus communicans

T11

White ramus communicans

Lesser splanchnic nerve

T12

Least splanchnic nerve

L1

Upper lumbar splanchnic nerves

L2

L3

Gray ramus communicans

L4

Testicular artery and plexus

Ductus deferens and plexus

Inferior extent of peritoneum

S1

Pelvic splanchnic nerves

S2

S3

S4

Sacral plexus

S5

Pudendal nerve

Inferior hypogastric (pelvic) plexus

Vesical plexus

Prostatic plexus

(Greater and lesser) cavernous nerves of penis

Celiac ganglia

Superior mesenteric ganglion

Left aorticorenal ganglion

Renal ganglion

Intermesenteric (aortic) plexus

Inferior mesenteric ganglion

Testicular artery and plexus

Superior hypogastric plexus

Hypogastric nerves

Ductus deferens and plexus

S1

Pelvic splanchnic nerves

S2

S3

Sacral plexus

S4

S5

Pudendal nerve

Dorsal nerves of penis

Epididymis

Testis

Sympathetic fibers	Preganglionic ———		Parasympathetic fibers	Preganglionic ———	Afferent fibers ———
	Postganglionic – – –			Postganglionic – – –	

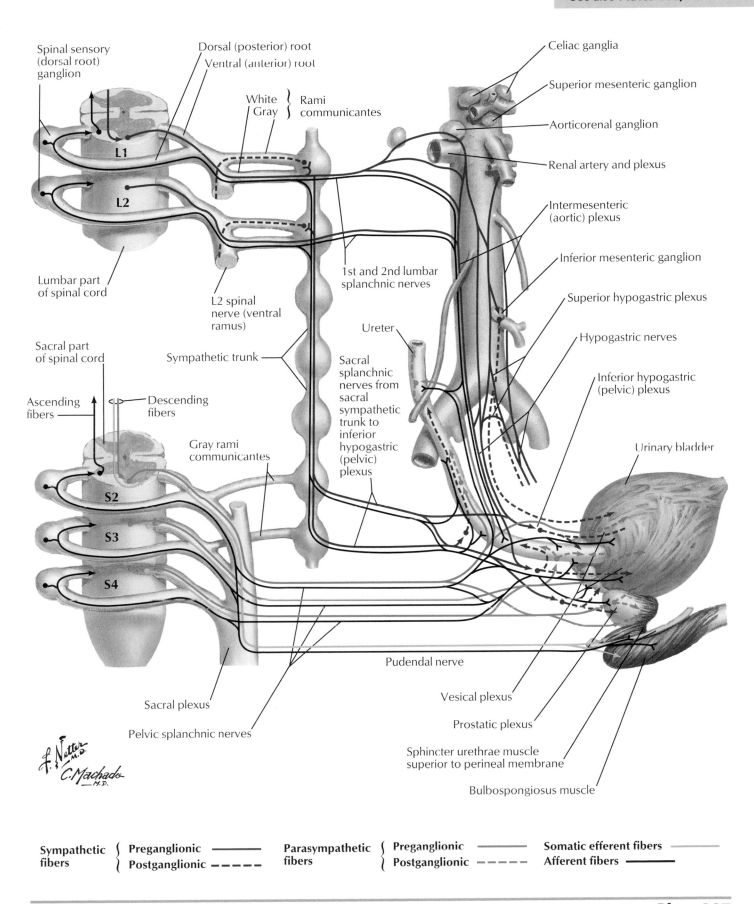

Spinal sensory (dorsal root) ganglion

Dorsal (posterior) root

Ventral (anterior) root

White / Gray } Rami communicantes

Celiac ganglia

Superior mesenteric ganglion

Aorticorenal ganglion

Renal artery and plexus

L1

L2

Lumbar part of spinal cord

L2 spinal nerve (ventral ramus)

1st and 2nd lumbar splanchnic nerves

Sympathetic trunk

Ureter

Sacral splanchnic nerves from sacral sympathetic trunk to inferior hypogastric (pelvic) plexus

Intermesenteric (aortic) plexus

Inferior mesenteric ganglion

Superior hypogastric plexus

Hypogastric nerves

Inferior hypogastric (pelvic) plexus

Sacral part of spinal cord

Ascending fibers

Descending fibers

Gray rami communicantes

S2

S3

S4

Urinary bladder

Pudendal nerve

Vesical plexus

Prostatic plexus

Sphincter urethrae muscle superior to perineal membrane

Bulbospongiosus muscle

Sacral plexus

Pelvic splanchnic nerves

f. Netter M.D.
C. Machado M.D.

Sympathetic fibers { Preganglionic ——— Postganglionic - - - -

Parasympathetic fibers { Preganglionic ——— Postganglionic - - - -

Somatic efferent fibers ———
Afferent fibers ———

Transverse Section: Pubic Crest, Femoral Heads, Coccyx

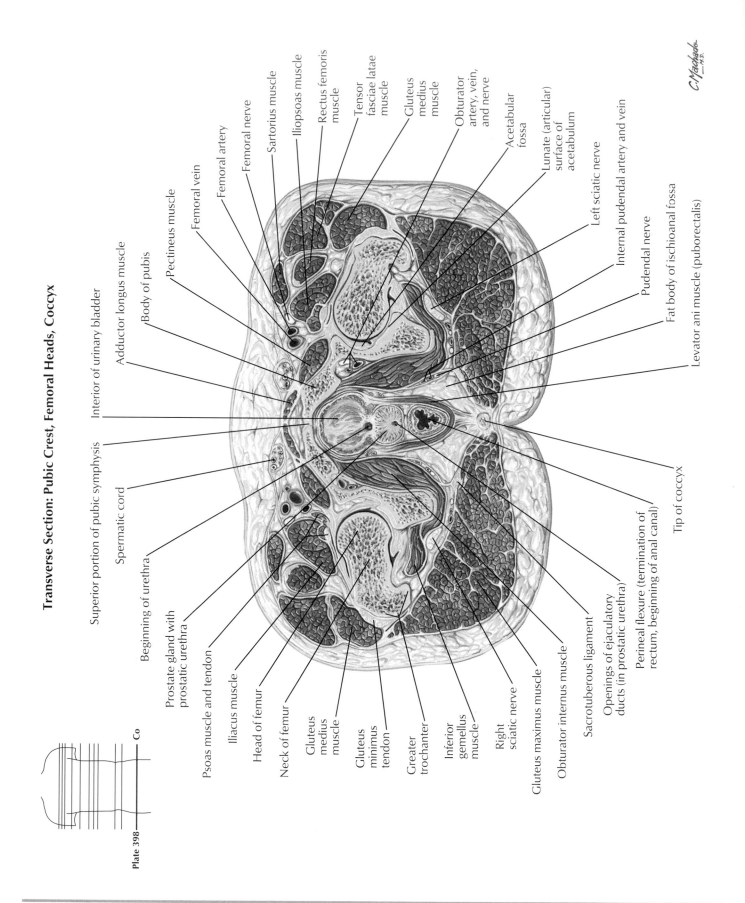

Superior portion of pubic symphysis

Interior of urinary bladder

Adductor longus muscle

Body of pubis

Pectineus muscle

Femoral vein

Femoral artery

Femoral nerve

Sartorius muscle

Iliopsoas muscle

Rectus femoris muscle

Tensor fasciae latae muscle

Gluteus medius muscle

Obturator artery, vein, and nerve

Acetabular fossa

Lunate (articular) surface of acetabulum

Left sciatic nerve

Internal pudendal artery and vein

Pudendal nerve

Fat body of ischioanal fossa

Levator ani muscle (puborectalis)

Spermatic cord

Beginning of urethra

Prostate gland with prostatic urethra

Psoas muscle and tendon

Iliacus muscle

Head of femur

Neck of femur

Gluteus medius muscle

Gluteus minimus tendon

Greater trochanter

Inferior gemellus muscle

Right sciatic nerve

Gluteus maximus muscle

Obturator internus muscle

Sacrotuberous ligament

Openings of ejaculatory ducts (in prostatic urethra)

Perineal flexure (termination of rectum, beginning of anal canal)

Tip of coccyx

Co

Plate 398

Plate 398

Cross-sectional Anatomy

Transverse Section: Vagina and Urethra

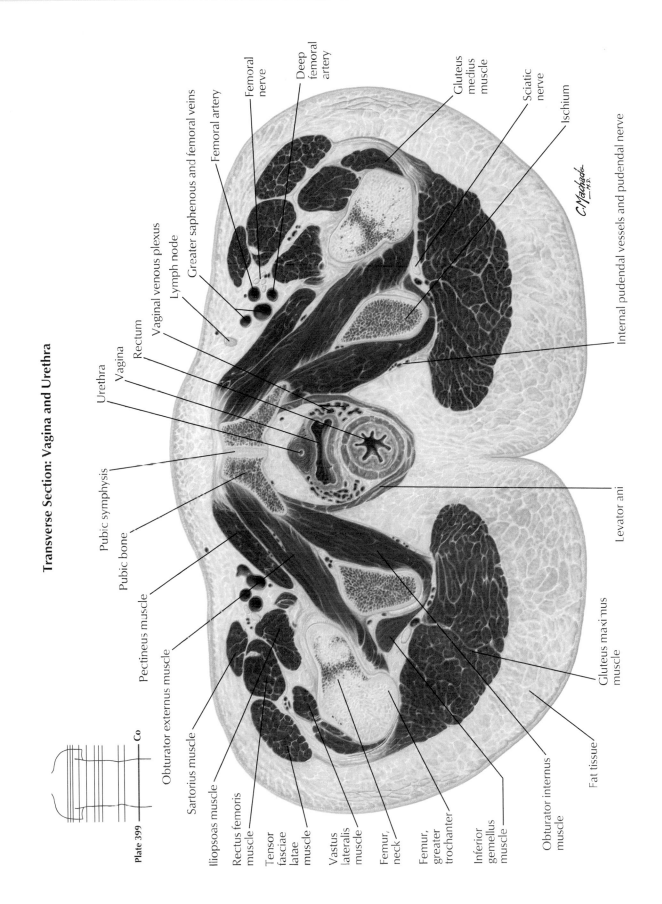

Femoral nerve

Deep femoral artery

Greater saphenous and femoral veins

Femoral artery

Gluteus medius muscle

Sciatic nerve

Ischium

Internal pudendal vessels and pudendal nerve

Vaginal venous plexus

Lymph node

Rectum

Vagina

Urethra

Pubic symphysis

Pubic bone

Levator ani

Pectineus muscle

Obturator externus muscle

Sartorius muscle

Iliopsoas muscle

Rectus femoris muscle

Tensor fasciae latae muscle

Vastus lateralis muscle

Femur, neck

Femur, greater trochanter

Inferior gemellus muscle

Obturator internus muscle

Fat tissue

Gluteus maximus muscle

Co

Plate 399

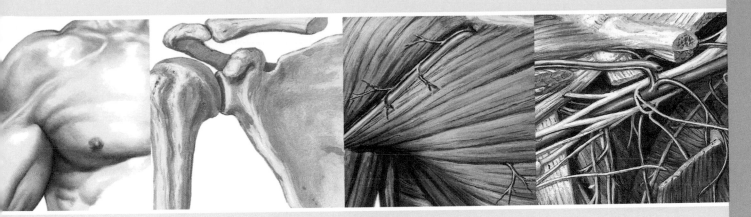

Section 6 UPPER LIMB

6 UPPER LIMB

Atlas of Human Anatomy

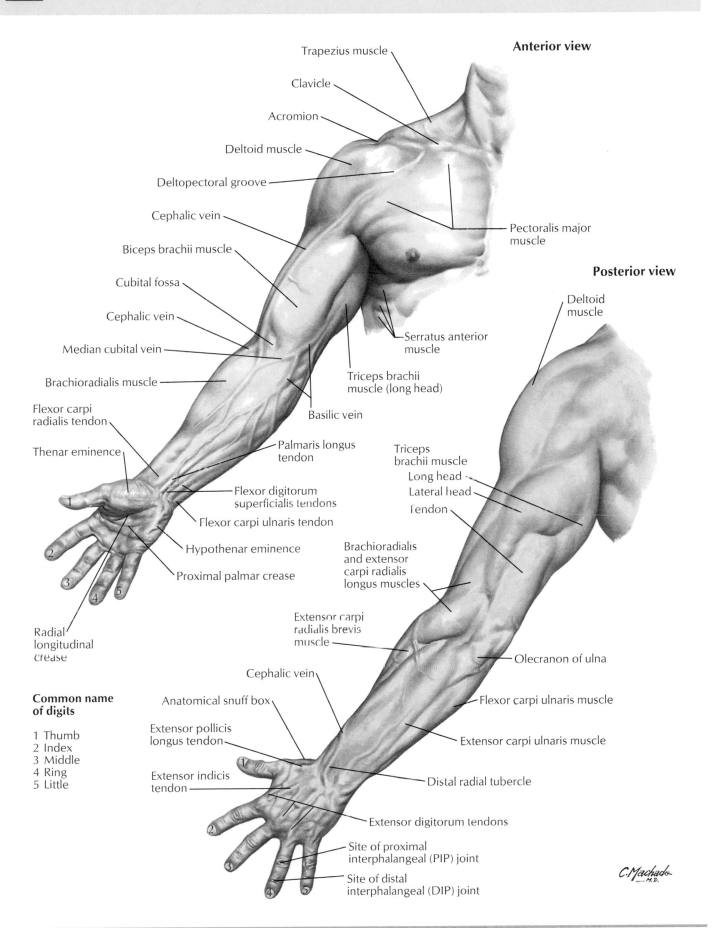

Anterior view

Trapezius muscle

Clavicle

Acromion

Deltoid muscle

Deltopectoral groove

Cephalic vein

Biceps brachii muscle

Cubital fossa

Cephalic vein

Median cubital vein

Brachioradialis muscle

Flexor carpi
radialis tendon

Thenar eminence

Pectoralis major
muscle

Serratus anterior
muscle

Triceps brachii
muscle (long head)

Basilic vein

Palmaris longus
tendon

Flexor digitorum
superficialis tendons

Flexor carpi ulnaris tendon

Hypothenar eminence

Proximal palmar crease

1

2

3   5

4

Radial
longitudinal
crease

**Common name
of digits**

1 Thumb
2 Index
3 Middle
4 Ring
5 Little

Anatomical snuff box

Extensor pollicis
longus tendon

Extensor indicis
tendon

Cephalic vein

Posterior view

Deltoid
muscle

Triceps
brachii muscle

Long head
Lateral head
Tendon

Brachioradialis
and extensor
carpi radialis
longus muscles

Extensor carpi
radialis brevis
muscle

Olecranon of ulna

Flexor carpi ulnaris muscle

Extensor carpi ulnaris muscle

Distal radial tubercle

Extensor digitorum tendons

Site of proximal
interphalangeal (PIP) joint

Site of distal
interphalangeal (DIP) joint

1

2

3

4   5

C. Machado
—M.D.

Note: Schematic demarcation of dermatomes (according to Keegan and Garrett) shown as distinct segments. There is actually considerable overlap between adjacent dermatomes. An alternative dermatome map is provided online.

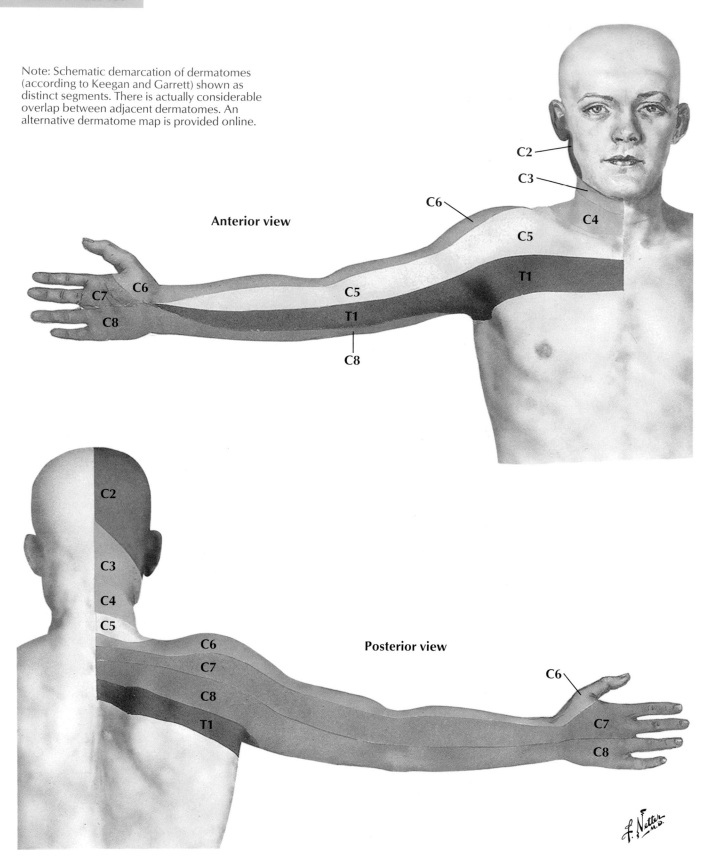

Anterior view

Posterior view

Plate 401

Cutaneous Anatomy

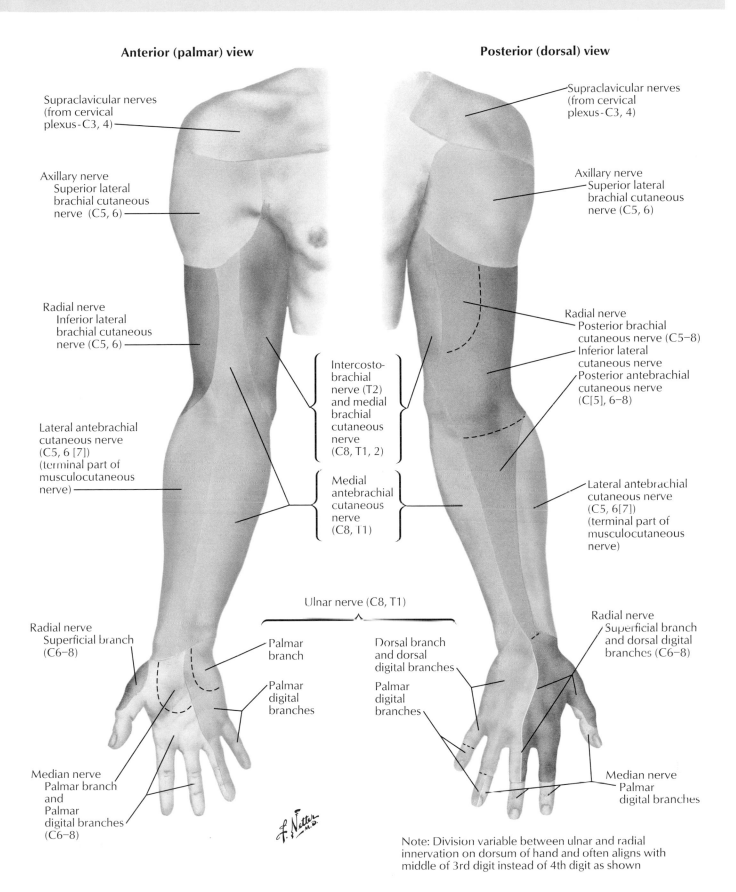

Anterior (palmar) view

Posterior (dorsal) view

Supraclavicular nerves
(from cervical
plexus-C3, 4)

Axillary nerve
Superior lateral
brachial cutaneous
nerve (C5, 6)

Radial nerve
Inferior lateral
brachial cutaneous
nerve (C5, 6)

Lateral antebrachial
cutaneous nerve
(C5, 6 [7])
(terminal part of
musculocutaneous
nerve)

Radial nerve
Superficial branch
(C6–8)

Median nerve
Palmar branch
and
Palmar
digital branches
(C6–8)

Intercosto-
brachial
nerve (T2)
and medial
brachial
cutaneous
nerve
(C8, T1, 2)

Medial
antebrachial
cutaneous
nerve
(C8, T1)

Ulnar nerve (C8, T1)

Palmar
branch

Palmar
digital
branches

Dorsal branch
and dorsal
digital branches

Palmar
digital
branches

Supraclavicular nerves
(from cervical
plexus-C3, 4)

Axillary nerve
Superior lateral
brachial cutaneous
nerve (C5, 6)

Radial nerve
Posterior brachial
cutaneous nerve (C5–8)
Inferior lateral
cutaneous nerve
Posterior antebrachial
cutaneous nerve
(C[5], 6–8)

Lateral antebrachial
cutaneous nerve
(C5, 6[7])
(terminal part of
musculocutaneous
nerve)

Radial nerve
Superficial branch
and dorsal digital
branches (C6–8)

Median nerve
Palmar
digital branches

Note: Division variable between ulnar and radial
innervation on dorsum of hand and often aligns with
middle of 3rd digit instead of 4th digit as shown

f. Netter M.D.

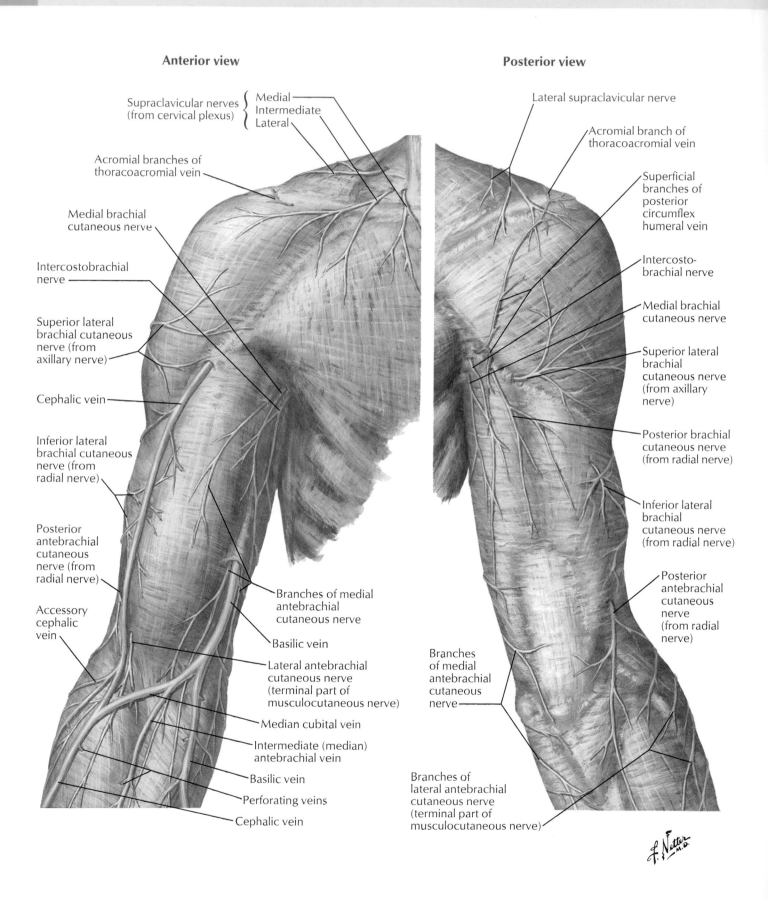

Anterior view

Supraclavicular nerves (from cervical plexus) { Medial / Intermediate / Lateral

Acromial branches of thoracoacromial vein

Medial brachial cutaneous nerve

Intercostobrachial nerve

Superior lateral brachial cutaneous nerve (from axillary nerve)

Cephalic vein

Inferior lateral brachial cutaneous nerve (from radial nerve)

Posterior antebrachial cutaneous nerve (from radial nerve)

Accessory cephalic vein

Branches of medial antebrachial cutaneous nerve

Basilic vein

Lateral antebrachial cutaneous nerve (terminal part of musculocutaneous nerve)

Median cubital vein

Intermediate (median) antebrachial vein

Basilic vein

Perforating veins

Cephalic vein

Posterior view

Lateral supraclavicular nerve

Acromial branch of thoracoacromial vein

Superficial branches of posterior circumflex humeral vein

Intercosto-brachial nerve

Medial brachial cutaneous nerve

Superior lateral brachial cutaneous nerve (from axillary nerve)

Posterior brachial cutaneous nerve (from radial nerve)

Inferior lateral brachial cutaneous nerve (from radial nerve)

Posterior antebrachial cutaneous nerve (from radial nerve)

Branches of medial antebrachial cutaneous nerve

Branches of lateral antebrachial cutaneous nerve (terminal part of musculocutaneous nerve)

Plate 403

Cutaneous Anatomy

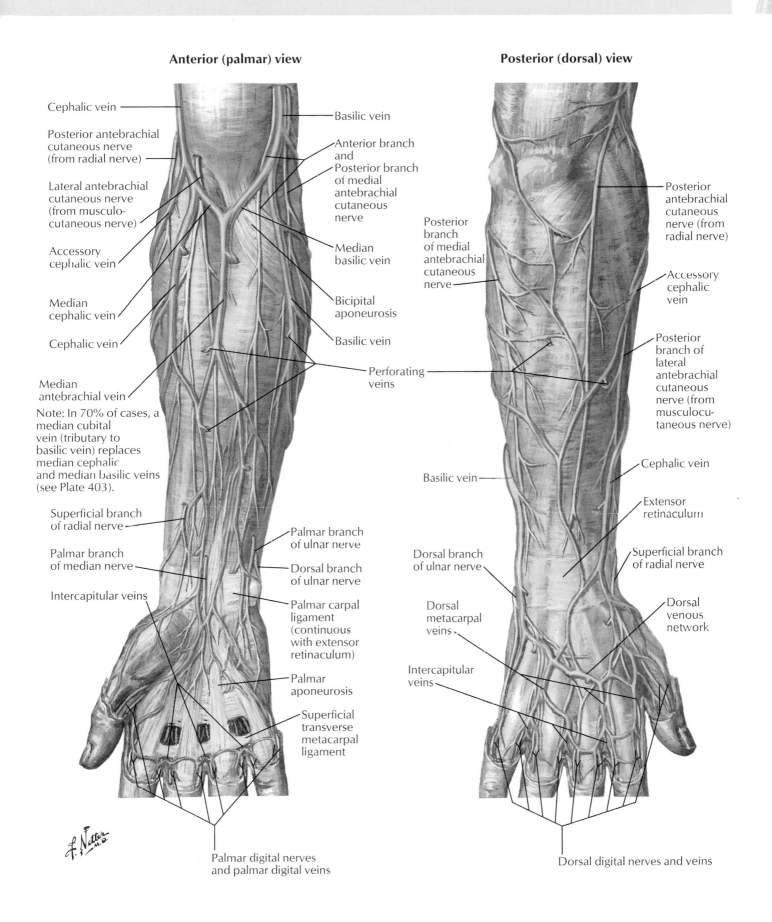

Anterior (palmar) view

Cephalic vein

Posterior antebrachial cutaneous nerve (from radial nerve)

Lateral antebrachial cutaneous nerve (from musculo-cutaneous nerve)

Accessory cephalic vein

Median cephalic vein

Cephalic vein

Median antebrachial vein

Note: In 70% of cases, a median cubital vein (tributary to basilic vein) replaces median cephalic and median basilic veins (see Plate 403).

Superficial branch of radial nerve

Palmar branch of median nerve

Intercapitular veins

Basilic vein

Anterior branch and Posterior branch of medial antebrachial cutaneous nerve

Median basilic vein

Bicipital aponeurosis

Basilic vein

Perforating veins

Palmar branch of ulnar nerve

Dorsal branch of ulnar nerve

Palmar carpal ligament (continuous with extensor retinaculum)

Palmar aponeurosis

Superficial transverse metacarpal ligament

Palmar digital nerves and palmar digital veins

Posterior (dorsal) view

Posterior branch of medial antebrachial cutaneous nerve

Posterior antebrachial cutaneous nerve (from radial nerve)

Accessory cephalic vein

Posterior branch of lateral antebrachial cutaneous nerve (from musculocutaneous nerve)

Cephalic vein

Extensor retinaculum

Superficial branch of radial nerve

Basilic vein

Dorsal branch of ulnar nerve

Dorsal metacarpal veins

Intercapitular veins

Dorsal venous network

Dorsal digital nerves and veins

Cutaneous Anatomy

Plate 404

Lymph Vessels and Nodes of Upper Limb

See also **Plates 178, 456**

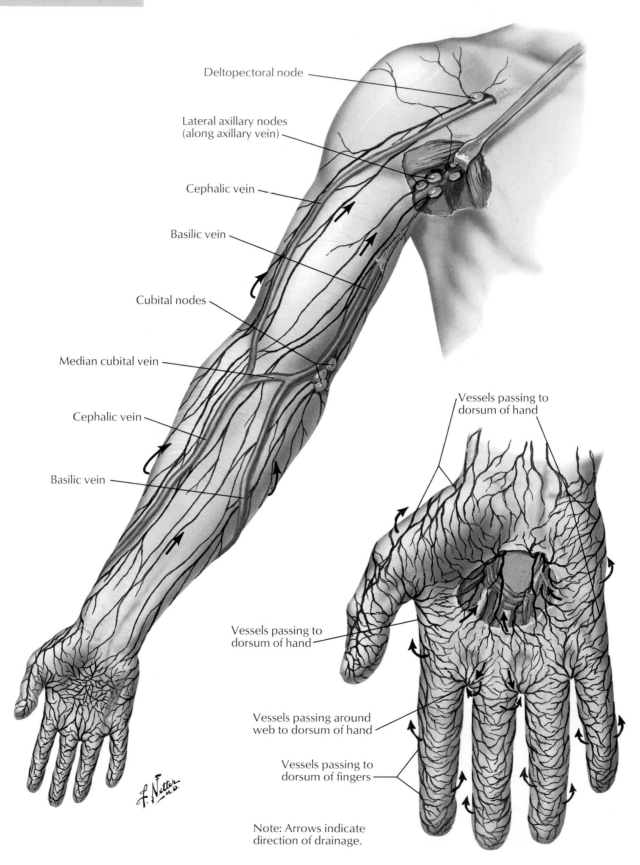

Deltopectoral node

Lateral axillary nodes
(along axillary vein)

Cephalic vein

Basilic vein

Cubital nodes

Median cubital vein

Cephalic vein

Basilic vein

Vessels passing to
dorsum of hand

Vessels passing to
dorsum of hand

Vessels passing around
web to dorsum of hand

Vessels passing to
dorsum of fingers

Note: Arrows indicate
direction of drainage.

Plate 405

Cutaneous Anatomy

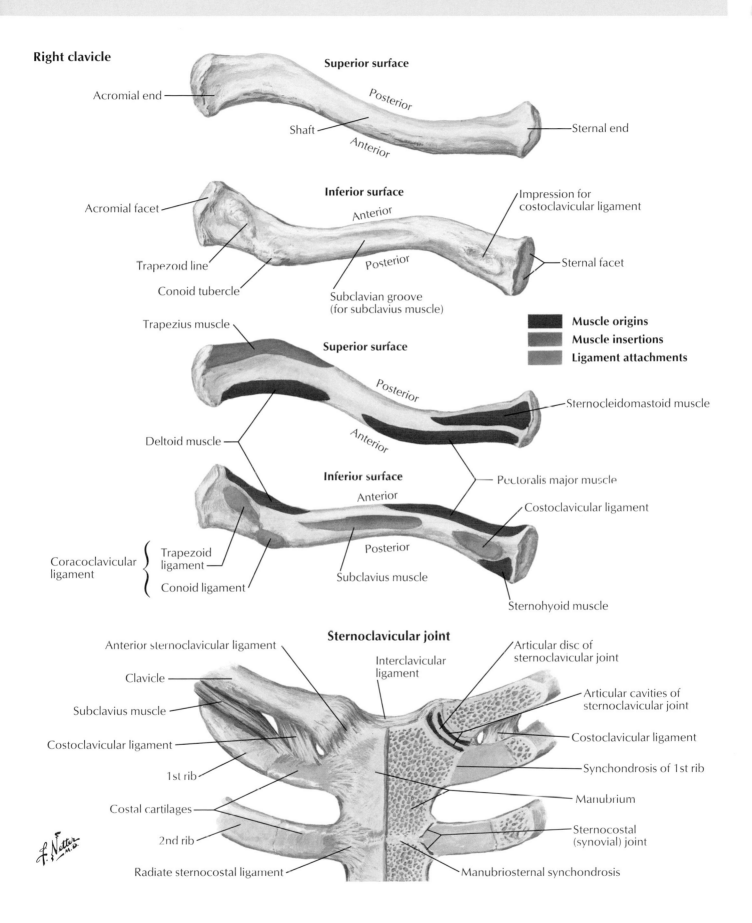

Right clavicle

Superior surface

Acromial end

Posterior

Shaft

Anterior

Sternal end

Inferior surface

Acromial facet

Anterior

Impression for costoclavicular ligament

Trapezoid line

Posterior

Sternal facet

Conoid tubercle

Subclavian groove (for subclavius muscle)

Muscle origins
Muscle insertions
Ligament attachments

Trapezius muscle

Superior surface

Posterior

Sternocleidomastoid muscle

Anterior

Deltoid muscle

Pectoralis major muscle

Inferior surface

Anterior

Costoclavicular ligament

Coracoclavicular ligament

Trapezoid ligament

Posterior

Conoid ligament

Subclavius muscle

Sternohyoid muscle

Sternoclavicular joint

Anterior sternoclavicular ligament

Interclavicular ligament

Articular disc of sternoclavicular joint

Clavicle

Articular cavities of sternoclavicular joint

Subclavius muscle

Costoclavicular ligament

Costoclavicular ligament

1st rib

Synchondrosis of 1st rib

Costal cartilages

Manubrium

2nd rib

Sternocostal (synovial) joint

Radiate sternocostal ligament

Manubriosternal synchondrosis

Humerus and Scapula: Anterior Views

See also **Plate 179**

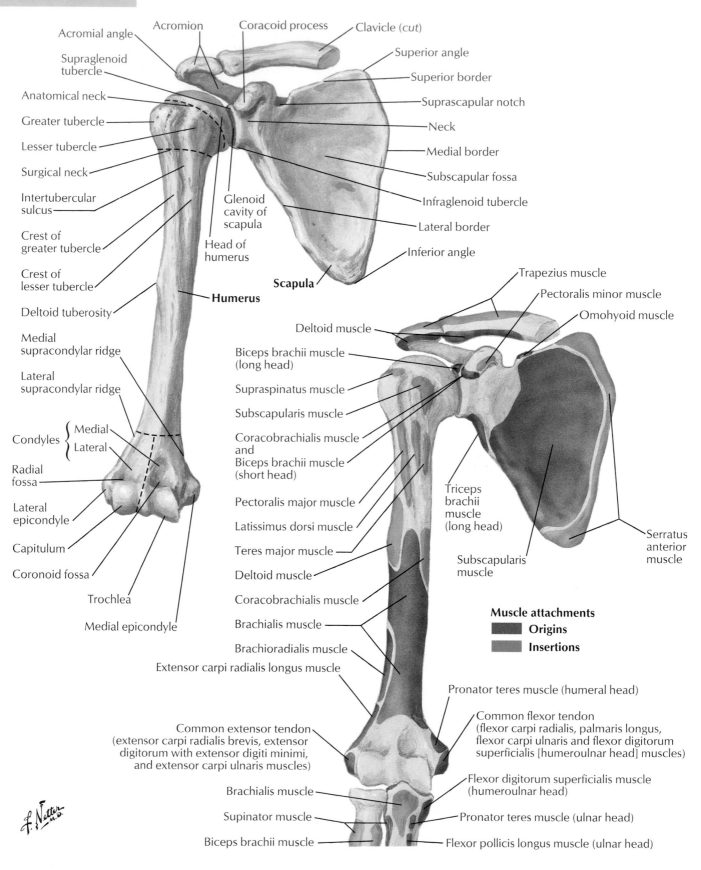

Acromial angle
Acromion
Coracoid process
Clavicle (cut)
Supraglenoid tubercle
Anatomical neck
Greater tubercle
Lesser tubercle
Surgical neck
Intertubercular sulcus
Crest of greater tubercle
Crest of lesser tubercle
Deltoid tuberosity
Medial supracondylar ridge
Lateral supracondylar ridge
Condyles { Medial / Lateral
Radial fossa
Lateral epicondyle
Capitulum
Coronoid fossa
Trochlea
Medial epicondyle

Superior angle
Superior border
Suprascapular notch
Neck
Medial border
Subscapular fossa
Infraglenoid tubercle
Lateral border
Inferior angle

Glenoid cavity of scapula
Head of humerus
Scapula
Humerus

Deltoid muscle
Biceps brachii muscle (long head)
Supraspinatus muscle
Subscapularis muscle
Coracobrachialis muscle and Biceps brachii muscle (short head)
Pectoralis major muscle
Latissimus dorsi muscle
Teres major muscle
Deltoid muscle
Coracobrachialis muscle
Brachialis muscle
Brachioradialis muscle
Extensor carpi radialis longus muscle

Trapezius muscle
Pectoralis minor muscle
Omohyoid muscle

Triceps brachii muscle (long head)
Subscapularis muscle
Serratus anterior muscle

Muscle attachments
■ **Origins**
■ **Insertions**

Pronator teres muscle (humeral head)
Common flexor tendon (flexor carpi radialis, palmaris longus, flexor carpi ulnaris and flexor digitorum superficialis [humeroulnar head] muscles)
Flexor digitorum superficialis muscle (humeroulnar head)
Pronator teres muscle (ulnar head)
Flexor pollicis longus muscle (ulnar head)

Common extensor tendon (extensor carpi radialis brevis, extensor digitorum with extensor digiti minimi, and extensor carpi ulnaris muscles)
Brachialis muscle
Supinator muscle
Biceps brachii muscle

Plate 407

Shoulder and Axilla

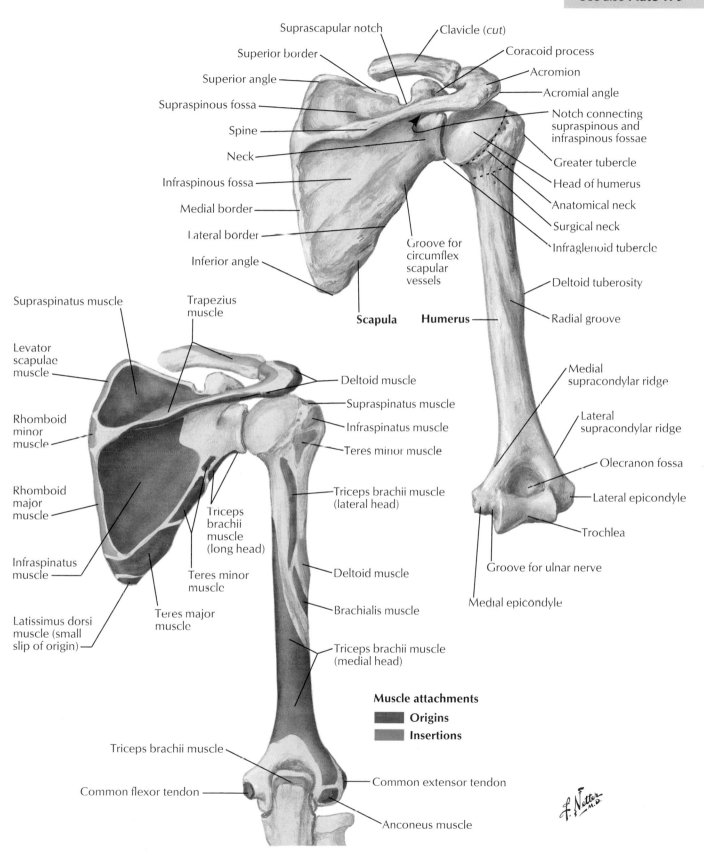

Suprascapular notch

Clavicle (*cut*)

Superior border

Coracoid process

Superior angle

Acromion

Supraspinous fossa

Acromial angle

Spine

Notch connecting supraspinous and infraspinous fossae

Neck

Greater tubercle

Infraspinous fossa

Head of humerus

Medial border

Anatomical neck

Lateral border

Surgical neck

Inferior angle

Infraglenoid tubercle

Groove for circumflex scapular vessels

Deltoid tuberosity

Scapula **Humerus**

Radial groove

Supraspinatus muscle

Trapezius muscle

Levator scapulae muscle

Medial supracondylar ridge

Deltoid muscle

Lateral supracondylar ridge

Rhomboid minor muscle

Supraspinatus muscle

Infraspinatus muscle

Olecranon fossa

Teres minor muscle

Lateral epicondyle

Rhomboid major muscle

Triceps brachii muscle (long head)

Triceps brachii muscle (lateral head)

Trochlea

Infraspinatus muscle

Teres minor muscle

Deltoid muscle

Groove for ulnar nerve

Latissimus dorsi muscle (small slip of origin)

Teres major muscle

Medial epicondyle

Brachialis muscle

Triceps brachii muscle (medial head)

Muscle attachments

■ **Origins**

■ **Insertions**

Triceps brachii muscle

Common flexor tendon

Common extensor tendon

Anconeus muscle

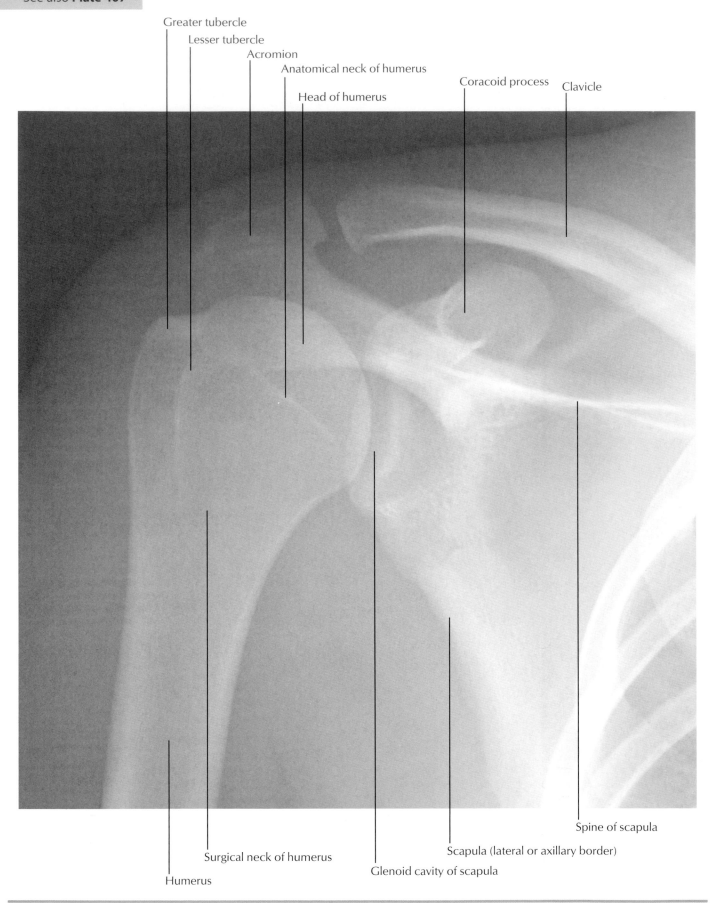

Greater tubercle

Lesser tubercle

Acromion

Anatomical neck of humerus

Coracoid process

Clavicle

Head of humerus

Surgical neck of humerus

Humerus

Glenoid cavity of scapula

Scapula (lateral or axillary border)

Spine of scapula

Plate 409   **Shoulder and Axilla**

Anterior view

Acromioclavicular joint capsule
(incorporating acromioclavicular ligament)

Acromion

Coracoacromial ligament

Supraspinatus tendon (cut)

Coracohumeral ligament

Greater tubercle and
Lesser tubercle
of humerus

Transverse humeral ligament

Intertubercular tendon sheath
(communicates with synovial cavity)

Subscapularis tendon (cut)

Biceps brachii tendon (long head)

Clavicle

Trapezoid
ligament

Conoid
ligament

} Coraco-
clavicular
ligament

Transverse scapular
ligament and
suprascapular foramen

Coracoid process

Communication of
subtendinous
bursa of subscapularis

Broken line indicates
position of subtendinous
bursa of subscapularis

Capsular
ligaments

F. Netter M.D.

**Anterior
view**

Deltoid
muscle
(reflected)

Capsular
ligament

Supraspinatus muscle

Subdeltoid bursa fused with
subacromial bursa

Subscapularis muscle

Subdeltoid bursa

Supraspinatus tendon

Capsular ligament

Synovial membrane

Acromion

Acromioclavicular
joint

Deltoid
muscle

Glenoid
labrum

Glenoid
cavity of
scapula

Axillary recess

Acromion

Supraspinatus tendon
(fused to capsule)

Subdeltoid bursa

Infraspinatus tendon
(fused to capsule)

Glenoid cavity
(articular cartilage)

Teres minor tendon
(fused to capsule)

Synovial membrane (cut edge)

Opening of subtendinous
bursa of subscapularis

Coracoacromial ligament

Coracoid process

Coracohumeral ligament

Biceps brachii tendon
(long head)

Superior glenohumeral
ligament

Subscapularis tendon
(fused to capsule)

Middle glenohumeral
ligament

Inferior glenohumeral
ligament

Joint opened: lateral view

Coronal section through joint

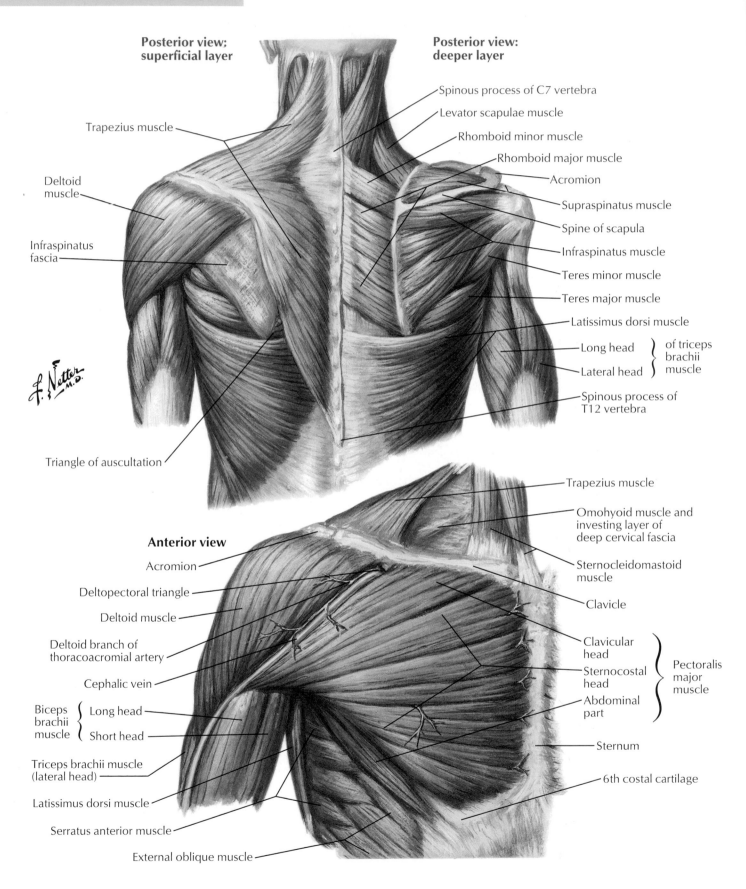

Posterior view: superficial layer

Trapezius muscle

Deltoid muscle

Infraspinatus fascia

Triangle of auscultation

Posterior view: deeper layer

Spinous process of C7 vertebra

Levator scapulae muscle

Rhomboid minor muscle

Rhomboid major muscle

Acromion

Supraspinatus muscle

Spine of scapula

Infraspinatus muscle

Teres minor muscle

Teres major muscle

Latissimus dorsi muscle

Long head ⎫ of triceps
⎬ brachii
Lateral head ⎭ muscle

Spinous process of T12 vertebra

Anterior view

Acromion

Deltopectoral triangle

Deltoid muscle

Deltoid branch of thoracoacromial artery

Cephalic vein

Biceps brachii muscle { Long head

Short head

Triceps brachii muscle (lateral head)

Latissimus dorsi muscle

Serratus anterior muscle

External oblique muscle

Trapezius muscle

Omohyoid muscle and investing layer of deep cervical fascia

Sternocleidomastoid muscle

Clavicle

Clavicular head ⎫
Sternocostal head ⎬ Pectoralis major muscle
Abdominal part ⎭

Sternum

6th costal cartilage

Plate 411   **Shoulder and Axilla**

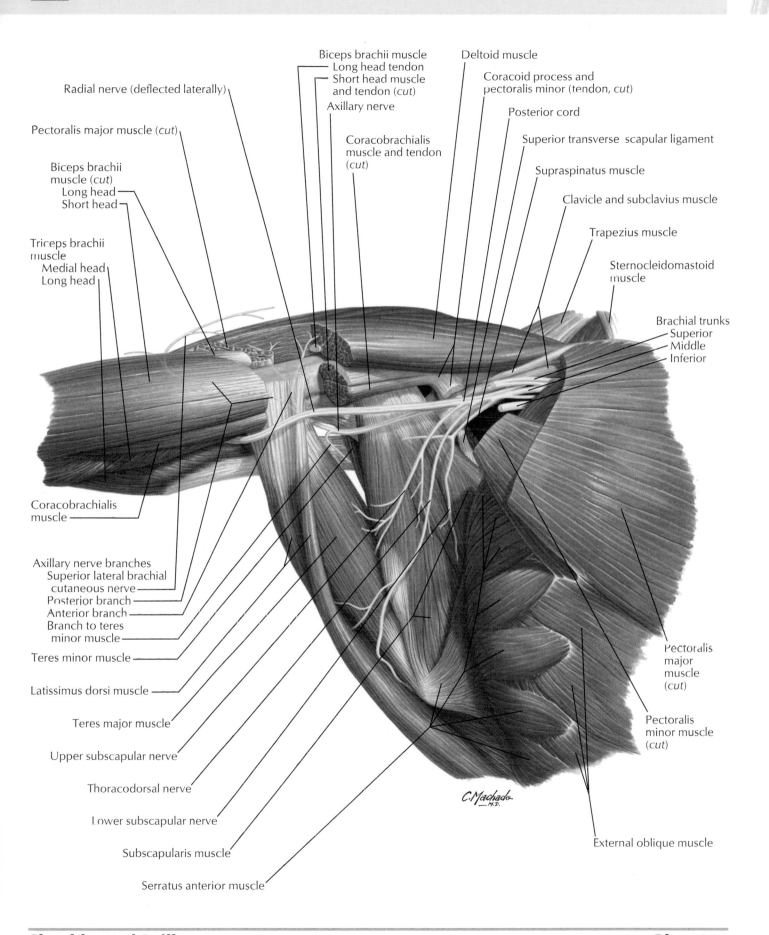

Radial nerve (deflected laterally)

Biceps brachii muscle
Long head tendon
Short head muscle and tendon (cut)
Axillary nerve

Deltoid muscle

Coracoid process and pectoralis minor (tendon, cut)

Posterior cord

Pectoralis major muscle (cut)

Coracobrachialis muscle and tendon (cut)

Superior transverse scapular ligament

Biceps brachii muscle (cut)
Long head
Short head

Supraspinatus muscle

Clavicle and subclavius muscle

Triceps brachii muscle
Medial head
Long head

Trapezius muscle

Sternocleidomastoid muscle

Brachial trunks
Superior
Middle
Inferior

Coracobrachialis muscle

Axillary nerve branches
Superior lateral brachial cutaneous nerve
Posterior branch
Anterior branch
Branch to teres minor muscle

Teres minor muscle

Latissimus dorsi muscle

Teres major muscle

Upper subscapular nerve

Thoracodorsal nerve

Lower subscapular nerve

Subscapularis muscle

Serratus anterior muscle

Pectoralis major muscle (cut)

Pectoralis minor muscle (cut)

External oblique muscle

C. Machado
M.D.

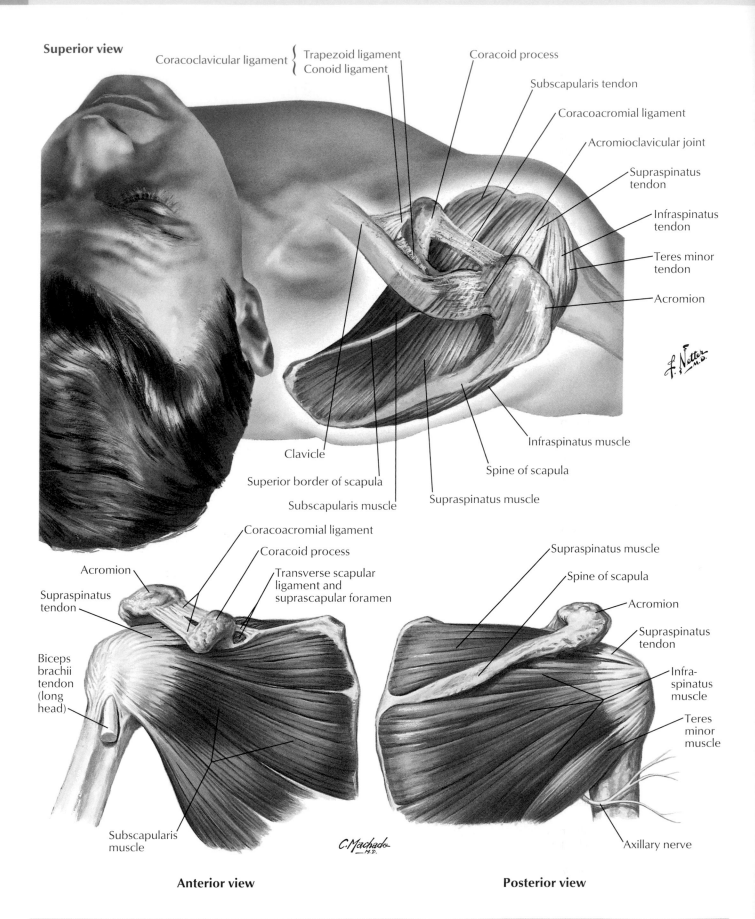

Superior view

Coracoclavicular ligament { Trapezoid ligament
Conoid ligament

Coracoid process

Subscapularis tendon

Coracoacromial ligament

Acromioclavicular joint

Supraspinatus tendon

Infraspinatus tendon

Teres minor tendon

Acromion

Infraspinatus muscle

Spine of scapula

Supraspinatus muscle

Clavicle

Superior border of scapula

Subscapularis muscle

Coracoacromial ligament

Coracoid process

Acromion

Transverse scapular ligament and suprascapular foramen

Supraspinatus tendon

Biceps brachii tendon (long head)

Subscapularis muscle

Anterior view

Supraspinatus muscle

Spine of scapula

Acromion

Supraspinatus tendon

Infraspinatus muscle

Teres minor muscle

Axillary nerve

Posterior view

Plate 413

Shoulder and Axilla

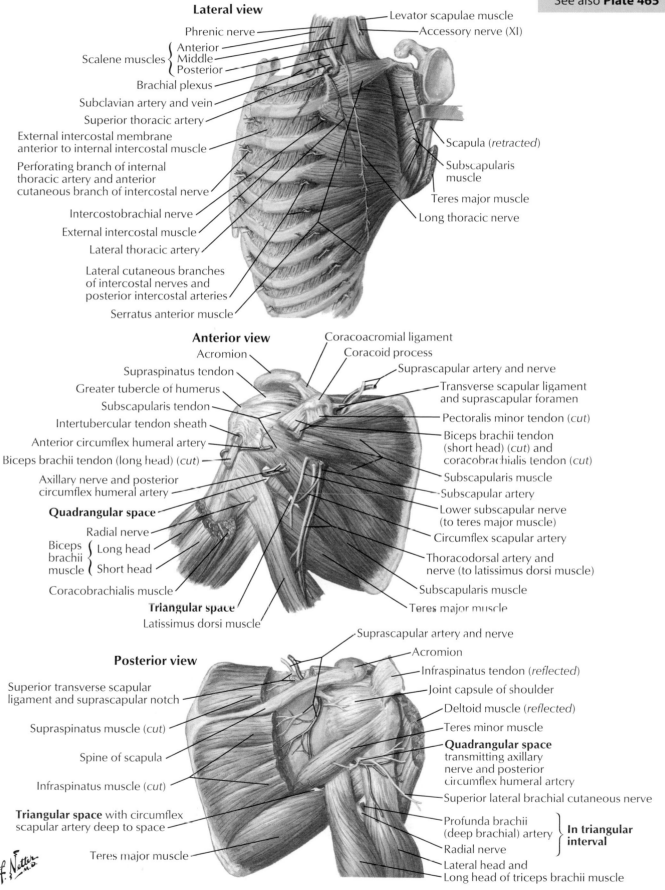

Lateral view

Phrenic nerve

Scalene muscles { Anterior / Middle / Posterior

Brachial plexus

Subclavian artery and vein

Superior thoracic artery

External intercostal membrane anterior to internal intercostal muscle

Perforating branch of internal thoracic artery and anterior cutaneous branch of intercostal nerve

Intercostobrachial nerve

External intercostal muscle

Lateral thoracic artery

Lateral cutaneous branches of intercostal nerves and posterior intercostal arteries

Serratus anterior muscle

Levator scapulae muscle

Accessory nerve (XI)

Scapula (*retracted*)

Subscapularis muscle

Teres major muscle

Long thoracic nerve

Anterior view

Acromion

Supraspinatus tendon

Greater tubercle of humerus

Subscapularis tendon

Intertubercular tendon sheath

Anterior circumflex humeral artery

Biceps brachii tendon (long head) (*cut*)

Axillary nerve and posterior circumflex humeral artery

Quadrangular space

Radial nerve

Biceps brachii muscle { Long head / Short head

Coracobrachialis muscle

Triangular space

Latissimus dorsi muscle

Coracoacromial ligament

Coracoid process

Suprascapular artery and nerve

Transverse scapular ligament and suprascapular foramen

Pectoralis minor tendon (*cut*)

Biceps brachii tendon (short head) (*cut*) and coracobrachialis tendon (*cut*)

Subscapularis muscle

Subscapular artery

Lower subscapular nerve (to teres major muscle)

Circumflex scapular artery

Thoracodorsal artery and nerve (to latissimus dorsi muscle)

Subscapularis muscle

Teres major muscle

Posterior view

Superior transverse scapular ligament and suprascapular notch

Supraspinatus muscle (*cut*)

Spine of scapula

Infraspinatus muscle (*cut*)

Triangular space with circumflex scapular artery deep to space

Teres major muscle

Suprascapular artery and nerve

Acromion

Infraspinatus tendon (*reflected*)

Joint capsule of shoulder

Deltoid muscle (*reflected*)

Teres minor muscle

Quadrangular space transmitting axillary nerve and posterior circumflex humeral artery

Superior lateral brachial cutaneous nerve

Profunda brachii (deep brachial) artery } **In triangular interval**

Radial nerve

Lateral head and Long head of triceps brachii muscle

See also **Plates 32, 422**

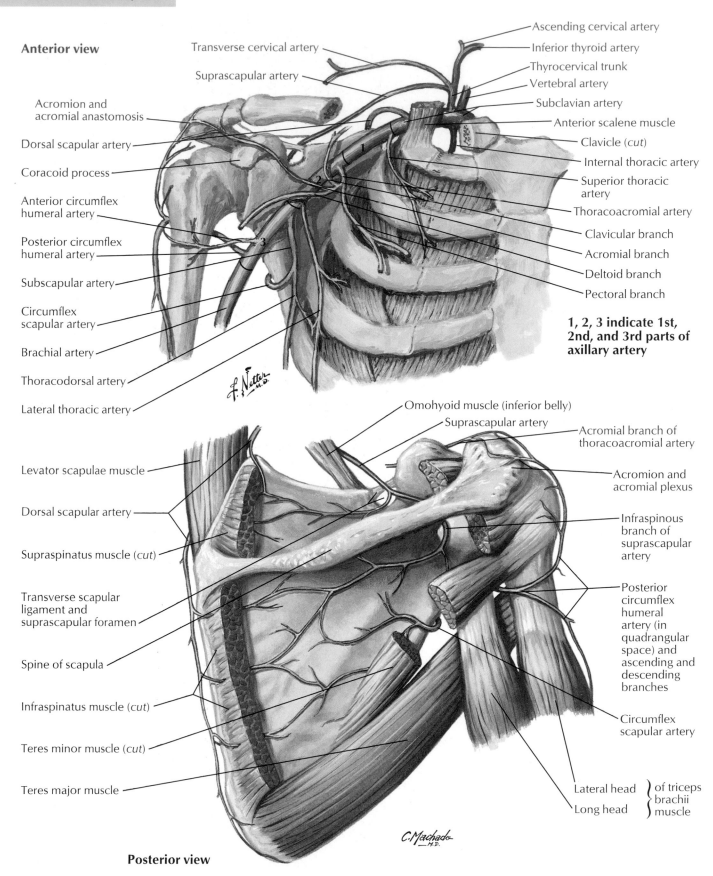

Anterior view

Transverse cervical artery

Suprascapular artery

Ascending cervical artery

Inferior thyroid artery

Thyrocervical trunk

Vertebral artery

Subclavian artery

Anterior scalene muscle

Clavicle (*cut*)

Internal thoracic artery

Superior thoracic artery

Thoracoacromial artery

Clavicular branch

Acromial branch

Deltoid branch

Pectoral branch

Acromion and acromial anastomosis

Dorsal scapular artery

Coracoid process

Anterior circumflex humeral artery

Posterior circumflex humeral artery

Subscapular artery

Circumflex scapular artery

Brachial artery

Thoracodorsal artery

Lateral thoracic artery

1, 2, 3 indicate 1st, 2nd, and 3rd parts of axillary artery

Omohyoid muscle (inferior belly)

Suprascapular artery

Acromial branch of thoracoacromial artery

Acromion and acromial plexus

Infraspinous branch of suprascapular artery

Posterior circumflex humeral artery (in quadrangular space) and ascending and descending branches

Circumflex scapular artery

Levator scapulae muscle

Dorsal scapular artery

Supraspinatus muscle (*cut*)

Transverse scapular ligament and suprascapular foramen

Spine of scapula

Infraspinatus muscle (*cut*)

Teres minor muscle (*cut*)

Teres major muscle

Lateral head ⎫ of triceps
Long head ⎭ brachii muscle

Posterior view

Plate 415   **Shoulder and Axilla**

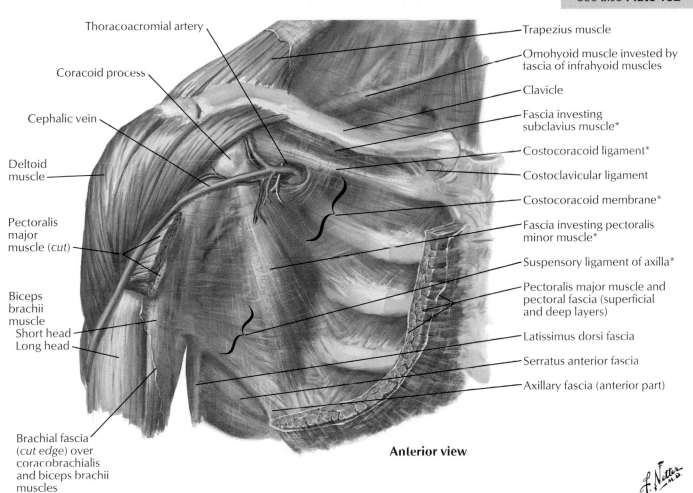

Thoracoacromial artery

Coracoid process

Cephalic vein

Deltoid muscle

Pectoralis major muscle (cut)

Biceps brachii muscle
Short head
Long head

Brachial fascia (cut edge) over coracobrachialis and biceps brachii muscles

Trapezius muscle

Omohyoid muscle invested by fascia of infrahyoid muscles

Clavicle

Fascia investing subclavius muscle*

Costocoracoid ligament*

Costoclavicular ligament

Costocoracoid membrane*

Fascia investing pectoralis minor muscle*

Suspensory ligament of axilla*

Pectoralis major muscle and pectoral fascia (superficial and deep layers)

Latissimus dorsi fascia

Serratus anterior fascia

Axillary fascia (anterior part)

Anterior view

f. Netter

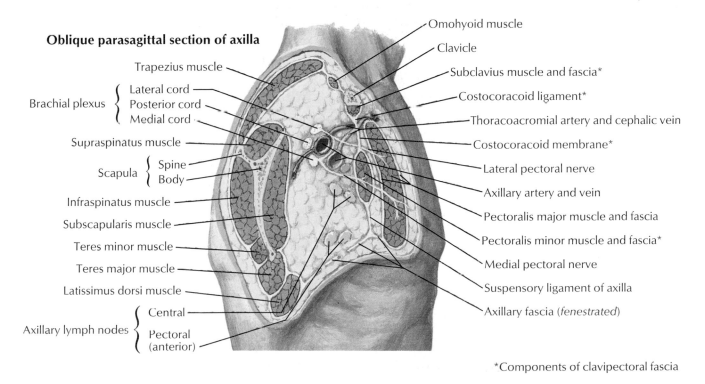

Oblique parasagittal section of axilla

Trapezius muscle

Brachial plexus {
Lateral cord
Posterior cord
Medial cord
}

Supraspinatus muscle

Scapula {
Spine
Body
}

Infraspinatus muscle

Subscapularis muscle

Teres minor muscle

Teres major muscle

Latissimus dorsi muscle

Axillary lymph nodes {
Central
Pectoral (anterior)
}

Omohyoid muscle

Clavicle

Subclavius muscle and fascia*

Costocoracoid ligament*

Thoracoacromial artery and cephalic vein

Costocoracoid membrane*

Lateral pectoral nerve

Axillary artery and vein

Pectoralis major muscle and fascia

Pectoralis minor muscle and fascia*

Medial pectoral nerve

Suspensory ligament of axilla

Axillary fascia (fenestrated)

*Components of clavipectoral fascia

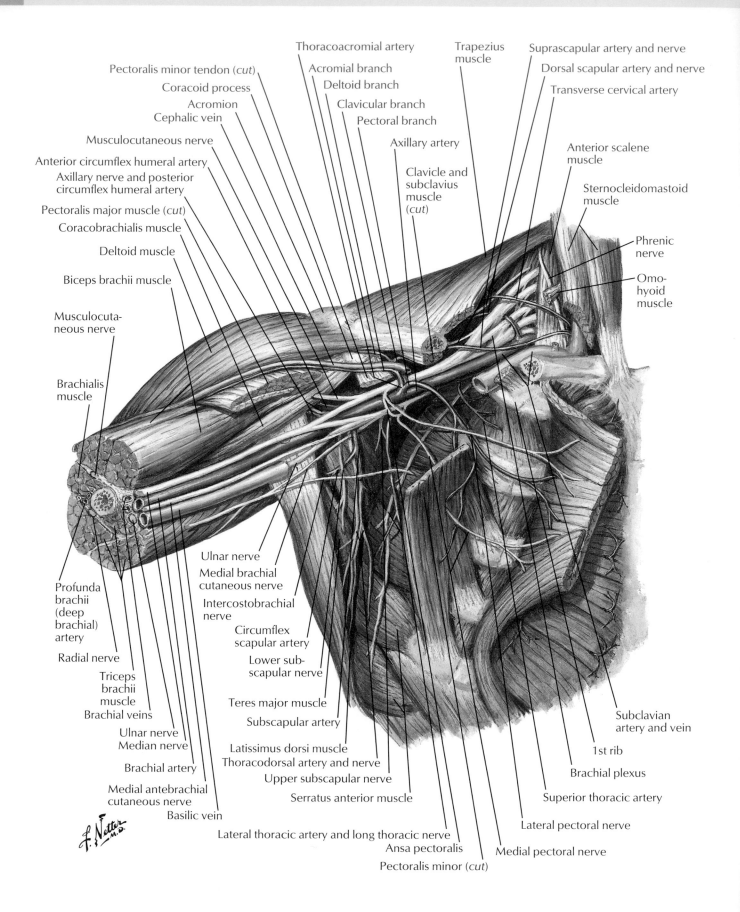

Pectoralis minor tendon (*cut*)
Coracoid process
Acromion
Cephalic vein
Musculocutaneous nerve
Anterior circumflex humeral artery
Axillary nerve and posterior circumflex humeral artery
Pectoralis major muscle (*cut*)
Coracobrachialis muscle
Deltoid muscle
Biceps brachii muscle
Musculocuta-neous nerve
Brachialis muscle

Thoracoacromial artery
Acromial branch
Deltoid branch
Clavicular branch
Pectoral branch
Axillary artery
Clavicle and subclavius muscle (*cut*)

Trapezius muscle

Suprascapular artery and nerve
Dorsal scapular artery and nerve
Transverse cervical artery

Anterior scalene muscle

Sternocleidomastoid muscle

Phrenic nerve

Omo-hyoid muscle

Profunda brachii (deep brachial) artery
Radial nerve
Triceps brachii muscle
Brachial veins
Ulnar nerve
Median nerve
Brachial artery
Medial antebrachial cutaneous nerve
Basilic vein

Ulnar nerve
Medial brachial cutaneous nerve
Intercostobrachial nerve
Circumflex scapular artery
Lower sub-scapular nerve
Teres major muscle
Subscapular artery
Latissimus dorsi muscle
Thoracodorsal artery and nerve
Upper subscapular nerve
Serratus anterior muscle

Lateral thoracic artery and long thoracic nerve
Ansa pectoralis
Pectoralis minor (*cut*)

Subclavian artery and vein
1st rib
Brachial plexus
Superior thoracic artery
Lateral pectoral nerve
Medial pectoral nerve

Plate 417

Shoulder and Axilla

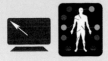

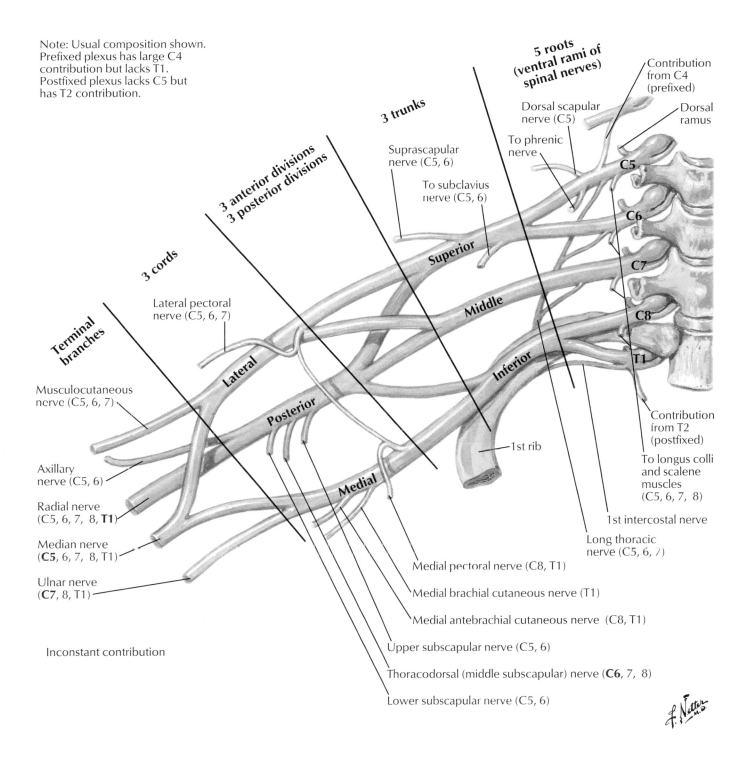

Note: Usual composition shown. Prefixed plexus has large C4 contribution but lacks T1. Postfixed plexus lacks C5 but has T2 contribution.

5 roots (ventral rami of spinal nerves)

Contribution from C4 (prefixed)

Dorsal scapular nerve (C5)

Dorsal ramus

To phrenic nerve

3 trunks

Suprascapular nerve (C5, 6)

To subclavius nerve (C5, 6)

C5

C6

C7

C8

T1

3 anterior divisions
3 posterior divisions

Superior

Middle

3 cords

Lateral pectoral nerve (C5, 6, 7)

Inferior

Terminal branches

Lateral

Musculocutaneous nerve (C5, 6, 7)

Posterior

Contribution from T2 (postfixed)

1st rib

To longus colli and scalene muscles (C5, 6, 7, 8)

Axillary nerve (C5, 6)

Medial

1st intercostal nerve

Radial nerve (C5, 6, 7, 8, **T1**)

Long thoracic nerve (C5, 6, 7)

Median nerve (**C5**, 6, 7, 8, T1)

Medial pectoral nerve (C8, T1)

Ulnar nerve (**C7**, 8, T1)

Medial brachial cutaneous nerve (T1)

Medial antebrachial cutaneous nerve (C8, T1)

Upper subscapular nerve (C5, 6)

Inconstant contribution

Thoracodorsal (middle subscapular) nerve (**C6**, 7, 8)

Lower subscapular nerve (C5, 6)

Muscles of Arm: Anterior Views

See also **Plate 462**

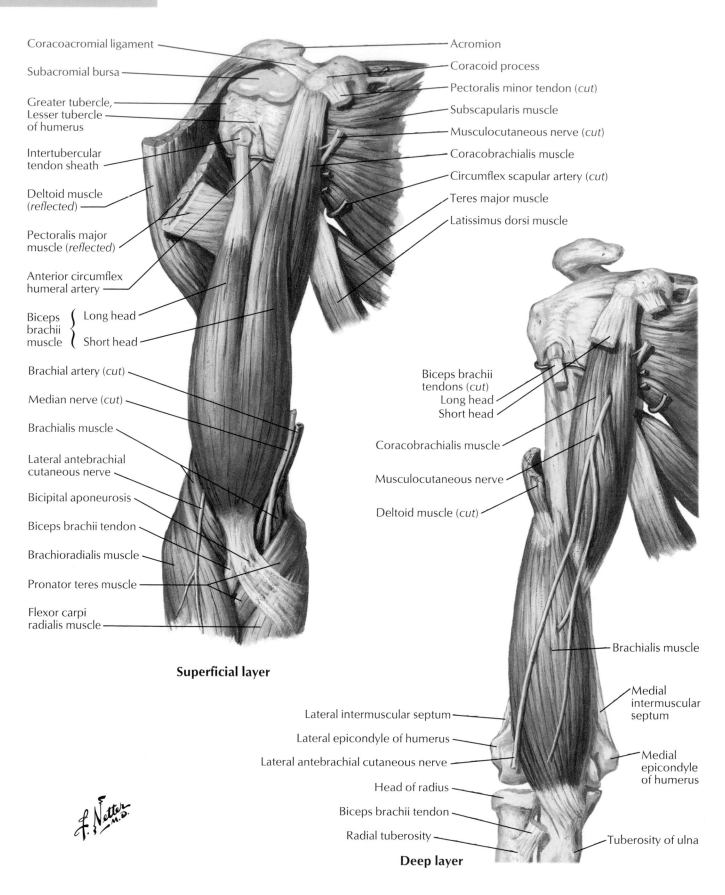

Coracoacromial ligament

Subacromial bursa

Greater tubercle,
Lesser tubercle
of humerus

Intertubercular
tendon sheath

Deltoid muscle
(reflected)

Pectoralis major
muscle (reflected)

Anterior circumflex
humeral artery

Biceps
brachii
muscle { Long head
Short head

Brachial artery (cut)

Median nerve (cut)

Brachialis muscle

Lateral antebrachial
cutaneous nerve

Bicipital aponeurosis

Biceps brachii tendon

Brachioradialis muscle

Pronator teres muscle

Flexor carpi
radialis muscle

Acromion

Coracoid process

Pectoralis minor tendon (cut)

Subscapularis muscle

Musculocutaneous nerve (cut)

Coracobrachialis muscle

Circumflex scapular artery (cut)

Teres major muscle

Latissimus dorsi muscle

Superficial layer

Biceps brachii
tendons (cut)
Long head
Short head

Coracobrachialis muscle

Musculocutaneous nerve

Deltoid muscle (cut)

Brachialis muscle

Medial
intermuscular
septum

Lateral intermuscular septum

Lateral epicondyle of humerus

Lateral antebrachial cutaneous nerve

Head of radius

Biceps brachii tendon

Radial tuberosity

Medial
epicondyle
of humerus

Tuberosity of ulna

Deep layer

F. Netter
M.D.

Plate 419

Superficial layer

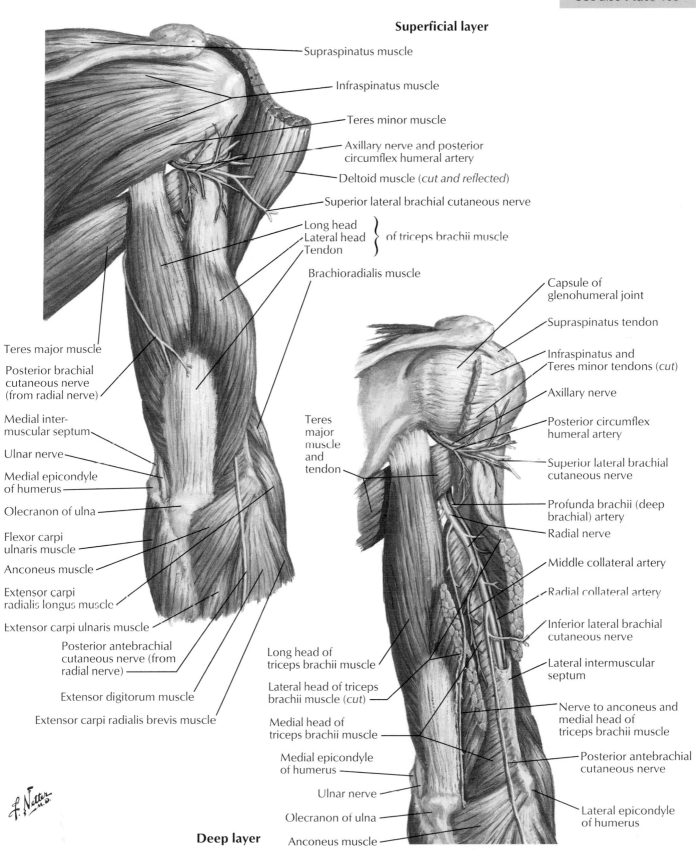

Supraspinatus muscle

Infraspinatus muscle

Teres minor muscle

Axillary nerve and posterior circumflex humeral artery

Deltoid muscle (*cut and reflected*)

Superior lateral brachial cutaneous nerve

Long head
Lateral head } of triceps brachii muscle
Tendon

Brachioradialis muscle

Teres major muscle

Posterior brachial cutaneous nerve (from radial nerve)

Medial inter-muscular septum

Ulnar nerve

Medial epicondyle of humerus

Olecranon of ulna

Flexor carpi ulnaris muscle

Anconeus muscle

Extensor carpi radialis longus muscle

Extensor carpi ulnaris muscle

Posterior antebrachial cutaneous nerve (from radial nerve)

Extensor digitorum muscle

Extensor carpi radialis brevis muscle

Teres major muscle and tendon

Capsule of glenohumeral joint

Supraspinatus tendon

Infraspinatus and Teres minor tendons (*cut*)

Axillary nerve

Posterior circumflex humeral artery

Superior lateral brachial cutaneous nerve

Profunda brachii (deep brachial) artery

Radial nerve

Middle collateral artery

Radial collateral artery

Inferior lateral brachial cutaneous nerve

Lateral intermuscular septum

Nerve to anconeus and medial head of triceps brachii muscle

Posterior antebrachial cutaneous nerve

Lateral epicondyle of humerus

Long head of triceps brachii muscle

Lateral head of triceps brachii muscle (*cut*)

Medial head of triceps brachii muscle

Medial epicondyle of humerus

Ulnar nerve

Olecranon of ulna

Anconeus muscle

Deep layer

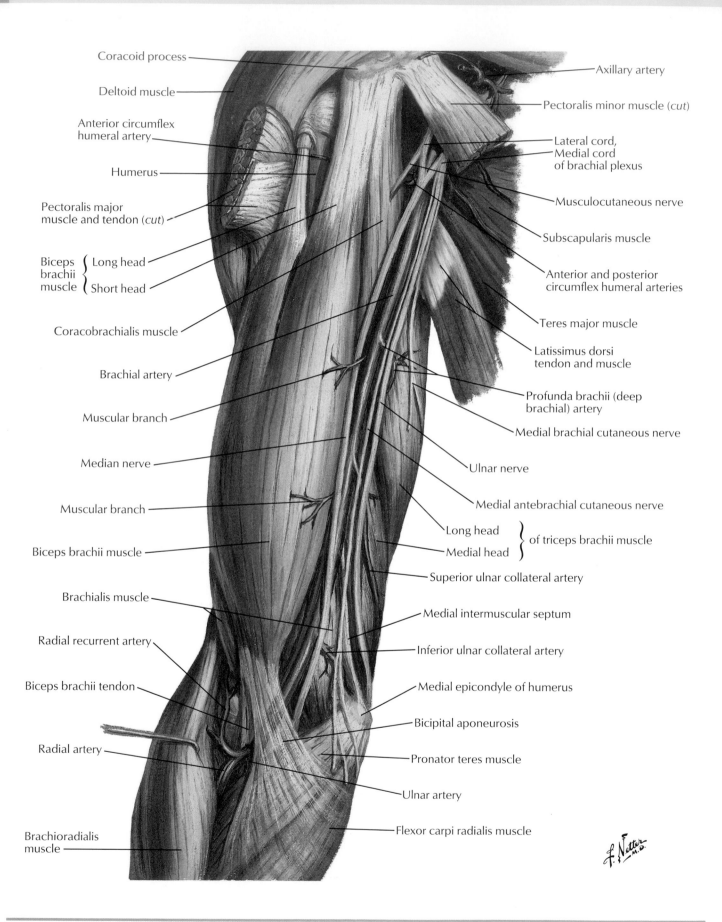

Coracoid process

Deltoid muscle

Anterior circumflex
humeral artery

Humerus

Pectoralis major
muscle and tendon (cut)

Biceps { Long head
brachii
muscle { Short head

Coracobrachialis muscle

Brachial artery

Muscular branch

Median nerve

Muscular branch

Biceps brachii muscle

Brachialis muscle

Radial recurrent artery

Biceps brachii tendon

Radial artery

Brachioradialis
muscle

Axillary artery

Pectoralis minor muscle (cut)

Lateral cord,
Medial cord
of brachial plexus

Musculocutaneous nerve

Subscapularis muscle

Anterior and posterior
circumflex humeral arteries

Teres major muscle

Latissimus dorsi
tendon and muscle

Profunda brachii (deep
brachial) artery

Medial brachial cutaneous nerve

Ulnar nerve

Medial antebrachial cutaneous nerve

Long head
} of triceps brachii muscle
Medial head

Superior ulnar collateral artery

Medial intermuscular septum

Inferior ulnar collateral artery

Medial epicondyle of humerus

Bicipital aponeurosis

Pronator teres muscle

Ulnar artery

Flexor carpi radialis muscle

Plate 421

Arm

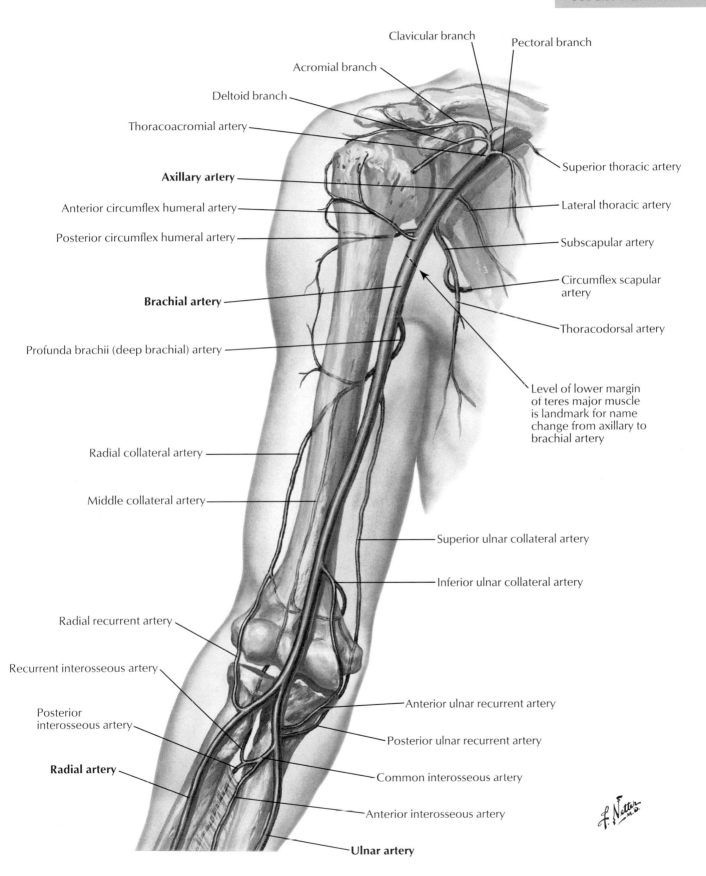

Clavicular branch

Pectoral branch

Acromial branch

Deltoid branch

Thoracoacromial artery

Axillary artery

Anterior circumflex humeral artery

Posterior circumflex humeral artery

Brachial artery

Profunda brachii (deep brachial) artery

Superior thoracic artery

Lateral thoracic artery

Subscapular artery

Circumflex scapular artery

Thoracodorsal artery

Level of lower margin of teres major muscle is landmark for name change from axillary to brachial artery

Radial collateral artery

Middle collateral artery

Superior ulnar collateral artery

Inferior ulnar collateral artery

Radial recurrent artery

Recurrent interosseous artery

Posterior interosseous artery

Radial artery

Anterior ulnar recurrent artery

Posterior ulnar recurrent artery

Common interosseous artery

Anterior interosseous artery

Ulnar artery

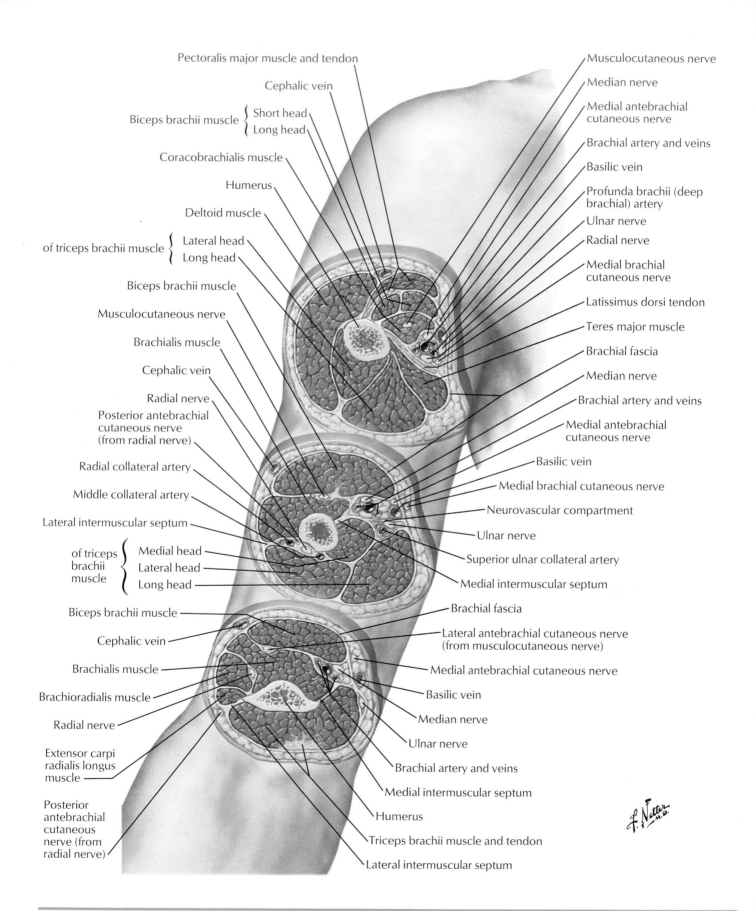

Pectoralis major muscle and tendon

Cephalic vein

Biceps brachii muscle { Short head / Long head

Coracobrachialis muscle

Humerus

Deltoid muscle

of triceps brachii muscle { Lateral head / Long head

Biceps brachii muscle

Musculocutaneous nerve

Brachialis muscle

Cephalic vein

Radial nerve

Posterior antebrachial cutaneous nerve (from radial nerve)

Radial collateral artery

Middle collateral artery

Lateral intermuscular septum

of triceps brachii muscle { Medial head / Lateral head / Long head

Biceps brachii muscle

Cephalic vein

Brachialis muscle

Brachioradialis muscle

Radial nerve

Extensor carpi radialis longus muscle

Posterior antebrachial cutaneous nerve (from radial nerve)

Musculocutaneous nerve

Median nerve

Medial antebrachial cutaneous nerve

Brachial artery and veins

Basilic vein

Profunda brachii (deep brachial) artery

Ulnar nerve

Radial nerve

Medial brachial cutaneous nerve

Latissimus dorsi tendon

Teres major muscle

Brachial fascia

Median nerve

Brachial artery and veins

Medial antebrachial cutaneous nerve

Basilic vein

Medial brachial cutaneous nerve

Neurovascular compartment

Ulnar nerve

Superior ulnar collateral artery

Medial intermuscular septum

Brachial fascia

Lateral antebrachial cutaneous nerve (from musculocutaneous nerve)

Medial antebrachial cutaneous nerve

Basilic vein

Median nerve

Ulnar nerve

Brachial artery and veins

Medial intermuscular septum

Humerus

Triceps brachii muscle and tendon

Lateral intermuscular septum

Plate 423

Arm

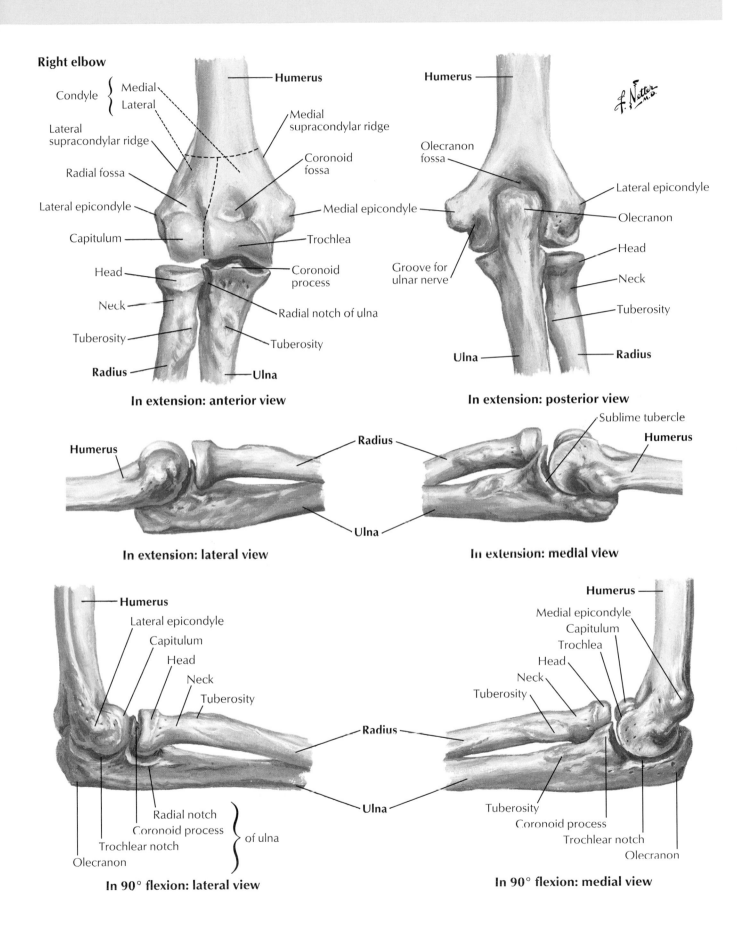

Right elbow

Condyle { Medial / Lateral

Lateral supracondylar ridge

Radial fossa

Lateral epicondyle

Capitulum

Head

Neck

Tuberosity

Radius

Humerus

Medial supracondylar ridge

Coronoid fossa

Medial epicondyle

Trochlea

Coronoid process

Radial notch of ulna

Tuberosity

Ulna

In extension: anterior view

Humerus

Olecranon fossa

Lateral epicondyle

Olecranon

Head

Neck

Tuberosity

Groove for ulnar nerve

Ulna

Radius

In extension: posterior view

Humerus

Radius

Ulna

In extension: lateral view

Sublime tubercle

Humerus

Radius

Ulna

In extension: medial view

Humerus

Lateral epicondyle

Capitulum

Head

Neck

Tuberosity

Radius

Radial notch

Coronoid process } of ulna

Trochlear notch

Olecranon

Ulna

In 90° flexion: lateral view

Humerus

Medial epicondyle

Capitulum

Trochlea

Head

Neck

Tuberosity

Radius

Tuberosity

Coronoid process

Trochlear notch

Olecranon

Ulna

In 90° flexion: medial view

Anteroposterior radiograph

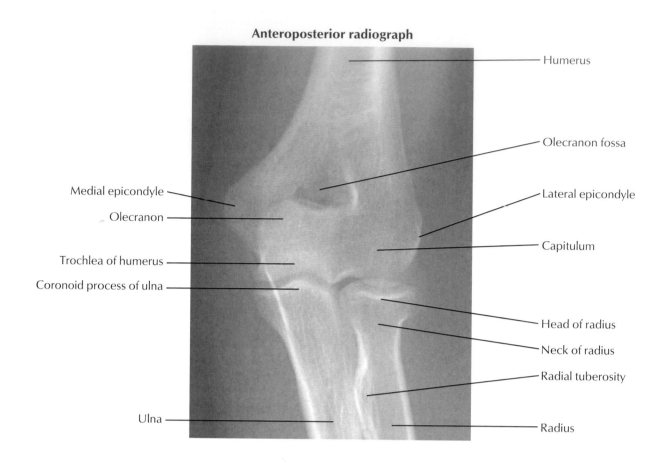

Humerus

Olecranon fossa

Medial epicondyle

Lateral epicondyle

Olecranon

Capitulum

Trochlea of humerus

Coronoid process of ulna

Head of radius

Neck of radius

Radial tuberosity

Ulna

Radius

Lateral radiograph

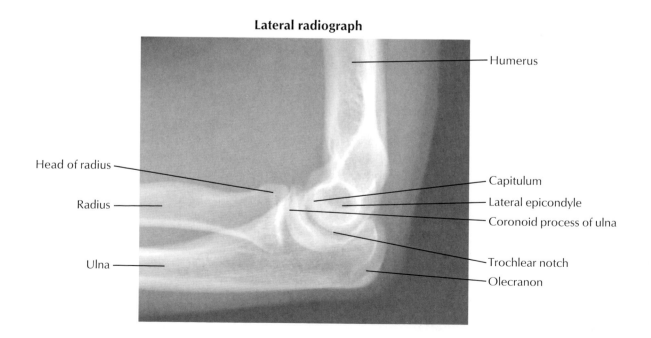

Humerus

Head of radius

Capitulum

Radius

Lateral epicondyle

Coronoid process of ulna

Ulna

Trochlear notch

Olecranon

Plate 425

Elbow and Forearm

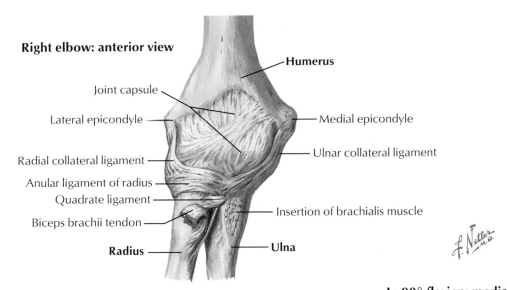

Right elbow: anterior view

Humerus

Joint capsule

Lateral epicondyle

Medial epicondyle

Radial collateral ligament

Ulnar collateral ligament

Anular ligament of radius

Quadrate ligament

Insertion of brachialis muscle

Biceps brachii tendon

Ulna

Radius

F. Netter M.D.

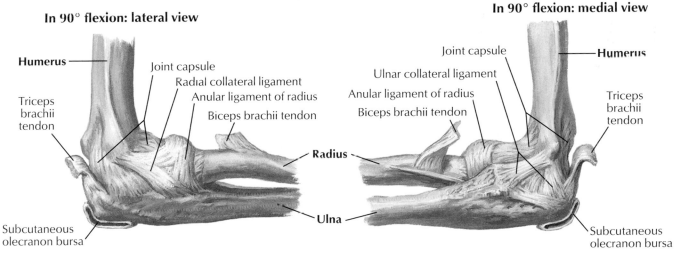

In 90° flexion: lateral view

Humerus

Joint capsule

Radial collateral ligament

Anular ligament of radius

Biceps brachii tendon

Triceps brachii tendon

Radius

Ulna

Subcutaneous olecranon bursa

In 90° flexion: medial view

Joint capsule

Humerus

Ulnar collateral ligament

Anular ligament of radius

Biceps brachii tendon

Triceps brachii tendon

Subcutaneous olecranon bursa

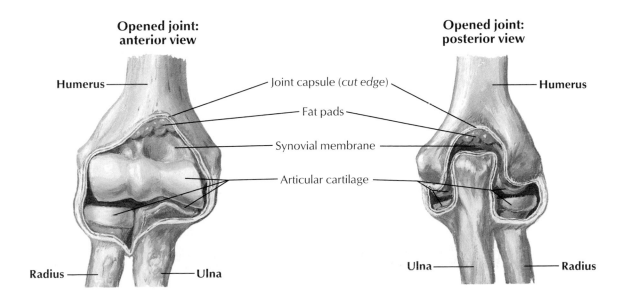

Opened joint: anterior view

Humerus

Joint capsule (*cut edge*)

Fat pads

Synovial membrane

Articular cartilage

Radius

Ulna

Opened joint: posterior view

Humerus

Ulna

Radius

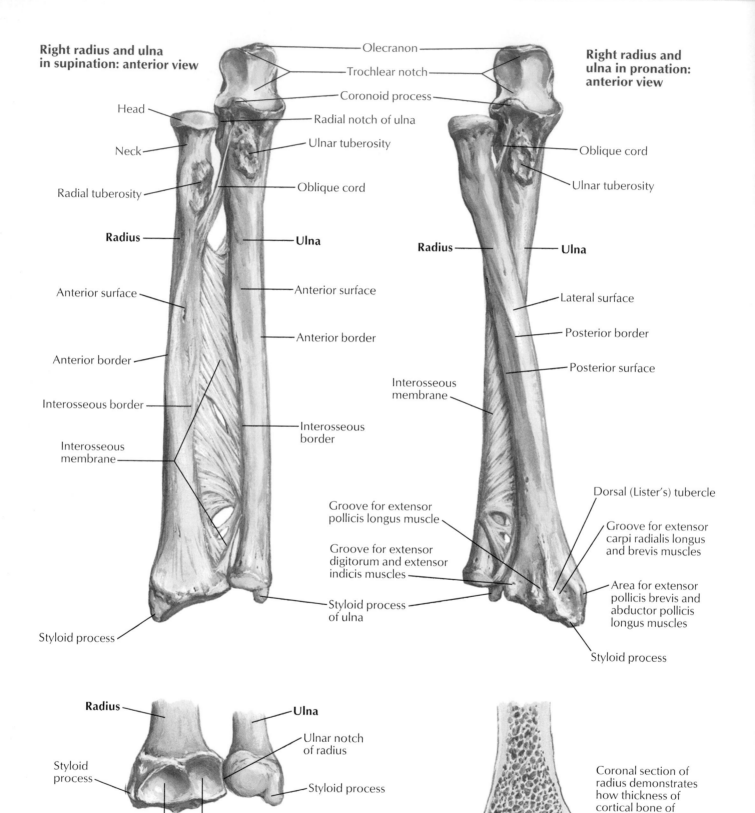

Right radius and ulna
in supination: anterior view

Olecranon

Trochlear notch

Coronoid process

Right radius and
ulna in pronation:
anterior view

Head

Radial notch of ulna

Neck

Ulnar tuberosity

Oblique cord

Radial tuberosity

Oblique cord

Ulnar tuberosity

Radius

Ulna

Radius

Ulna

Anterior surface

Anterior surface

Lateral surface

Anterior border

Posterior border

Anterior border

Interosseous
membrane

Posterior surface

Interosseous border

Interosseous
border

Interosseous
membrane

Dorsal (Lister's) tubercle

Groove for extensor
pollicis longus muscle

Groove for extensor
carpi radialis longus
and brevis muscles

Groove for extensor
digitorum and extensor
indicis muscles

Area for extensor
pollicis brevis and
abductor pollicis
longus muscles

Styloid process
of ulna

Styloid process

Styloid process

Radius

Ulna

Styloid
process

Ulnar notch
of radius

Styloid process

Articulation with
scaphoid bone

Articulation with
lunate bone

Coronal section of
radius demonstrates
how thickness of
cortical bone of
shaft diminishes
to thin layer over
cancellous bone
at distal end

Carpal articular surface

F. Netter M.D.

Plate 427

Elbow and Forearm

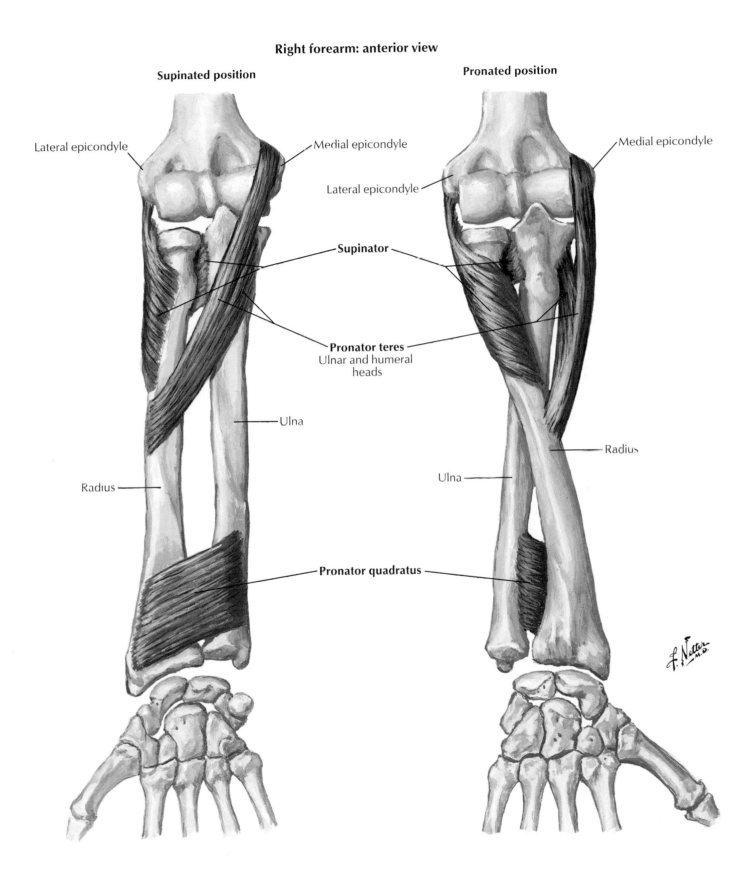

Right forearm: anterior view

Supinated position

Lateral epicondyle

Medial epicondyle

Supinator

Pronator teres
Ulnar and humeral heads

Ulna

Radius

Pronator quadratus

Pronated position

Medial epicondyle

Lateral epicondyle

Radius

Ulna

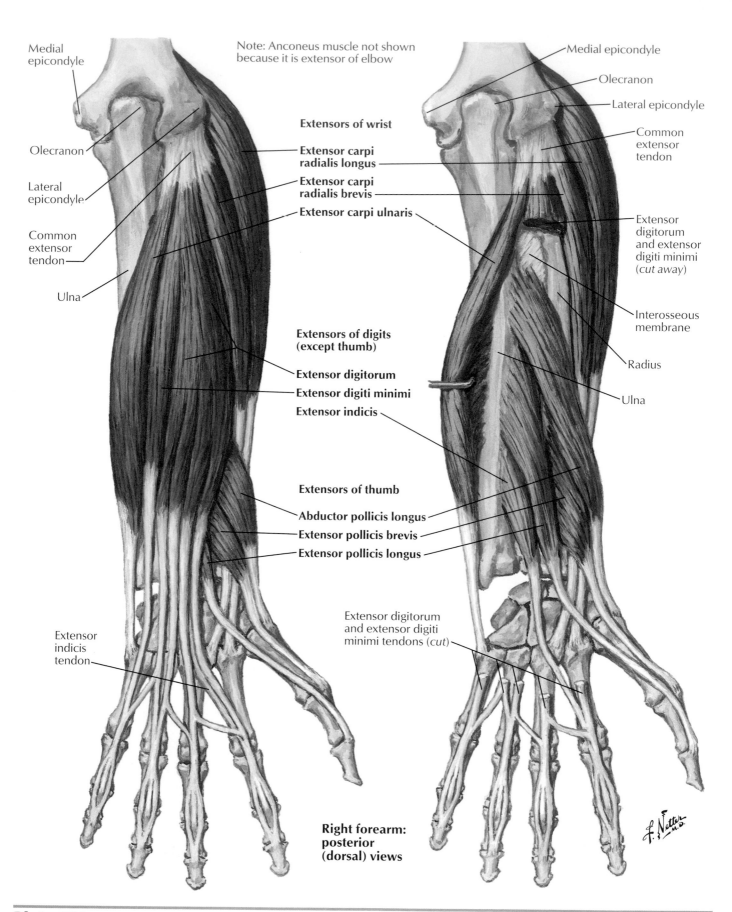

Medial epicondyle

Note: Anconeus muscle not shown because it is extensor of elbow

Medial epicondyle

Olecranon

Lateral epicondyle

Olecranon

Common extensor tendon

Extensors of wrist

Lateral epicondyle

Extensor carpi radialis longus

Common extensor tendon

Extensor carpi radialis brevis

Extensor digitorum and extensor digiti minimi (*cut away*)

Common extensor tendon

Extensor carpi ulnaris

Ulna

Interosseous membrane

Extensors of digits (except thumb)

Radius

Extensor digitorum

Extensor digiti minimi

Ulna

Extensor indicis

Extensors of thumb

Abductor pollicis longus

Extensor pollicis brevis

Extensor pollicis longus

Extensor digitorum and extensor digiti minimi tendons (*cut*)

Extensor indicis tendon

Right forearm: posterior (dorsal) views

f. Netter
M.D.

Plate 429

Elbow and Forearm

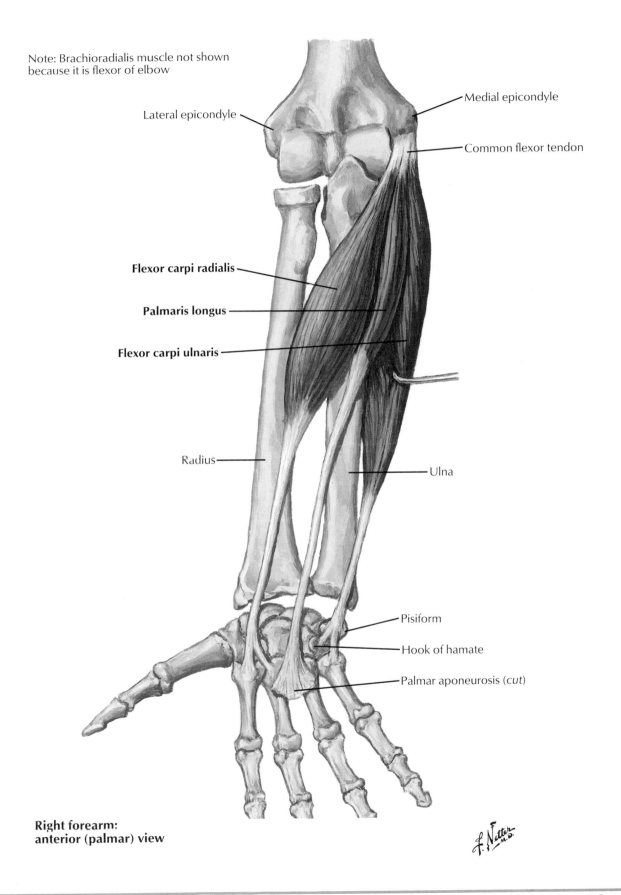

Note: Brachioradialis muscle not shown because it is flexor of elbow

Lateral epicondyle

Medial epicondyle

Common flexor tendon

Flexor carpi radialis

Palmaris longus

Flexor carpi ulnaris

Radius

Ulna

Pisiform

Hook of hamate

Palmar aponeurosis (*cut*)

**Right forearm:
anterior (palmar) view**

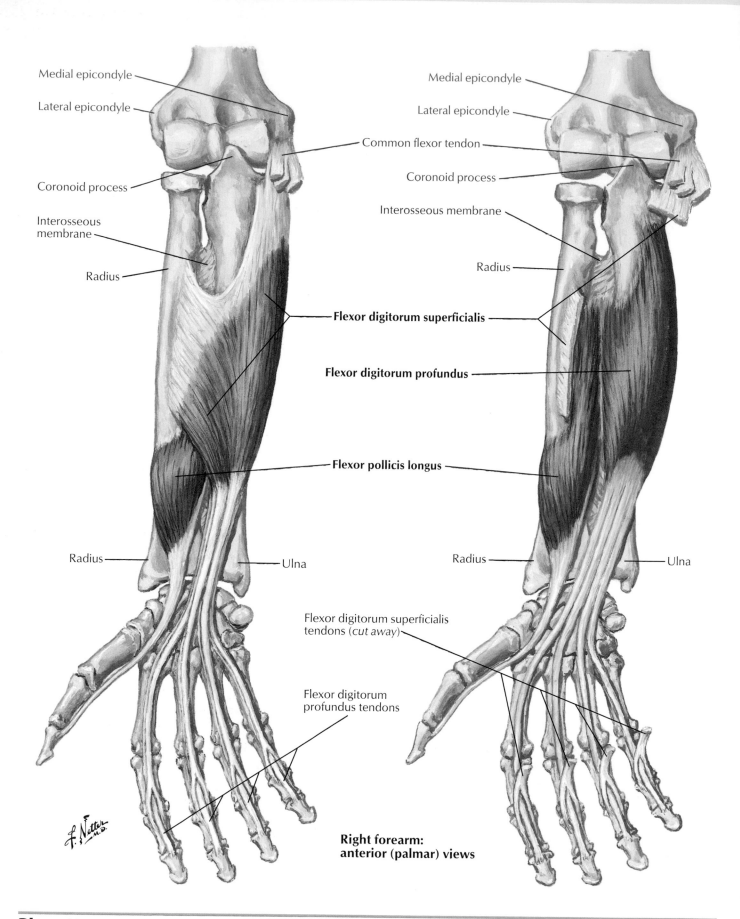

Medial epicondyle

Lateral epicondyle

Coronoid process

Interosseous membrane

Radius

Medial epicondyle

Lateral epicondyle

Common flexor tendon

Coronoid process

Interosseous membrane

Radius

Flexor digitorum superficialis

Flexor digitorum profundus

Flexor pollicis longus

Radius

Ulna

Radius

Ulna

Flexor digitorum superficialis tendons (*cut away*)

Flexor digitorum profundus tendons

Right forearm: anterior (palmar) views

Plate 431

Elbow and Forearm

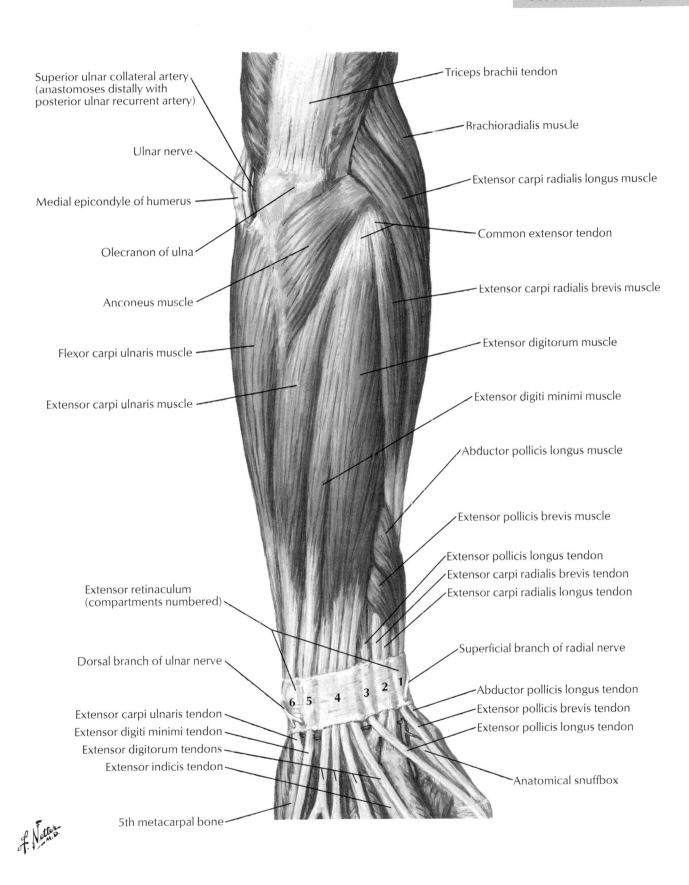

Superior ulnar collateral artery (anastomoses distally with posterior ulnar recurrent artery)

Triceps brachii tendon

Brachioradialis muscle

Ulnar nerve

Extensor carpi radialis longus muscle

Medial epicondyle of humerus

Common extensor tendon

Olecranon of ulna

Extensor carpi radialis brevis muscle

Anconeus muscle

Extensor digitorum muscle

Flexor carpi ulnaris muscle

Extensor digiti minimi muscle

Extensor carpi ulnaris muscle

Abductor pollicis longus muscle

Extensor pollicis brevis muscle

Extensor pollicis longus tendon
Extensor carpi radialis brevis tendon
Extensor carpi radialis longus tendon

Extensor retinaculum (compartments numbered)

Superficial branch of radial nerve

Dorsal branch of ulnar nerve

6 5   4   3   2 1

Abductor pollicis longus tendon
Extensor pollicis brevis tendon
Extensor pollicis longus tendon

Extensor carpi ulnaris tendon
Extensor digiti minimi tendon
Extensor digitorum tendons
Extensor indicis tendon

Anatomical snuffbox

5th metacarpal bone

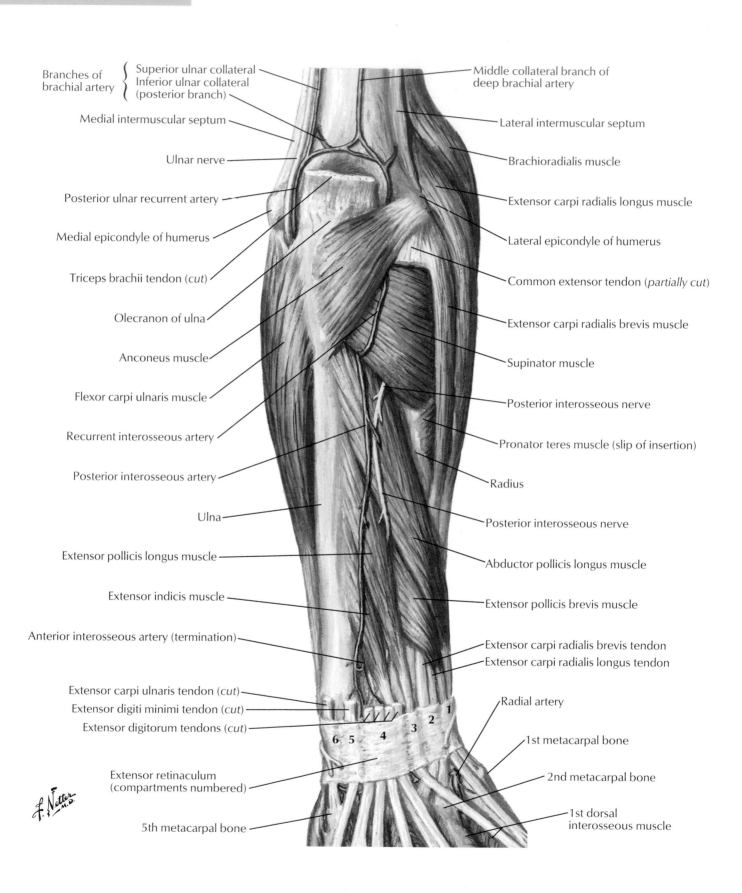

Branches of brachial artery {
Superior ulnar collateral
Inferior ulnar collateral (posterior branch)

Middle collateral branch of deep brachial artery

Medial intermuscular septum

Lateral intermuscular septum

Ulnar nerve

Brachioradialis muscle

Posterior ulnar recurrent artery

Extensor carpi radialis longus muscle

Medial epicondyle of humerus

Lateral epicondyle of humerus

Triceps brachii tendon (*cut*)

Common extensor tendon (*partially cut*)

Olecranon of ulna

Extensor carpi radialis brevis muscle

Anconeus muscle

Supinator muscle

Flexor carpi ulnaris muscle

Posterior interosseous nerve

Recurrent interosseous artery

Pronator teres muscle (slip of insertion)

Posterior interosseous artery

Radius

Ulna

Posterior interosseous nerve

Extensor pollicis longus muscle

Abductor pollicis longus muscle

Extensor indicis muscle

Extensor pollicis brevis muscle

Anterior interosseous artery (termination)

Extensor carpi radialis brevis tendon
Extensor carpi radialis longus tendon

Extensor carpi ulnaris tendon (*cut*)
Extensor digiti minimi tendon (*cut*)
Extensor digitorum tendons (*cut*)

Radial artery

1st metacarpal bone

Extensor retinaculum (compartments numbered)

2nd metacarpal bone

1st dorsal interosseous muscle

5th metacarpal bone

Plate 433

Elbow and Forearm

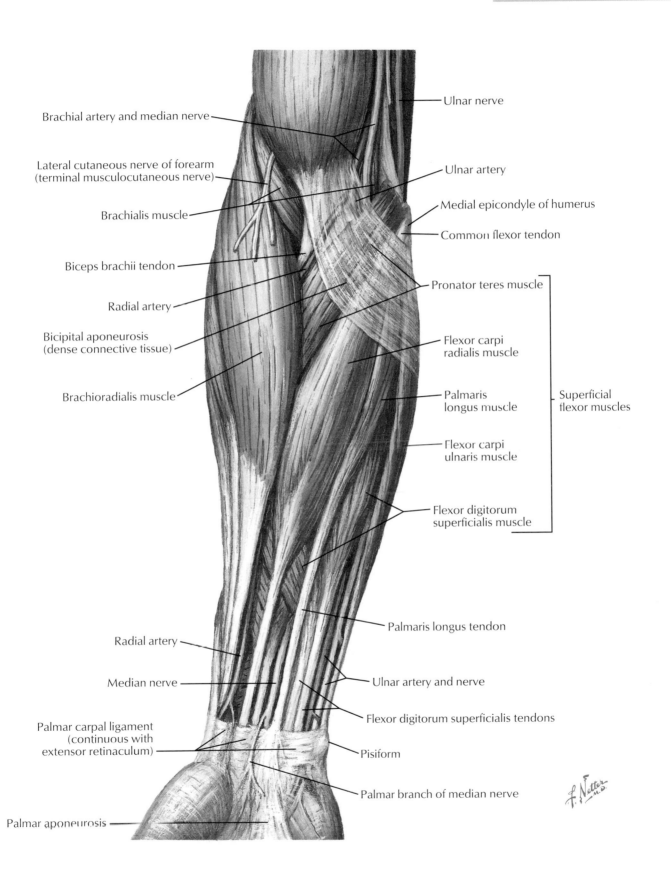

Brachial artery and median nerve

Lateral cutaneous nerve of forearm (terminal musculocutaneous nerve)

Brachialis muscle

Biceps brachii tendon

Radial artery

Bicipital aponeurosis (dense connective tissue)

Brachioradialis muscle

Radial artery

Median nerve

Palmar carpal ligament (continuous with extensor retinaculum)

Palmar aponeurosis

Ulnar nerve

Ulnar artery

Medial epicondyle of humerus

Common flexor tendon

Pronator teres muscle

Flexor carpi radialis muscle

Palmaris longus muscle

Flexor carpi ulnaris muscle

Flexor digitorum superficialis muscle

Superficial flexor muscles

Palmaris longus tendon

Ulnar artery and nerve

Flexor digitorum superficialis tendons

Pisiform

Palmar branch of median nerve

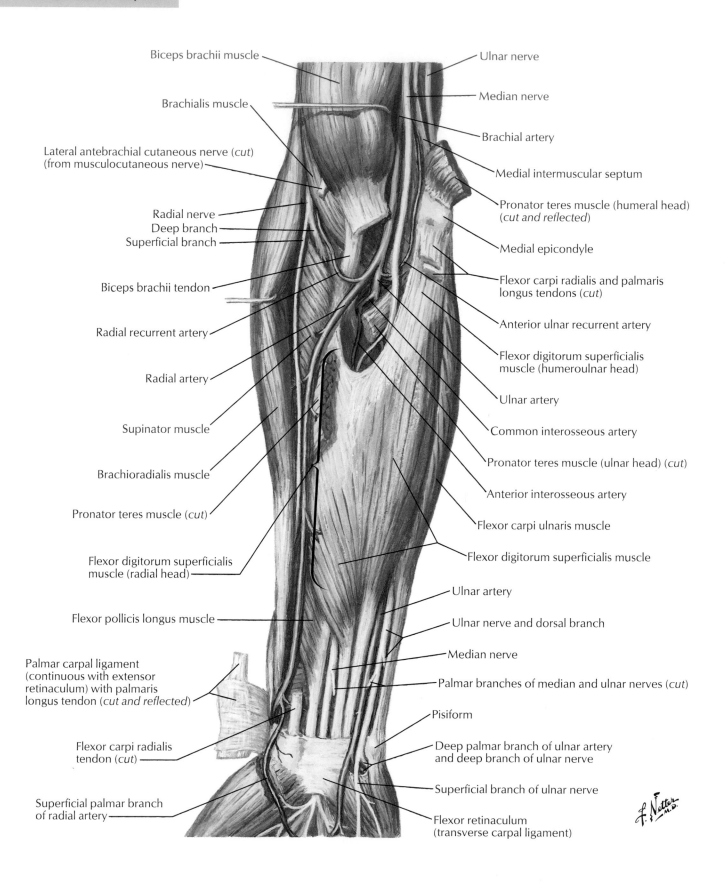

Biceps brachii muscle

Brachialis muscle

Lateral antebrachial cutaneous nerve (cut)
(from musculocutaneous nerve)

Radial nerve
Deep branch
Superficial branch

Biceps brachii tendon

Radial recurrent artery

Radial artery

Supinator muscle

Brachioradialis muscle

Pronator teres muscle (cut)

Flexor digitorum superficialis
muscle (radial head)

Flexor pollicis longus muscle

Palmar carpal ligament
(continuous with extensor
retinaculum) with palmaris
longus tendon (cut and reflected)

Flexor carpi radialis
tendon (cut)

Superficial palmar branch
of radial artery

Ulnar nerve

Median nerve

Brachial artery

Medial intermuscular septum

Pronator teres muscle (humeral head)
(cut and reflected)

Medial epicondyle

Flexor carpi radialis and palmaris
longus tendons (cut)

Anterior ulnar recurrent artery

Flexor digitorum superficialis
muscle (humeroulnar head)

Ulnar artery

Common interosseous artery

Pronator teres muscle (ulnar head) (cut)

Anterior interosseous artery

Flexor carpi ulnaris muscle

Flexor digitorum superficialis muscle

Ulnar artery

Ulnar nerve and dorsal branch

Median nerve

Palmar branches of median and ulnar nerves (cut)

Pisiform

Deep palmar branch of ulnar artery
and deep branch of ulnar nerve

Superficial branch of ulnar nerve

Flexor retinaculum
(transverse carpal ligament)

Plate 435   **Elbow and Forearm**

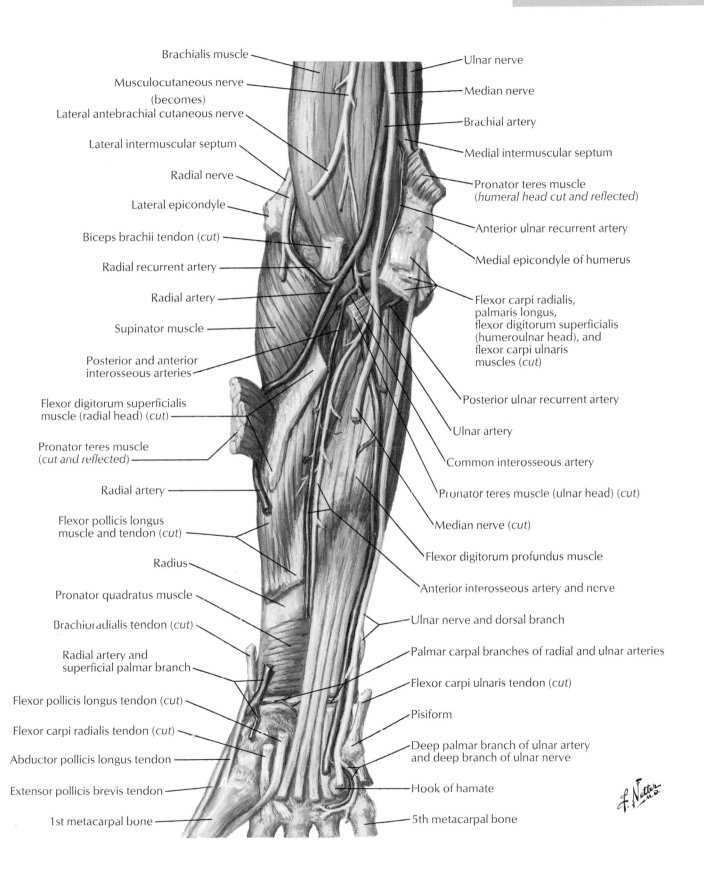

Brachialis muscle

Musculocutaneous nerve (becomes)

Lateral antebrachial cutaneous nerve

Lateral intermuscular septum

Radial nerve

Lateral epicondyle

Biceps brachii tendon (cut)

Radial recurrent artery

Radial artery

Supinator muscle

Posterior and anterior interosseous arteries

Flexor digitorum superficialis muscle (radial head) (cut)

Pronator teres muscle (cut and reflected)

Radial artery

Flexor pollicis longus muscle and tendon (cut)

Radius

Pronator quadratus muscle

Brachioradialis tendon (cut)

Radial artery and superficial palmar branch

Flexor pollicis longus tendon (cut)

Flexor carpi radialis tendon (cut)

Abductor pollicis longus tendon

Extensor pollicis brevis tendon

1st metacarpal bone

Ulnar nerve

Median nerve

Brachial artery

Medial intermuscular septum

Pronator teres muscle (humeral head cut and reflected)

Anterior ulnar recurrent artery

Medial epicondyle of humerus

Flexor carpi radialis, palmaris longus, flexor digitorum superficialis (humeroulnar head), and flexor carpi ulnaris muscles (cut)

Posterior ulnar recurrent artery

Ulnar artery

Common interosseous artery

Pronator teres muscle (ulnar head) (cut)

Median nerve (cut)

Flexor digitorum profundus muscle

Anterior interosseous artery and nerve

Ulnar nerve and dorsal branch

Palmar carpal branches of radial and ulnar arteries

Flexor carpi ulnaris tendon (cut)

Pisiform

Deep palmar branch of ulnar artery and deep branch of ulnar nerve

Hook of hamate

5th metacarpal bone

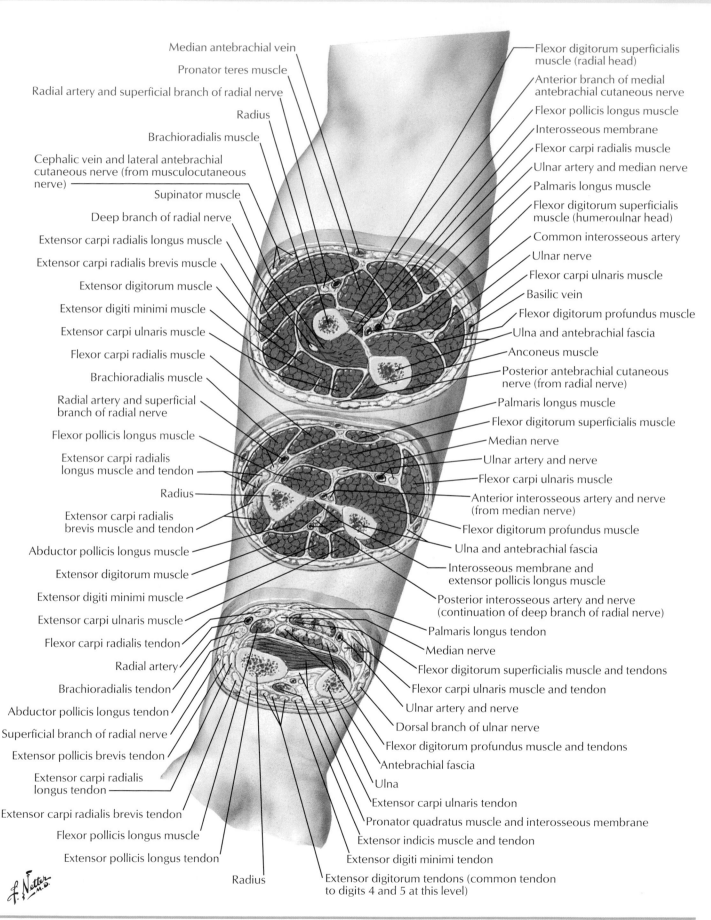

Median antebrachial vein

Pronator teres muscle

Radial artery and superficial branch of radial nerve

Radius

Brachioradialis muscle

Cephalic vein and lateral antebrachial cutaneous nerve (from musculocutaneous nerve)

Supinator muscle

Deep branch of radial nerve

Extensor carpi radialis longus muscle

Extensor carpi radialis brevis muscle

Extensor digitorum muscle

Extensor digiti minimi muscle

Extensor carpi ulnaris muscle

Flexor carpi radialis muscle

Brachioradialis muscle

Radial artery and superficial branch of radial nerve

Flexor pollicis longus muscle

Extensor carpi radialis longus muscle and tendon

Radius

Extensor carpi radialis brevis muscle and tendon

Abductor pollicis longus muscle

Extensor digitorum muscle

Extensor digiti minimi muscle

Extensor carpi ulnaris muscle

Flexor carpi radialis tendon

Radial artery

Brachioradialis tendon

Abductor pollicis longus tendon

Superficial branch of radial nerve

Extensor pollicis brevis tendon

Extensor carpi radialis longus tendon

Extensor carpi radialis brevis tendon

Flexor pollicis longus muscle

Extensor pollicis longus tendon

Radius

Flexor digitorum superficialis muscle (radial head)

Anterior branch of medial antebrachial cutaneous nerve

Flexor pollicis longus muscle

Interosseous membrane

Flexor carpi radialis muscle

Ulnar artery and median nerve

Palmaris longus muscle

Flexor digitorum superficialis muscle (humeroulnar head)

Common interosseous artery

Ulnar nerve

Flexor carpi ulnaris muscle

Basilic vein

Flexor digitorum profundus muscle

Ulna and antebrachial fascia

Anconeus muscle

Posterior antebrachial cutaneous nerve (from radial nerve)

Palmaris longus muscle

Flexor digitorum superficialis muscle

Median nerve

Ulnar artery and nerve

Flexor carpi ulnaris muscle

Anterior interosseous artery and nerve (from median nerve)

Flexor digitorum profundus muscle

Ulna and antebrachial fascia

Interosseous membrane and extensor pollicis longus muscle

Posterior interosseous artery and nerve (continuation of deep branch of radial nerve)

Palmaris longus tendon

Median nerve

Flexor digitorum superficialis muscle and tendons

Flexor carpi ulnaris muscle and tendon

Ulnar artery and nerve

Dorsal branch of ulnar nerve

Flexor digitorum profundus muscle and tendons

Antebrachial fascia

Ulna

Extensor carpi ulnaris tendon

Pronator quadratus muscle and interosseous membrane

Extensor indicis muscle and tendon

Extensor digiti minimi tendon

Extensor digitorum tendons (common tendon to digits 4 and 5 at this level)

F. Netter M.D.

Plate 437 **Elbow and Forearm**

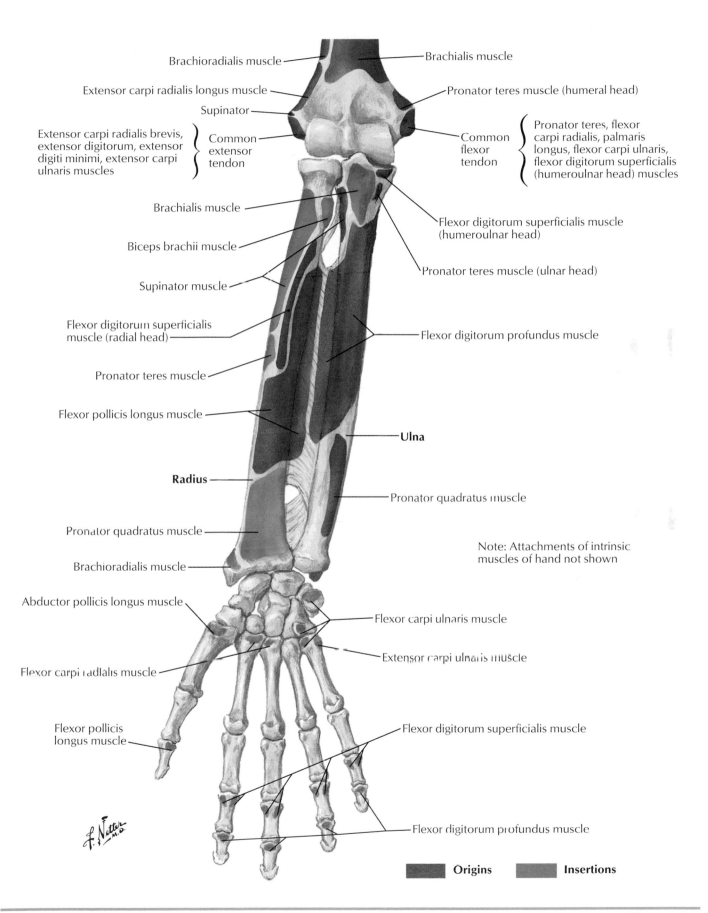

Brachioradialis muscle

Extensor carpi radialis longus muscle

Supinator

Extensor carpi radialis brevis, extensor digitorum, extensor digiti minimi, extensor carpi ulnaris muscles

Common extensor tendon

Brachialis muscle

Biceps brachii muscle

Supinator muscle

Flexor digitorum superficialis muscle (radial head)

Pronator teres muscle

Flexor pollicis longus muscle

Radius

Pronator quadratus muscle

Brachioradialis muscle

Abductor pollicis longus muscle

Flexor carpi radialis muscle

Flexor pollicis longus muscle

Brachialis muscle

Pronator teres muscle (humeral head)

Common flexor tendon

Pronator teres, flexor carpi radialis, palmaris longus, flexor carpi ulnaris, flexor digitorum superficialis (humeroulnar head) muscles

Flexor digitorum superficialis muscle (humeroulnar head)

Pronator teres muscle (ulnar head)

Flexor digitorum profundus muscle

Ulna

Pronator quadratus muscle

Note: Attachments of intrinsic muscles of hand not shown

Flexor carpi ulnaris muscle

Extensor carpi ulnaris muscle

Flexor digitorum superficialis muscle

Flexor digitorum profundus muscle

Origins   Insertions

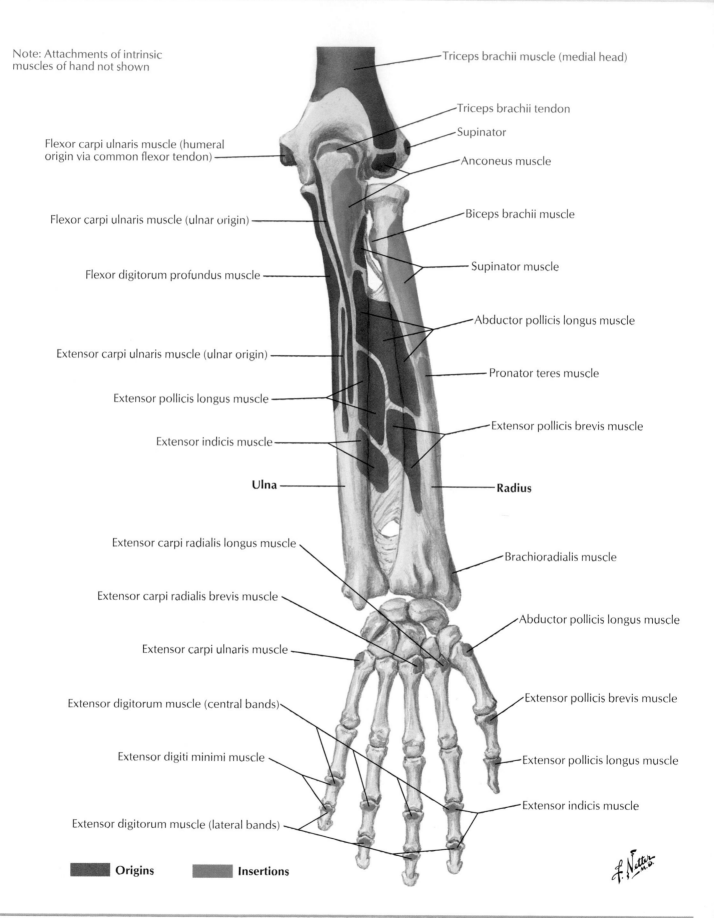

Note: Attachments of intrinsic muscles of hand not shown

Triceps brachii muscle (medial head)

Triceps brachii tendon

Supinator

Flexor carpi ulnaris muscle (humeral origin via common flexor tendon)

Anconeus muscle

Flexor carpi ulnaris muscle (ulnar origin)

Biceps brachii muscle

Supinator muscle

Flexor digitorum profundus muscle

Abductor pollicis longus muscle

Extensor carpi ulnaris muscle (ulnar origin)

Pronator teres muscle

Extensor pollicis longus muscle

Extensor pollicis brevis muscle

Extensor indicis muscle

Ulna

Radius

Extensor carpi radialis longus muscle

Brachioradialis muscle

Extensor carpi radialis brevis muscle

Abductor pollicis longus muscle

Extensor carpi ulnaris muscle

Extensor pollicis brevis muscle

Extensor digitorum muscle (central bands)

Extensor pollicis longus muscle

Extensor digiti minimi muscle

Extensor indicis muscle

Extensor digitorum muscle (lateral bands)

Origins   Insertions

Plate 439

Elbow and Forearm

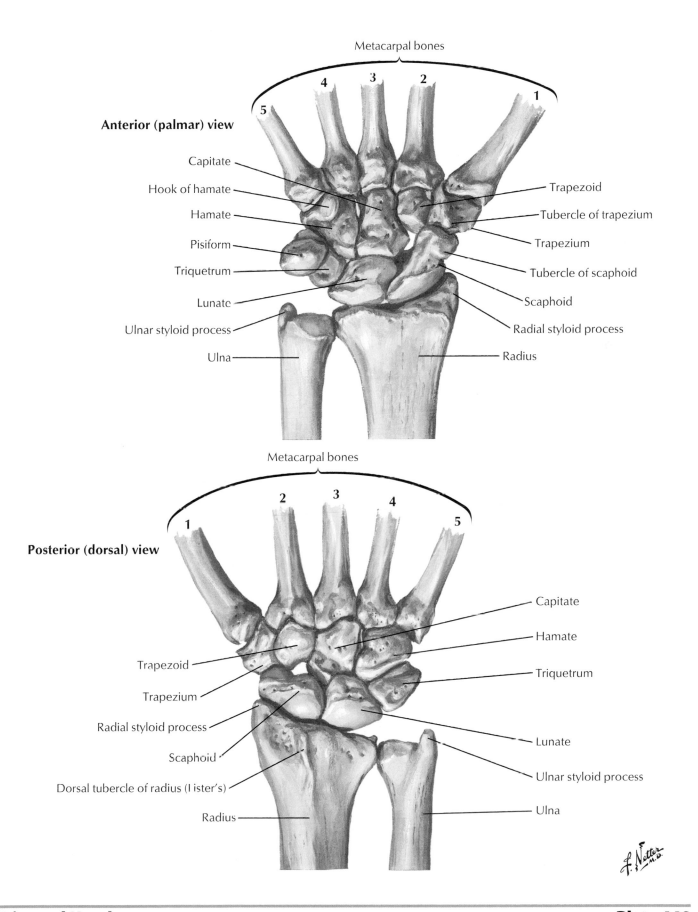

Metacarpal bones

4   3   2

5   1

Anterior (palmar) view

Capitate
Hook of hamate
Hamate
Pisiform
Triquetrum
Lunate
Ulnar styloid process
Ulna

Trapezoid
Tubercle of trapezium
Trapezium
Tubercle of scaphoid
Scaphoid
Radial styloid process
Radius

Metacarpal bones

2   3   4

1   5

Posterior (dorsal) view

Trapezoid
Trapezium
Radial styloid process
Scaphoid
Dorsal tubercle of radius (Lister's)
Radius

Capitate
Hamate
Triquetrum
Lunate
Ulnar styloid process
Ulna

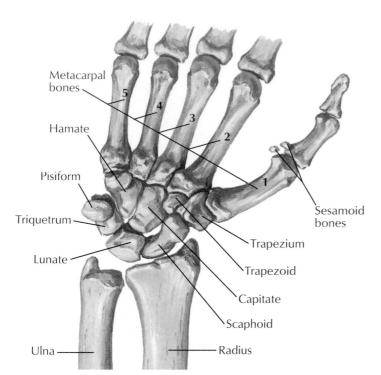

Metacarpal bones

5

4

3

2

Hamate

Pisiform

Triquetrum

Lunate

Ulna

Radius

1

Sesamoid bones

Trapezium

Trapezoid

Capitate

Scaphoid

Position of carpal bones with hand in abduction: anterior (palmar) view

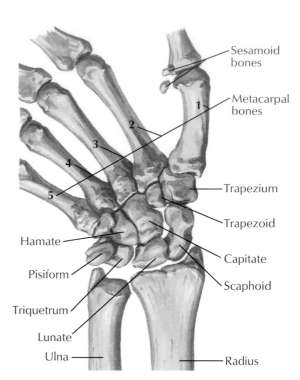

Sesamoid bones

Metacarpal bones

1

2

3

4

5

Trapezium

Trapezoid

Capitate

Scaphoid

Hamate

Pisiform

Triquetrum

Lunate

Ulna

Radius

Position of carpal bones with hand in adduction: anterior (palmar) view

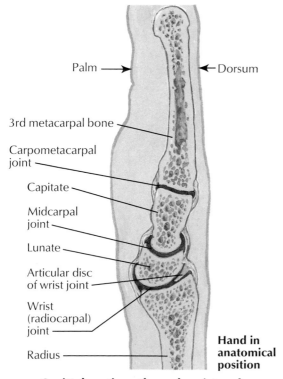

Palm

Dorsum

3rd metacarpal bone

Carpometacarpal joint

Capitate

Midcarpal joint

Lunate

Articular disc of wrist joint

Wrist (radiocarpal) joint

Radius

Hand in anatomical position

Sagittal sections through wrist and middle finger

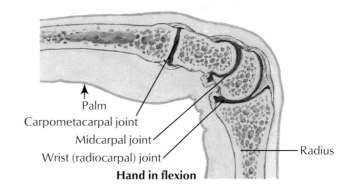

Palm

Carpometacarpal joint

Midcarpal joint

Wrist (radiocarpal) joint

Radius

Hand in flexion

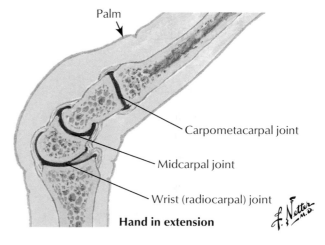

Palm

Carpometacarpal joint

Midcarpal joint

Wrist (radiocarpal) joint

Hand in extension

Plate 441

Wrist and Hand

Carpal tunnel: palmar view

Metacarpal bones

5 4 3 2 1

Hook of hamate

Deep palmar branch of ulnar artery and deep branch of ulnar nerve

Pisiform

Flexor digitorum superficialis tendons

Flexor digitorum profundus tendons

Flexor carpi ulnaris tendon

Ulnar artery and nerve

Interosseous membrane

Ulna

Flexor retinaculum (transverse carpal ligament)

Tubercle of trapezium

Tubercle of scaphoid

Palmar aponeurosis

Median nerve

Flexor pollicis longus tendon

Flexor carpi radialis tendon

Radial artery and superficial palmar branch

Palmar carpal ligament (thickening of deep antebrachial fascia) (*cut and reflected*)

Palmaris longus tendon

Radius

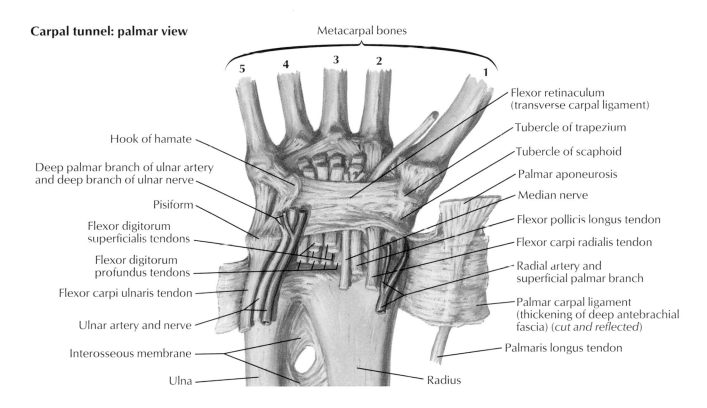

Flexor retinaculum removed: palmar view

Metacarpal bones

5 4 3 2 1

Palmar metacarpal ligaments

Hook of hamate

Pisohamate ligament

Pisometacarpal ligament

Lunate

Pisiform

Flexor carpi ulnaris tendon (*cut*)

Ulnar collateral ligament

Palmar ulno-carpal ligament { Ulnotriquetral part
{ Ulnolunate part

Area of articular disc

Palmar radioulnar ligament

Ulna

Palmar carpometacarpal ligaments

Capitotriquetral ligament (part of radiate capitate ligament)

Capitate

Articular capsule of carpometacarpal joint of thumb

Tubercle of trapezium

Tubercle of scaphoid

Radial collateral ligament

Space (of Poirier)

Radiocapitate part }
Radioscapholunate part } Palmar radiocarpal ligament

Interosseous membrane

Radius

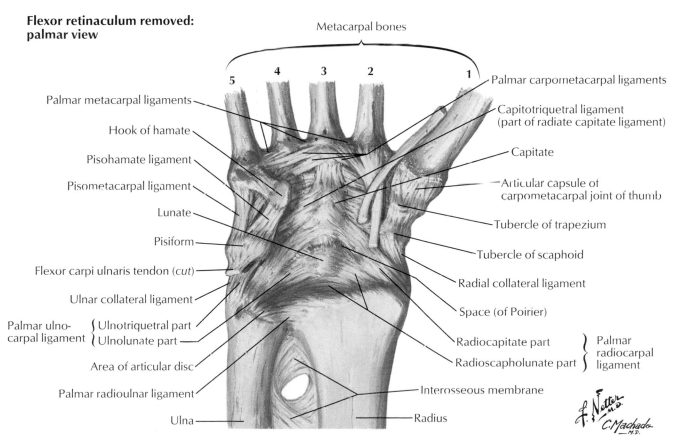

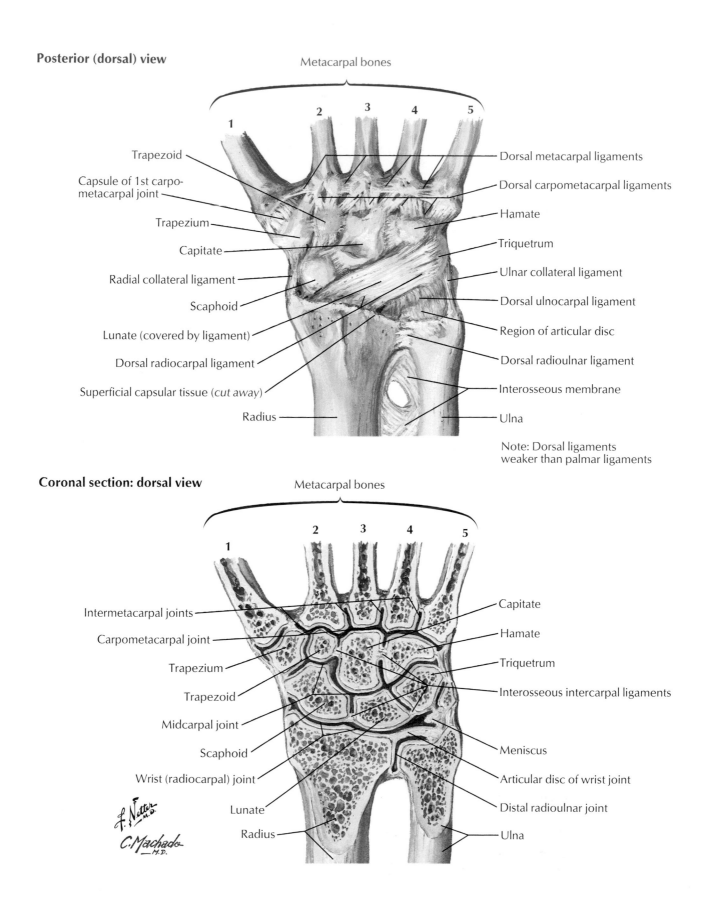

Posterior (dorsal) view

Metacarpal bones

1   2   3   4   5

Trapezoid

Capsule of 1st carpo-metacarpal joint

Trapezium

Capitate

Radial collateral ligament

Scaphoid

Lunate (covered by ligament)

Dorsal radiocarpal ligament

Superficial capsular tissue (*cut away*)

Radius

Dorsal metacarpal ligaments

Dorsal carpometacarpal ligaments

Hamate

Triquetrum

Ulnar collateral ligament

Dorsal ulnocarpal ligament

Region of articular disc

Dorsal radioulnar ligament

Interosseous membrane

Ulna

Note: Dorsal ligaments weaker than palmar ligaments

Coronal section: dorsal view

Metacarpal bones

1   2   3   4   5

Intermetacarpal joints

Carpometacarpal joint

Trapezium

Trapezoid

Midcarpal joint

Scaphoid

Wrist (radiocarpal) joint

Lunate

Radius

Capitate

Hamate

Triquetrum

Interosseous intercarpal ligaments

Meniscus

Articular disc of wrist joint

Distal radioulnar joint

Ulna

Plate 443   **Wrist and Hand**

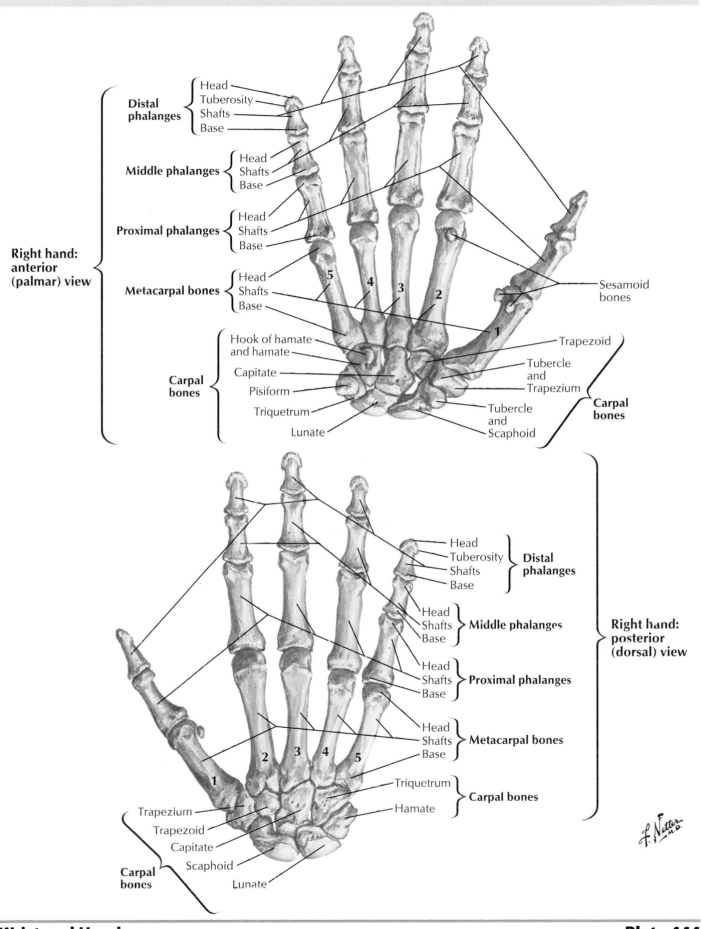

Head
Tuberosity
Shafts
Base
Distal phalanges

Head
Shafts
Base
Middle phalanges

Head
Shafts
Base
Proximal phalanges

Head
Shafts
Base
Metacarpal bones

Right hand: anterior (palmar) view

5   4   3   2   1

Hook of hamate and hamate
Capitate
Pisiform
Triquetrum
Lunate
Carpal bones

Sesamoid bones

Trapezoid
Tubercle and Trapezium
Tubercle and Scaphoid
Carpal bones

Head
Tuberosity
Shafts
Base
Distal phalanges

Head
Shafts
Base
Middle phalanges

Head
Shafts
Base
Proximal phalanges

Head
Shafts
Base
Metacarpal bones

Right hand: posterior (dorsal) view

1   2   3   4   5

Triquetrum
Hamate
Carpal bones

Trapezium
Trapezoid
Capitate
Scaphoid
Lunate
Carpal bones

Anteroposterior view

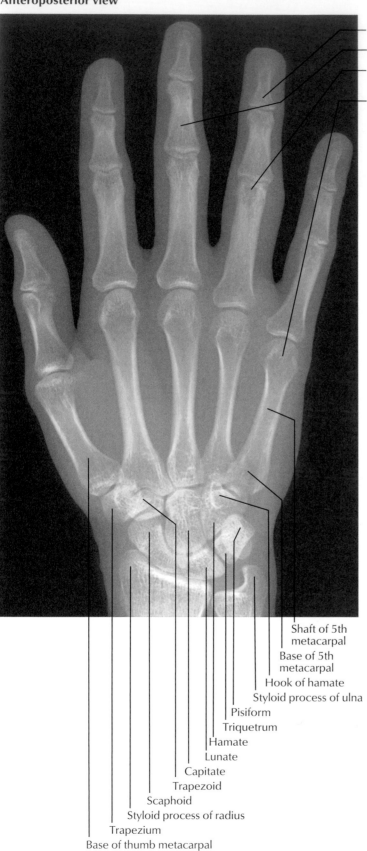

- Distal phalanx of ring finger
- Middle phalanx of middle finger
- Head of proximal phalanx
- Head of 5th metacarpal

Shaft of 5th metacarpal
Base of 5th metacarpal
Hook of hamate
Styloid process of ulna
Pisiform
Triquetrum
Hamate
Lunate
Capitate
Trapezoid
Scaphoid
Styloid process of radius
Trapezium
Base of thumb metacarpal

Lateral view

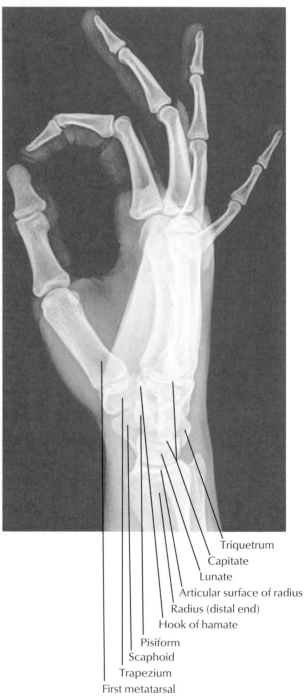

Triquetrum
Capitate
Lunate
Articular surface of radius
Radius (distal end)
Hook of hamate
Pisiform
Scaphoid
Trapezium
First metatarsal

Plate 445

Wrist and Hand

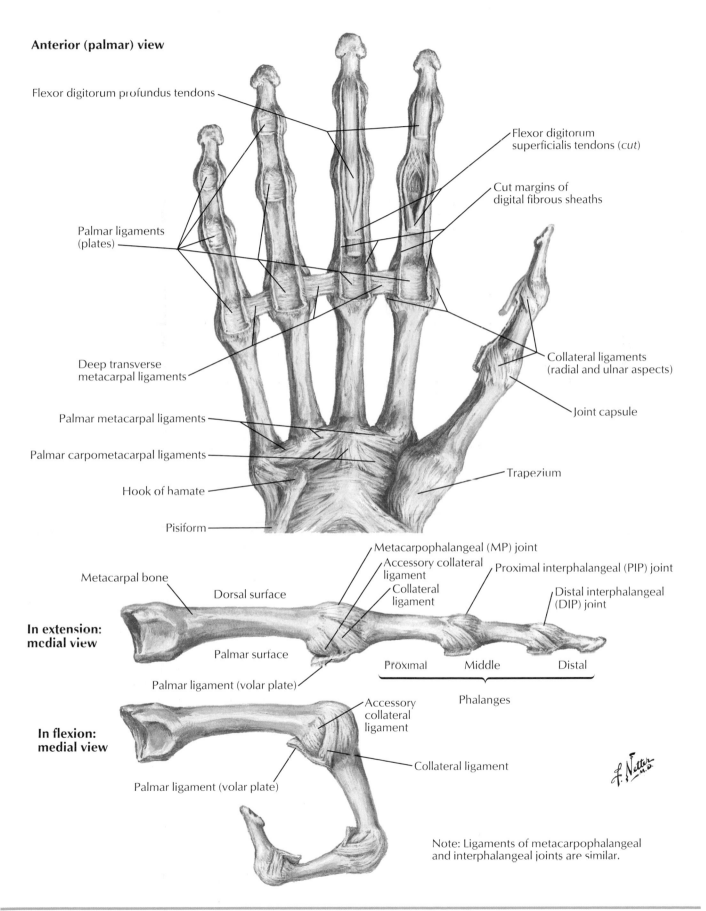

Anterior (palmar) view

Flexor digitorum profundus tendons

Flexor digitorum superficialis tendons (*cut*)

Cut margins of digital fibrous sheaths

Palmar ligaments (plates)

Collateral ligaments (radial and ulnar aspects)

Deep transverse metacarpal ligaments

Joint capsule

Palmar metacarpal ligaments

Palmar carpometacarpal ligaments

Trapezium

Hook of hamate

Pisiform

Metacarpophalangeal (MP) joint

Accessory collateral ligament

Proximal interphalangeal (PIP) joint

Collateral ligament

Distal interphalangeal (DIP) joint

Metacarpal bone

Dorsal surface

In extension: medial view

Palmar surface

Proximal   Middle   Distal

Palmar ligament (volar plate)

Phalanges

Accessory collateral ligament

In flexion: medial view

Collateral ligament

Palmar ligament (volar plate)

Note: Ligaments of metacarpophalangeal and interphalangeal joints are similar.

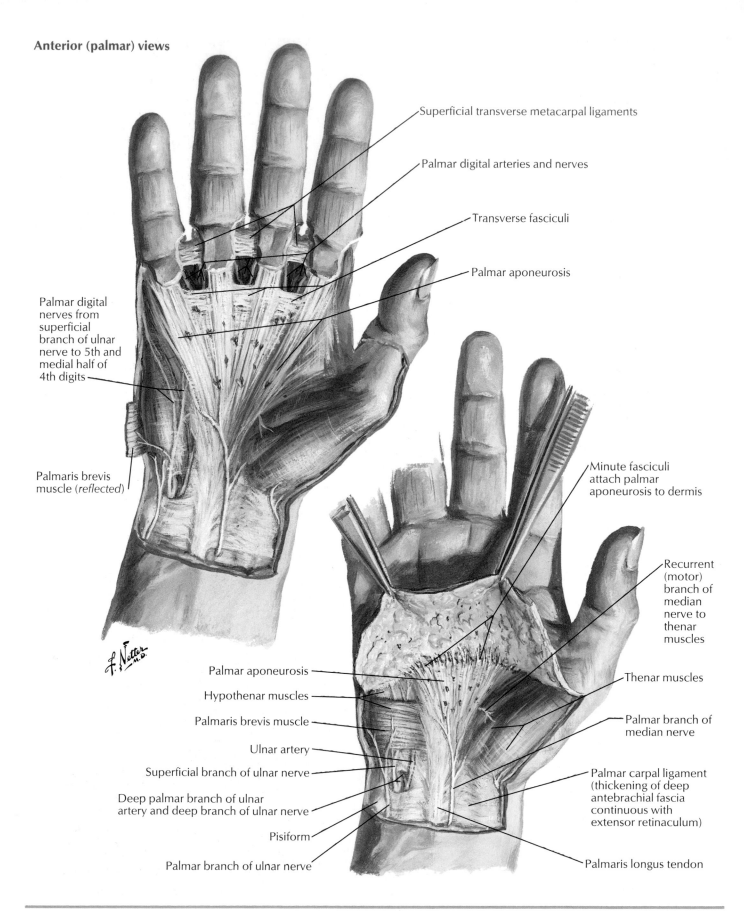

Anterior (palmar) views

Superficial transverse metacarpal ligaments

Palmar digital arteries and nerves

Transverse fasciculi

Palmar aponeurosis

Palmar digital nerves from superficial branch of ulnar nerve to 5th and medial half of 4th digits

Palmaris brevis muscle (*reflected*)

Minute fasciculi attach palmar aponeurosis to dermis

Recurrent (motor) branch of median nerve to thenar muscles

Thenar muscles

Palmar branch of median nerve

Palmar carpal ligament (thickening of deep antebrachial fascia continuous with extensor retinaculum)

Palmaris longus tendon

Palmar aponeurosis

Hypothenar muscles

Palmaris brevis muscle

Ulnar artery

Superficial branch of ulnar nerve

Deep palmar branch of ulnar artery and deep branch of ulnar nerve

Pisiform

Palmar branch of ulnar nerve

Plate 447   **Wrist and Hand**

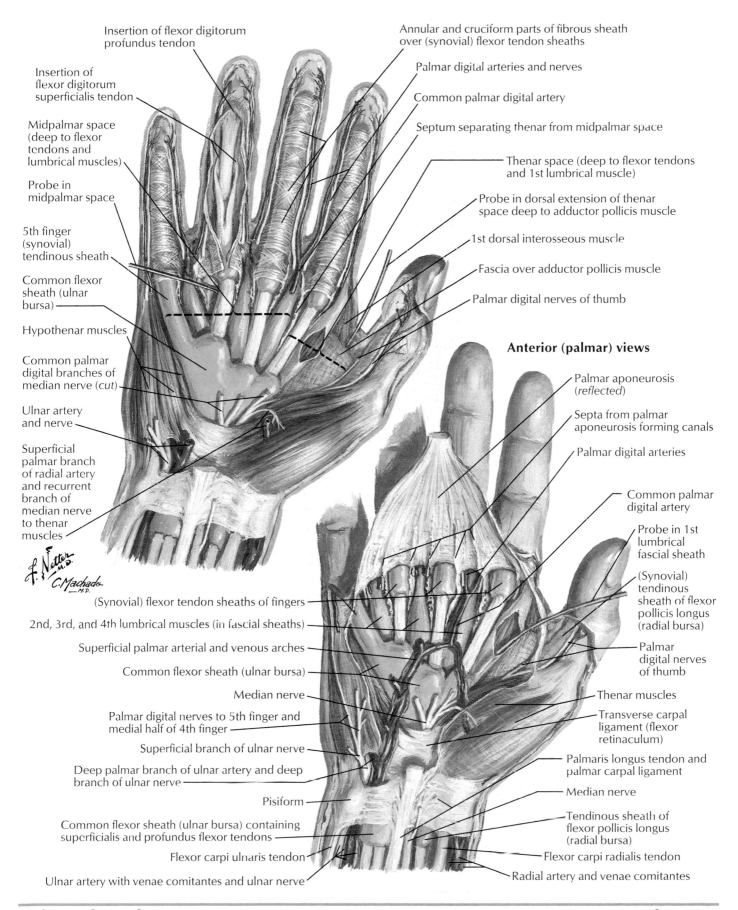

Insertion of flexor digitorum profundus tendon

Insertion of flexor digitorum superficialis tendon

Midpalmar space (deep to flexor tendons and lumbrical muscles)

Probe in midpalmar space

5th finger (synovial) tendinous sheath

Common flexor sheath (ulnar bursa)

Hypothenar muscles

Common palmar digital branches of median nerve (cut)

Ulnar artery and nerve

Superficial palmar branch of radial artery and recurrent branch of median nerve to thenar muscles

Annular and cruciform parts of fibrous sheath over (synovial) flexor tendon sheaths

Palmar digital arteries and nerves

Common palmar digital artery

Septum separating thenar from midpalmar space

Thenar space (deep to flexor tendons and 1st lumbrical muscle)

Probe in dorsal extension of thenar space deep to adductor pollicis muscle

1st dorsal interosseous muscle

Fascia over adductor pollicis muscle

Palmar digital nerves of thumb

Anterior (palmar) views

Palmar aponeurosis (reflected)

Septa from palmar aponeurosis forming canals

Palmar digital arteries

Common palmar digital artery

Probe in 1st lumbrical fascial sheath

(Synovial) tendinous sheath of flexor pollicis longus (radial bursa)

Palmar digital nerves of thumb

Thenar muscles

Transverse carpal ligament (flexor retinaculum)

Palmaris longus tendon and palmar carpal ligament

Median nerve

Tendinous sheath of flexor pollicis longus (radial bursa)

Flexor carpi radialis tendon

Radial artery and venae comitantes

(Synovial) flexor tendon sheaths of fingers

2nd, 3rd, and 4th lumbrical muscles (in fascial sheaths)

Superficial palmar arterial and venous arches

Common flexor sheath (ulnar bursa)

Median nerve

Palmar digital nerves to 5th finger and medial half of 4th finger

Superficial branch of ulnar nerve

Deep palmar branch of ulnar artery and deep branch of ulnar nerve

Pisiform

Common flexor sheath (ulnar bursa) containing superficialis and profundus flexor tendons

Flexor carpi ulnaris tendon

Ulnar artery with venae comitantes and ulnar nerve

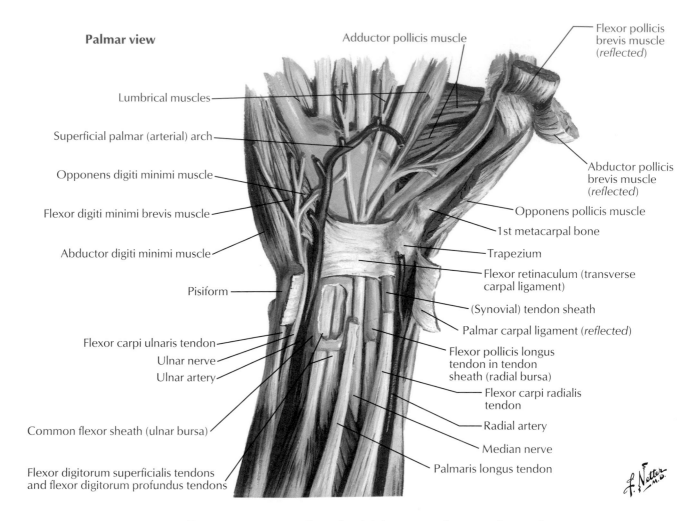

Palmar view

Adductor pollicis muscle

Flexor pollicis brevis muscle (*reflected*)

Lumbrical muscles

Superficial palmar (arterial) arch

Opponens digiti minimi muscle

Flexor digiti minimi brevis muscle

Abductor digiti minimi muscle

Pisiform

Flexor carpi ulnaris tendon

Ulnar nerve

Ulnar artery

Common flexor sheath (ulnar bursa)

Flexor digitorum superficialis tendons and flexor digitorum profundus tendons

Abductor pollicis brevis muscle (*reflected*)

Opponens pollicis muscle

1st metacarpal bone

Trapezium

Flexor retinaculum (transverse carpal ligament)

(Synovial) tendon sheath

Palmar carpal ligament (*reflected*)

Flexor pollicis longus tendon in tendon sheath (radial bursa)

Flexor carpi radialis tendon

Radial artery

Median nerve

Palmaris longus tendon

Transverse cross section of wrist demonstrating carpal tunnel

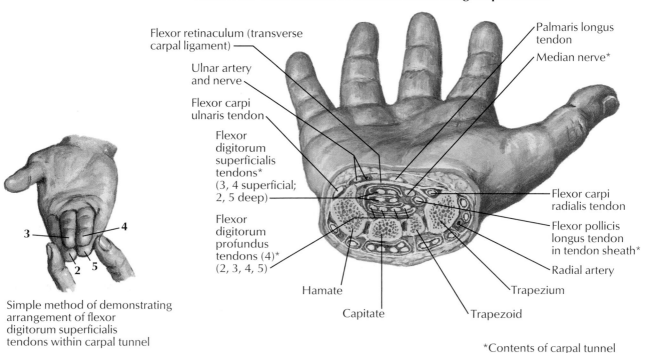

Flexor retinaculum (transverse carpal ligament)

Ulnar artery and nerve

Flexor carpi ulnaris tendon

Flexor digitorum superficialis tendons* (3, 4 superficial; 2, 5 deep)

Flexor digitorum profundus tendons (4)* (2, 3, 4, 5)

Palmaris longus tendon

Median nerve*

Flexor carpi radialis tendon

Flexor pollicis longus tendon in tendon sheath*

Radial artery

Trapezium

Trapezoid

Capitate

Hamate

Simple method of demonstrating arrangement of flexor digitorum superficialis tendons within carpal tunnel

*Contents of carpal tunnel

3 4

2 5

Plate 449　　　　　　　　　　　　　　　　　　　　　　　　**Wrist and Hand**

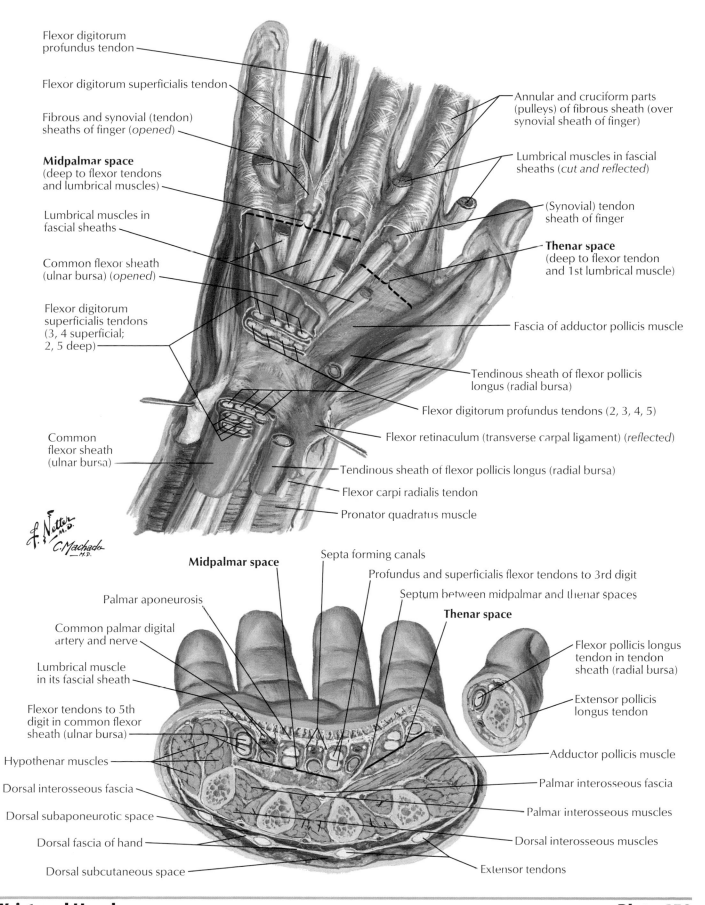

Flexor digitorum profundus tendon

Flexor digitorum superficialis tendon

Fibrous and synovial (tendon) sheaths of finger (*opened*)

Midpalmar space (deep to flexor tendons and lumbrical muscles)

Lumbrical muscles in fascial sheaths

Common flexor sheath (ulnar bursa) (*opened*)

Flexor digitorum superficialis tendons (3, 4 superficial; 2, 5 deep)

Common flexor sheath (ulnar bursa)

Annular and cruciform parts (pulleys) of fibrous sheath (over synovial sheath of finger)

Lumbrical muscles in fascial sheaths (*cut and reflected*)

(Synovial) tendon sheath of finger

Thenar space (deep to flexor tendon and 1st lumbrical muscle)

Fascia of adductor pollicis muscle

Tendinous sheath of flexor pollicis longus (radial bursa)

Flexor digitorum profundus tendons (2, 3, 4, 5)

Flexor retinaculum (transverse carpal ligament) (*reflected*)

Tendinous sheath of flexor pollicis longus (radial bursa)

Flexor carpi radialis tendon

Pronator quadratus muscle

Midpalmar space

Palmar aponeurosis

Common palmar digital artery and nerve

Lumbrical muscle in its fascial sheath

Flexor tendons to 5th digit in common flexor sheath (ulnar bursa)

Hypothenar muscles

Dorsal interosseous fascia

Dorsal subaponeurotic space

Dorsal fascia of hand

Dorsal subcutaneous space

Septa forming canals

Profundus and superficialis flexor tendons to 3rd digit

Septum between midpalmar and thenar spaces

Thenar space

Flexor pollicis longus tendon in tendon sheath (radial bursa)

Extensor pollicis longus tendon

Adductor pollicis muscle

Palmar interosseous fascia

Palmar interosseous muscles

Dorsal interosseous muscles

Extensor tendons

Lumbrical Muscles and Bursae, Spaces, and Sheaths: Schema

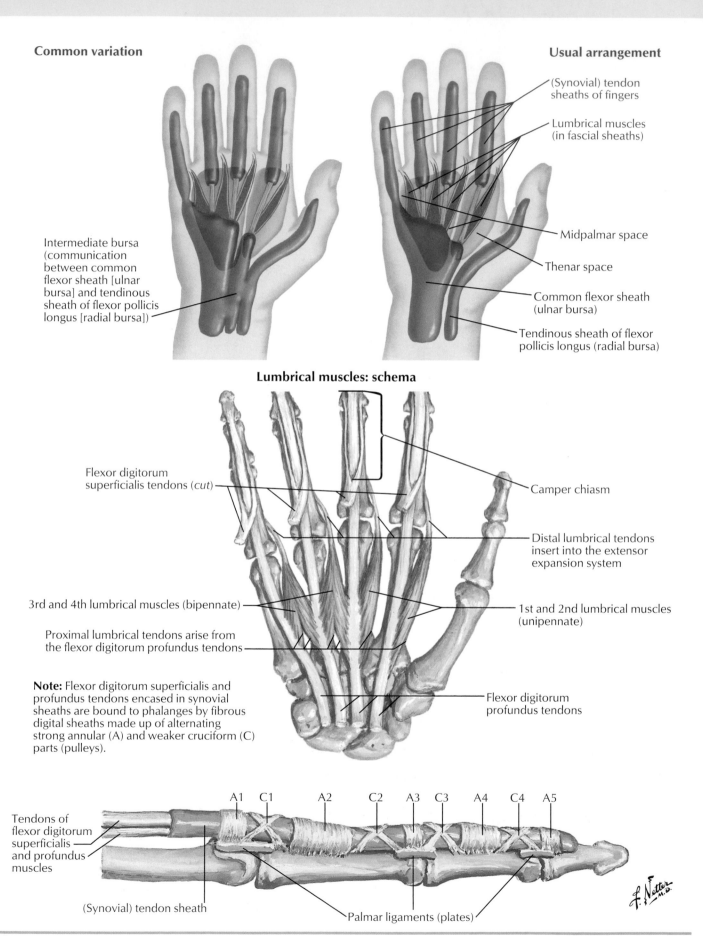

Common variation

Usual arrangement

(Synovial) tendon sheaths of fingers

Lumbrical muscles (in fascial sheaths)

Intermediate bursa (communication between common flexor sheath [ulnar bursa] and tendinous sheath of flexor pollicis longus [radial bursa])

Midpalmar space

Thenar space

Common flexor sheath (ulnar bursa)

Tendinous sheath of flexor pollicis longus (radial bursa)

Lumbrical muscles: schema

Flexor digitorum superficialis tendons (*cut*)

Camper chiasm

Distal lumbrical tendons insert into the extensor expansion system

3rd and 4th lumbrical muscles (bipennate)

1st and 2nd lumbrical muscles (unipennate)

Proximal lumbrical tendons arise from the flexor digitorum profundus tendons

Note: Flexor digitorum superficialis and profundus tendons encased in synovial sheaths are bound to phalanges by fibrous digital sheaths made up of alternating strong annular (A) and weaker cruciform (C) parts (pulleys).

Flexor digitorum profundus tendons

A1   C1   A2   C2   A3   C3   A4   C4   A5

Tendons of flexor digitorum superficialis and profundus muscles

(Synovial) tendon sheath

Palmar ligaments (plates)

F. Netter M.D.

Plate 451

Wrist and Hand

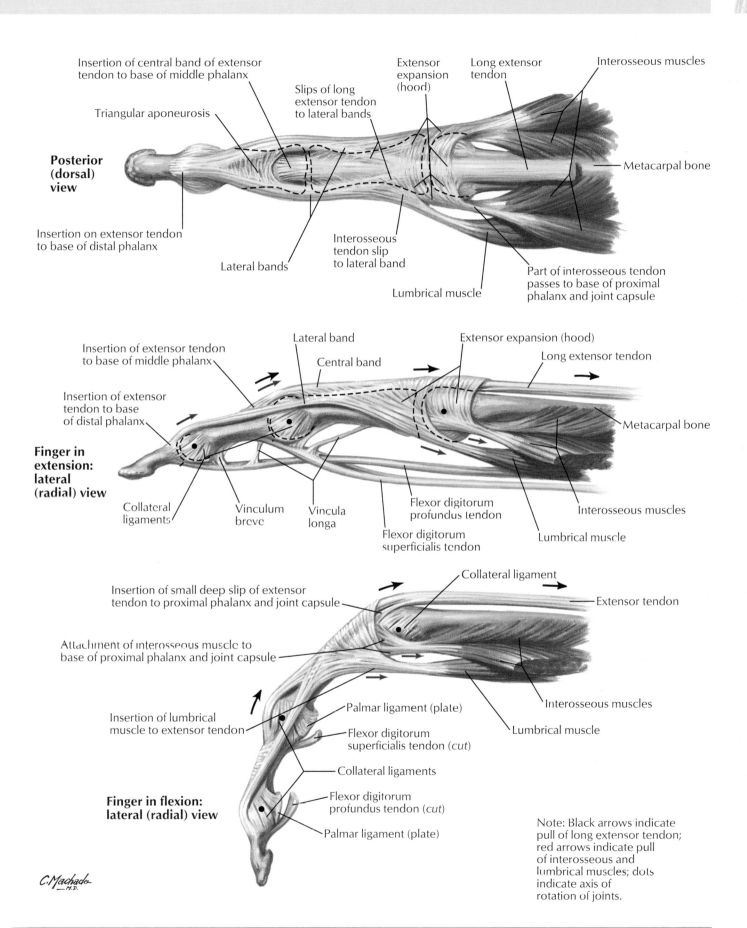

Posterior (dorsal) view

Insertion of central band of extensor tendon to base of middle phalanx

Triangular aponeurosis

Slips of long extensor tendon to lateral bands

Extensor expansion (hood)

Long extensor tendon

Interosseous muscles

Metacarpal bone

Insertion on extensor tendon to base of distal phalanx

Interosseous tendon slip to lateral band

Lateral bands

Lumbrical muscle

Part of interosseous tendon passes to base of proximal phalanx and joint capsule

Finger in extension: lateral (radial) view

Insertion of extensor tendon to base of middle phalanx

Lateral band

Central band

Extensor expansion (hood)

Long extensor tendon

Insertion of extensor tendon to base of distal phalanx

Metacarpal bone

Collateral ligaments

Vinculum breve

Vincula longa

Flexor digitorum profundus tendon

Interosseous muscles

Flexor digitorum superficialis tendon

Lumbrical muscle

Finger in flexion: lateral (radial) view

Insertion of small deep slip of extensor tendon to proximal phalanx and joint capsule

Collateral ligament

Extensor tendon

Attachment of interosseous muscle to base of proximal phalanx and joint capsule

Insertion of lumbrical muscle to extensor tendon

Palmar ligament (plate)

Flexor digitorum superficialis tendon (cut)

Collateral ligaments

Flexor digitorum profundus tendon (cut)

Palmar ligament (plate)

Interosseous muscles

Lumbrical muscle

Note: Black arrows indicate pull of long extensor tendon; red arrows indicate pull of interosseous and lumbrical muscles; dots indicate axis of rotation of joints.

C. Machado —M.D.

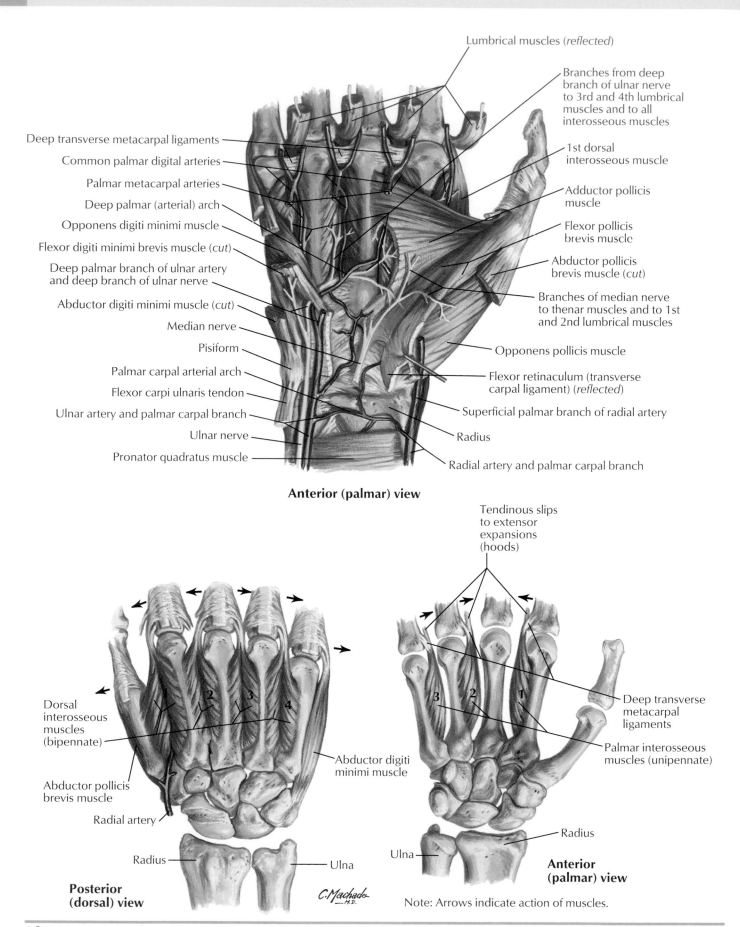

Lumbrical muscles (*reflected*)

Branches from deep branch of ulnar nerve to 3rd and 4th lumbrical muscles and to all interosseous muscles

Deep transverse metacarpal ligaments

Common palmar digital arteries

Palmar metacarpal arteries

Deep palmar (arterial) arch

Opponens digiti minimi muscle

Flexor digiti minimi brevis muscle (*cut*)

Deep palmar branch of ulnar artery and deep branch of ulnar nerve

Abductor digiti minimi muscle (*cut*)

Median nerve

Pisiform

Palmar carpal arterial arch

Flexor carpi ulnaris tendon

Ulnar artery and palmar carpal branch

Ulnar nerve

Pronator quadratus muscle

1st dorsal interosseous muscle

Adductor pollicis muscle

Flexor pollicis brevis muscle

Abductor pollicis brevis muscle (*cut*)

Branches of median nerve to thenar muscles and to 1st and 2nd lumbrical muscles

Opponens pollicis muscle

Flexor retinaculum (transverse carpal ligament) (*reflected*)

Superficial palmar branch of radial artery

Radius

Radial artery and palmar carpal branch

Anterior (palmar) view

Tendinous slips to extensor expansions (hoods)

Dorsal interosseous muscles (bipennate)

Abductor pollicis brevis muscle

Radial artery

Radius

Ulna

Abductor digiti minimi muscle

Deep transverse metacarpal ligaments

Palmar interosseous muscles (unipennate)

Radius

Ulna

Posterior (dorsal) view

Anterior (palmar) view

Note: Arrows indicate action of muscles.

C. Machado M.D.

Plate 453 **Wrist and Hand**

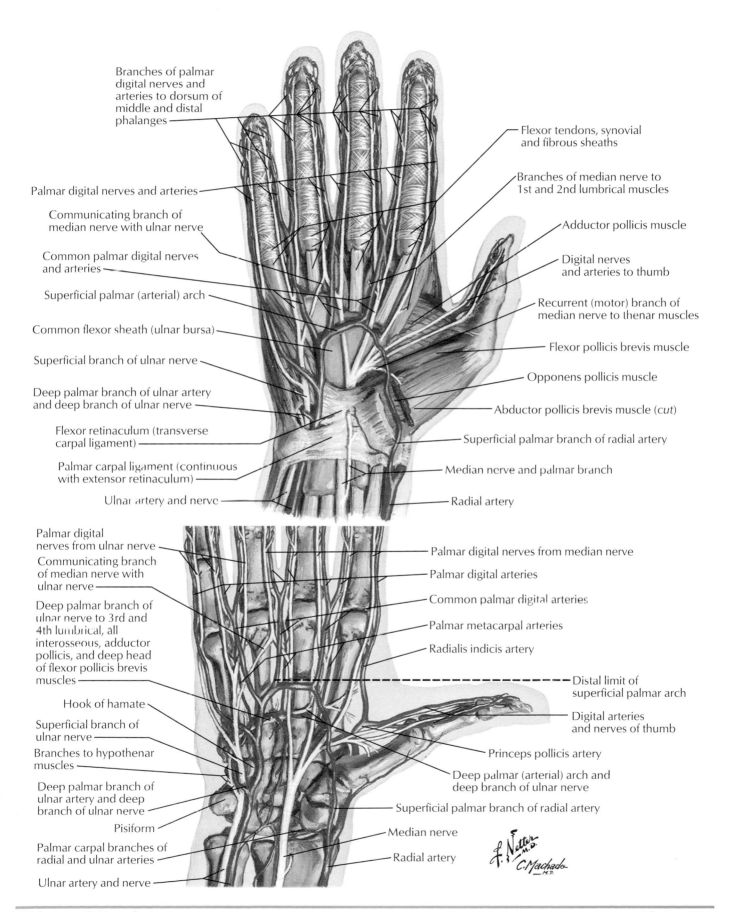

Branches of palmar digital nerves and arteries to dorsum of middle and distal phalanges

Palmar digital nerves and arteries

Communicating branch of median nerve with ulnar nerve

Common palmar digital nerves and arteries

Superficial palmar (arterial) arch

Common flexor sheath (ulnar bursa)

Superficial branch of ulnar nerve

Deep palmar branch of ulnar artery and deep branch of ulnar nerve

Flexor retinaculum (transverse carpal ligament)

Palmar carpal ligament (continuous with extensor retinaculum)

Ulnar artery and nerve

Flexor tendons, synovial and fibrous sheaths

Branches of median nerve to 1st and 2nd lumbrical muscles

Adductor pollicis muscle

Digital nerves and arteries to thumb

Recurrent (motor) branch of median nerve to thenar muscles

Flexor pollicis brevis muscle

Opponens pollicis muscle

Abductor pollicis brevis muscle (cut)

Superficial palmar branch of radial artery

Median nerve and palmar branch

Radial artery

Palmar digital nerves from ulnar nerve

Communicating branch of median nerve with ulnar nerve

Deep palmar branch of ulnar nerve to 3rd and 4th lumbrical, all interosseous, adductor pollicis, and deep head of flexor pollicis brevis muscles

Hook of hamate

Superficial branch of ulnar nerve

Branches to hypothenar muscles

Deep palmar branch of ulnar artery and deep branch of ulnar nerve

Pisiform

Palmar carpal branches of radial and ulnar arteries

Ulnar artery and nerve

Palmar digital nerves from median nerve

Palmar digital arteries

Common palmar digital arteries

Palmar metacarpal arteries

Radialis indicis artery

Distal limit of superficial palmar arch

Digital arteries and nerves of thumb

Princeps pollicis artery

Deep palmar (arterial) arch and deep branch of ulnar nerve

Superficial palmar branch of radial artery

Median nerve

Radial artery

Wrist and Hand

Plate 454

Lateral (radial) view

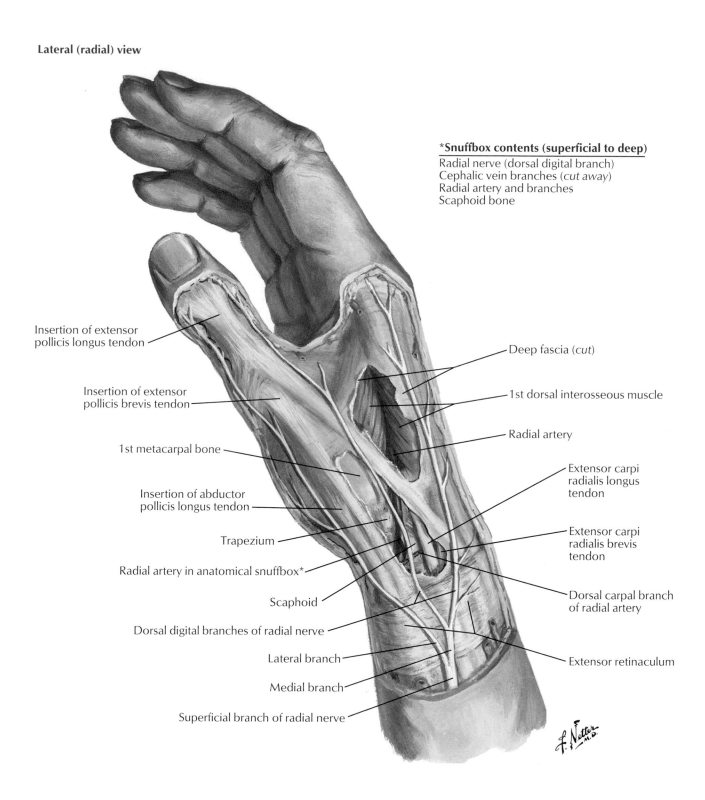

*Snuffbox contents (superficial to deep)
Radial nerve (dorsal digital branch)
Cephalic vein branches (*cut away*)
Radial artery and branches
Scaphoid bone

Insertion of extensor
pollicis longus tendon

Insertion of extensor
pollicis brevis tendon

1st metacarpal bone

Insertion of abductor
pollicis longus tendon

Trapezium

Radial artery in anatomical snuffbox*

Scaphoid

Dorsal digital branches of radial nerve

Lateral branch

Medial branch

Superficial branch of radial nerve

Deep fascia (*cut*)

1st dorsal interosseous muscle

Radial artery

Extensor carpi
radialis longus
tendon

Extensor carpi
radialis brevis
tendon

Dorsal carpal branch
of radial artery

Extensor retinaculum

Plate 455

Wrist and Hand

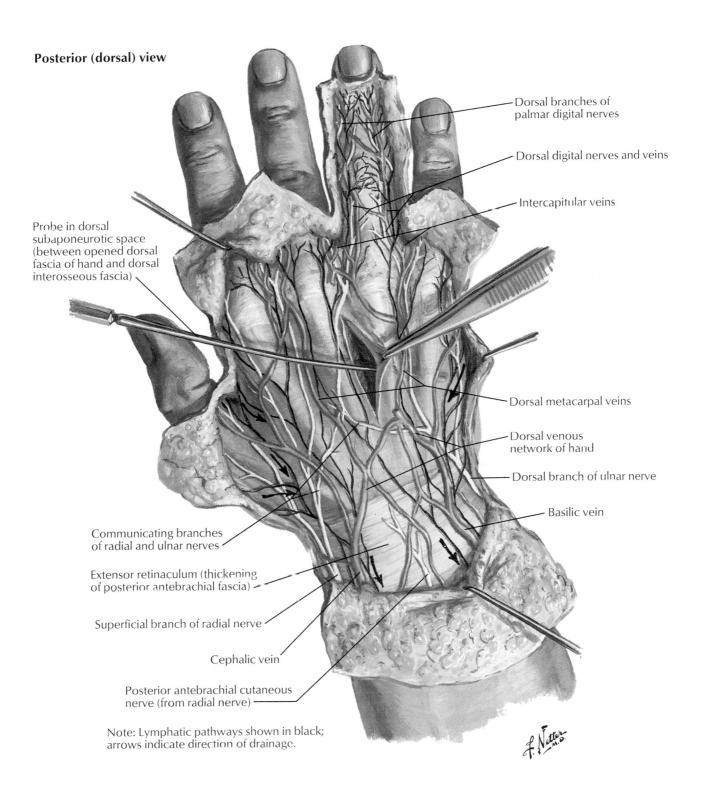

Posterior (dorsal) view

Dorsal branches of palmar digital nerves

Dorsal digital nerves and veins

Intercapitular veins

Probe in dorsal subaponeurotic space (between opened dorsal fascia of hand and dorsal interosseous fascia)

Dorsal metacarpal veins

Dorsal venous network of hand

Dorsal branch of ulnar nerve

Basilic vein

Communicating branches of radial and ulnar nerves

Extensor retinaculum (thickening of posterior antebrachial fascia)

Superficial branch of radial nerve

Cephalic vein

Posterior antebrachial cutaneous nerve (from radial nerve)

Note: Lymphatic pathways shown in black; arrows indicate direction of drainage.

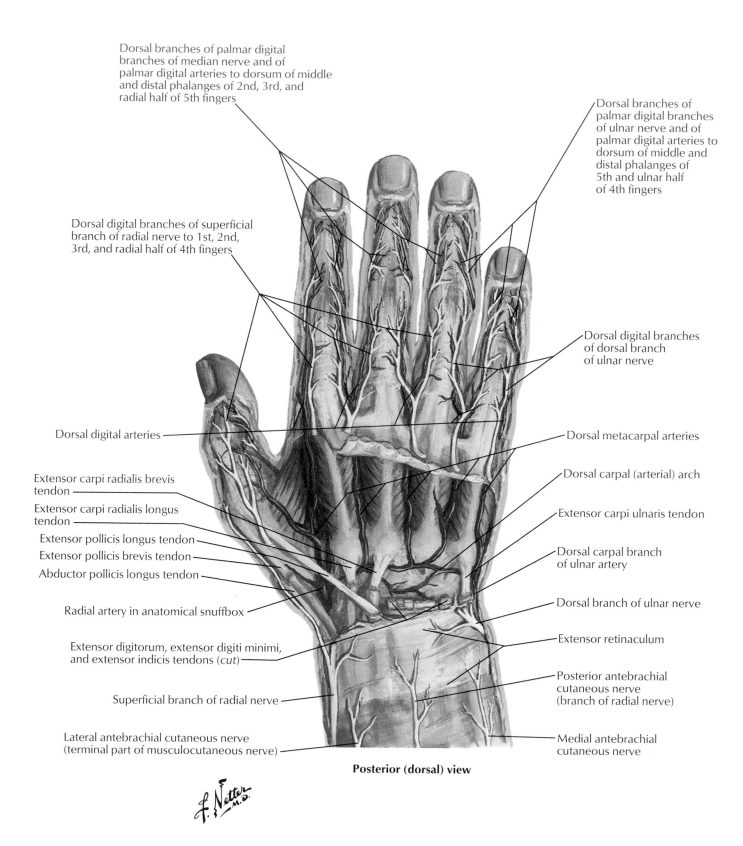

Dorsal branches of palmar digital branches of median nerve and of palmar digital arteries to dorsum of middle and distal phalanges of 2nd, 3rd, and radial half of 5th fingers

Dorsal branches of palmar digital branches of ulnar nerve and of palmar digital arteries to dorsum of middle and distal phalanges of 5th and ulnar half of 4th fingers

Dorsal digital branches of superficial branch of radial nerve to 1st, 2nd, 3rd, and radial half of 4th fingers

Dorsal digital branches of dorsal branch of ulnar nerve

Dorsal digital arteries

Dorsal metacarpal arteries

Extensor carpi radialis brevis tendon

Dorsal carpal (arterial) arch

Extensor carpi radialis longus tendon

Extensor carpi ulnaris tendon

Extensor pollicis longus tendon

Extensor pollicis brevis tendon

Dorsal carpal branch of ulnar artery

Abductor pollicis longus tendon

Radial artery in anatomical snuffbox

Dorsal branch of ulnar nerve

Extensor retinaculum

Extensor digitorum, extensor digiti minimi, and extensor indicis tendons (*cut*)

Posterior antebrachial cutaneous nerve (branch of radial nerve)

Superficial branch of radial nerve

Lateral antebrachial cutaneous nerve (terminal part of musculocutaneous nerve)

Medial antebrachial cutaneous nerve

Posterior (dorsal) view

Plate 457

Wrist and Hand

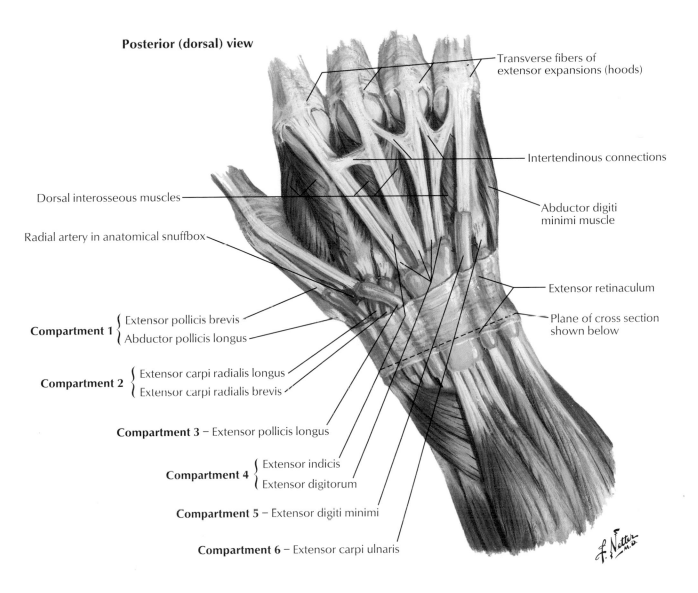

Posterior (dorsal) view

Transverse fibers of extensor expansions (hoods)

Intertendinous connections

Dorsal interosseous muscles

Abductor digiti minimi muscle

Radial artery in anatomical snuffbox

Extensor retinaculum

Plane of cross section shown below

Compartment 1 { Extensor pollicis brevis
Abductor pollicis longus

Compartment 2 { Extensor carpi radialis longus
Extensor carpi radialis brevis

Compartment 3 – Extensor pollicis longus

Compartment 4 { Extensor indicis
Extensor digitorum

Compartment 5 – Extensor digiti minimi

Compartment 6 – Extensor carpi ulnaris

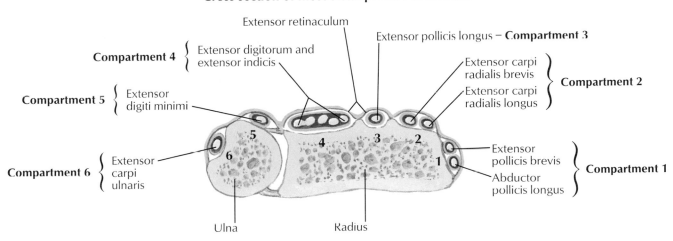

Cross section of most distal portion of forearm

Extensor retinaculum

Extensor pollicis longus – **Compartment 3**

Compartment 4 { Extensor digitorum and extensor indicis

Extensor carpi radialis brevis
Extensor carpi radialis longus } **Compartment 2**

Compartment 5 { Extensor digiti minimi

Compartment 6 { Extensor carpi ulnaris

Extensor pollicis brevis
Abductor pollicis longus } **Compartment 1**

Ulna

Radius

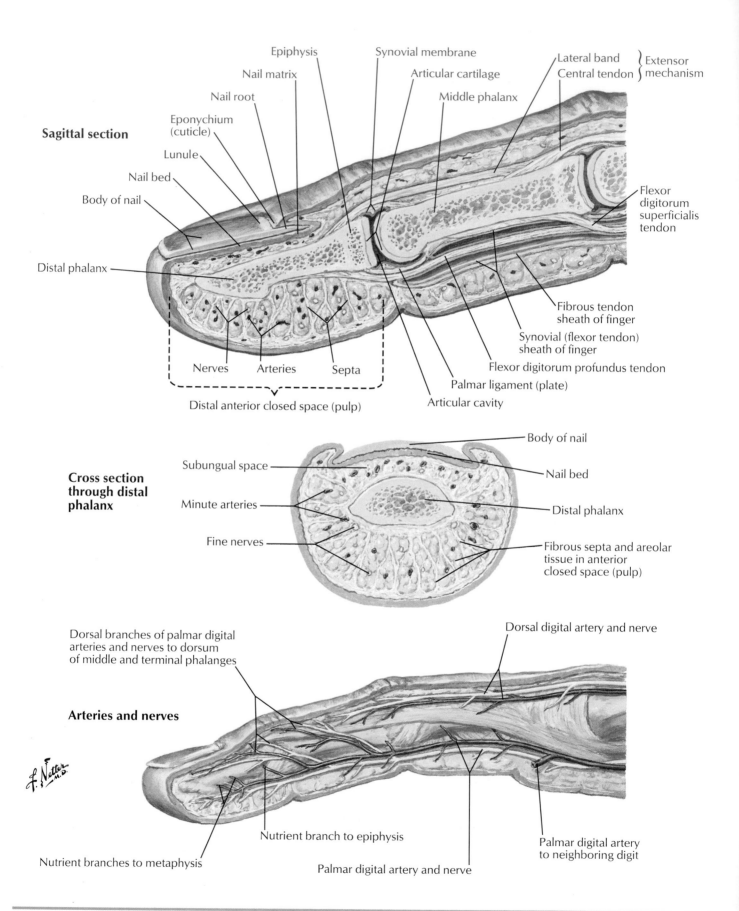

Sagittal section

Epiphysis

Nail matrix

Nail root

Eponychium (cuticle)

Lunule

Nail bed

Body of nail

Synovial membrane

Articular cartilage

Middle phalanx

Lateral band

Central tendon } Extensor mechanism

Distal phalanx

Flexor digitorum superficialis tendon

Fibrous tendon sheath of finger

Synovial (flexor tendon) sheath of finger

Flexor digitorum profundus tendon

Palmar ligament (plate)

Articular cavity

Nerves   Arteries   Septa

Distal anterior closed space (pulp)

Cross section through distal phalanx

Subungual space

Minute arteries

Fine nerves

Body of nail

Nail bed

Distal phalanx

Fibrous septa and areolar tissue in anterior closed space (pulp)

Arteries and nerves

Dorsal branches of palmar digital arteries and nerves to dorsum of middle and terminal phalanges

Dorsal digital artery and nerve

Nutrient branches to metaphysis

Nutrient branch to epiphysis

Palmar digital artery and nerve

Palmar digital artery to neighboring digit

Plate 459

Wrist and Hand

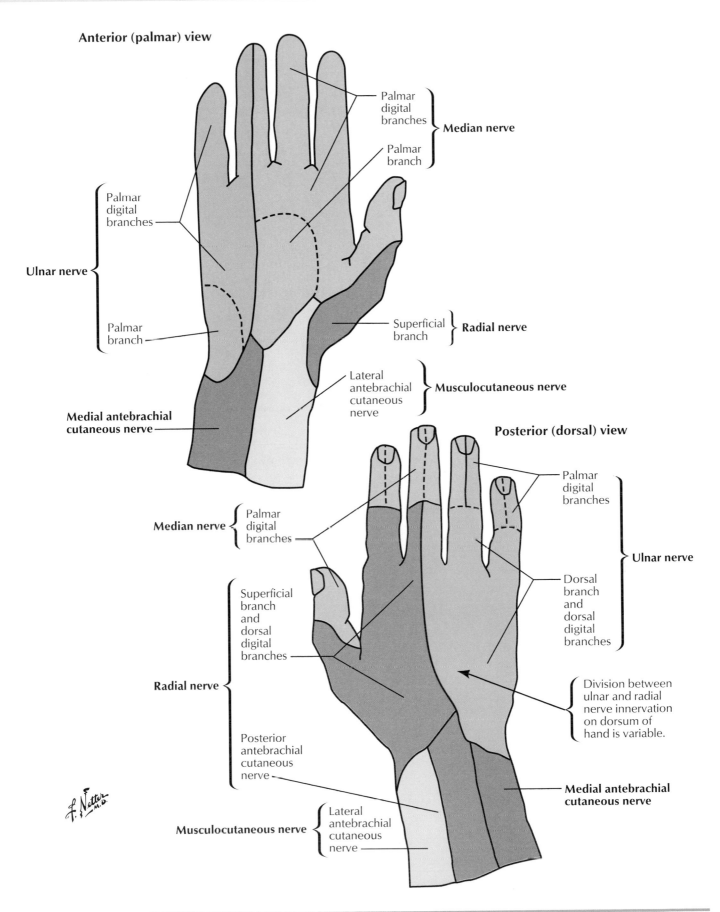

Anterior (palmar) view

Palmar
digital
branches
} **Median nerve**

Palmar
branch

Palmar
digital
branches

Ulnar nerve

Palmar
branch

Superficial
branch } **Radial nerve**

Lateral
antebrachial
cutaneous
nerve } **Musculocutaneous nerve**

**Medial antebrachial
cutaneous nerve**

Posterior (dorsal) view

Median nerve { Palmar
digital
branches

Palmar
digital
branches

Dorsal
branch
and
dorsal
digital
branches

} **Ulnar nerve**

**Superficial
branch
and
dorsal
digital
branches**

Radial nerve {

{ Division between
ulnar and radial
nerve innervation
on dorsum of
hand is variable.

Posterior
antebrachial
cutaneous
nerve

**Medial antebrachial
cutaneous nerve**

Lateral
antebrachial
cutaneous
nerve

Musculocutaneous nerve

Anterior view

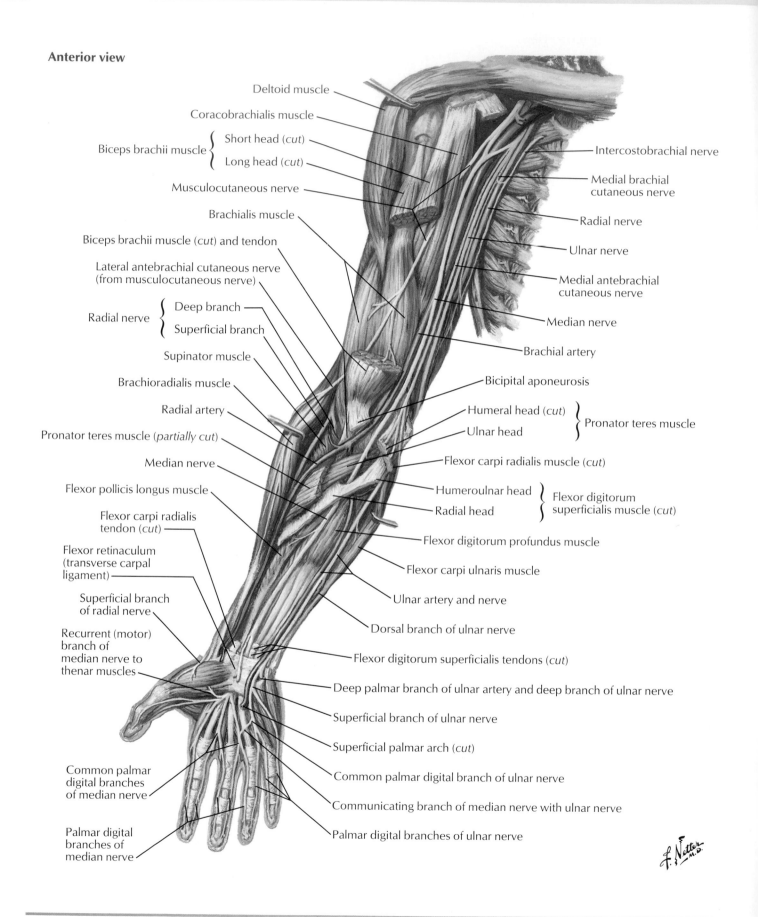

Deltoid muscle

Coracobrachialis muscle

Biceps brachii muscle { Short head (*cut*)

Long head (*cut*)

Musculocutaneous nerve

Brachialis muscle

Biceps brachii muscle (*cut*) and tendon

Lateral antebrachial cutaneous nerve (from musculocutaneous nerve)

Radial nerve { Deep branch

Superficial branch

Supinator muscle

Brachioradialis muscle

Radial artery

Pronator teres muscle (*partially cut*)

Median nerve

Flexor pollicis longus muscle

Flexor carpi radialis tendon (*cut*)

Flexor retinaculum (transverse carpal ligament)

Superficial branch of radial nerve

Recurrent (motor) branch of median nerve to thenar muscles

Common palmar digital branches of median nerve

Palmar digital branches of median nerve

Intercostobrachial nerve

Medial brachial cutaneous nerve

Radial nerve

Ulnar nerve

Medial antebrachial cutaneous nerve

Median nerve

Brachial artery

Bicipital aponeurosis

Humeral head (*cut*) } Pronator teres muscle

Ulnar head

Flexor carpi radialis muscle (*cut*)

Humeroulnar head } Flexor digitorum superficialis muscle (*cut*)

Radial head

Flexor digitorum profundus muscle

Flexor carpi ulnaris muscle

Ulnar artery and nerve

Dorsal branch of ulnar nerve

Flexor digitorum superficialis tendons (*cut*)

Deep palmar branch of ulnar artery and deep branch of ulnar nerve

Superficial branch of ulnar nerve

Superficial palmar arch (*cut*)

Common palmar digital branch of ulnar nerve

Communicating branch of median nerve with ulnar nerve

Palmar digital branches of ulnar nerve

Plate 461

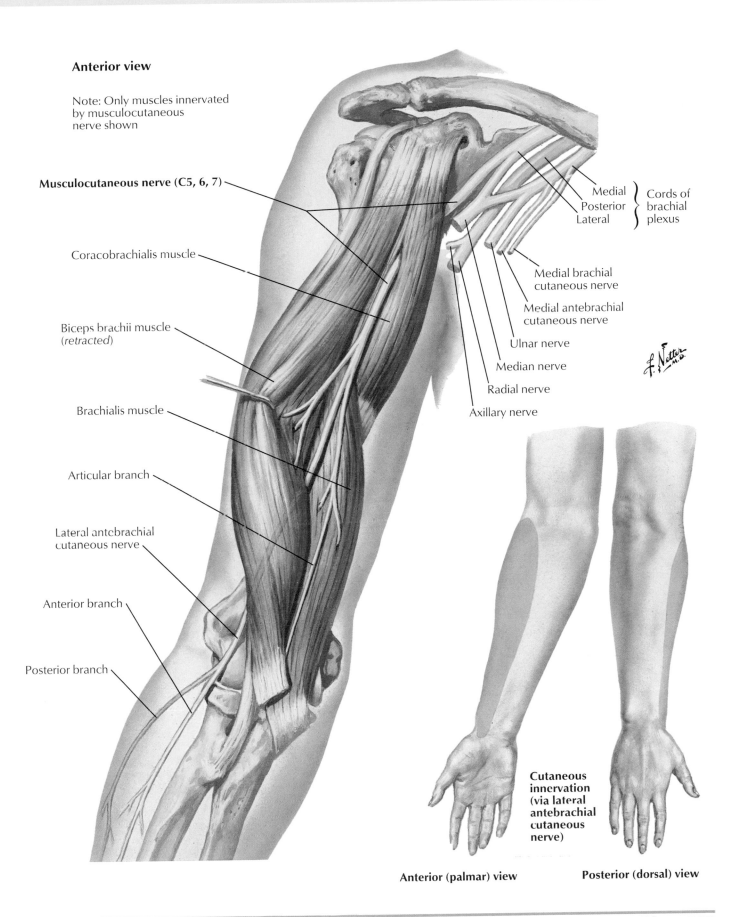

Anterior view

Note: Only muscles innervated by musculocutaneous nerve shown

Musculocutaneous nerve (C5, 6, 7)

Coracobrachialis muscle

Biceps brachii muscle (*retracted*)

Brachialis muscle

Articular branch

Lateral antebrachial cutaneous nerve

Anterior branch

Posterior branch

Medial
Posterior } Cords of
Lateral } brachial plexus

Medial brachial cutaneous nerve

Medial antebrachial cutaneous nerve

Ulnar nerve

Median nerve

Radial nerve

Axillary nerve

Cutaneous innervation (via lateral antebrachial cutaneous nerve)

Anterior (palmar) view   Posterior (dorsal) view

Anterior view

Note: Only muscles innervated by median nerve shown

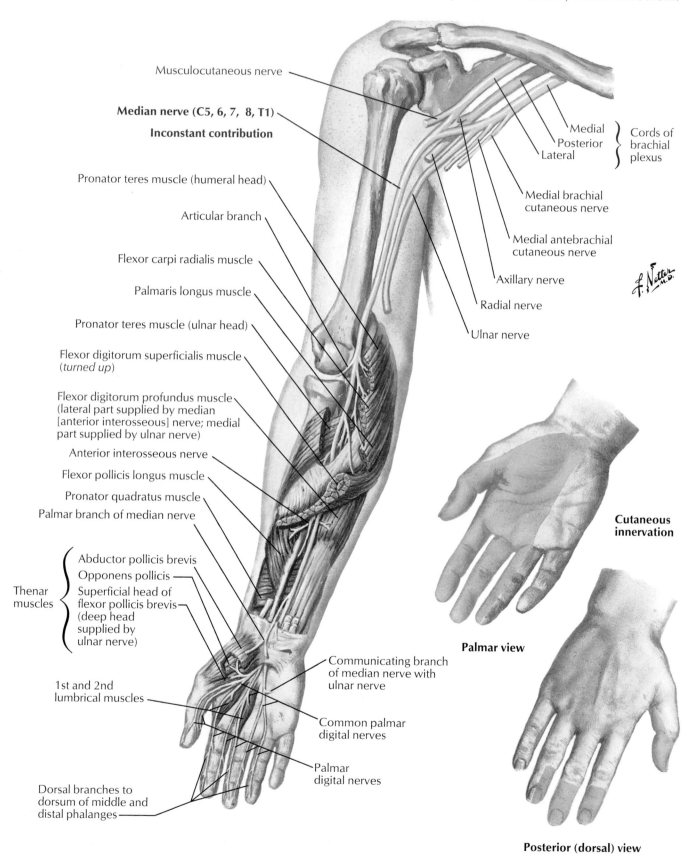

Musculocutaneous nerve

Median nerve (C5, 6, 7, 8, T1)

Inconstant contribution

Pronator teres muscle (humeral head)

Articular branch

Flexor carpi radialis muscle

Palmaris longus muscle

Pronator teres muscle (ulnar head)

Flexor digitorum superficialis muscle (*turned up*)

Flexor digitorum profundus muscle (lateral part supplied by median [anterior interosseous] nerve; medial part supplied by ulnar nerve)

Anterior interosseous nerve

Flexor pollicis longus muscle

Pronator quadratus muscle

Palmar branch of median nerve

Thenar muscles
- Abductor pollicis brevis
- Opponens pollicis
- Superficial head of flexor pollicis brevis (deep head supplied by ulnar nerve)

1st and 2nd lumbrical muscles

Dorsal branches to dorsum of middle and distal phalanges

Medial
Posterior
Lateral
Cords of brachial plexus

Medial brachial cutaneous nerve

Medial antebrachial cutaneous nerve

Axillary nerve

Radial nerve

Ulnar nerve

Communicating branch of median nerve with ulnar nerve

Common palmar digital nerves

Palmar digital nerves

Cutaneous innervation

Palmar view

Posterior (dorsal) view

Plate 463

Neurovasculature

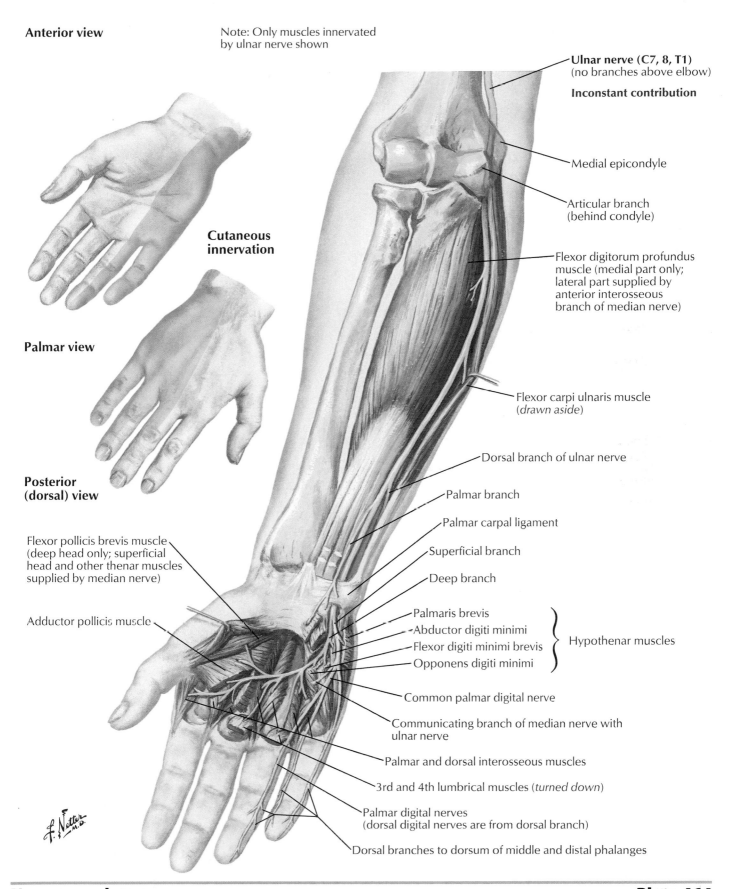

Anterior view

Note: Only muscles innervated by ulnar nerve shown

Ulnar nerve (C7, 8, T1)
(no branches above elbow)

Inconstant contribution

Medial epicondyle

Articular branch
(behind condyle)

Flexor digitorum profundus muscle (medial part only; lateral part supplied by anterior interosseous branch of median nerve)

Cutaneous innervation

Palmar view

Flexor carpi ulnaris muscle (*drawn aside*)

Posterior (dorsal) view

Dorsal branch of ulnar nerve

Palmar branch

Palmar carpal ligament

Superficial branch

Deep branch

Flexor pollicis brevis muscle (deep head only; superficial head and other thenar muscles supplied by median nerve)

Adductor pollicis muscle

Palmaris brevis

Abductor digiti minimi

Flexor digiti minimi brevis

Opponens digiti minimi

} Hypothenar muscles

Common palmar digital nerve

Communicating branch of median nerve with ulnar nerve

Palmar and dorsal interosseous muscles

3rd and 4th lumbrical muscles (*turned down*)

Palmar digital nerves (dorsal digital nerves are from dorsal branch)

Dorsal branches to dorsum of middle and distal phalanges

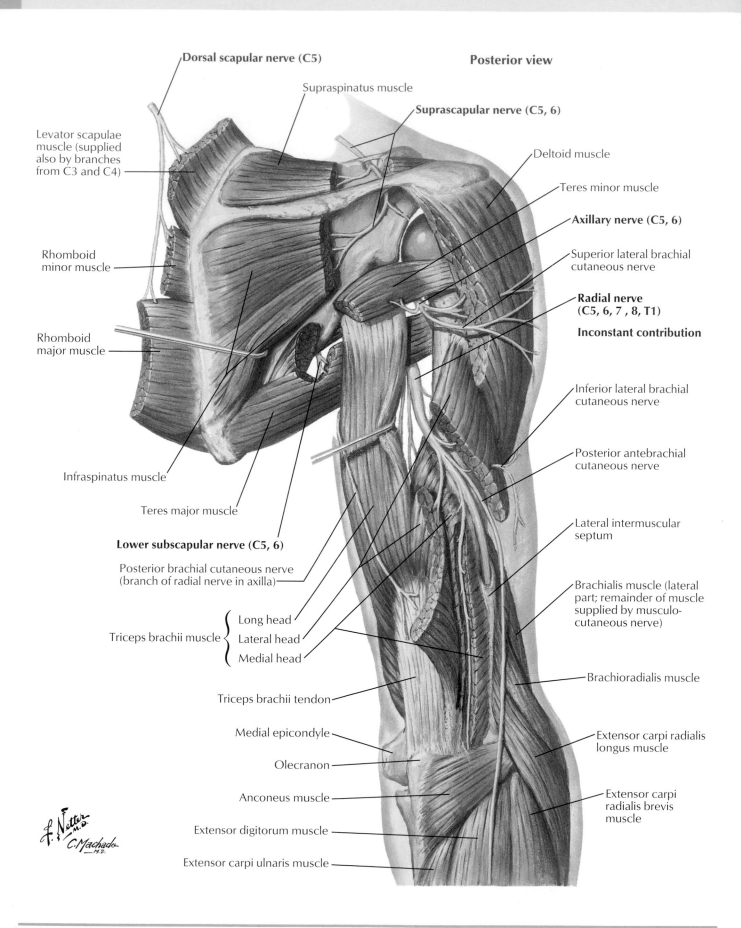

Dorsal scapular nerve (C5)

Supraspinatus muscle

Posterior view

Suprascapular nerve (C5, 6)

Levator scapulae muscle (supplied also by branches from C3 and C4)

Deltoid muscle

Teres minor muscle

Axillary nerve (C5, 6)

Rhomboid minor muscle

Superior lateral brachial cutaneous nerve

Radial nerve (C5, 6, 7 , 8, T1)

Inconstant contribution

Rhomboid major muscle

Inferior lateral brachial cutaneous nerve

Posterior antebrachial cutaneous nerve

Infraspinatus muscle

Teres major muscle

Lateral intermuscular septum

Lower subscapular nerve (C5, 6)

Posterior brachial cutaneous nerve (branch of radial nerve in axilla)

Brachialis muscle (lateral part; remainder of muscle supplied by musculo-cutaneous nerve)

Triceps brachii muscle { Long head / Lateral head / Medial head

Brachioradialis muscle

Triceps brachii tendon

Medial epicondyle

Extensor carpi radialis longus muscle

Olecranon

Anconeus muscle

Extensor carpi radialis brevis muscle

Extensor digitorum muscle

Extensor carpi ulnaris muscle

Plate 465

Neurovasculature

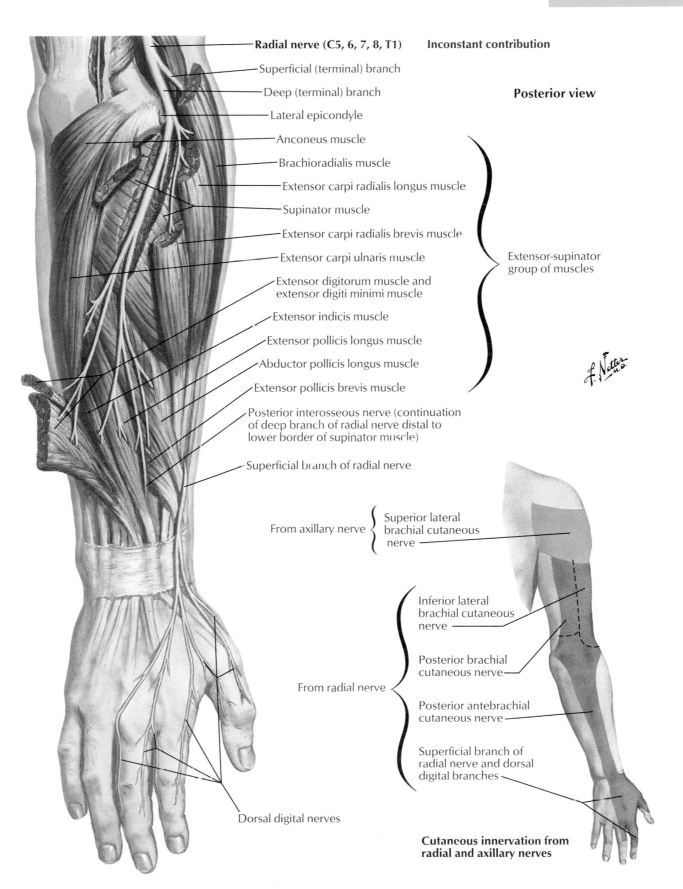

Radial nerve (C5, 6, 7, 8, T1)   Inconstant contribution

Superficial (terminal) branch

Deep (terminal) branch   **Posterior view**

Lateral epicondyle

Anconeus muscle

Brachioradialis muscle

Extensor carpi radialis longus muscle

Supinator muscle

Extensor carpi radialis brevis muscle

Extensor carpi ulnaris muscle   Extensor-supinator group of muscles

Extensor digitorum muscle and extensor digiti minimi muscle

Extensor indicis muscle

Extensor pollicis longus muscle

Abductor pollicis longus muscle

Extensor pollicis brevis muscle

Posterior interosseous nerve (continuation of deep branch of radial nerve distal to lower border of supinator muscle)

Superficial branch of radial nerve

From axillary nerve { Superior lateral brachial cutaneous nerve

Inferior lateral brachial cutaneous nerve

Posterior brachial cutaneous nerve

From radial nerve

Posterior antebrachial cutaneous nerve

Superficial branch of radial nerve and dorsal digital branches

Dorsal digital nerves

Cutaneous innervation from radial and axillary nerves

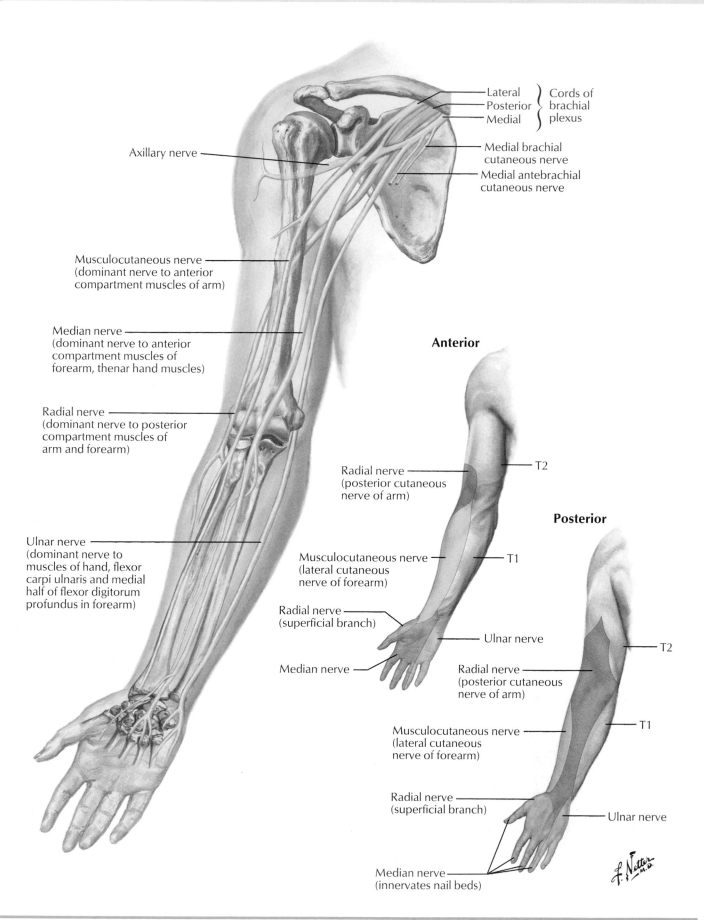

Lateral ⎫
Posterior ⎬ Cords of brachial plexus
Medial ⎭

Axillary nerve

Medial brachial cutaneous nerve

Medial antebrachial cutaneous nerve

Musculocutaneous nerve (dominant nerve to anterior compartment muscles of arm)

Median nerve (dominant nerve to anterior compartment muscles of forearm, thenar hand muscles)

Radial nerve (dominant nerve to posterior compartment muscles of arm and forearm)

Ulnar nerve (dominant nerve to muscles of hand, flexor carpi ulnaris and medial half of flexor digitorum profundus in forearm)

Anterior

Radial nerve (posterior cutaneous nerve of arm) — T2

Musculocutaneous nerve (lateral cutaneous nerve of forearm) — T1

Radial nerve (superficial branch)

Ulnar nerve

Median nerve

Posterior

Radial nerve (posterior cutaneous nerve of arm) — T2

Musculocutaneous nerve (lateral cutaneous nerve of forearm) — T1

Radial nerve (superficial branch)

Ulnar nerve

Median nerve (innervates nail beds)

Plate 467

Neurovasculature

Arthrogram: glenohumeral joint

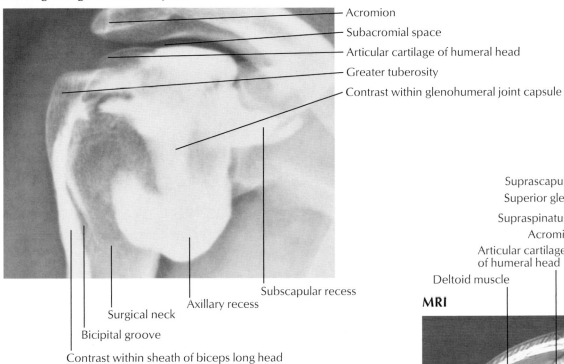

- Acromion
- Subacromial space
- Articular cartilage of humeral head
- Greater tuberosity
- Contrast within glenohumeral joint capsule
- Subscapular recess
- Axillary recess
- Surgical neck
- Bicipital groove
- Contrast within sheath of biceps long head

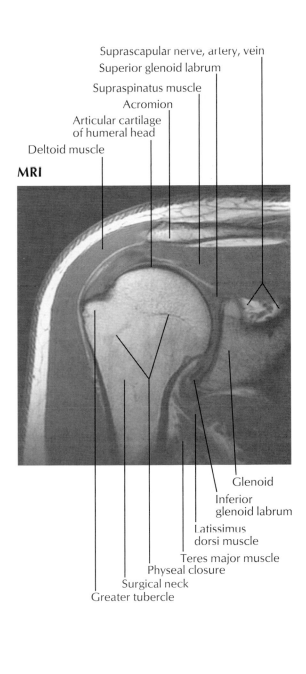

- Suprascapular nerve, artery, vein
- Superior glenoid labrum
- Supraspinatus muscle
- Acromion
- Articular cartilage of humeral head
- Deltoid muscle

MRI

- Glenoid
- Inferior glenoid labrum
- Latissimus dorsi muscle
- Teres major muscle
- Physeal closure
- Surgical neck
- Greater tubercle

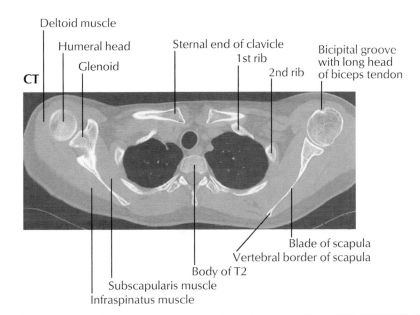

- Deltoid muscle
- Humeral head
- Glenoid

CT

- Sternal end of clavicle
- 1st rib
- 2nd rib
- Bicipital groove with long head of biceps tendon
- Blade of scapula
- Vertebral border of scapula
- Body of T2
- Subscapularis muscle
- Infraspinatus muscle

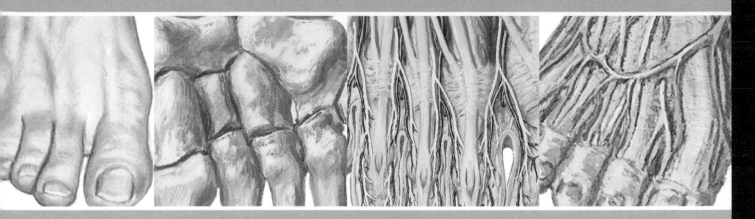

Section 7 LOWER LIMB

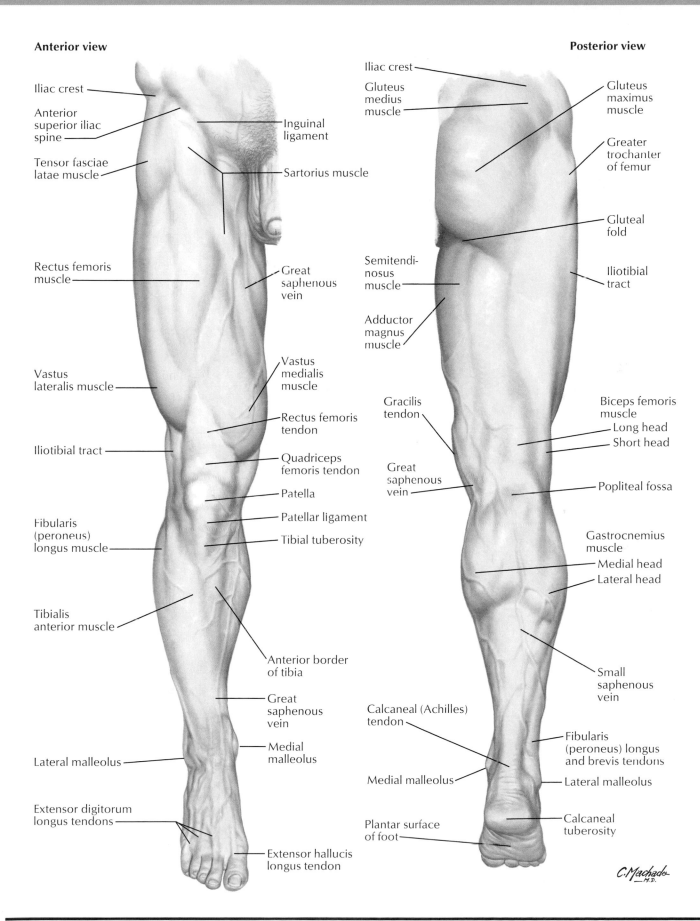

Anterior view

Iliac crest

Anterior superior iliac spine

Tensor fasciae latae muscle

Rectus femoris muscle

Vastus lateralis muscle

Iliotibial tract

Fibularis (peroneus) longus muscle

Tibialis anterior muscle

Lateral malleolus

Extensor digitorum longus tendons

Inguinal ligament

Sartorius muscle

Great saphenous vein

Vastus medialis muscle

Rectus femoris tendon

Quadriceps femoris tendon

Patella

Patellar ligament

Tibial tuberosity

Anterior border of tibia

Great saphenous vein

Medial malleolus

Extensor hallucis longus tendon

Posterior view

Iliac crest

Gluteus medius muscle

Semitendinosus muscle

Adductor magnus muscle

Gracilis tendon

Great saphenous vein

Calcaneal (Achilles) tendon

Medial malleolus

Plantar surface of foot

Gluteus maximus muscle

Greater trochanter of femur

Gluteal fold

Iliotibial tract

Biceps femoris muscle
Long head
Short head

Popliteal fossa

Gastrocnemius muscle
Medial head
Lateral head

Small saphenous vein

Fibularis (peroneus) longus and brevis tendons

Lateral malleolus

Calcaneal tuberosity

C. Machado
_M.D.

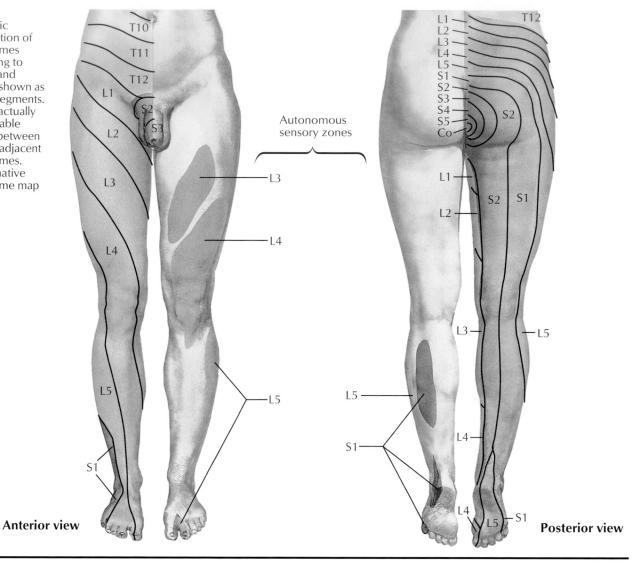

Schematic demarcation of dermatomes (according to Keegan and Garrett) shown as distinct segments. There is actually considerable overlap between any two adjacent dermatomes. An alternative dermatome map is online.

Autonomous sensory zones

Anterior view

Posterior view

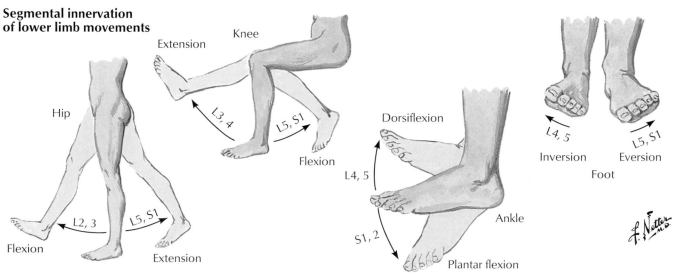

Segmental innervation of lower limb movements

Hip

Flexion — L2, 3

Extension — L5, S1

Knee

Extension

L3, 4

L5, S1

Flexion

Dorsiflexion

L4, 5

S1, 2

Plantar flexion

Ankle

Inversion — L4, 5

Eversion — L5, S1

Foot

Plate 470

Cutaneous Anatomy

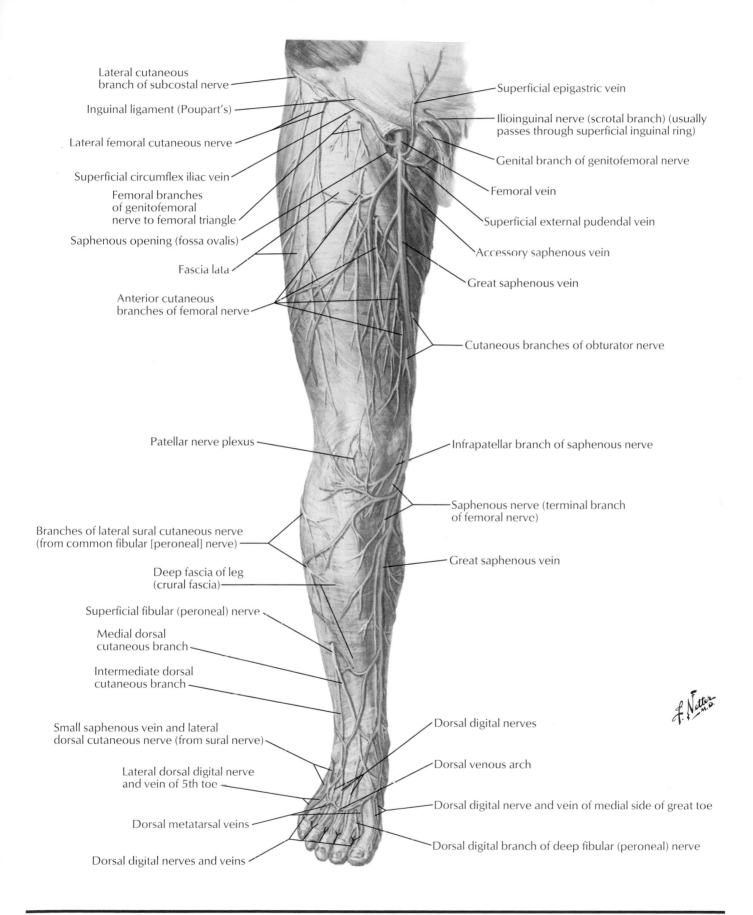

Lateral cutaneous branch of subcostal nerve

Inguinal ligament (Poupart's)

Lateral femoral cutaneous nerve

Superficial circumflex iliac vein

Femoral branches of genitofemoral nerve to femoral triangle

Saphenous opening (fossa ovalis)

Fascia lata

Anterior cutaneous branches of femoral nerve

Patellar nerve plexus

Branches of lateral sural cutaneous nerve (from common fibular [peroneal] nerve)

Deep fascia of leg (crural fascia)

Superficial fibular (peroneal) nerve

Medial dorsal cutaneous branch

Intermediate dorsal cutaneous branch

Small saphenous vein and lateral dorsal cutaneous nerve (from sural nerve)

Lateral dorsal digital nerve and vein of 5th toe

Dorsal metatarsal veins

Dorsal digital nerves and veins

Superficial epigastric vein

Ilioinguinal nerve (scrotal branch) (usually passes through superficial inguinal ring)

Genital branch of genitofemoral nerve

Femoral vein

Superficial external pudendal vein

Accessory saphenous vein

Great saphenous vein

Cutaneous branches of obturator nerve

Infrapatellar branch of saphenous nerve

Saphenous nerve (terminal branch of femoral nerve)

Great saphenous vein

Dorsal digital nerves

Dorsal venous arch

Dorsal digital nerve and vein of medial side of great toe

Dorsal digital branch of deep fibular (peroneal) nerve

7

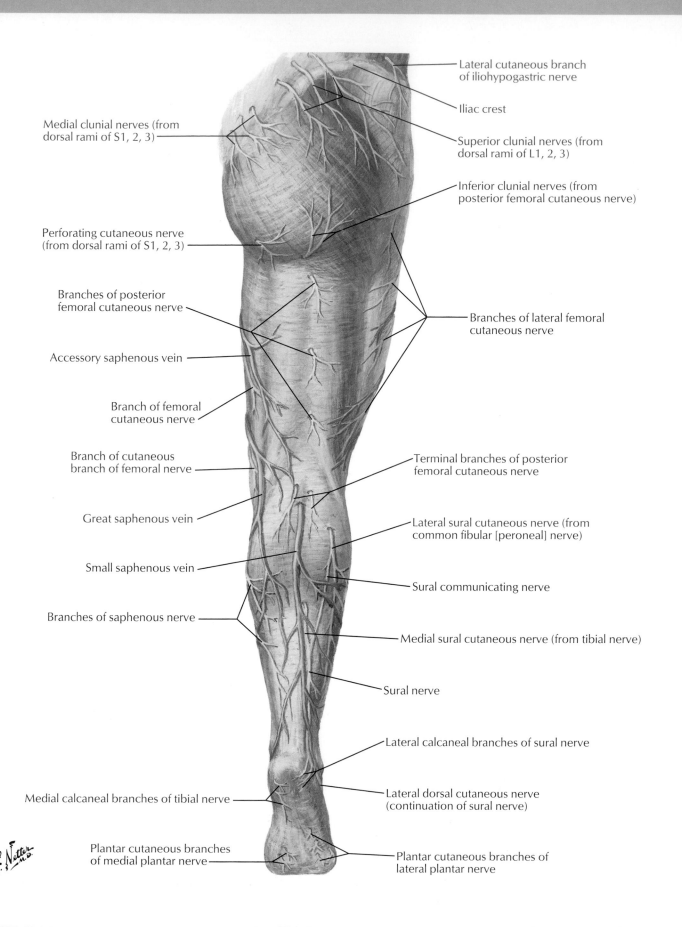

Lateral cutaneous branch of iliohypogastric nerve

Iliac crest

Medial clunial nerves (from dorsal rami of S1, 2, 3)

Superior clunial nerves (from dorsal rami of L1, 2, 3)

Inferior clunial nerves (from posterior femoral cutaneous nerve)

Perforating cutaneous nerve (from dorsal rami of S1, 2, 3)

Branches of posterior femoral cutaneous nerve

Branches of lateral femoral cutaneous nerve

Accessory saphenous vein

Branch of femoral cutaneous nerve

Branch of cutaneous branch of femoral nerve

Terminal branches of posterior femoral cutaneous nerve

Great saphenous vein

Lateral sural cutaneous nerve (from common fibular [peroneal] nerve)

Small saphenous vein

Sural communicating nerve

Branches of saphenous nerve

Medial sural cutaneous nerve (from tibial nerve)

Sural nerve

Lateral calcaneal branches of sural nerve

Medial calcaneal branches of tibial nerve

Lateral dorsal cutaneous nerve (continuation of sural nerve)

Plantar cutaneous branches of medial plantar nerve

Plantar cutaneous branches of lateral plantar nerve

Plate 472   **Cutaneous Anatomy**

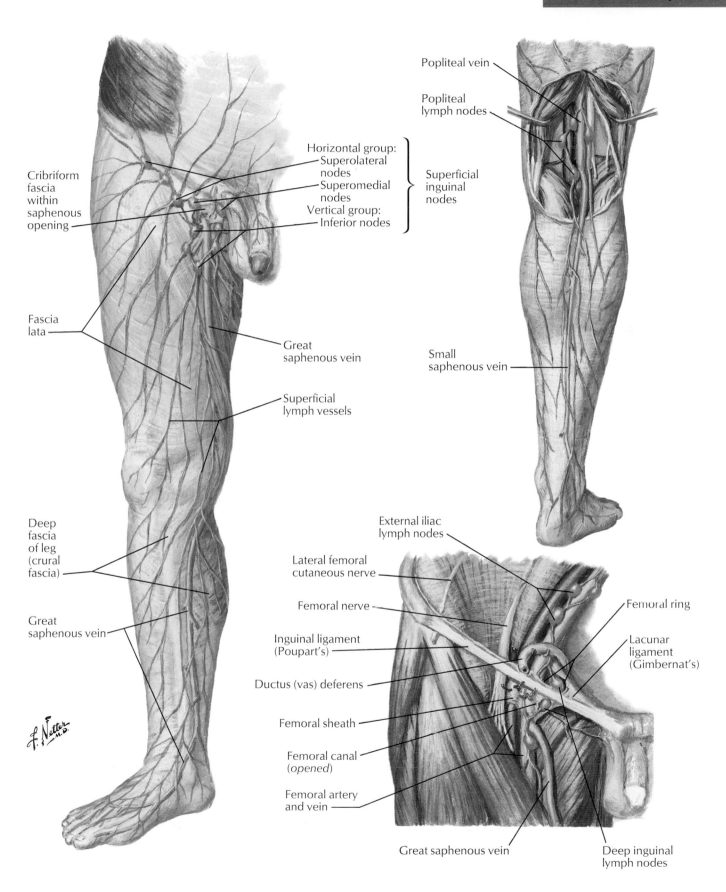

Cribriform fascia within saphenous opening

Horizontal group:
Superolateral nodes
Superomedial nodes
Vertical group:
Inferior nodes

Superficial inguinal nodes

Fascia lata

Great saphenous vein

Superficial lymph vessels

Deep fascia of leg (crural fascia)

Great saphenous vein

Popliteal vein

Popliteal lymph nodes

Superficial inguinal nodes

Small saphenous vein

External iliac lymph nodes

Lateral femoral cutaneous nerve

Femoral nerve

Inguinal ligament (Poupart's)

Ductus (vas) deferens

Femoral sheath

Femoral canal (opened)

Femoral artery and vein

Femoral ring

Lacunar ligament (Gimbernat's)

Great saphenous vein

Deep inguinal lymph nodes

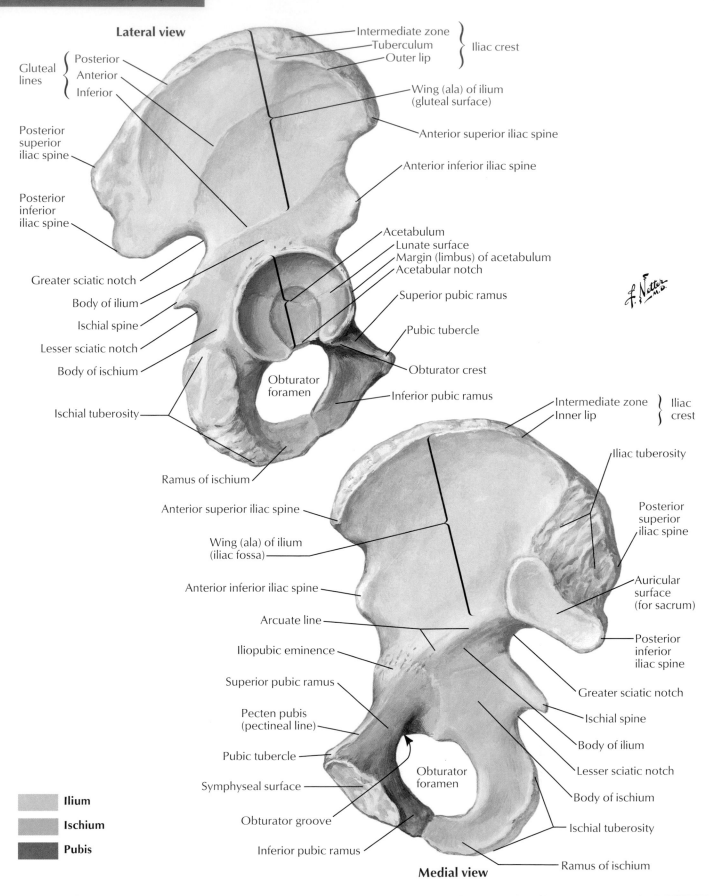

Lateral view

Intermediate zone
Tuberculum
Outer lip
} Iliac crest

Gluteal lines {
Posterior
Anterior
Inferior

Wing (ala) of ilium (gluteal surface)

Anterior superior iliac spine

Posterior superior iliac spine

Anterior inferior iliac spine

Posterior inferior iliac spine

Acetabulum
Lunate surface
Margin (limbus) of acetabulum
Acetabular notch

Greater sciatic notch

Superior pubic ramus

Body of ilium

Pubic tubercle

Ischial spine

Lesser sciatic notch

Obturator crest

Body of ischium

Obturator foramen

Inferior pubic ramus

Ischial tuberosity

Ramus of ischium

Intermediate zone
Inner lip
} Iliac crest

Iliac tuberosity

Anterior superior iliac spine

Posterior superior iliac spine

Wing (ala) of ilium (iliac fossa)

Auricular surface (for sacrum)

Anterior inferior iliac spine

Arcuate line

Posterior inferior iliac spine

Iliopubic eminence

Greater sciatic notch

Superior pubic ramus

Ischial spine

Pecten pubis (pectineal line)

Body of ilium

Pubic tubercle

Lesser sciatic notch

Symphyseal surface

Obturator foramen

Body of ischium

Obturator groove

Ischial tuberosity

Inferior pubic ramus

Ramus of ischium

Medial view

Ilium

Ischium

Pubis

Plate 474

Hip and Thigh

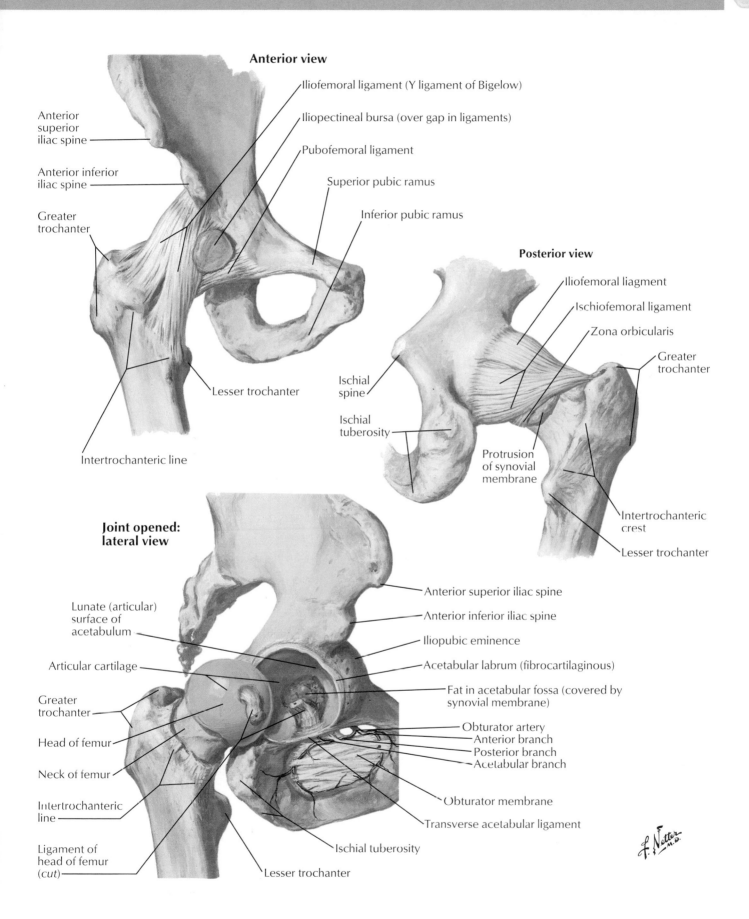

Anterior view

Iliofemoral ligament (Y ligament of Bigelow)

Iliopectineal bursa (over gap in ligaments)

Pubofemoral ligament

Superior pubic ramus

Inferior pubic ramus

Anterior superior iliac spine

Anterior inferior iliac spine

Greater trochanter

Lesser trochanter

Intertrochanteric line

Posterior view

Iliofemoral liagment

Ischiofemoral ligament

Zona orbicularis

Greater trochanter

Ischial spine

Ischial tuberosity

Protrusion of synovial membrane

Intertrochanteric crest

Lesser trochanter

Joint opened: lateral view

Lunate (articular) surface of acetabulum

Articular cartilage

Greater trochanter

Head of femur

Neck of femur

Intertrochanteric line

Ligament of head of femur (*cut*)

Lesser trochanter

Ischial tuberosity

Anterior superior iliac spine

Anterior inferior iliac spine

Iliopubic eminence

Acetabular labrum (fibrocartilaginous)

Fat in acetabular fossa (covered by synovial membrane)

Obturator artery
Anterior branch
Posterior branch
Acetabular branch

Obturator membrane

Transverse acetabular ligament

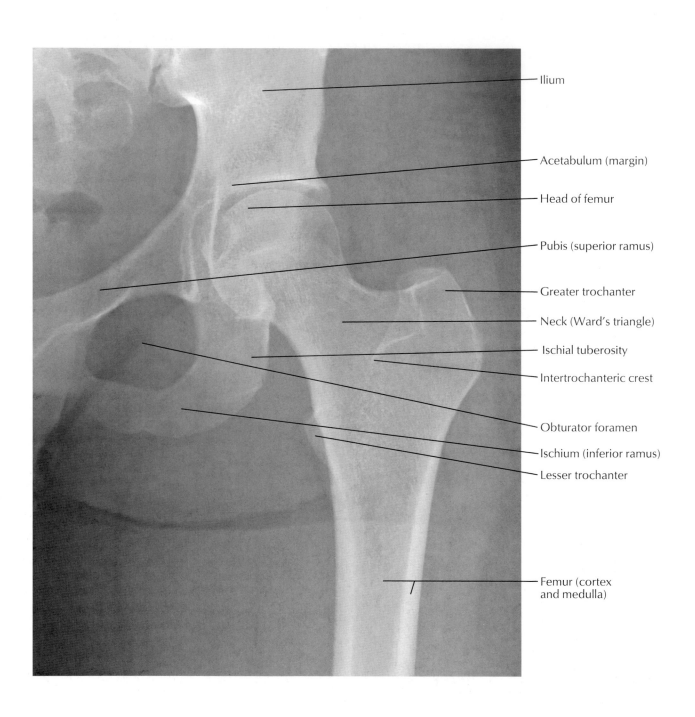

Ilium

Acetabulum (margin)

Head of femur

Pubis (superior ramus)

Greater trochanter

Neck (Ward's triangle)

Ischial tuberosity

Intertrochanteric crest

Obturator foramen

Ischium (inferior ramus)

Lesser trochanter

Femur (cortex and medulla)

Plate 476

Hip and Thigh

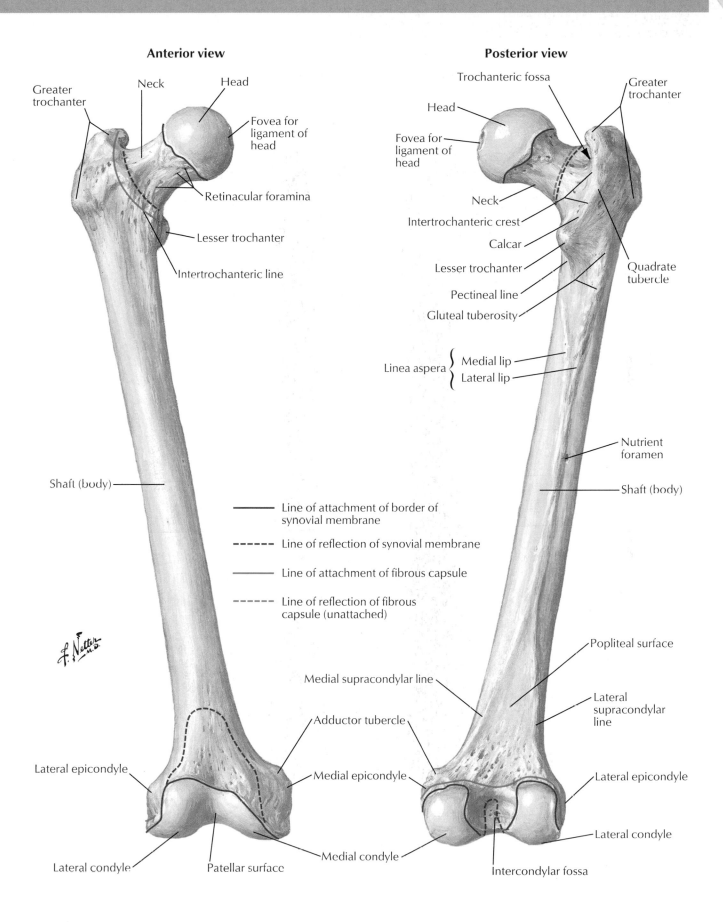

Anterior view

Greater trochanter
Neck
Head
Fovea for ligament of head
Retinacular foramina
Lesser trochanter
Intertrochanteric line
Shaft (body)

Line of attachment of border of synovial membrane

Line of reflection of synovial membrane

Line of attachment of fibrous capsule

Line of reflection of fibrous capsule (unattached)

Lateral epicondyle
Lateral condyle
Patellar surface
Adductor tubercle
Medial epicondyle
Medial condyle

Posterior view

Trochanteric fossa
Greater trochanter
Head
Fovea for ligament of head
Neck
Intertrochanteric crest
Calcar
Lesser trochanter
Pectineal line
Gluteal tuberosity
Quadrate tubercle
Linea aspera { Medial lip / Lateral lip
Nutrient foramen
Shaft (body)
Popliteal surface
Medial supracondylar line
Lateral supracondylar line
Lateral epicondyle
Lateral condyle
Intercondylar fossa

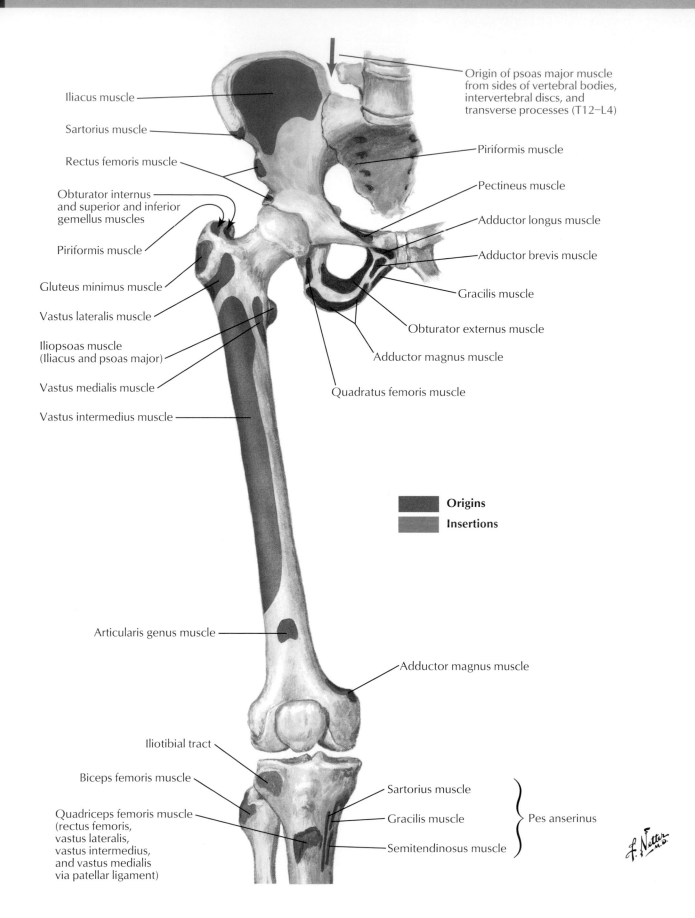

Iliacus muscle

Sartorius muscle

Rectus femoris muscle

Obturator internus
and superior and inferior
gemellus muscles

Piriformis muscle

Gluteus minimus muscle

Vastus lateralis muscle

Iliopsoas muscle
(Iliacus and psoas major)

Vastus medialis muscle

Vastus intermedius muscle

Origin of psoas major muscle
from sides of vertebral bodies,
intervertebral discs, and
transverse processes (T12–L4)

Piriformis muscle

Pectineus muscle

Adductor longus muscle

Adductor brevis muscle

Gracilis muscle

Obturator externus muscle

Adductor magnus muscle

Quadratus femoris muscle

Origins
Insertions

Articularis genus muscle

Adductor magnus muscle

Iliotibial tract

Biceps femoris muscle

Sartorius muscle

Gracilis muscle

Pes anserinus

Quadriceps femoris muscle
(rectus femoris,
vastus lateralis,
vastus intermedius,
and vastus medialis
via patellar ligament)

Semitendinosus muscle

Plate 478

Hip and Thigh

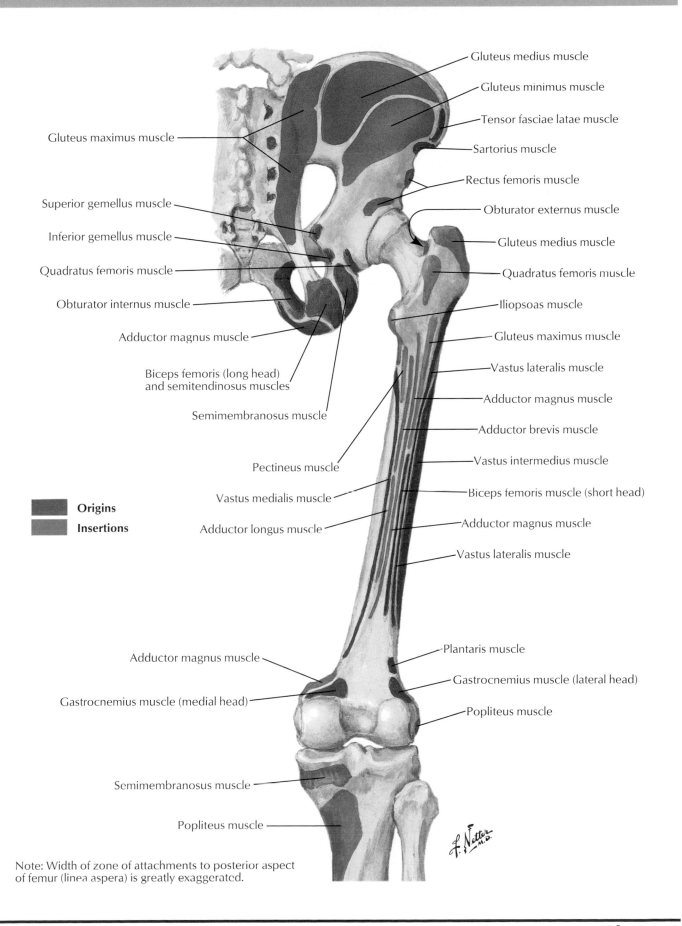

Gluteus medius muscle

Gluteus minimus muscle

Tensor fasciae latae muscle

Sartorius muscle

Rectus femoris muscle

Obturator externus muscle

Gluteus medius muscle

Quadratus femoris muscle

Iliopsoas muscle

Gluteus maximus muscle

Vastus lateralis muscle

Adductor magnus muscle

Adductor brevis muscle

Vastus intermedius muscle

Biceps femoris muscle (short head)

Adductor magnus muscle

Vastus lateralis muscle

Gluteus maximus muscle

Superior gemellus muscle

Inferior gemellus muscle

Quadratus femoris muscle

Obturator internus muscle

Adductor magnus muscle

Biceps femoris (long head) and semitendinosus muscles

Semimembranosus muscle

Pectineus muscle

Vastus medialis muscle

Adductor longus muscle

Origins

Insertions

Adductor magnus muscle

Gastrocnemius muscle (medial head)

Plantaris muscle

Gastrocnemius muscle (lateral head)

Popliteus muscle

Semimembranosus muscle

Popliteus muscle

Note: Width of zone of attachments to posterior aspect of femur (linea aspera) is greatly exaggerated.

Hip and Thigh

Plate 479

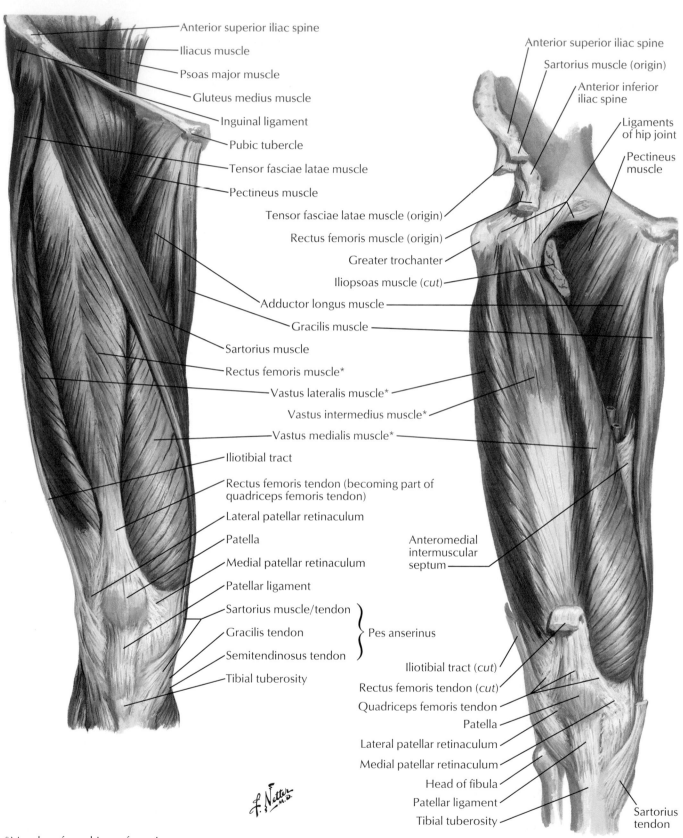

Anterior superior iliac spine

Iliacus muscle

Psoas major muscle

Gluteus medius muscle

Inguinal ligament

Pubic tubercle

Tensor fasciae latae muscle

Pectineus muscle

Tensor fasciae latae muscle (origin)

Rectus femoris muscle (origin)

Greater trochanter

Iliopsoas muscle (*cut*)

Adductor longus muscle

Gracilis muscle

Sartorius muscle

Rectus femoris muscle*

Vastus lateralis muscle*

Vastus intermedius muscle*

Vastus medialis muscle*

Iliotibial tract

Rectus femoris tendon (becoming part of quadriceps femoris tendon)

Lateral patellar retinaculum

Patella

Medial patellar retinaculum

Patellar ligament

Sartorius muscle/tendon

Gracilis tendon

Semitendinosus tendon

Tibial tuberosity

Pes anserinus

Anterior superior iliac spine

Sartorius muscle (origin)

Anterior inferior iliac spine

Ligaments of hip joint

Pectineus muscle

Anteromedial intermuscular septum

Iliotibial tract (*cut*)

Rectus femoris tendon (*cut*)

Quadriceps femoris tendon

Patella

Lateral patellar retinaculum

Medial patellar retinaculum

Head of fibula

Patellar ligament

Tibial tuberosity

Sartorius tendon

*Muscles of quadriceps femoris

Plate 480

Hip and Thigh

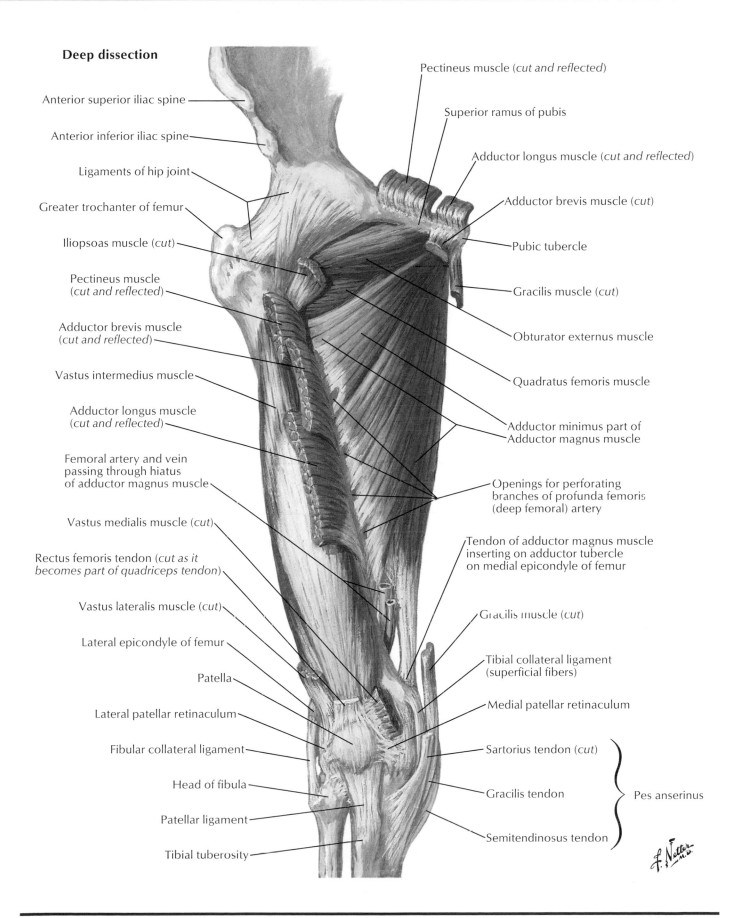

Deep dissection

Anterior superior iliac spine

Anterior inferior iliac spine

Ligaments of hip joint

Greater trochanter of femur

Iliopsoas muscle (*cut*)

Pectineus muscle
(*cut and reflected*)

Adductor brevis muscle
(*cut and reflected*)

Vastus intermedius muscle

Adductor longus muscle
(*cut and reflected*)

Femoral artery and vein
passing through hiatus
of adductor magnus muscle

Vastus medialis muscle (*cut*)

Rectus femoris tendon (*cut as it
becomes part of quadriceps tendon*)

Vastus lateralis muscle (*cut*)

Lateral epicondyle of femur

Patella

Lateral patellar retinaculum

Fibular collateral ligament

Head of fibula

Patellar ligament

Tibial tuberosity

Pectineus muscle (*cut and reflected*)

Superior ramus of pubis

Adductor longus muscle (*cut and reflected*)

Adductor brevis muscle (*cut*)

Pubic tubercle

Gracilis muscle (*cut*)

Obturator externus muscle

Quadratus femoris muscle

Adductor minimus part of
Adductor magnus muscle

Openings for perforating
branches of profunda femoris
(deep femoral) artery

Tendon of adductor magnus muscle
inserting on adductor tubercle
on medial epicondyle of femur

Gracilis muscle (*cut*)

Tibial collateral ligament
(superficial fibers)

Medial patellar retinaculum

Sartorius tendon (*cut*)

Gracilis tendon

Semitendinosus tendon

Pes anserinus

f. Netter

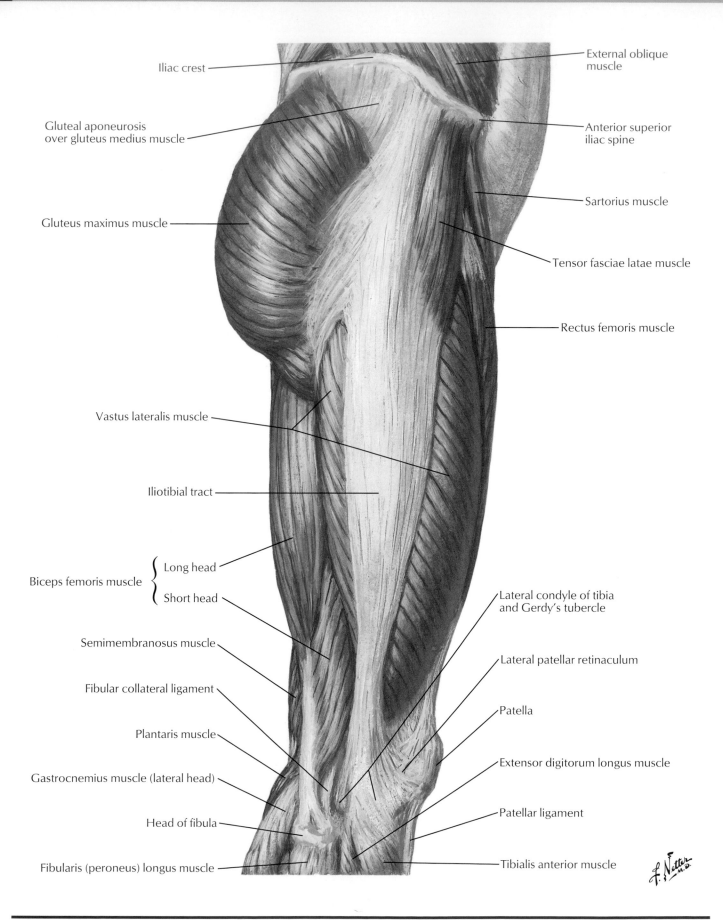

Iliac crest

External oblique muscle

Gluteal aponeurosis over gluteus medius muscle

Anterior superior iliac spine

Sartorius muscle

Gluteus maximus muscle

Tensor fasciae latae muscle

Rectus femoris muscle

Vastus lateralis muscle

Iliotibial tract

Biceps femoris muscle
{ Long head
{ Short head

Lateral condyle of tibia and Gerdy's tubercle

Semimembranosus muscle

Lateral patellar retinaculum

Fibular collateral ligament

Patella

Plantaris muscle

Extensor digitorum longus muscle

Gastrocnemius muscle (lateral head)

Patellar ligament

Head of fibula

Fibularis (peroneus) longus muscle

Tibialis anterior muscle

Plate 482   **Hip and Thigh**

Superficial dissection

Deeper dissection

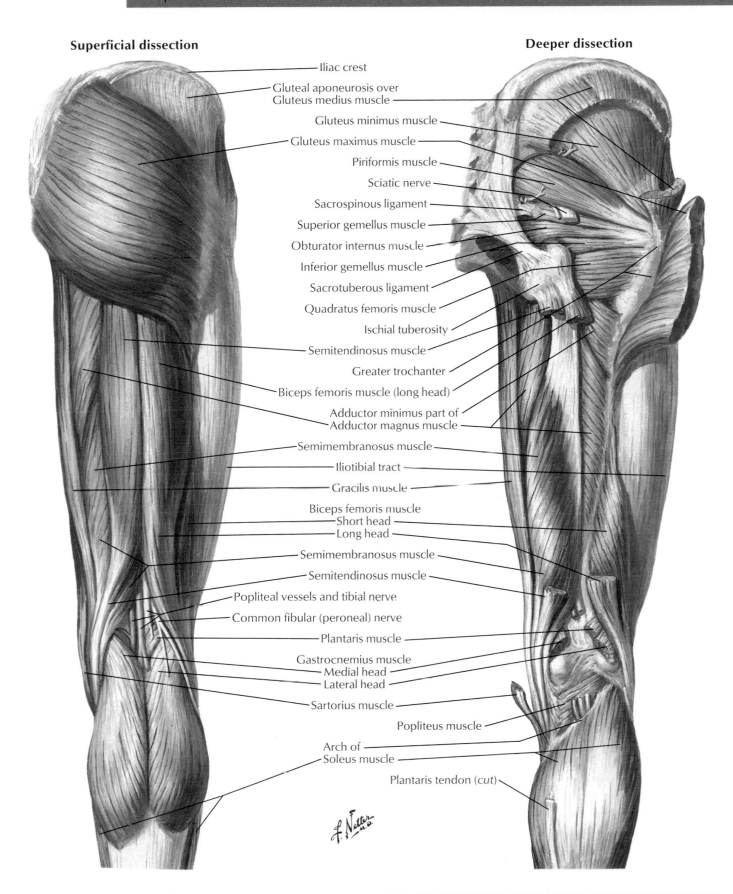

Iliac crest

Gluteal aponeurosis over
Gluteus medius muscle

Gluteus minimus muscle

Gluteus maximus muscle

Piriformis muscle

Sciatic nerve

Sacrospinous ligament

Superior gemellus muscle

Obturator internus muscle

Inferior gemellus muscle

Sacrotuberous ligament

Quadratus femoris muscle

Ischial tuberosity

Semitendinosus muscle

Greater trochanter

Biceps femoris muscle (long head)

Adductor minimus part of
Adductor magnus muscle

Semimembranosus muscle

Iliotibial tract

Gracilis muscle

Biceps femoris muscle
Short head
Long head

Semimembranosus muscle

Semitendinosus muscle

Popliteal vessels and tibial nerve

Common fibular (peroneal) nerve

Plantaris muscle

Gastrocnemius muscle
Medial head
Lateral head

Sartorius muscle

Popliteus muscle

Arch of
Soleus muscle

Plantaris tendon (*cut*)

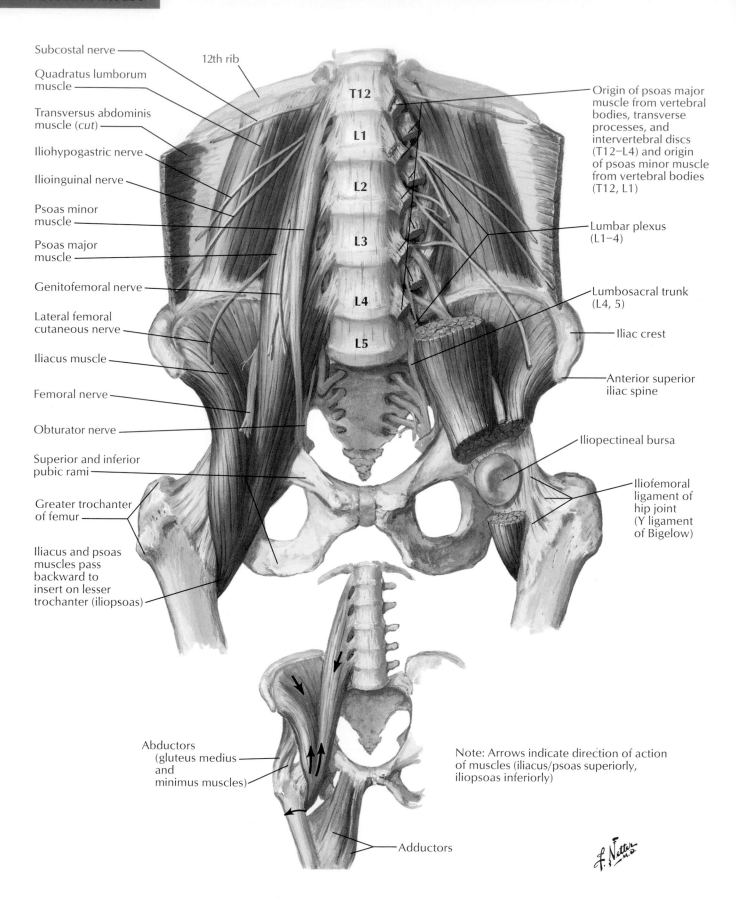

Subcostal nerve

Quadratus lumborum muscle

Transversus abdominis muscle (*cut*)

Iliohypogastric nerve

Ilioinguinal nerve

Psoas minor muscle

Psoas major muscle

Genitofemoral nerve

Lateral femoral cutaneous nerve

Iliacus muscle

Femoral nerve

Obturator nerve

Superior and inferior pubic rami

Greater trochanter of femur

Iliacus and psoas muscles pass backward to insert on lesser trochanter (iliopsoas)

12th rib

T12

L1

L2

L3

L4

L5

Origin of psoas major muscle from vertebral bodies, transverse processes, and intervertebral discs (T12–L4) and origin of psoas minor muscle from vertebral bodies (T12, L1)

Lumbar plexus (L1–4)

Lumbosacral trunk (L4, 5)

Iliac crest

Anterior superior iliac spine

Iliopectineal bursa

Iliofemoral ligament of hip joint (Y ligament of Bigelow)

Abductors (gluteus medius and minimus muscles)

Note: Arrows indicate direction of action of muscles (iliacus/psoas superiorly, iliopsoas inferiorly)

Adductors

Plate 484

Hip and Thigh

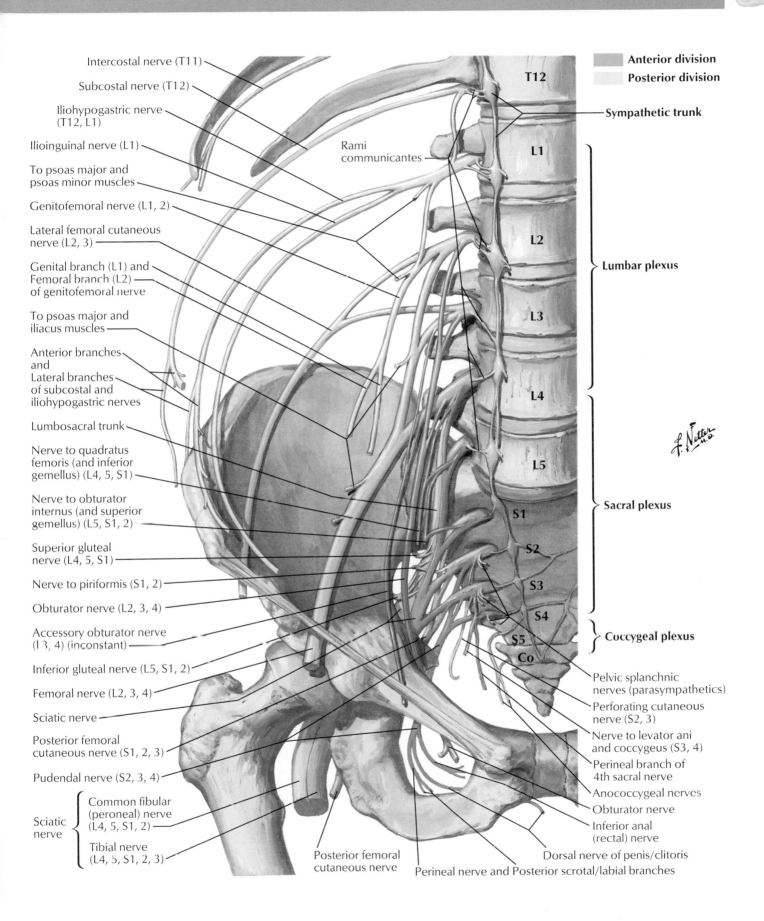

Intercostal nerve (T11)

Subcostal nerve (T12)

Iliohypogastric nerve (T12, L1)

Ilioinguinal nerve (L1)

To psoas major and psoas minor muscles

Genitofemoral nerve (L1, 2)

Lateral femoral cutaneous nerve (L2, 3)

Genital branch (L1) and Femoral branch (L2) of genitofemoral nerve

To psoas major and iliacus muscles

Anterior branches and Lateral branches of subcostal and iliohypogastric nerves

Lumbosacral trunk

Nerve to quadratus femoris (and inferior gemellus) (L4, 5, S1)

Nerve to obturator internus (and superior gemellus) (L5, S1, 2)

Superior gluteal nerve (L4, 5, S1)

Nerve to piriformis (S1, 2)

Obturator nerve (L2, 3, 4)

Accessory obturator nerve (L3, 4) (inconstant)

Inferior gluteal nerve (L5, S1, 2)

Femoral nerve (L2, 3, 4)

Sciatic nerve

Posterior femoral cutaneous nerve (S1, 2, 3)

Pudendal nerve (S2, 3, 4)

Sciatic nerve {
Common fibular (peroneal) nerve (L4, 5, S1, 2)

Tibial nerve (L4, 5, S1, 2, 3)
}

Rami communicantes

T12

L1

L2

L3

L4

L5

S1

S2

S3

S4

S5

Co

Anterior division

Posterior division

Sympathetic trunk

Lumbar plexus

Sacral plexus

Coccygeal plexus

Pelvic splanchnic nerves (parasympathetics)

Perforating cutaneous nerve (S2, 3)

Nerve to levator ani and coccygeus (S3, 4)

Perineal branch of 4th sacral nerve

Anococcygeal nerves

Obturator nerve

Inferior anal (rectal) nerve

Dorsal nerve of penis/clitoris

Posterior femoral cutaneous nerve

Perineal nerve and Posterior scrotal/labial branches

F. Netter M.D.

Schema

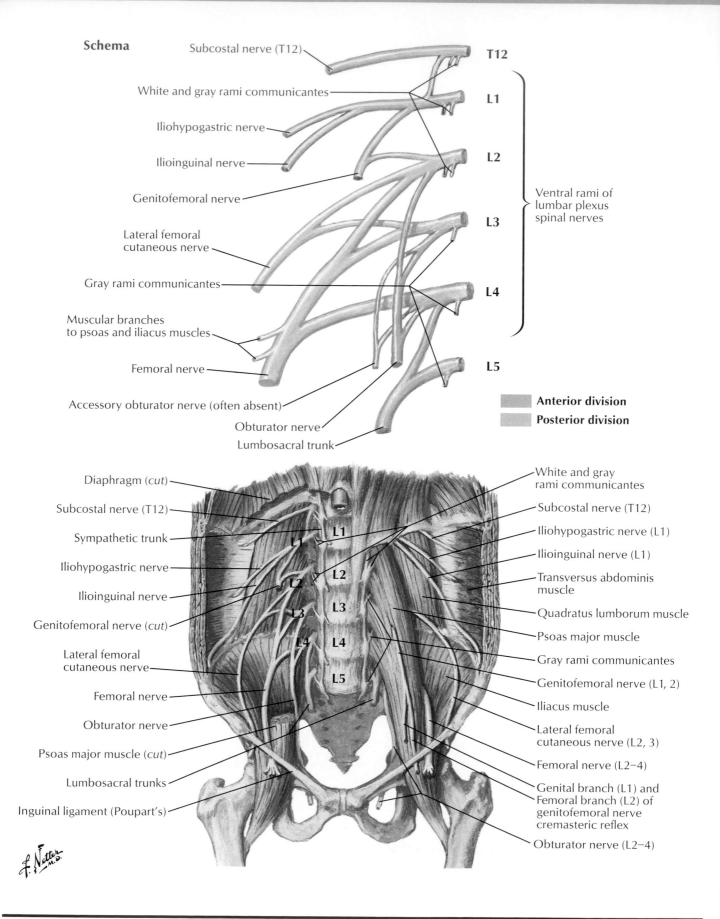

Subcostal nerve (T12)

White and gray rami communicantes

Iliohypogastric nerve

Ilioinguinal nerve

Genitofemoral nerve

Lateral femoral cutaneous nerve

Gray rami communicantes

Muscular branches to psoas and iliacus muscles

Femoral nerve

Accessory obturator nerve (often absent)

Obturator nerve

Lumbosacral trunk

T12

L1

L2

L3

L4

L5

Ventral rami of lumbar plexus spinal nerves

Anterior division
Posterior division

Diaphragm (*cut*)

Subcostal nerve (T12)

Sympathetic trunk

Iliohypogastric nerve

Ilioinguinal nerve

Genitofemoral nerve (*cut*)

Lateral femoral cutaneous nerve

Femoral nerve

Obturator nerve

Psoas major muscle (*cut*)

Lumbosacral trunks

Inguinal ligament (Poupart's)

White and gray rami communicantes

Subcostal nerve (T12)

Iliohypogastric nerve (L1)

Ilioinguinal nerve (L1)

Transversus abdominis muscle

Quadratus lumborum muscle

Psoas major muscle

Gray rami communicantes

Genitofemoral nerve (L1, 2)

Iliacus muscle

Lateral femoral cutaneous nerve (L2, 3)

Femoral nerve (L2–4)

Genital branch (L1) and Femoral branch (L2) of genitofemoral nerve cremasteric reflex

Obturator nerve (L2–4)

L1

L2

L3

L4

L5

Plate 486

Hip and Thigh

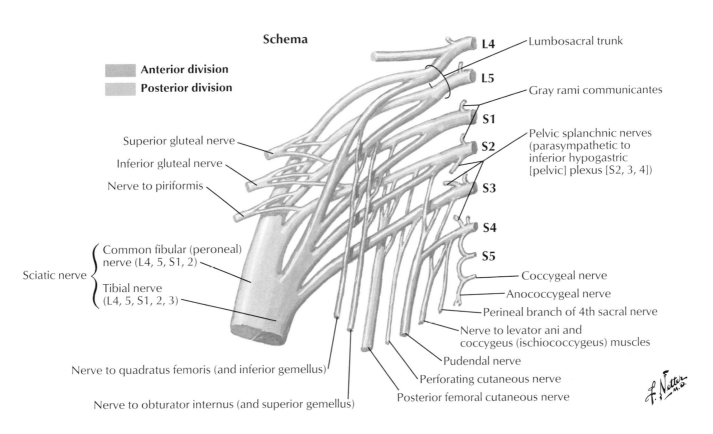

Schema

Anterior division
Posterior division

Superior gluteal nerve

Inferior gluteal nerve

Nerve to piriformis

L4 — Lumbosacral trunk

L5

S1 — Gray rami communicantes

S2 — Pelvic splanchnic nerves (parasympathetic to inferior hypogastric [pelvic] plexus [S2, 3, 4])

S3

S4

S5

Sciatic nerve {
Common fibular (peroneal) nerve (L4, 5, S1, 2)
Tibial nerve (L4, 5, S1, 2, 3)
}

Coccygeal nerve
Anococcygeal nerve
Perineal branch of 4th sacral nerve
Nerve to levator ani and coccygeus (ischiococcygeus) muscles
Pudendal nerve

Nerve to quadratus femoris (and inferior gemellus)

Perforating cutaneous nerve
Posterior femoral cutaneous nerve

Nerve to obturator internus (and superior gemellus)

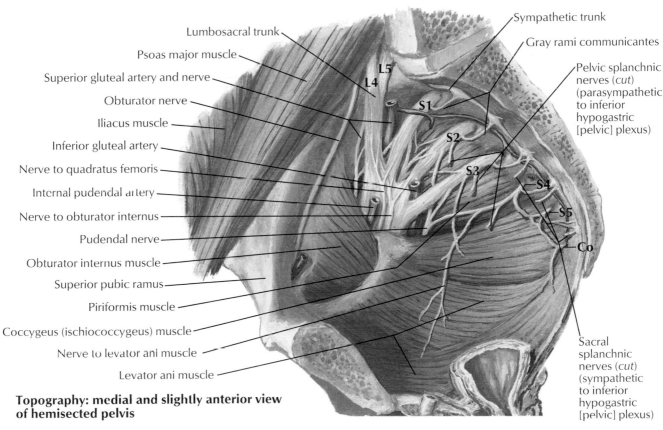

Lumbosacral trunk
Psoas major muscle
Superior gluteal artery and nerve
Obturator nerve
Iliacus muscle
Inferior gluteal artery
Nerve to quadratus femoris
Internal pudendal artery
Nerve to obturator internus
Pudendal nerve
Obturator internus muscle
Superior pubic ramus
Piriformis muscle
Coccygeus (ischiococcygeus) muscle
Nerve to levator ani muscle
Levator ani muscle

Sympathetic trunk
Gray rami communicantes
Pelvic splanchnic nerves (cut) (parasympathetic to inferior hypogastric [pelvic] plexus)

L5
L4
S1
S2
S3
S4
S5
Co

Sacral splanchnic nerves (cut) (sympathetic to inferior hypogastric [pelvic] plexus)

Topography: medial and slightly anterior view of hemisected pelvis

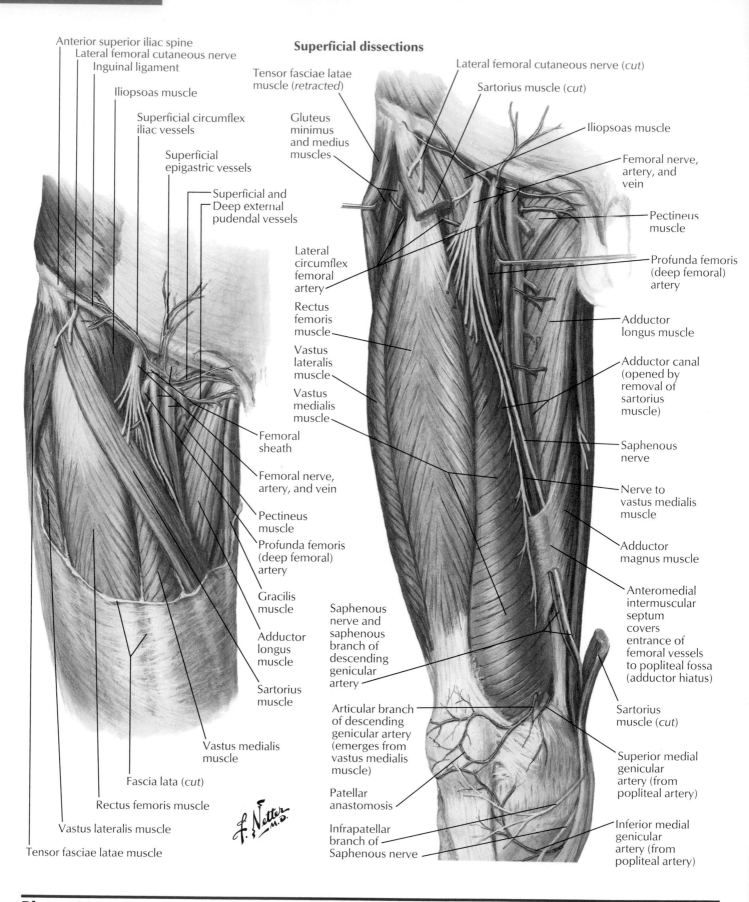

Superficial dissections

Anterior superior iliac spine

Lateral femoral cutaneous nerve

Inguinal ligament

Iliopsoas muscle

Superficial circumflex iliac vessels

Superficial epigastric vessels

Superficial and Deep external pudendal vessels

Tensor fasciae latae muscle (*retracted*)

Gluteus minimus and medius muscles

Lateral circumflex femoral artery

Rectus femoris muscle

Vastus lateralis muscle

Vastus medialis muscle

Femoral sheath

Femoral nerve, artery, and vein

Pectineus muscle

Profunda femoris (deep femoral) artery

Gracilis muscle

Adductor longus muscle

Sartorius muscle

Vastus medialis muscle

Fascia lata (*cut*)

Rectus femoris muscle

Vastus lateralis muscle

Tensor fasciae latae muscle

Saphenous nerve and saphenous branch of descending genicular artery

Articular branch of descending genicular artery (emerges from vastus medialis muscle)

Patellar anastomosis

Infrapatellar branch of Saphenous nerve

Lateral femoral cutaneous nerve (*cut*)

Sartorius muscle (*cut*)

Iliopsoas muscle

Femoral nerve, artery, and vein

Pectineus muscle

Profunda femoris (deep femoral) artery

Adductor longus muscle

Adductor canal (opened by removal of sartorius muscle)

Saphenous nerve

Nerve to vastus medialis muscle

Adductor magnus muscle

Anteromedial intermuscular septum covers entrance of femoral vessels to popliteal fossa (adductor hiatus)

Sartorius muscle (*cut*)

Superior medial genicular artery (from popliteal artery)

Inferior medial genicular artery (from popliteal artery)

Plate 488

Hip and Thigh

Deep dissection

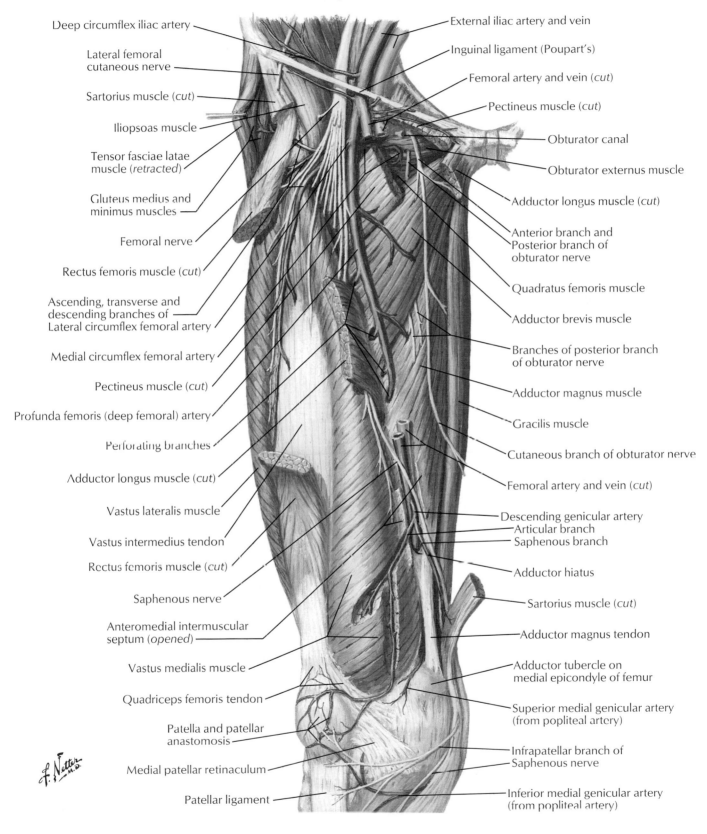

Deep circumflex iliac artery

Lateral femoral cutaneous nerve

Sartorius muscle (*cut*)

Iliopsoas muscle

Tensor fasciae latae muscle (*retracted*)

Gluteus medius and minimus muscles

Femoral nerve

Rectus femoris muscle (*cut*)

Ascending, transverse and descending branches of Lateral circumflex femoral artery

Medial circumflex femoral artery

Pectineus muscle (*cut*)

Profunda femoris (deep femoral) artery

Perforating branches

Adductor longus muscle (*cut*)

Vastus lateralis muscle

Vastus intermedius tendon

Rectus femoris muscle (*cut*)

Saphenous nerve

Anteromedial intermuscular septum (*opened*)

Vastus medialis muscle

Quadriceps femoris tendon

Patella and patellar anastomosis

Medial patellar retinaculum

Patellar ligament

External iliac artery and vein

Inguinal ligament (Poupart's)

Femoral artery and vein (*cut*)

Pectineus muscle (*cut*)

Obturator canal

Obturator externus muscle

Adductor longus muscle (*cut*)

Anterior branch and Posterior branch of obturator nerve

Quadratus femoris muscle

Adductor brevis muscle

Branches of posterior branch of obturator nerve

Adductor magnus muscle

Gracilis muscle

Cutaneous branch of obturator nerve

Femoral artery and vein (*cut*)

Descending genicular artery
Articular branch
Saphenous branch

Adductor hiatus

Sartorius muscle (*cut*)

Adductor magnus tendon

Adductor tubercle on medial epicondyle of femur

Superior medial genicular artery (from popliteal artery)

Infrapatellar branch of Saphenous nerve

Inferior medial genicular artery (from popliteal artery)

Deep dissection

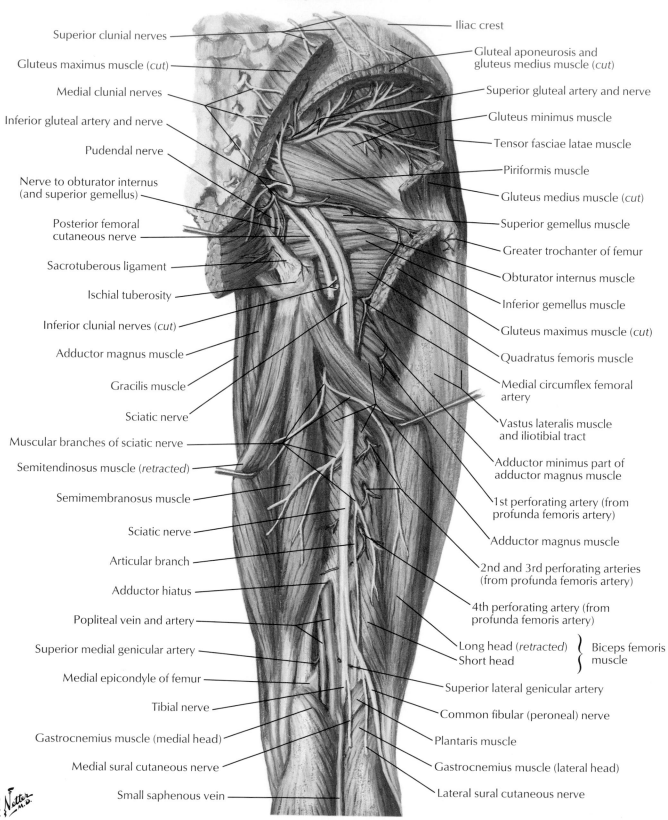

Superior clunial nerves

Gluteus maximus muscle (*cut*)

Medial clunial nerves

Inferior gluteal artery and nerve

Pudendal nerve

Nerve to obturator internus (and superior gemellus)

Posterior femoral cutaneous nerve

Sacrotuberous ligament

Ischial tuberosity

Inferior clunial nerves (*cut*)

Adductor magnus muscle

Gracilis muscle

Sciatic nerve

Muscular branches of sciatic nerve

Semitendinosus muscle (*retracted*)

Semimembranosus muscle

Sciatic nerve

Articular branch

Adductor hiatus

Popliteal vein and artery

Superior medial genicular artery

Medial epicondyle of femur

Tibial nerve

Gastrocnemius muscle (medial head)

Medial sural cutaneous nerve

Small saphenous vein

Iliac crest

Gluteal aponeurosis and gluteus medius muscle (*cut*)

Superior gluteal artery and nerve

Gluteus minimus muscle

Tensor fasciae latae muscle

Piriformis muscle

Gluteus medius muscle (*cut*)

Superior gemellus muscle

Greater trochanter of femur

Obturator internus muscle

Inferior gemellus muscle

Gluteus maximus muscle (*cut*)

Quadratus femoris muscle

Medial circumflex femoral artery

Vastus lateralis muscle and iliotibial tract

Adductor minimus part of adductor magnus muscle

1st perforating artery (from profunda femoris artery)

Adductor magnus muscle

2nd and 3rd perforating arteries (from profunda femoris artery)

4th perforating artery (from profunda femoris artery)

Long head (*retracted*) } Biceps femoris
Short head   } muscle

Superior lateral genicular artery

Common fibular (peroneal) nerve

Plantaris muscle

Gastrocnemius muscle (lateral head)

Lateral sural cutaneous nerve

Plate 490

Hip and Thigh

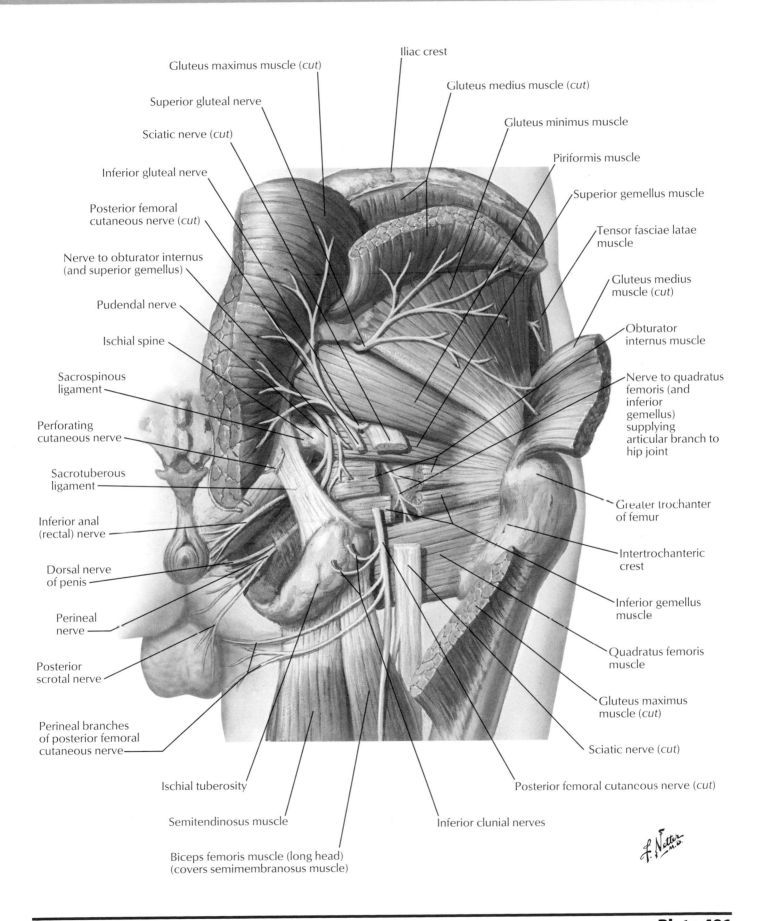

Gluteus maximus muscle (*cut*)

Superior gluteal nerve

Sciatic nerve (*cut*)

Inferior gluteal nerve

Posterior femoral cutaneous nerve (*cut*)

Nerve to obturator internus (and superior gemellus)

Pudendal nerve

Ischial spine

Sacrospinous ligament

Perforating cutaneous nerve

Sacrotuberous ligament

Inferior anal (rectal) nerve

Dorsal nerve of penis

Perineal nerve

Posterior scrotal nerve

Perineal branches of posterior femoral cutaneous nerve

Ischial tuberosity

Semitendinosus muscle

Biceps femoris muscle (long head) (covers semimembranosus muscle)

Iliac crest

Gluteus medius muscle (*cut*)

Gluteus minimus muscle

Piriformis muscle

Superior gemellus muscle

Tensor fasciae latae muscle

Gluteus medius muscle (*cut*)

Obturator internus muscle

Nerve to quadratus femoris (and inferior gemellus) supplying articular branch to hip joint

Greater trochanter of femur

Intertrochanteric crest

Inferior gemellus muscle

Quadratus femoris muscle

Gluteus maximus muscle (*cut*)

Sciatic nerve (*cut*)

Posterior femoral cutaneous nerve (*cut*)

Inferior clunial nerves

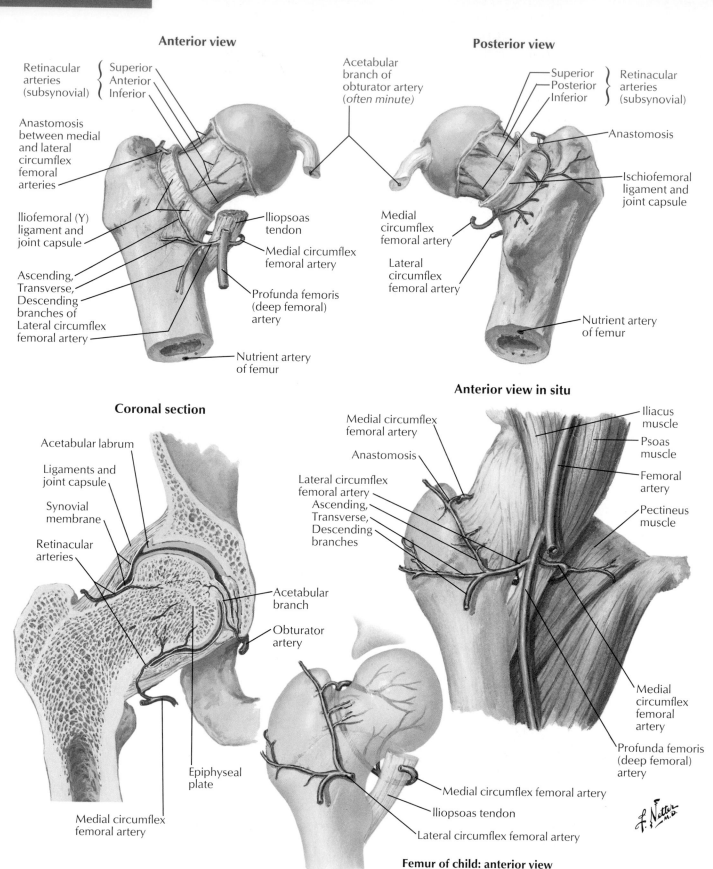

Anterior view

Retinacular arteries (subsynovial) { Superior Anterior Inferior

Anastomosis between medial and lateral circumflex femoral arteries

Iliofemoral (Y) ligament and joint capsule

Ascending, Transverse, Descending branches of Lateral circumflex femoral artery

Iliopsoas tendon

Medial circumflex femoral artery

Profunda femoris (deep femoral) artery

Nutrient artery of femur

Acetabular branch of obturator artery (often minute)

Posterior view

Superior Posterior Inferior } Retinacular arteries (subsynovial)

Anastomosis

Ischiofemoral ligament and joint capsule

Medial circumflex femoral artery

Lateral circumflex femoral artery

Nutrient artery of femur

Coronal section

Acetabular labrum

Ligaments and joint capsule

Synovial membrane

Retinacular arteries

Acetabular branch

Obturator artery

Epiphyseal plate

Medial circumflex femoral artery

Anterior view in situ

Medial circumflex femoral artery

Anastomosis

Lateral circumflex femoral artery

Ascending, Transverse, Descending branches

Iliacus muscle

Psoas muscle

Femoral artery

Pectineus muscle

Medial circumflex femoral artery

Profunda femoris (deep femoral) artery

Medial circumflex femoral artery

Iliopsoas tendon

Lateral circumflex femoral artery

Femur of child: anterior view

Plate 492

Hip and Thigh

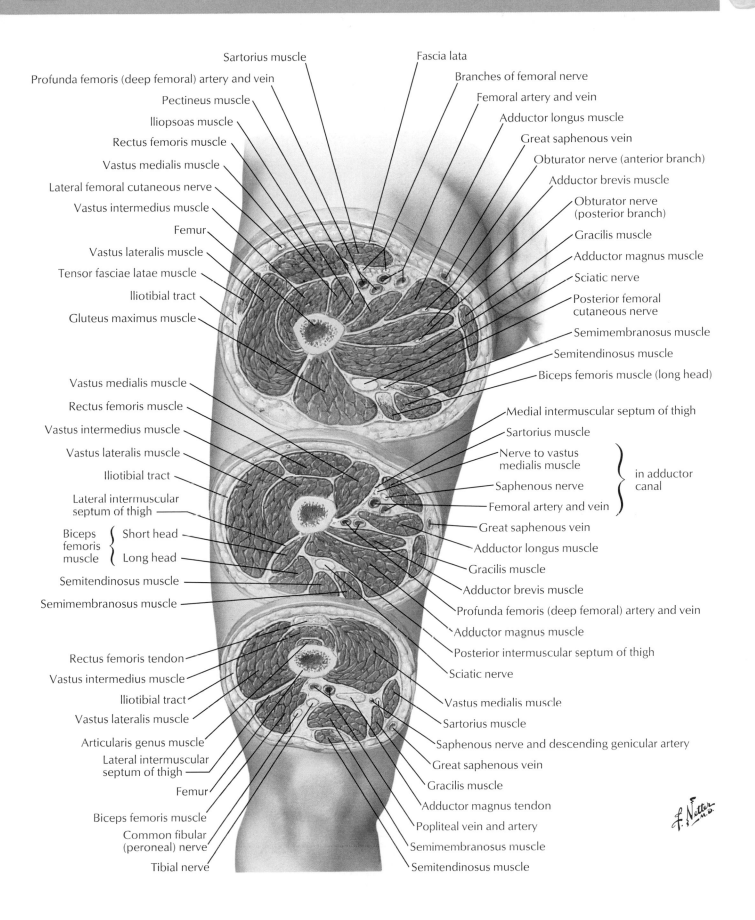

Sartorius muscle

Profunda femoris (deep femoral) artery and vein

Pectineus muscle

Iliopsoas muscle

Rectus femoris muscle

Vastus medialis muscle

Lateral femoral cutaneous nerve

Vastus intermedius muscle

Femur

Vastus lateralis muscle

Tensor fasciae latae muscle

Iliotibial tract

Gluteus maximus muscle

Vastus medialis muscle

Rectus femoris muscle

Vastus intermedius muscle

Vastus lateralis muscle

Iliotibial tract

Lateral intermuscular septum of thigh

Biceps femoris muscle { Short head / Long head }

Semitendinosus muscle

Semimembranosus muscle

Rectus femoris tendon

Vastus intermedius muscle

Iliotibial tract

Vastus lateralis muscle

Articularis genus muscle

Lateral intermuscular septum of thigh

Femur

Biceps femoris muscle

Common fibular (peroneal) nerve

Tibial nerve

Fascia lata

Branches of femoral nerve

Femoral artery and vein

Adductor longus muscle

Great saphenous vein

Obturator nerve (anterior branch)

Adductor brevis muscle

Obturator nerve (posterior branch)

Gracilis muscle

Adductor magnus muscle

Sciatic nerve

Posterior femoral cutaneous nerve

Semimembranosus muscle

Semitendinosus muscle

Biceps femoris muscle (long head)

Medial intermuscular septum of thigh

Sartorius muscle

Nerve to vastus medialis muscle

Saphenous nerve

Femoral artery and vein

} in adductor canal

Great saphenous vein

Adductor longus muscle

Gracilis muscle

Adductor brevis muscle

Profunda femoris (deep femoral) artery and vein

Adductor magnus muscle

Posterior intermuscular septum of thigh

Sciatic nerve

Vastus medialis muscle

Sartorius muscle

Saphenous nerve and descending genicular artery

Great saphenous vein

Gracilis muscle

Adductor magnus tendon

Popliteal vein and artery

Semimembranosus muscle

Semitendinosus muscle

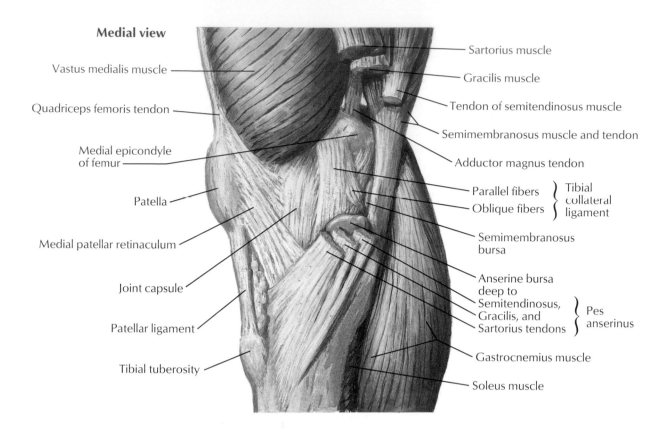

Medial view

Vastus medialis muscle

Quadriceps femoris tendon

Medial epicondyle of femur

Patella

Medial patellar retinaculum

Joint capsule

Patellar ligament

Tibial tuberosity

Sartorius muscle

Gracilis muscle

Tendon of semitendinosus muscle

Semimembranosus muscle and tendon

Adductor magnus tendon

Parallel fibers } Tibial collateral ligament
Oblique fibers }

Semimembranosus bursa

Anserine bursa deep to Semitendinosus, Gracilis, and Sartorius tendons } Pes anserinus

Gastrocnemius muscle

Soleus muscle

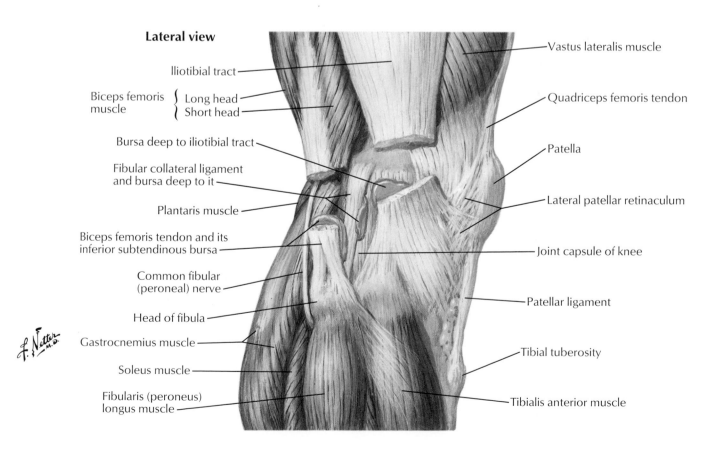

Lateral view

Iliotibial tract

Biceps femoris muscle { Long head / Short head

Bursa deep to iliotibial tract

Fibular collateral ligament and bursa deep to it

Plantaris muscle

Biceps femoris tendon and its inferior subtendinous bursa

Common fibular (peroneal) nerve

Head of fibula

Gastrocnemius muscle

Soleus muscle

Fibularis (peroneus) longus muscle

Vastus lateralis muscle

Quadriceps femoris tendon

Patella

Lateral patellar retinaculum

Joint capsule of knee

Patellar ligament

Tibial tuberosity

Tibialis anterior muscle

Plate 494

Knee

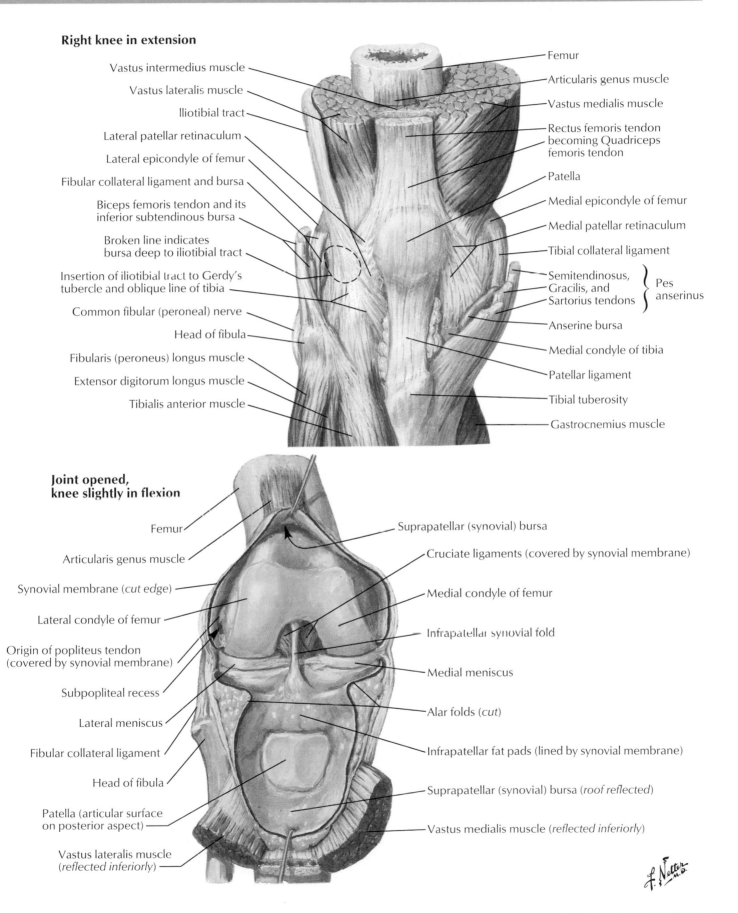

Right knee in extension

Vastus intermedius muscle

Vastus lateralis muscle

Iliotibial tract

Lateral patellar retinaculum

Lateral epicondyle of femur

Fibular collateral ligament and bursa

Biceps femoris tendon and its inferior subtendinous bursa

Broken line indicates bursa deep to iliotibial tract

Insertion of iliotibial tract to Gerdy's tubercle and oblique line of tibia

Common fibular (peroneal) nerve

Head of fibula

Fibularis (peroneus) longus muscle

Extensor digitorum longus muscle

Tibialis anterior muscle

Femur

Articularis genus muscle

Vastus medialis muscle

Rectus femoris tendon becoming Quadriceps femoris tendon

Patella

Medial epicondyle of femur

Medial patellar retinaculum

Tibial collateral ligament

Semitendinosus, Gracilis, and Sartorius tendons } Pes anserinus

Anserine bursa

Medial condyle of tibia

Patellar ligament

Tibial tuberosity

Gastrocnemius muscle

Joint opened, knee slightly in flexion

Femur

Articularis genus muscle

Synovial membrane (*cut edge*)

Lateral condyle of femur

Origin of popliteus tendon (covered by synovial membrane)

Subpopliteal recess

Lateral meniscus

Fibular collateral ligament

Head of fibula

Patella (articular surface on posterior aspect)

Vastus lateralis muscle (*reflected inferiorly*)

Suprapatellar (synovial) bursa

Cruciate ligaments (covered by synovial membrane)

Medial condyle of femur

Infrapatellar synovial fold

Medial meniscus

Alar folds (*cut*)

Infrapatellar fat pads (lined by synovial membrane)

Suprapatellar (synovial) bursa (*roof reflected*)

Vastus medialis muscle (*reflected inferiorly*)

Inferior view

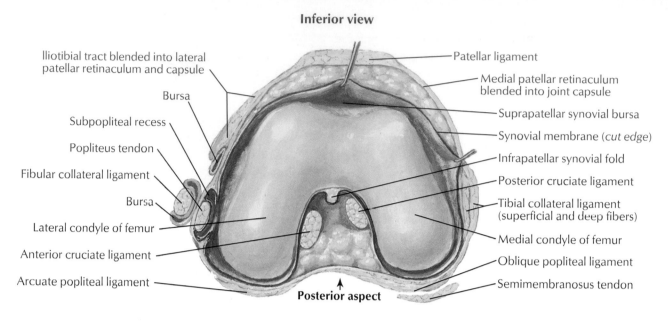

Iliotibial tract blended into lateral patellar retinaculum and capsule

Bursa

Subpopliteal recess

Popliteus tendon

Fibular collateral ligament

Bursa

Lateral condyle of femur

Anterior cruciate ligament

Arcuate popliteal ligament

Patellar ligament

Medial patellar retinaculum blended into joint capsule

Suprapatellar synovial bursa

Synovial membrane (*cut edge*)

Infrapatellar synovial fold

Posterior cruciate ligament

Tibial collateral ligament (superficial and deep fibers)

Medial condyle of femur

Oblique popliteal ligament

Semimembranosus tendon

Posterior aspect

Superior view

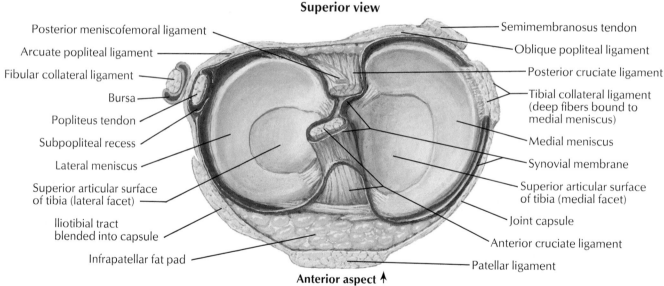

Posterior meniscofemoral ligament

Arcuate popliteal ligament

Fibular collateral ligament

Bursa

Popliteus tendon

Subpopliteal recess

Lateral meniscus

Superior articular surface of tibia (lateral facet)

Iliotibial tract blended into capsule

Infrapatellar fat pad

Semimembranosus tendon

Oblique popliteal ligament

Posterior cruciate ligament

Tibial collateral ligament (deep fibers bound to medial meniscus)

Medial meniscus

Synovial membrane

Superior articular surface of tibia (medial facet)

Joint capsule

Anterior cruciate ligament

Patellar ligament

Anterior aspect

Superior view: ligaments and cartilage removed

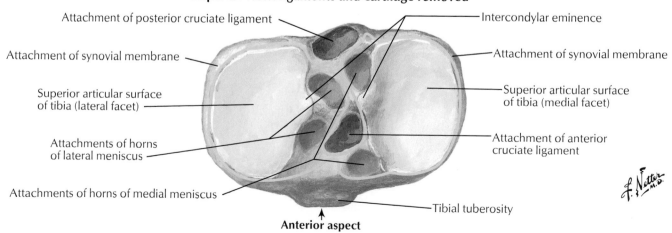

Attachment of posterior cruciate ligament

Attachment of synovial membrane

Superior articular surface of tibia (lateral facet)

Attachments of horns of lateral meniscus

Attachments of horns of medial meniscus

Intercondylar eminence

Attachment of synovial membrane

Superior articular surface of tibia (medial facet)

Attachment of anterior cruciate ligament

Tibial tuberosity

Anterior aspect

Plate 496

Knee

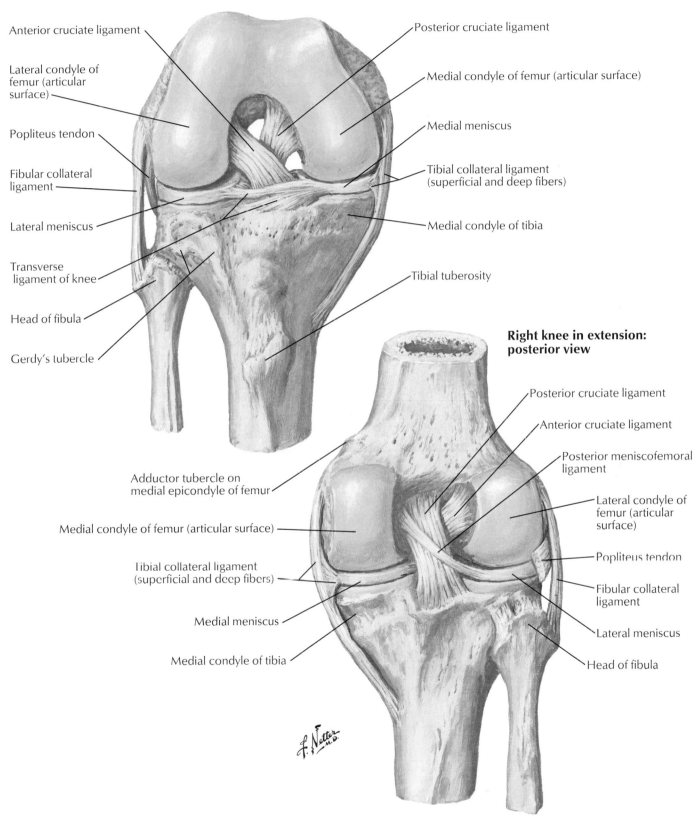

Right knee in flexion: anterior view

Anterior cruciate ligament

Lateral condyle of femur (articular surface)

Popliteus tendon

Fibular collateral ligament

Lateral meniscus

Transverse ligament of knee

Head of fibula

Gerdy's tubercle

Posterior cruciate ligament

Medial condyle of femur (articular surface)

Medial meniscus

Tibial collateral ligament (superficial and deep fibers)

Medial condyle of tibia

Tibial tuberosity

Right knee in extension: posterior view

Posterior cruciate ligament

Anterior cruciate ligament

Posterior meniscofemoral ligament

Lateral condyle of femur (articular surface)

Popliteus tendon

Fibular collateral ligament

Lateral meniscus

Head of fibula

Adductor tubercle on medial epicondyle of femur

Medial condyle of femur (articular surface)

Tibial collateral ligament (superficial and deep fibers)

Medial meniscus

Medial condyle of tibia

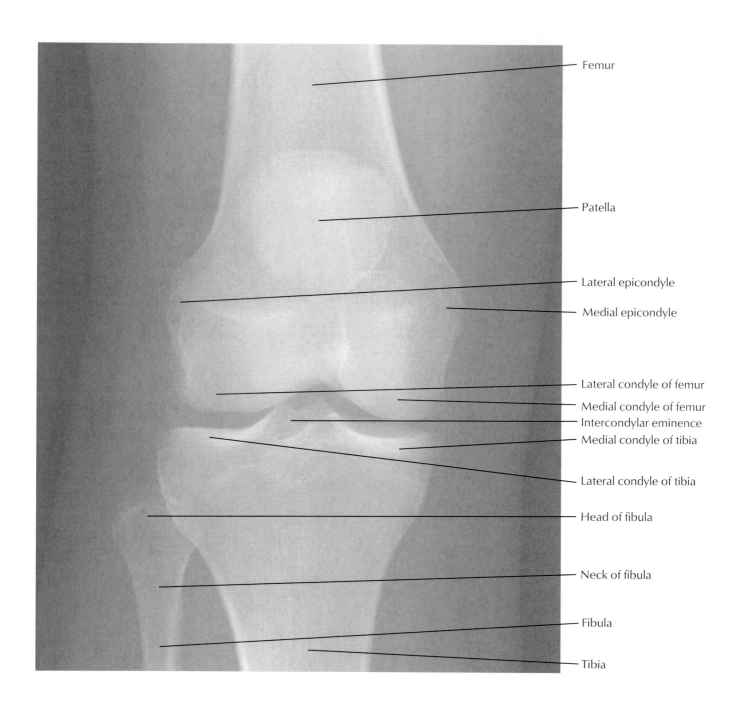

Femur

Patella

Lateral epicondyle

Medial epicondyle

Lateral condyle of femur

Medial condyle of femur

Intercondylar eminence

Medial condyle of tibia

Lateral condyle of tibia

Head of fibula

Neck of fibula

Fibula

Tibia

Plate 498

Knee

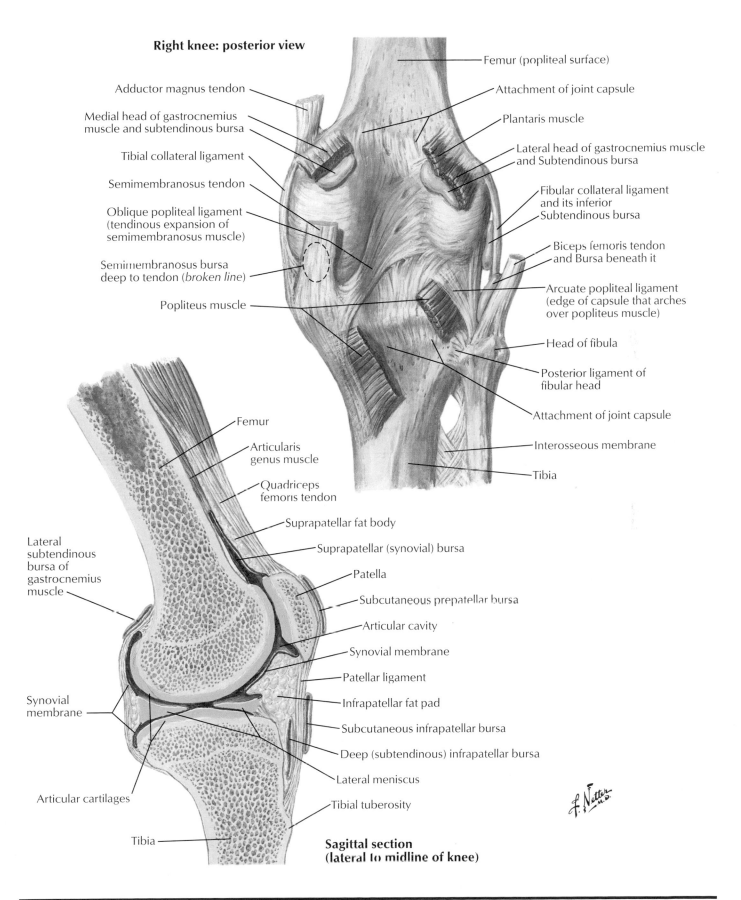

Right knee: posterior view

Adductor magnus tendon

Medial head of gastrocnemius muscle and subtendinous bursa

Tibial collateral ligament

Semimembranosus tendon

Oblique popliteal ligament (tendinous expansion of semimembranosus muscle)

Semimembranosus bursa deep to tendon (*broken line*)

Popliteus muscle

Femur (popliteal surface)

Attachment of joint capsule

Plantaris muscle

Lateral head of gastrocnemius muscle and Subtendinous bursa

Fibular collateral ligament and its inferior Subtendinous bursa

Biceps femoris tendon and Bursa beneath it

Arcuate popliteal ligament (edge of capsule that arches over popliteus muscle)

Head of fibula

Posterior ligament of fibular head

Attachment of joint capsule

Interosseous membrane

Tibia

Femur

Articularis genus muscle

Quadriceps femoris tendon

Suprapatellar fat body

Suprapatellar (synovial) bursa

Patella

Subcutaneous prepatellar bursa

Articular cavity

Synovial membrane

Patellar ligament

Infrapatellar fat pad

Subcutaneous infrapatellar bursa

Deep (subtendinous) infrapatellar bursa

Lateral meniscus

Tibial tuberosity

Lateral subtendinous bursa of gastrocnemius muscle

Synovial membrane

Articular cartilages

Tibia

Sagittal section (lateral to midline of knee)

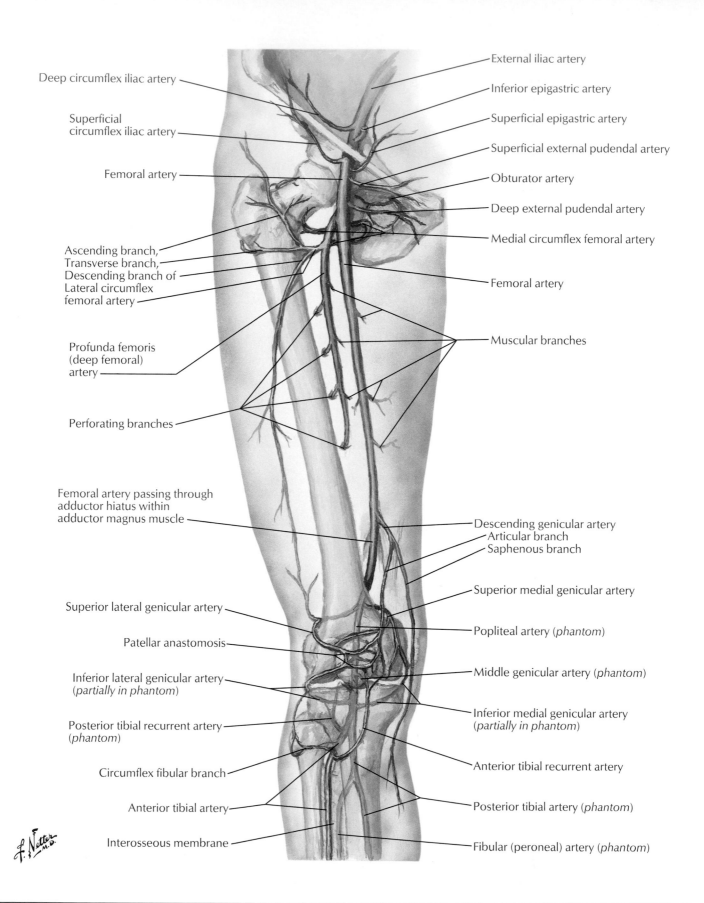

Deep circumflex iliac artery

Superficial circumflex iliac artery

Femoral artery

Ascending branch,
Transverse branch,
Descending branch of
Lateral circumflex
femoral artery

Profunda femoris
(deep femoral)
artery

Perforating branches

Femoral artery passing through
adductor hiatus within
adductor magnus muscle

Superior lateral genicular artery

Patellar anastomosis

Inferior lateral genicular artery
(*partially in phantom*)

Posterior tibial recurrent artery
(*phantom*)

Circumflex fibular branch

Anterior tibial artery

Interosseous membrane

External iliac artery

Inferior epigastric artery

Superficial epigastric artery

Superficial external pudendal artery

Obturator artery

Deep external pudendal artery

Medial circumflex femoral artery

Femoral artery

Muscular branches

Descending genicular artery
Articular branch
Saphenous branch

Superior medial genicular artery

Popliteal artery (*phantom*)

Middle genicular artery (*phantom*)

Inferior medial genicular artery
(*partially in phantom*)

Anterior tibial recurrent artery

Posterior tibial artery (*phantom*)

Fibular (peroneal) artery (*phantom*)

Plate 500

Knee

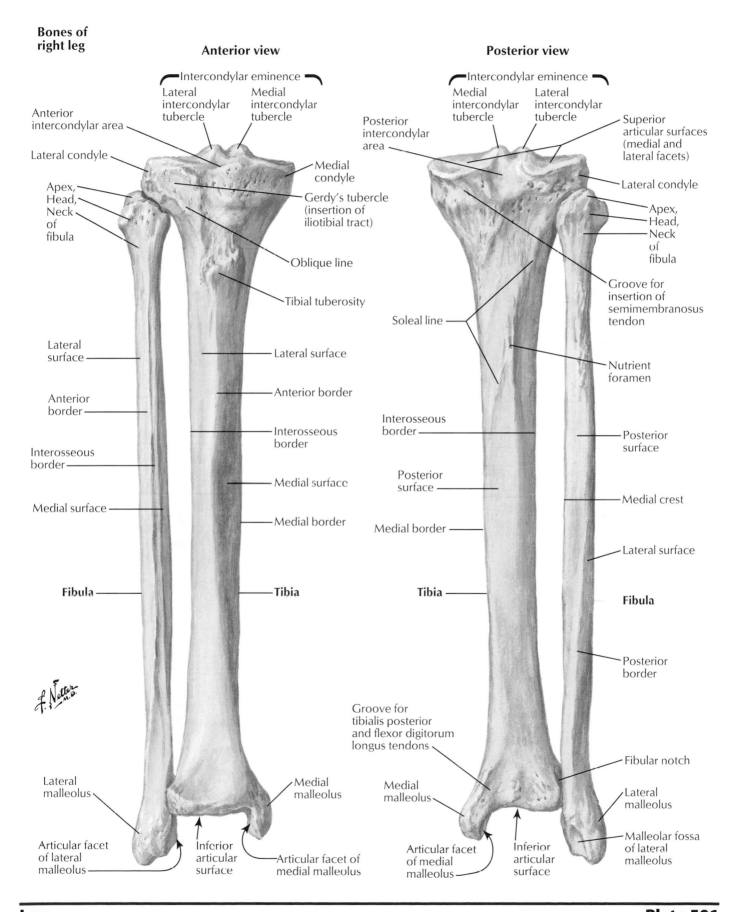

Bones of right leg

Anterior view

Posterior view

Intercondylar eminence

Lateral intercondylar tubercle

Medial intercondylar tubercle

Anterior intercondylar area

Lateral condyle

Apex, Head, Neck of fibula

Medial condyle

Gerdy's tubercle (insertion of iliotibial tract)

Oblique line

Tibial tuberosity

Lateral surface

Anterior border

Lateral surface

Anterior border

Interosseous border

Interosseous border

Medial surface

Medial surface

Medial border

Fibula

Tibia

Lateral malleolus

Medial malleolus

Articular facet of lateral malleolus

Inferior articular surface

Articular facet of medial malleolus

Intercondylar eminence

Medial intercondylar tubercle

Lateral intercondylar tubercle

Posterior intercondylar area

Superior articular surfaces (medial and lateral facets)

Lateral condyle

Apex, Head, Neck of fibula

Groove for insertion of semimembranosus tendon

Soleal line

Nutrient foramen

Interosseous border

Posterior surface

Posterior surface

Medial crest

Medial border

Lateral surface

Tibia

Fibula

Posterior border

Groove for tibialis posterior and flexor digitorum longus tendons

Medial malleolus

Fibular notch

Lateral malleolus

Articular facet of medial malleolus

Inferior articular surface

Malleolar fossa of lateral malleolus

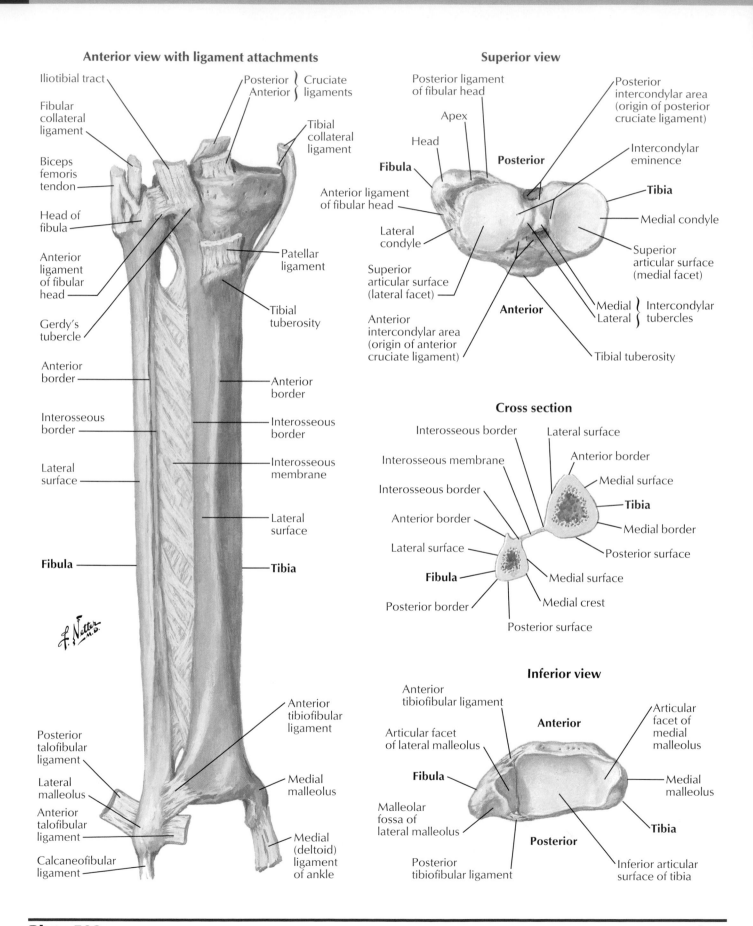

Anterior view with ligament attachments

Iliotibial tract

Fibular collateral ligament

Biceps femoris tendon

Head of fibula

Anterior ligament of fibular head

Gerdy's tubercle

Anterior border

Interosseous border

Lateral surface

Fibula

Posterior talofibular ligament

Lateral malleolus

Anterior talofibular ligament

Calcaneofibular ligament

Posterior } Cruciate
Anterior } ligaments

Tibial collateral ligament

Patellar ligament

Tibial tuberosity

Anterior border

Interosseous border

Interosseous membrane

Lateral surface

Tibia

Anterior tibiofibular ligament

Medial malleolus

Medial (deltoid) ligament of ankle

Superior view

Posterior ligament of fibular head

Apex

Head

Fibula

Anterior ligament of fibular head

Lateral condyle

Superior articular surface (lateral facet)

Anterior

Anterior intercondylar area (origin of anterior cruciate ligament)

Posterior intercondylar area (origin of posterior cruciate ligament)

Posterior

Intercondylar eminence

Tibia

Medial condyle

Superior articular surface (medial facet)

Medial } Intercondylar
Lateral } tubercles

Tibial tuberosity

Cross section

Interosseous border

Interosseous membrane

Interosseous border

Anterior border

Lateral surface

Fibula

Posterior border

Lateral surface

Anterior border

Medial surface

Tibia

Medial border

Posterior surface

Medial surface

Medial crest

Posterior surface

Inferior view

Anterior tibiofibular ligament

Articular facet of lateral malleolus

Fibula

Malleolar fossa of lateral malleolus

Posterior tibiofibular ligament

Anterior

Articular facet of medial malleolus

Medial malleolus

Tibia

Posterior

Inferior articular surface of tibia

Plate 502 | **Leg**

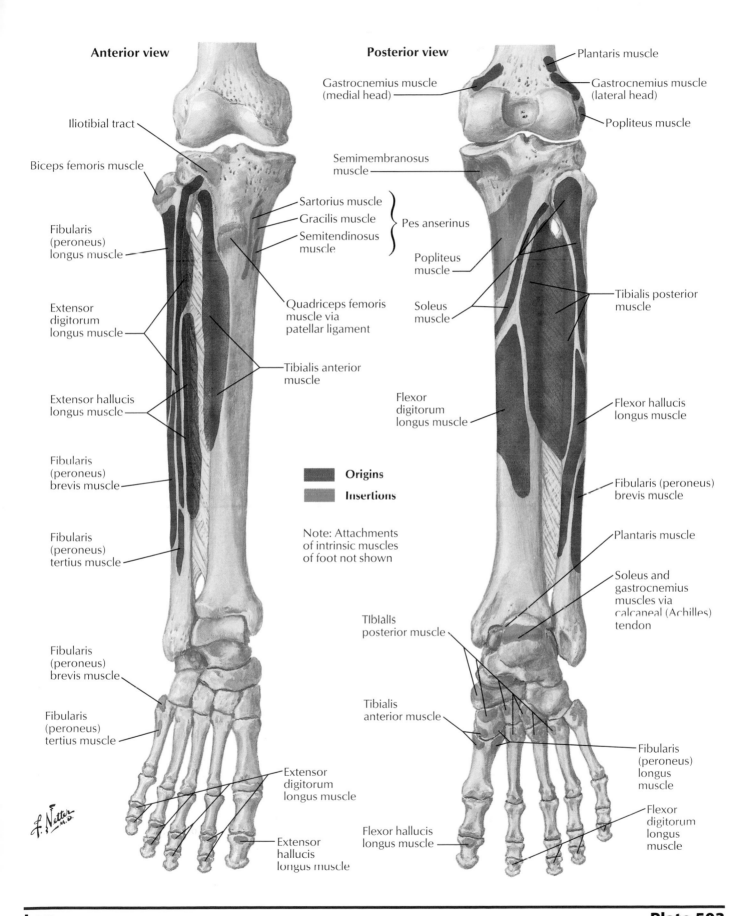

Anterior view

Iliotibial tract

Biceps femoris muscle

Fibularis (peroneus) longus muscle

Extensor digitorum longus muscle

Extensor hallucis longus muscle

Fibularis (peroneus) brevis muscle

Fibularis (peroneus) tertius muscle

Fibularis (peroneus) brevis muscle

Fibularis (peroneus) tertius muscle

Extensor digitorum longus muscle

Extensor hallucis longus muscle

Posterior view

Gastrocnemius muscle (medial head)

Semimembranosus muscle

Sartorius muscle
Gracilis muscle
Semitendinosus muscle
} Pes anserinus

Quadriceps femoris muscle via patellar ligament

Tibialis anterior muscle

Popliteus muscle

Soleus muscle

Flexor digitorum longus muscle

Tibialis posterior muscle

Tibialis anterior muscle

Flexor hallucis longus muscle

Flexor digitorum longus muscle

Plantaris muscle

Gastrocnemius muscle (lateral head)

Popliteus muscle

Tibialis posterior muscle

Flexor hallucis longus muscle

Fibularis (peroneus) brevis muscle

Plantaris muscle

Soleus and gastrocnemius muscles via calcaneal (Achilles) tendon

Fibularis (peroneus) longus muscle

Flexor digitorum longus muscle

■ **Origins**

■ **Insertions**

Note: Attachments of intrinsic muscles of foot not shown

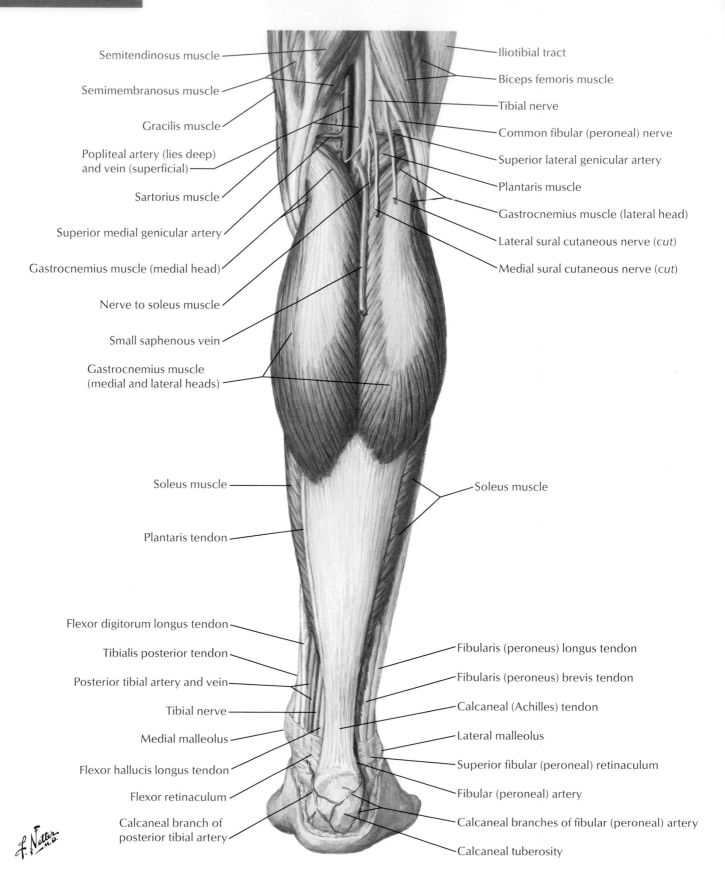

Semitendinosus muscle

Semimembranosus muscle

Gracilis muscle

Popliteal artery (lies deep) and vein (superficial)

Sartorius muscle

Superior medial genicular artery

Gastrocnemius muscle (medial head)

Nerve to soleus muscle

Small saphenous vein

Gastrocnemius muscle (medial and lateral heads)

Soleus muscle

Plantaris tendon

Flexor digitorum longus tendon

Tibialis posterior tendon

Posterior tibial artery and vein

Tibial nerve

Medial malleolus

Flexor hallucis longus tendon

Flexor retinaculum

Calcaneal branch of posterior tibial artery

Iliotibial tract

Biceps femoris muscle

Tibial nerve

Common fibular (peroneal) nerve

Superior lateral genicular artery

Plantaris muscle

Gastrocnemius muscle (lateral head)

Lateral sural cutaneous nerve (*cut*)

Medial sural cutaneous nerve (*cut*)

Soleus muscle

Fibularis (peroneus) longus tendon

Fibularis (peroneus) brevis tendon

Calcaneal (Achilles) tendon

Lateral malleolus

Superior fibular (peroneal) retinaculum

Fibular (peroneal) artery

Calcaneal branches of fibular (peroneal) artery

Calcaneal tuberosity

Plate 504

Leg

See also **Plate 529**

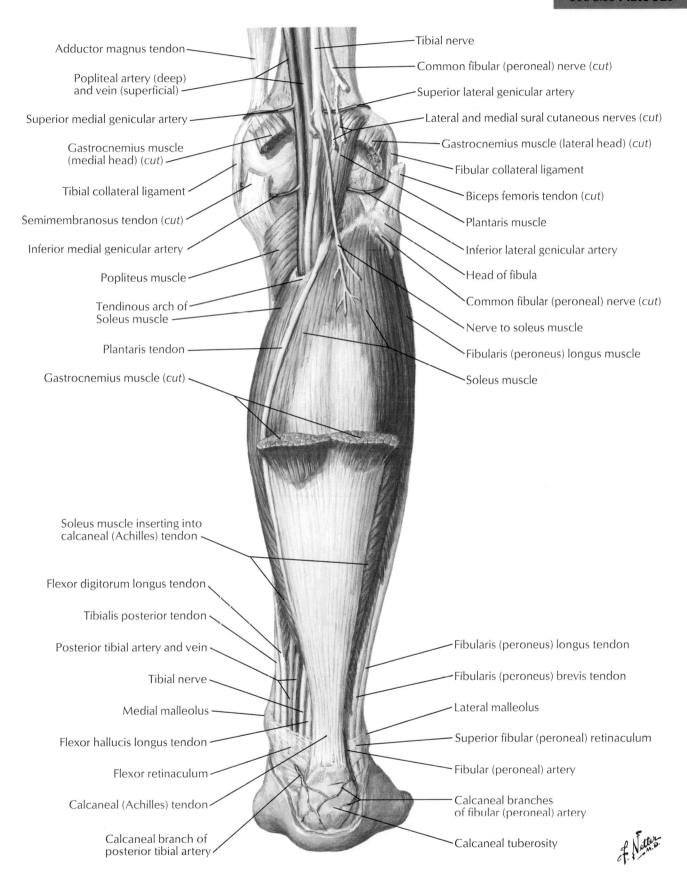

Adductor magnus tendon

Popliteal artery (deep) and vein (superficial)

Superior medial genicular artery

Gastrocnemius muscle (medial head) (*cut*)

Tibial collateral ligament

Semimembranosus tendon (*cut*)

Inferior medial genicular artery

Popliteus muscle

Tendinous arch of Soleus muscle

Plantaris tendon

Gastrocnemius muscle (*cut*)

Soleus muscle inserting into calcaneal (Achilles) tendon

Flexor digitorum longus tendon

Tibialis posterior tendon

Posterior tibial artery and vein

Tibial nerve

Medial malleolus

Flexor hallucis longus tendon

Flexor retinaculum

Calcaneal (Achilles) tendon

Calcaneal branch of posterior tibial artery

Tibial nerve

Common fibular (peroneal) nerve (*cut*)

Superior lateral genicular artery

Lateral and medial sural cutaneous nerves (*cut*)

Gastrocnemius muscle (lateral head) (*cut*)

Fibular collateral ligament

Biceps femoris tendon (*cut*)

Plantaris muscle

Inferior lateral genicular artery

Head of fibula

Common fibular (peroneal) nerve (*cut*)

Nerve to soleus muscle

Fibularis (peroneus) longus muscle

Soleus muscle

Fibularis (peroneus) longus tendon

Fibularis (peroneus) brevis tendon

Lateral malleolus

Superior fibular (peroneal) retinaculum

Fibular (peroneal) artery

Calcaneal branches of fibular (peroneal) artery

Calcaneal tuberosity

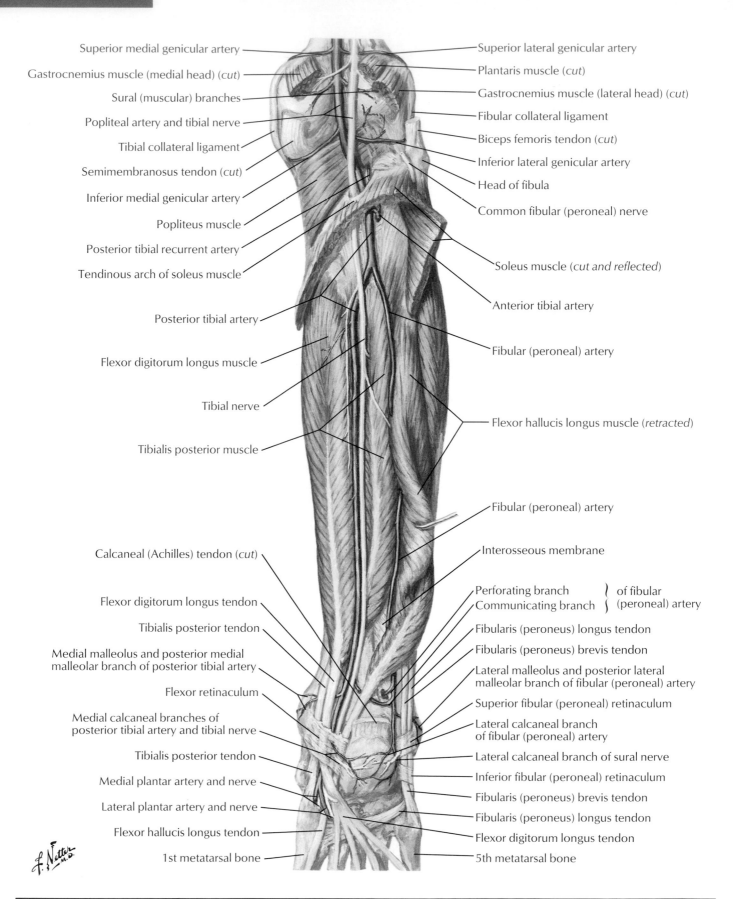

Superior medial genicular artery

Gastrocnemius muscle (medial head) (*cut*)

Sural (muscular) branches

Popliteal artery and tibial nerve

Tibial collateral ligament

Semimembranosus tendon (*cut*)

Inferior medial genicular artery

Popliteus muscle

Posterior tibial recurrent artery

Tendinous arch of soleus muscle

Posterior tibial artery

Flexor digitorum longus muscle

Tibial nerve

Tibialis posterior muscle

Calcaneal (Achilles) tendon (*cut*)

Flexor digitorum longus tendon

Tibialis posterior tendon

Medial malleolus and posterior medial malleolar branch of posterior tibial artery

Flexor retinaculum

Medial calcaneal branches of posterior tibial artery and tibial nerve

Tibialis posterior tendon

Medial plantar artery and nerve

Lateral plantar artery and nerve

Flexor hallucis longus tendon

1st metatarsal bone

Superior lateral genicular artery

Plantaris muscle (*cut*)

Gastrocnemius muscle (lateral head) (*cut*)

Fibular collateral ligament

Biceps femoris tendon (*cut*)

Inferior lateral genicular artery

Head of fibula

Common fibular (peroneal) nerve

Soleus muscle (*cut and reflected*)

Anterior tibial artery

Fibular (peroneal) artery

Flexor hallucis longus muscle (*retracted*)

Fibular (peroneal) artery

Interosseous membrane

Perforating branch } of fibular
Communicating branch } (peroneal) artery

Fibularis (peroneus) longus tendon

Fibularis (peroneus) brevis tendon

Lateral malleolus and posterior lateral malleolar branch of fibular (peroneal) artery

Superior fibular (peroneal) retinaculum

Lateral calcaneal branch of fibular (peroneal) artery

Lateral calcaneal branch of sural nerve

Inferior fibular (peroneal) retinaculum

Fibularis (peroneus) brevis tendon

Fibularis (peroneus) longus tendon

Flexor digitorum longus tendon

5th metatarsal bone

f. Netter
M.D.

Plate 506

Leg

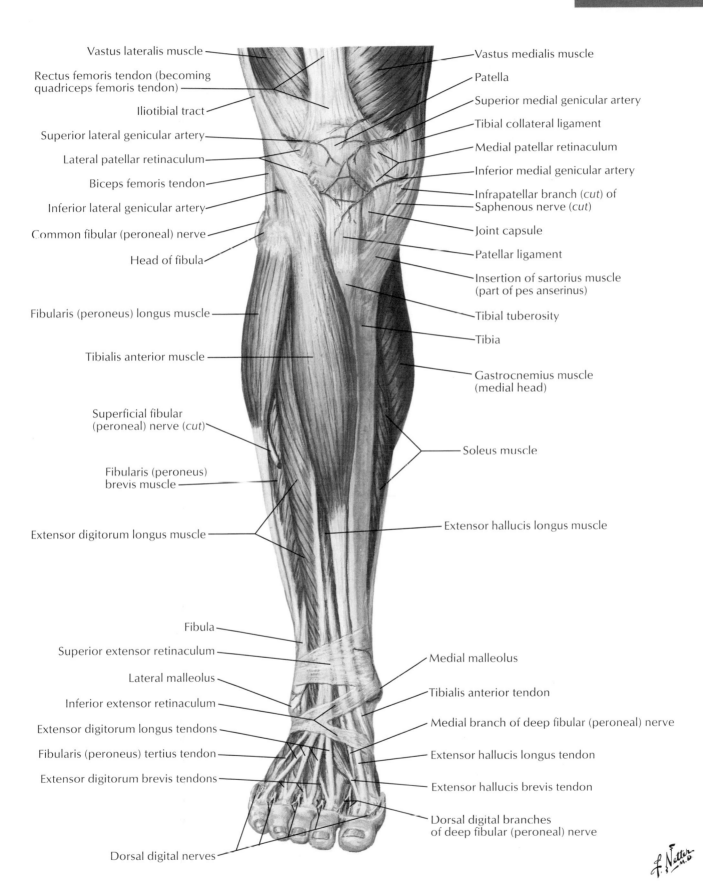

Vastus lateralis muscle

Rectus femoris tendon (becoming quadriceps femoris tendon)

Iliotibial tract

Superior lateral genicular artery

Lateral patellar retinaculum

Biceps femoris tendon

Inferior lateral genicular artery

Common fibular (peroneal) nerve

Head of fibula

Fibularis (peroneus) longus muscle

Tibialis anterior muscle

Superficial fibular (peroneal) nerve (*cut*)

Fibularis (peroneus) brevis muscle

Extensor digitorum longus muscle

Fibula

Superior extensor retinaculum

Lateral malleolus

Inferior extensor retinaculum

Extensor digitorum longus tendons

Fibularis (peroneus) tertius tendon

Extensor digitorum brevis tendons

Dorsal digital nerves

Vastus medialis muscle

Patella

Superior medial genicular artery

Tibial collateral ligament

Medial patellar retinaculum

Inferior medial genicular artery

Infrapatellar branch (*cut*) of Saphenous nerve (*cut*)

Joint capsule

Patellar ligament

Insertion of sartorius muscle (part of pes anserinus)

Tibial tuberosity

Tibia

Gastrocnemius muscle (medial head)

Soleus muscle

Extensor hallucis longus muscle

Medial malleolus

Tibialis anterior tendon

Medial branch of deep fibular (peroneal) nerve

Extensor hallucis longus tendon

Extensor hallucis brevis tendon

Dorsal digital branches of deep fibular (peroneal) nerve

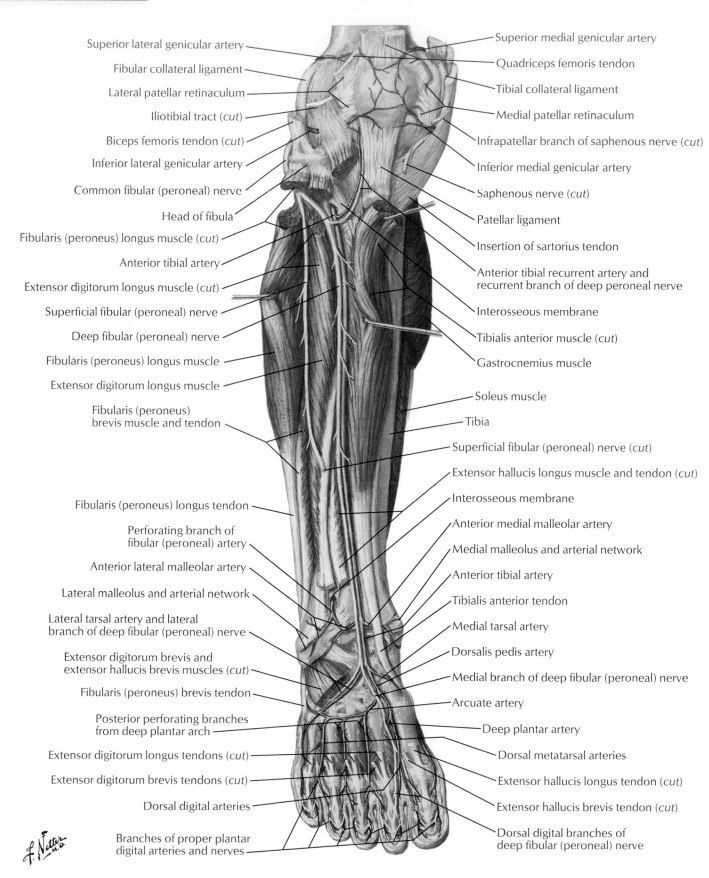

Superior lateral genicular artery

Fibular collateral ligament

Lateral patellar retinaculum

Iliotibial tract (*cut*)

Biceps femoris tendon (*cut*)

Inferior lateral genicular artery

Common fibular (peroneal) nerve

Head of fibula

Fibularis (peroneus) longus muscle (*cut*)

Anterior tibial artery

Extensor digitorum longus muscle (*cut*)

Superficial fibular (peroneal) nerve

Deep fibular (peroneal) nerve

Fibularis (peroneus) longus muscle

Extensor digitorum longus muscle

Fibularis (peroneus) brevis muscle and tendon

Fibularis (peroneus) longus tendon

Perforating branch of fibular (peroneal) artery

Anterior lateral malleolar artery

Lateral malleolus and arterial network

Lateral tarsal artery and lateral branch of deep fibular (peroneal) nerve

Extensor digitorum brevis and extensor hallucis brevis muscles (*cut*)

Fibularis (peroneus) brevis tendon

Posterior perforating branches from deep plantar arch

Extensor digitorum longus tendons (*cut*)

Extensor digitorum brevis tendons (*cut*)

Dorsal digital arteries

Branches of proper plantar digital arteries and nerves

Superior medial genicular artery

Quadriceps femoris tendon

Tibial collateral ligament

Medial patellar retinaculum

Infrapatellar branch of saphenous nerve (*cut*)

Inferior medial genicular artery

Saphenous nerve (*cut*)

Patellar ligament

Insertion of sartorius tendon

Anterior tibial recurrent artery and recurrent branch of deep peroneal nerve

Interosseous membrane

Tibialis anterior muscle (*cut*)

Gastrocnemius muscle

Soleus muscle

Tibia

Superficial fibular (peroneal) nerve (*cut*)

Extensor hallucis longus muscle and tendon (*cut*)

Interosseous membrane

Anterior medial malleolar artery

Medial malleolus and arterial network

Anterior tibial artery

Tibialis anterior tendon

Medial tarsal artery

Dorsalis pedis artery

Medial branch of deep fibular (peroneal) nerve

Arcuate artery

Deep plantar artery

Dorsal metatarsal arteries

Extensor hallucis longus tendon (*cut*)

Extensor hallucis brevis tendon (*cut*)

Dorsal digital branches of deep fibular (peroneal) nerve

Plate 508

Leg

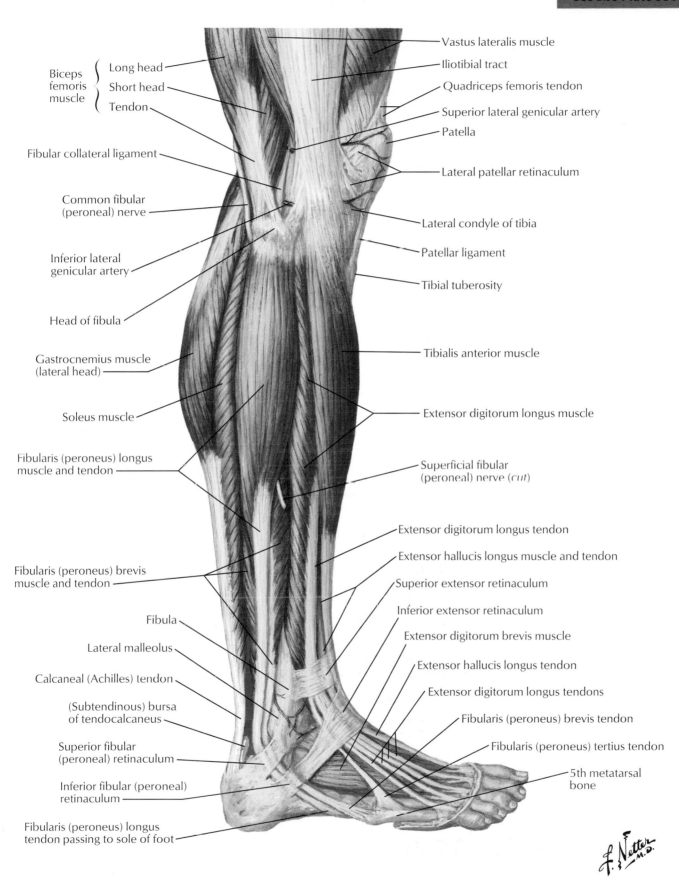

Biceps femoris muscle
{ Long head
Short head
Tendon

Fibular collateral ligament

Common fibular (peroneal) nerve

Inferior lateral genicular artery

Head of fibula

Gastrocnemius muscle (lateral head)

Soleus muscle

Fibularis (peroneus) longus muscle and tendon

Fibularis (peroneus) brevis muscle and tendon

Fibula

Lateral malleolus

Calcaneal (Achilles) tendon

(Subtendinous) bursa of tendocalcaneus

Superior fibular (peroneal) retinaculum

Inferior fibular (peroneal) retinaculum

Fibularis (peroneus) longus tendon passing to sole of foot

Vastus lateralis muscle

Iliotibial tract

Quadriceps femoris tendon

Superior lateral genicular artery

Patella

Lateral patellar retinaculum

Lateral condyle of tibia

Patellar ligament

Tibial tuberosity

Tibialis anterior muscle

Extensor digitorum longus muscle

Superficial fibular (peroneal) nerve (cut)

Extensor digitorum longus tendon

Extensor hallucis longus muscle and tendon

Superior extensor retinaculum

Inferior extensor retinaculum

Extensor digitorum brevis muscle

Extensor hallucis longus tendon

Extensor digitorum longus tendons

Fibularis (peroneus) brevis tendon

Fibularis (peroneus) tertius tendon

5th metatarsal bone

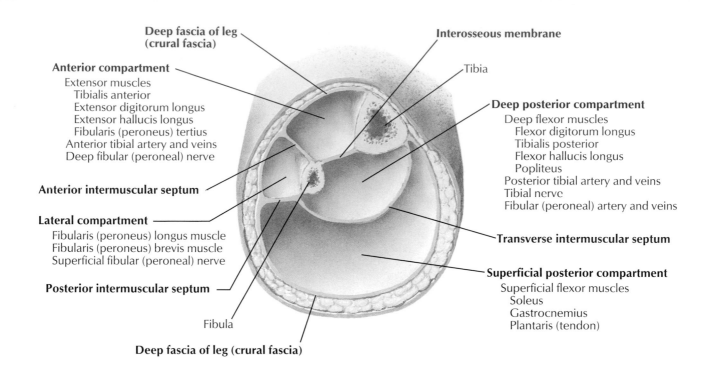

Deep fascia of leg (crural fascia)

Interosseous membrane

Tibia

Anterior compartment
 Extensor muscles
  Tibialis anterior
  Extensor digitorum longus
  Extensor hallucis longus
  Fibularis (peroneus) tertius
 Anterior tibial artery and veins
 Deep fibular (peroneal) nerve

Anterior intermuscular septum

Lateral compartment
 Fibularis (peroneus) longus muscle
 Fibularis (peroneus) brevis muscle
 Superficial fibular (peroneal) nerve

Posterior intermuscular septum

Fibula

Deep fascia of leg (crural fascia)

Deep posterior compartment
 Deep flexor muscles
  Flexor digitorum longus
  Tibialis posterior
  Flexor hallucis longus
  Popliteus
 Posterior tibial artery and veins
 Tibial nerve
 Fibular (peroneal) artery and veins

Transverse intermuscular septum

Superficial posterior compartment
 Superficial flexor muscles
  Soleus
  Gastrocnemius
  Plantaris (tendon)

Cross section just above middle of leg

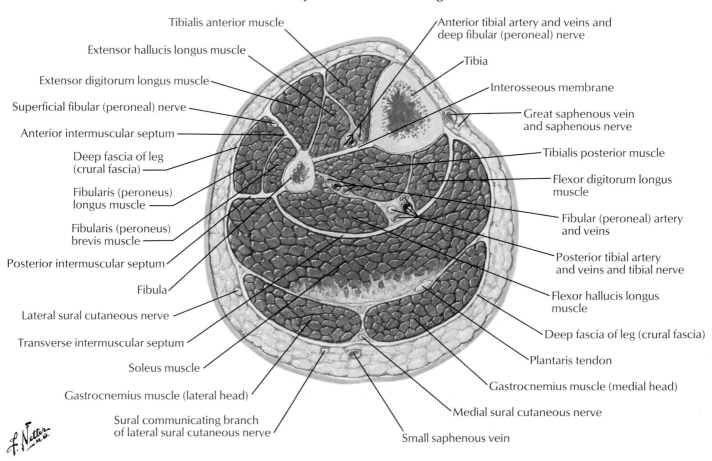

Tibialis anterior muscle

Extensor hallucis longus muscle

Extensor digitorum longus muscle

Superficial fibular (peroneal) nerve

Anterior intermuscular septum

Deep fascia of leg (crural fascia)

Fibularis (peroneus) longus muscle

Fibularis (peroneus) brevis muscle

Posterior intermuscular septum

Fibula

Lateral sural cutaneous nerve

Transverse intermuscular septum

Soleus muscle

Gastrocnemius muscle (lateral head)

Sural communicating branch of lateral sural cutaneous nerve

Anterior tibial artery and veins and deep fibular (peroneal) nerve

Tibia

Interosseous membrane

Great saphenous vein and saphenous nerve

Tibialis posterior muscle

Flexor digitorum longus muscle

Fibular (peroneal) artery and veins

Posterior tibial artery and veins and tibial nerve

Flexor hallucis longus muscle

Deep fascia of leg (crural fascia)

Plantaris tendon

Gastrocnemius muscle (medial head)

Medial sural cutaneous nerve

Small saphenous vein

Plate 510

Leg

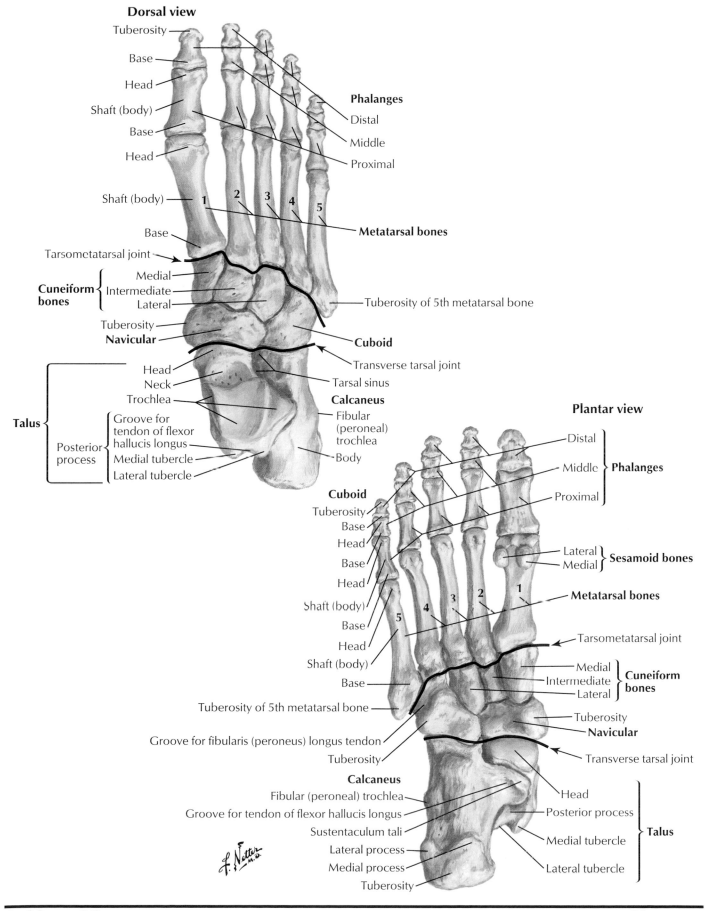

Dorsal view

Tuberosity

Base

Head

Shaft (body)

Base

Head

Phalanges

Distal

Middle

Proximal

Shaft (body)

1 2 3 4 5

Metatarsal bones

Base

Tarsometatarsal joint

Cuneiform bones { Medial / Intermediate / Lateral

Tuberosity of 5th metatarsal bone

Tuberosity

Navicular

Cuboid

Transverse tarsal joint

Head

Neck

Trochlea

Tarsal sinus

Calcaneus

Talus {

Posterior process {
Groove for tendon of flexor hallucis longus
Medial tubercle
Lateral tubercle

Fibular (peroneal) trochlea

Body

Cuboid

Tuberosity

Base

Head

Base

Head

Shaft (body)

Base

Head

Shaft (body)

Base

Tuberosity of 5th metatarsal bone

Groove for fibularis (peroneus) longus tendon

Tuberosity

Calcaneus

Fibular (peroneal) trochlea

Groove for tendon of flexor hallucis longus

Sustentaculum tali

Lateral process

Medial process

Tuberosity

Plantar view

Distal

Middle } **Phalanges**

Proximal

Lateral } **Sesamoid bones**
Medial

5 4 3 2 1

Metatarsal bones

Tarsometatarsal joint

Medial } **Cuneiform bones**
Intermediate
Lateral

Tuberosity

Navicular

Transverse tarsal joint

Head

Posterior process

Medial tubercle } **Talus**

Lateral tubercle

f. Netter M.D.

Plate 511

Lateral view

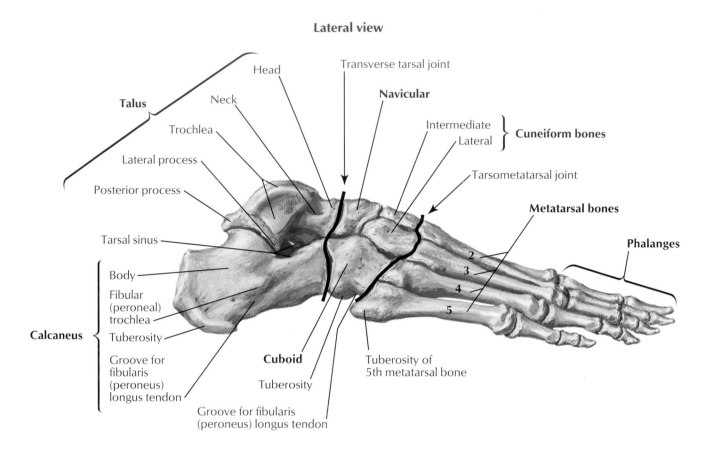

Head
Neck
Talus
Trochlea
Lateral process
Posterior process
Tarsal sinus
Body
Fibular (peroneal) trochlea
Tuberosity
Calcaneus
Groove for fibularis (peroneus) longus tendon

Transverse tarsal joint
Navicular
Intermediate
Lateral
Cuneiform bones
Tarsometatarsal joint
Metatarsal bones
2
3
4
5
Phalanges
Cuboid
Tuberosity of 5th metatarsal bone
Tuberosity
Groove for fibularis (peroneus) longus tendon

Medial view

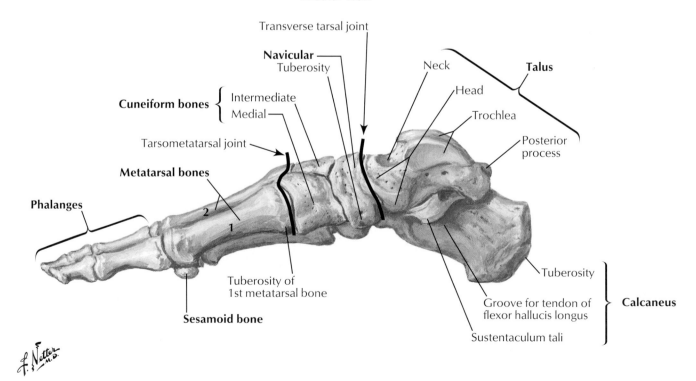

Transverse tarsal joint
Navicular
Tuberosity
Cuneiform bones
Intermediate
Medial
Tarsometatarsal joint
Metatarsal bones
Phalanges
2
1
Tuberosity of 1st metatarsal bone
Sesamoid bone

Neck
Head
Trochlea
Talus
Posterior process
Tuberosity
Groove for tendon of flexor hallucis longus
Calcaneus
Sustentaculum tali

Plate 512 **Ankle and Foot**

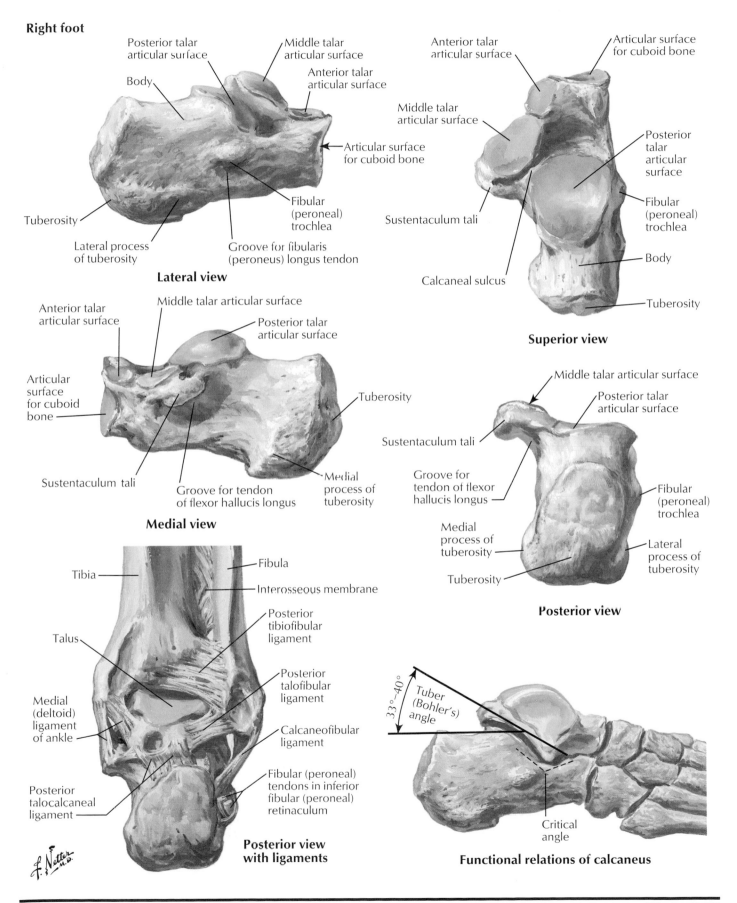

Right foot

Lateral view

Posterior talar articular surface

Body

Middle talar articular surface

Anterior talar articular surface

Articular surface for cuboid bone

Fibular (peroneal) trochlea

Groove for fibularis (peroneus) longus tendon

Lateral process of tuberosity

Tuberosity

Lateral view

Anterior talar articular surface

Articular surface for cuboid bone

Middle talar articular surface

Posterior talar articular surface

Tuberosity

Sustentaculum tali

Groove for tendon of flexor hallucis longus

Medial process of tuberosity

Medial view

Anterior talar articular surface

Middle talar articular surface

Articular surface for cuboid bone

Posterior talar articular surface

Sustentaculum tali

Fibular (peroneal) trochlea

Body

Calcaneal sulcus

Tuberosity

Superior view

Middle talar articular surface

Posterior talar articular surface

Sustentaculum tali

Groove for tendon of flexor hallucis longus

Medial process of tuberosity

Tuberosity

Fibular (peroneal) trochlea

Lateral process of tuberosity

Posterior view

Tibia

Fibula

Interosseous membrane

Talus

Posterior tibiofibular ligament

Posterior talofibular ligament

Medial (deltoid) ligament of ankle

Calcaneofibular ligament

Fibular (peroneal) tendons in inferior fibular (peroneal) retinaculum

Posterior talocalcaneal ligament

Posterior view with ligaments

33°–40°

Tuber (Bohler's) angle

Critical angle

Functional relations of calcaneus

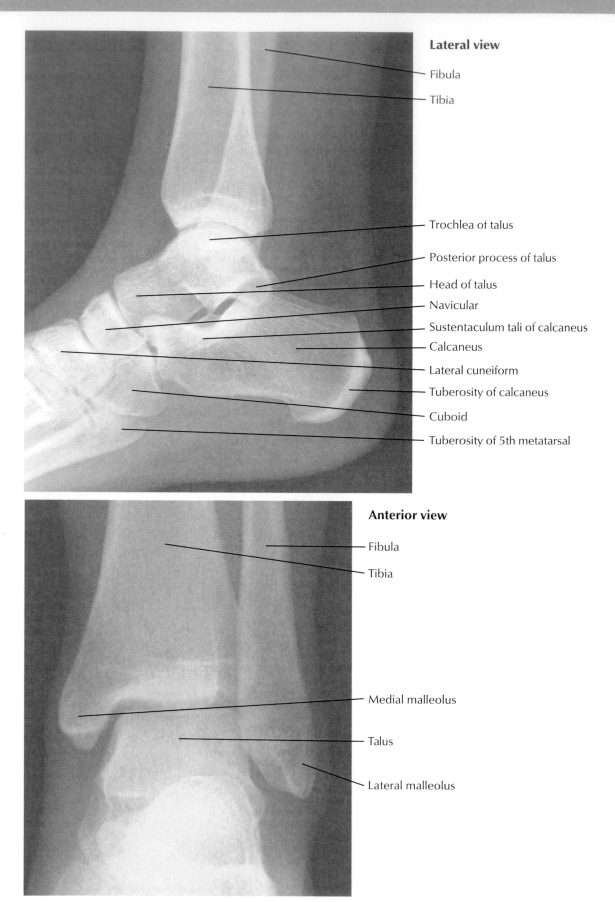

Lateral view

Fibula

Tibia

Trochlea of talus

Posterior process of talus

Head of talus

Navicular

Sustentaculum tali of calcaneus

Calcaneus

Lateral cuneiform

Tuberosity of calcaneus

Cuboid

Tuberosity of 5th metatarsal

Anterior view

Fibula

Tibia

Medial malleolus

Talus

Lateral malleolus

Plate 514 **Ankle and Foot**

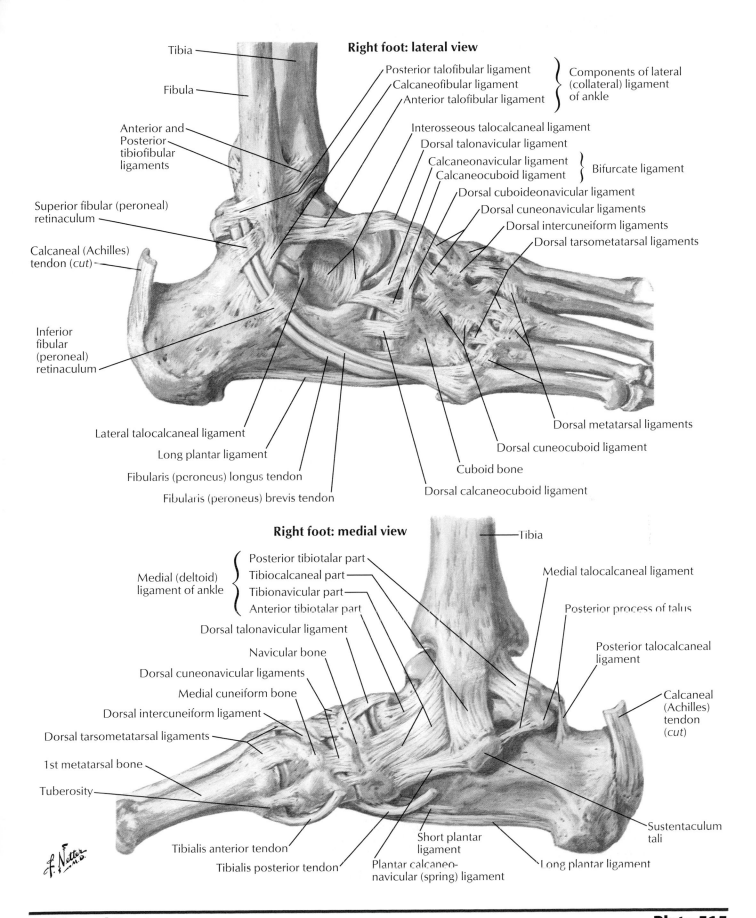

Right foot: lateral view

Tibia

Fibula

Anterior and Posterior tibiofibular ligaments

Superior fibular (peroneal) retinaculum

Calcaneal (Achilles) tendon (*cut*)

Inferior fibular (peroneal) retinaculum

Posterior talofibular ligament
Calcaneofibular ligament
Anterior talofibular ligament

Components of lateral (collateral) ligament of ankle

Interosseous talocalcaneal ligament
Dorsal talonavicular ligament
Calcaneonavicular ligament
Calcaneocuboid ligament

Bifurcate ligament

Dorsal cuboideonavicular ligament
Dorsal cuneonavicular ligaments
Dorsal intercuneiform ligaments
Dorsal tarsometatarsal ligaments

Dorsal metatarsal ligaments

Lateral talocalcaneal ligament

Long plantar ligament

Fibularis (peroneus) longus tendon

Fibularis (peroneus) brevis tendon

Dorsal cuneocuboid ligament

Cuboid bone

Dorsal calcaneocuboid ligament

Right foot: medial view

Medial (deltoid) ligament of ankle
Posterior tibiotalar part
Tibiocalcaneal part
Tibionavicular part
Anterior tibiotalar part

Dorsal talonavicular ligament

Navicular bone

Dorsal cuneonavicular ligaments

Medial cuneiform bone

Dorsal intercuneiform ligament

Dorsal tarsometatarsal ligaments

1st metatarsal bone

Tuberosity

Tibia

Medial talocalcaneal ligament

Posterior process of talus

Posterior talocalcaneal ligament

Calcaneal (Achilles) tendon (*cut*)

Sustentaculum tali

Tibialis anterior tendon

Tibialis posterior tendon

Short plantar ligament

Plantar calcaneonavicular (spring) ligament

Long plantar ligament

Ankle and Foot

Plate 515

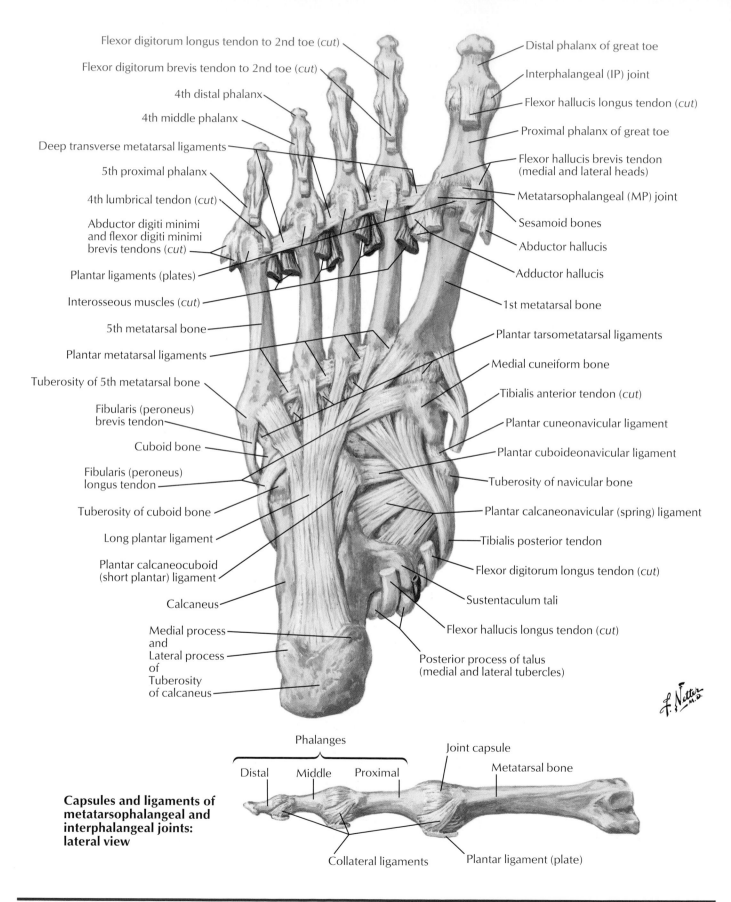

Flexor digitorum longus tendon to 2nd toe (*cut*)

Flexor digitorum brevis tendon to 2nd toe (*cut*)

4th distal phalanx

4th middle phalanx

Deep transverse metatarsal ligaments

5th proximal phalanx

4th lumbrical tendon (*cut*)

Abductor digiti minimi and flexor digiti minimi brevis tendons (*cut*)

Plantar ligaments (plates)

Interosseous muscles (*cut*)

5th metatarsal bone

Plantar metatarsal ligaments

Tuberosity of 5th metatarsal bone

Fibularis (peroneus) brevis tendon

Cuboid bone

Fibularis (peroneus) longus tendon

Tuberosity of cuboid bone

Long plantar ligament

Plantar calcaneocuboid (short plantar) ligament

Calcaneus

Medial process and Lateral process of Tuberosity of calcaneus

Distal phalanx of great toe

Interphalangeal (IP) joint

Flexor hallucis longus tendon (*cut*)

Proximal phalanx of great toe

Flexor hallucis brevis tendon (medial and lateral heads)

Metatarsophalangeal (MP) joint

Sesamoid bones

Abductor hallucis

Adductor hallucis

1st metatarsal bone

Plantar tarsometatarsal ligaments

Medial cuneiform bone

Tibialis anterior tendon (*cut*)

Plantar cuneonavicular ligament

Plantar cuboideonavicular ligament

Tuberosity of navicular bone

Plantar calcaneonavicular (spring) ligament

Tibialis posterior tendon

Flexor digitorum longus tendon (*cut*)

Sustentaculum tali

Flexor hallucis longus tendon (*cut*)

Posterior process of talus (medial and lateral tubercles)

Phalanges

Distal   Middle   Proximal

Joint capsule

Metatarsal bone

Capsules and ligaments of metatarsophalangeal and interphalangeal joints: lateral view

Collateral ligaments

Plantar ligament (plate)

Plate 516   **Ankle and Foot**

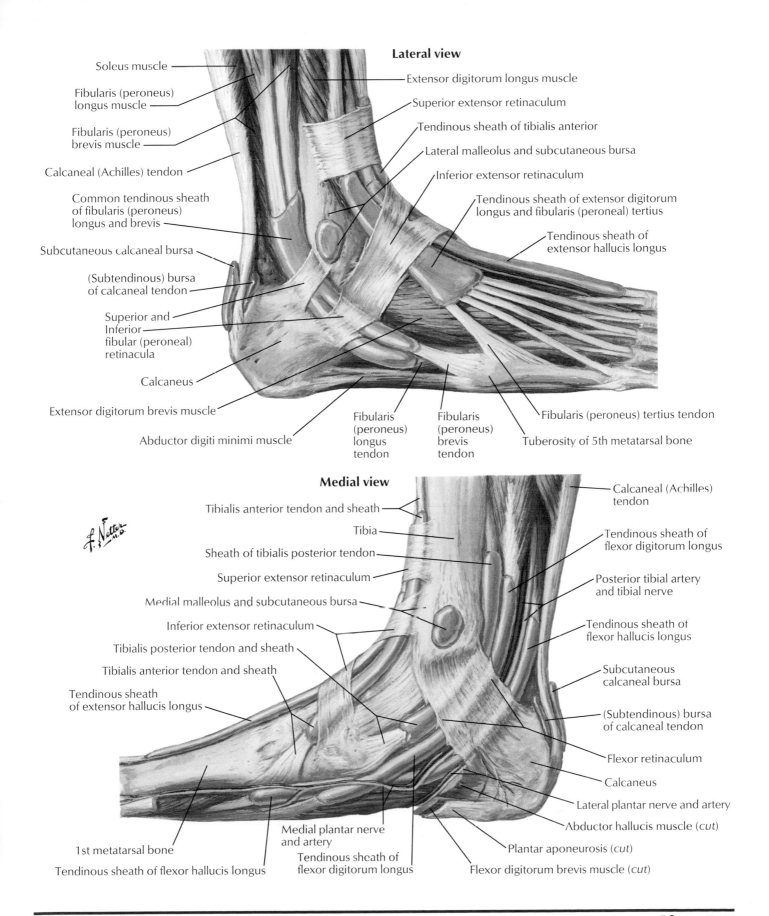

Lateral view

Soleus muscle

Fibularis (peroneus) longus muscle

Fibularis (peroneus) brevis muscle

Calcaneal (Achilles) tendon

Common tendinous sheath of fibularis (peroneus) longus and brevis

Subcutaneous calcaneal bursa

(Subtendinous) bursa of calcaneal tendon

Superior and Inferior fibular (peroneal) retinacula

Calcaneus

Extensor digitorum brevis muscle

Abductor digiti minimi muscle

Extensor digitorum longus muscle

Superior extensor retinaculum

Tendinous sheath of tibialis anterior

Lateral malleolus and subcutaneous bursa

Inferior extensor retinaculum

Tendinous sheath of extensor digitorum longus and fibularis (peroneal) tertius

Tendinous sheath of extensor hallucis longus

Fibularis (peroneus) longus tendon

Fibularis (peroneus) brevis tendon

Fibularis (peroneus) tertius tendon

Tuberosity of 5th metatarsal bone

Medial view

Tibialis anterior tendon and sheath

Tibia

Sheath of tibialis posterior tendon

Superior extensor retinaculum

Medial malleolus and subcutaneous bursa

Inferior extensor retinaculum

Tibialis posterior tendon and sheath

Tibialis anterior tendon and sheath

Tendinous sheath of extensor hallucis longus

1st metatarsal bone

Tendinous sheath of flexor hallucis longus

Medial plantar nerve and artery

Tendinous sheath of flexor digitorum longus

Calcaneal (Achilles) tendon

Tendinous sheath of flexor digitorum longus

Posterior tibial artery and tibial nerve

Tendinous sheath of flexor hallucis longus

Subcutaneous calcaneal bursa

(Subtendinous) bursa of calcaneal tendon

Flexor retinaculum

Calcaneus

Lateral plantar nerve and artery

Abductor hallucis muscle (cut)

Plantar aponeurosis (cut)

Flexor digitorum brevis muscle (cut)

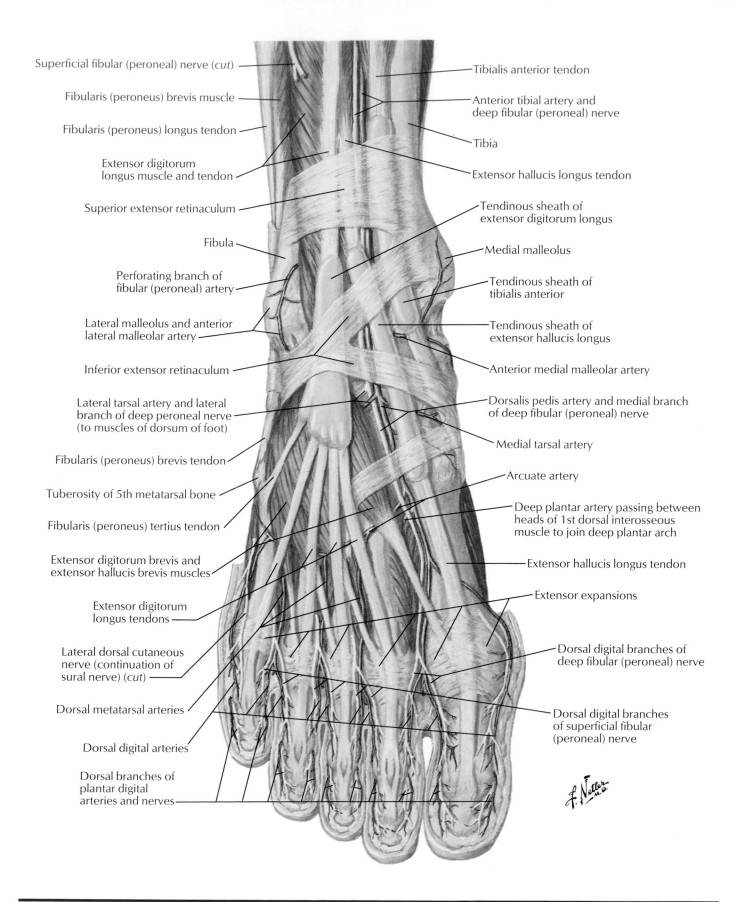

Superficial fibular (peroneal) nerve (*cut*)

Fibularis (peroneus) brevis muscle

Fibularis (peroneus) longus tendon

Extensor digitorum longus muscle and tendon

Superior extensor retinaculum

Fibula

Perforating branch of fibular (peroneal) artery

Lateral malleolus and anterior lateral malleolar artery

Inferior extensor retinaculum

Lateral tarsal artery and lateral branch of deep peroneal nerve (to muscles of dorsum of foot)

Fibularis (peroneus) brevis tendon

Tuberosity of 5th metatarsal bone

Fibularis (peroneus) tertius tendon

Extensor digitorum brevis and extensor hallucis brevis muscles

Extensor digitorum longus tendons

Lateral dorsal cutaneous nerve (continuation of sural nerve) (*cut*)

Dorsal metatarsal arteries

Dorsal digital arteries

Dorsal branches of plantar digital arteries and nerves

Tibialis anterior tendon

Anterior tibial artery and deep fibular (peroneal) nerve

Tibia

Extensor hallucis longus tendon

Tendinous sheath of extensor digitorum longus

Medial malleolus

Tendinous sheath of tibialis anterior

Tendinous sheath of extensor hallucis longus

Anterior medial malleolar artery

Dorsalis pedis artery and medial branch of deep fibular (peroneal) nerve

Medial tarsal artery

Arcuate artery

Deep plantar artery passing between heads of 1st dorsal interosseous muscle to join deep plantar arch

Extensor hallucis longus tendon

Extensor expansions

Dorsal digital branches of deep fibular (peroneal) nerve

Dorsal digital branches of superficial fibular (peroneal) nerve

Plate 518

Ankle and Foot

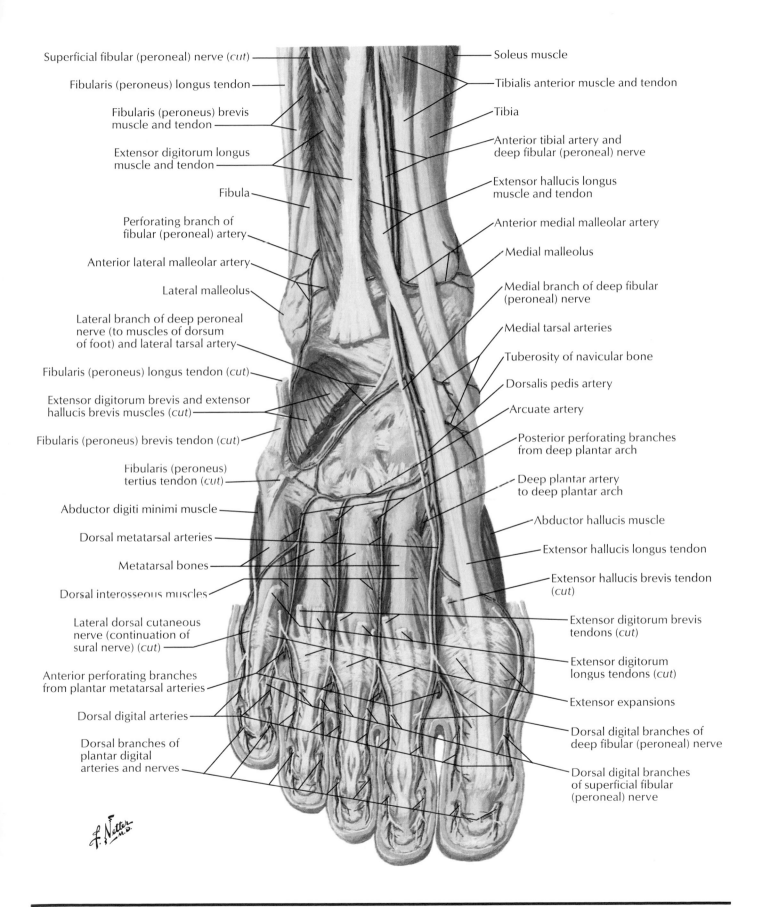

Superficial fibular (peroneal) nerve (cut)

Fibularis (peroneus) longus tendon

Fibularis (peroneus) brevis muscle and tendon

Extensor digitorum longus muscle and tendon

Fibula

Perforating branch of fibular (peroneal) artery

Anterior lateral malleolar artery

Lateral malleolus

Lateral branch of deep peroneal nerve (to muscles of dorsum of foot) and lateral tarsal artery

Fibularis (peroneus) longus tendon (cut)

Extensor digitorum brevis and extensor hallucis brevis muscles (cut)

Fibularis (peroneus) brevis tendon (cut)

Fibularis (peroneus) tertius tendon (cut)

Abductor digiti minimi muscle

Dorsal metatarsal arteries

Metatarsal bones

Dorsal interosseous muscles

Lateral dorsal cutaneous nerve (continuation of sural nerve) (cut)

Anterior perforating branches from plantar metatarsal arteries

Dorsal digital arteries

Dorsal branches of plantar digital arteries and nerves

Soleus muscle

Tibialis anterior muscle and tendon

Tibia

Anterior tibial artery and deep fibular (peroneal) nerve

Extensor hallucis longus muscle and tendon

Anterior medial malleolar artery

Medial malleolus

Medial branch of deep fibular (peroneal) nerve

Medial tarsal arteries

Tuberosity of navicular bone

Dorsalis pedis artery

Arcuate artery

Posterior perforating branches from deep plantar arch

Deep plantar artery to deep plantar arch

Abductor hallucis muscle

Extensor hallucis longus tendon

Extensor hallucis brevis tendon (cut)

Extensor digitorum brevis tendons (cut)

Extensor digitorum longus tendons (cut)

Extensor expansions

Dorsal digital branches of deep fibular (peroneal) nerve

Dorsal digital branches of superficial fibular (peroneal) nerve

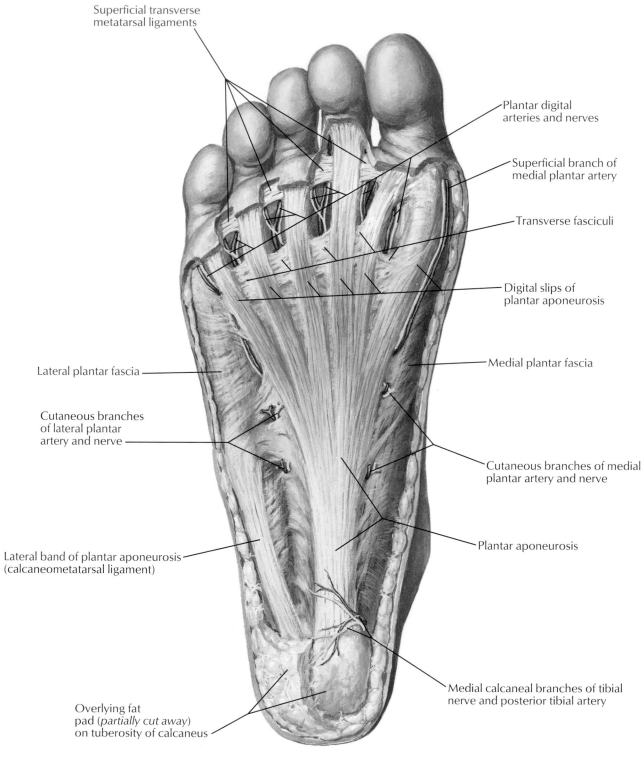

Superficial transverse
metatarsal ligaments

Plantar digital
arteries and nerves

Superficial branch of
medial plantar artery

Transverse fasciculi

Digital slips of
plantar aponeurosis

Medial plantar fascia

Cutaneous branches of medial
plantar artery and nerve

Plantar aponeurosis

Medial calcaneal branches of tibial
nerve and posterior tibial artery

Lateral plantar fascia

Cutaneous branches
of lateral plantar
artery and nerve

Lateral band of plantar aponeurosis
(calcaneometatarsal ligament)

Overlying fat
pad (*partially cut away*)
on tuberosity of calcaneus

Plate 520

Ankle and Foot

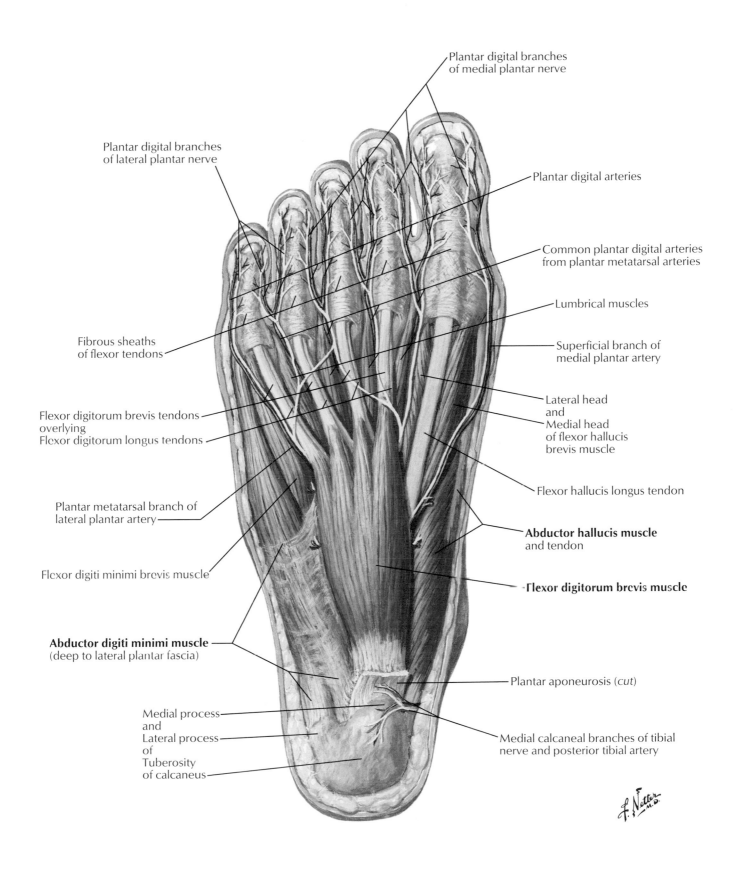

Plantar digital branches
of medial plantar nerve

Plantar digital branches
of lateral plantar nerve

Plantar digital arteries

Common plantar digital arteries
from plantar metatarsal arteries

Lumbrical muscles

Fibrous sheaths
of flexor tendons

Superficial branch of
medial plantar artery

Flexor digitorum brevis tendons
overlying
Flexor digitorum longus tendons

Lateral head
and
Medial head
of flexor hallucis
brevis muscle

Flexor hallucis longus tendon

Plantar metatarsal branch of
lateral plantar artery

Abductor hallucis muscle
and tendon

Flexor digiti minimi brevis muscle

Flexor digitorum brevis muscle

Abductor digiti minimi muscle
(deep to lateral plantar fascia)

Plantar aponeurosis (cut)

Medial process
and
Lateral process
of
Tuberosity
of calcaneus

Medial calcaneal branches of tibial
nerve and posterior tibial artery

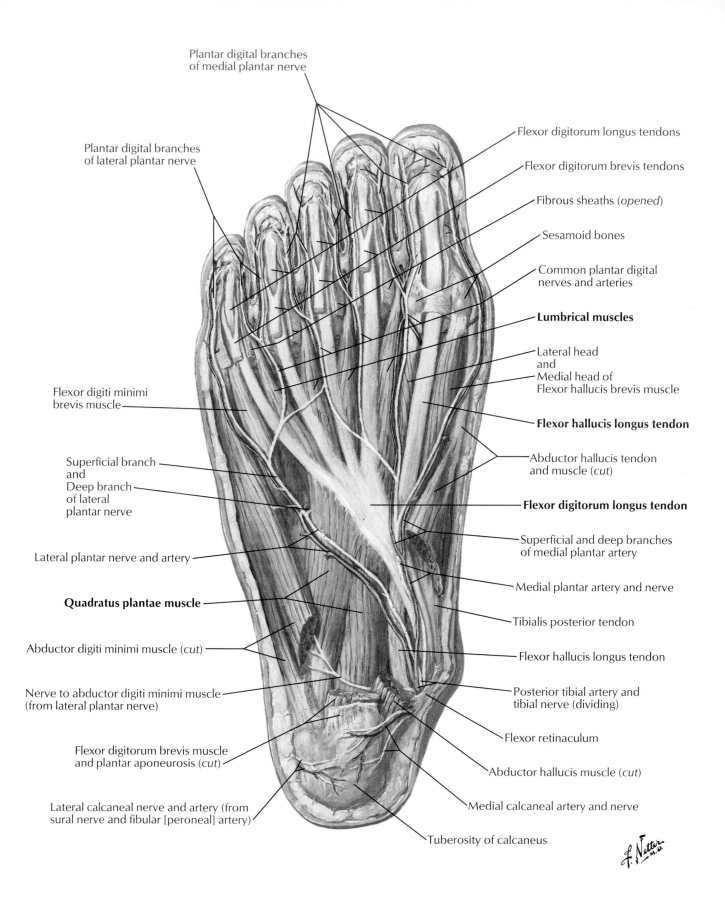

Plantar digital branches
of medial plantar nerve

Plantar digital branches
of lateral plantar nerve

Flexor digitorum longus tendons

Flexor digitorum brevis tendons

Fibrous sheaths (*opened*)

Sesamoid bones

Common plantar digital
nerves and arteries

Lumbrical muscles

Lateral head
and
Medial head of
Flexor hallucis brevis muscle

Flexor hallucis longus tendon

Abductor hallucis tendon
and muscle (*cut*)

Flexor digitorum longus tendon

Superficial and deep branches
of medial plantar artery

Medial plantar artery and nerve

Tibialis posterior tendon

Flexor hallucis longus tendon

Posterior tibial artery and
tibial nerve (dividing)

Flexor retinaculum

Abductor hallucis muscle (*cut*)

Medial calcaneal artery and nerve

Flexor digiti minimi
brevis muscle

Superficial branch
and
Deep branch
of lateral
plantar nerve

Lateral plantar nerve and artery

Quadratus plantae muscle

Abductor digiti minimi muscle (*cut*)

Nerve to abductor digiti minimi muscle
(from lateral plantar nerve)

Flexor digitorum brevis muscle
and plantar aponeurosis (*cut*)

Lateral calcaneal nerve and artery (from
sural nerve and fibular [peroneal] artery)

Tuberosity of calcaneus

Plate 522

Ankle and Foot

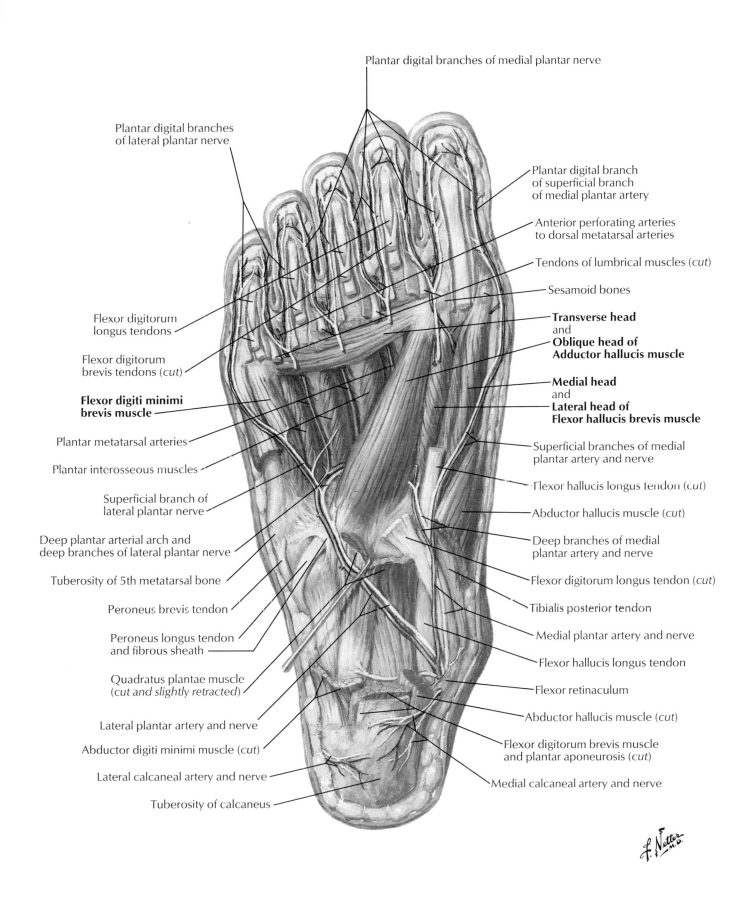

Plantar digital branches of medial plantar nerve

Plantar digital branches of lateral plantar nerve

Plantar digital branch of superficial branch of medial plantar artery

Anterior perforating arteries to dorsal metatarsal arteries

Tendons of lumbrical muscles (cut)

Sesamoid bones

Flexor digitorum longus tendons

Transverse head and **Oblique head of Adductor hallucis muscle**

Flexor digitorum brevis tendons (cut)

Medial head and **Lateral head of Flexor hallucis brevis muscle**

Flexor digiti minimi brevis muscle

Superficial branches of medial plantar artery and nerve

Plantar metatarsal arteries

Flexor hallucis longus tendon (cut)

Plantar interosseous muscles

Abductor hallucis muscle (cut)

Superficial branch of lateral plantar nerve

Deep branches of medial plantar artery and nerve

Deep plantar arterial arch and deep branches of lateral plantar nerve

Flexor digitorum longus tendon (cut)

Tuberosity of 5th metatarsal bone

Tibialis posterior tendon

Peroneus brevis tendon

Medial plantar artery and nerve

Peroneus longus tendon and fibrous sheath

Flexor hallucis longus tendon

Quadratus plantae muscle (cut and slightly retracted)

Flexor retinaculum

Lateral plantar artery and nerve

Abductor hallucis muscle (cut)

Abductor digiti minimi muscle (cut)

Flexor digitorum brevis muscle and plantar aponeurosis (cut)

Lateral calcaneal artery and nerve

Medial calcaneal artery and nerve

Tuberosity of calcaneus

Dorsal view

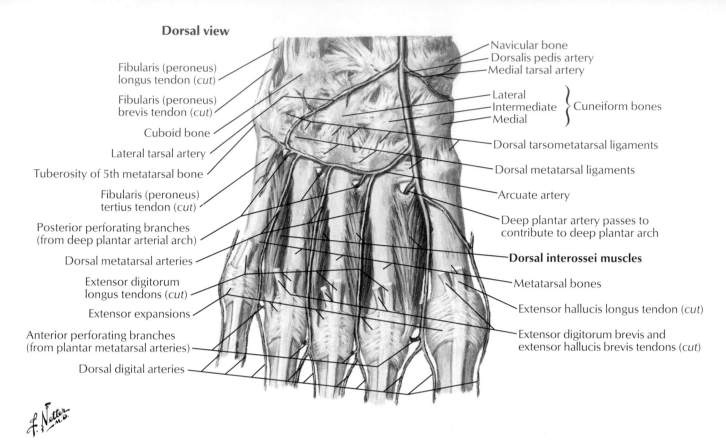

Fibularis (peroneus) longus tendon (*cut*)

Fibularis (peroneus) brevis tendon (*cut*)

Cuboid bone

Lateral tarsal artery

Tuberosity of 5th metatarsal bone

Fibularis (peroneus) tertius tendon (*cut*)

Posterior perforating branches (from deep plantar arterial arch)

Dorsal metatarsal arteries

Extensor digitorum longus tendons (*cut*)

Extensor expansions

Anterior perforating branches (from plantar metatarsal arteries)

Dorsal digital arteries

Navicular bone
Dorsalis pedis artery
Medial tarsal artery

Lateral
Intermediate } Cuneiform bones
Medial

Dorsal tarsometatarsal ligaments

Dorsal metatarsal ligaments

Arcuate artery

Deep plantar artery passes to contribute to deep plantar arch

Dorsal interossei muscles

Metatarsal bones

Extensor hallucis longus tendon (*cut*)

Extensor digitorum brevis and extensor hallucis brevis tendons (*cut*)

Plantar view

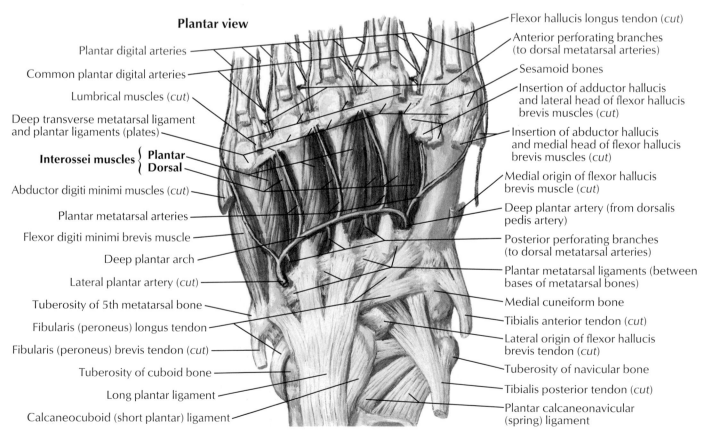

Plantar digital arteries

Common plantar digital arteries

Lumbrical muscles (*cut*)

Deep transverse metatarsal ligament and plantar ligaments (plates)

Interossei muscles { **Plantar**
Dorsal

Abductor digiti minimi muscles (*cut*)

Plantar metatarsal arteries

Flexor digiti minimi brevis muscle

Deep plantar arch

Lateral plantar artery (*cut*)

Tuberosity of 5th metatarsal bone

Fibularis (peroneus) longus tendon

Fibularis (peroneus) brevis tendon (*cut*)

Tuberosity of cuboid bone

Long plantar ligament

Calcaneocuboid (short plantar) ligament

Flexor hallucis longus tendon (*cut*)

Anterior perforating branches (to dorsal metatarsal arteries)

Sesamoid bones

Insertion of adductor hallucis and lateral head of flexor hallucis brevis muscles (*cut*)

Insertion of abductor hallucis and medial head of flexor hallucis brevis muscles (*cut*)

Medial origin of flexor hallucis brevis muscle (*cut*)

Deep plantar artery (from dorsalis pedis artery)

Posterior perforating branches (to dorsal metatarsal arteries)

Plantar metatarsal ligaments (between bases of metatarsal bones)

Medial cuneiform bone

Tibialis anterior tendon (*cut*)

Lateral origin of flexor hallucis brevis tendon (*cut*)

Tuberosity of navicular bone

Tibialis posterior tendon (*cut*)

Plantar calcaneonavicular (spring) ligament

Plate 524 **Ankle and Foot**

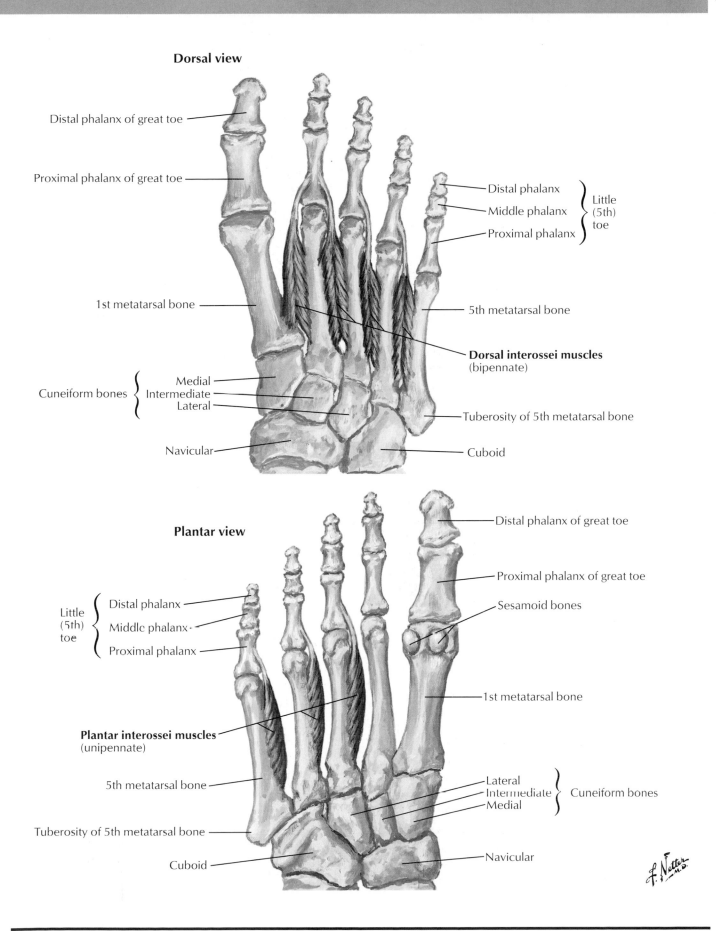

Dorsal view

Distal phalanx of great toe

Proximal phalanx of great toe

Distal phalanx
Middle phalanx
Proximal phalanx

Little (5th) toe

1st metatarsal bone

5th metatarsal bone

Dorsal interossei muscles (bipennate)

Cuneiform bones {
Medial
Intermediate
Lateral
}

Tuberosity of 5th metatarsal bone

Navicular

Cuboid

Plantar view

Distal phalanx of great toe

Proximal phalanx of great toe

Little (5th) toe {
Distal phalanx
Middle phalanx
Proximal phalanx
}

Sesamoid bones

1st metatarsal bone

Plantar interossei muscles (unipennate)

5th metatarsal bone

Lateral
Intermediate
Medial

Cuneiform bones

Tuberosity of 5th metatarsal bone

Cuboid

Navicular

f. Netter M.D.

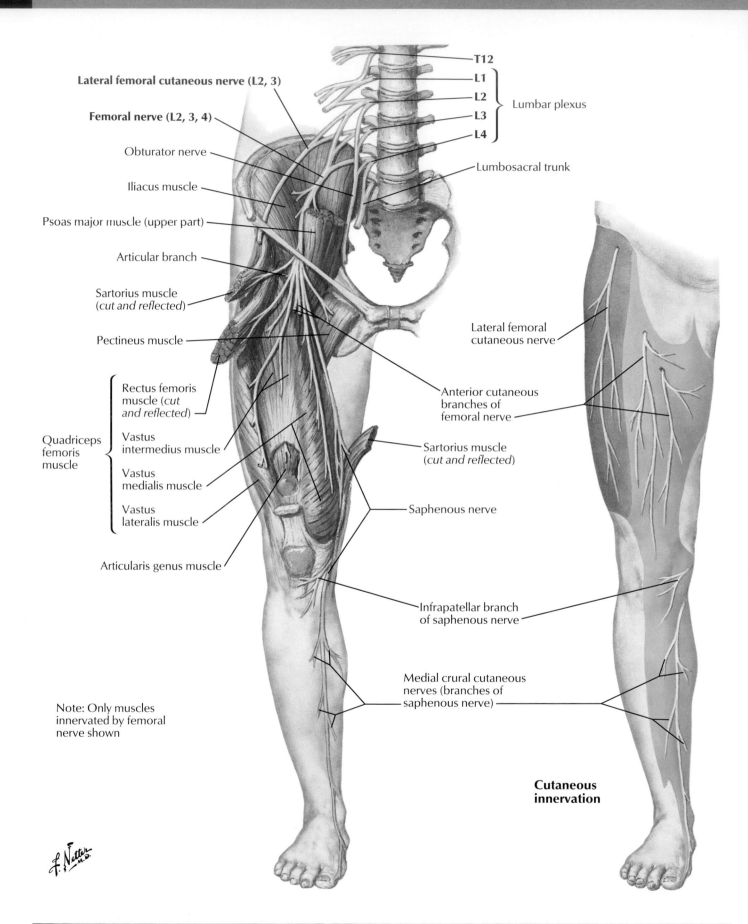

Lateral femoral cutaneous nerve (L2, 3)

Femoral nerve (L2, 3, 4)

Obturator nerve

Iliacus muscle

Psoas major muscle (upper part)

Articular branch

Sartorius muscle
(*cut and reflected*)

Pectineus muscle

Rectus femoris
muscle (*cut
and reflected*)

Quadriceps
femoris
muscle

Vastus
intermedius muscle

Vastus
medialis muscle

Vastus
lateralis muscle

Articularis genus muscle

T12

L1

L2   Lumbar plexus

L3

L4

Lumbosacral trunk

Lateral femoral
cutaneous nerve

Anterior cutaneous
branches of
femoral nerve

Sartorius muscle
(*cut and reflected*)

Saphenous nerve

Infrapatellar branch
of saphenous nerve

Medial crural cutaneous
nerves (branches of
saphenous nerve)

Note: Only muscles
innervated by femoral
nerve shown

**Cutaneous
innervation**

Plate 526   **Neurovasculature**

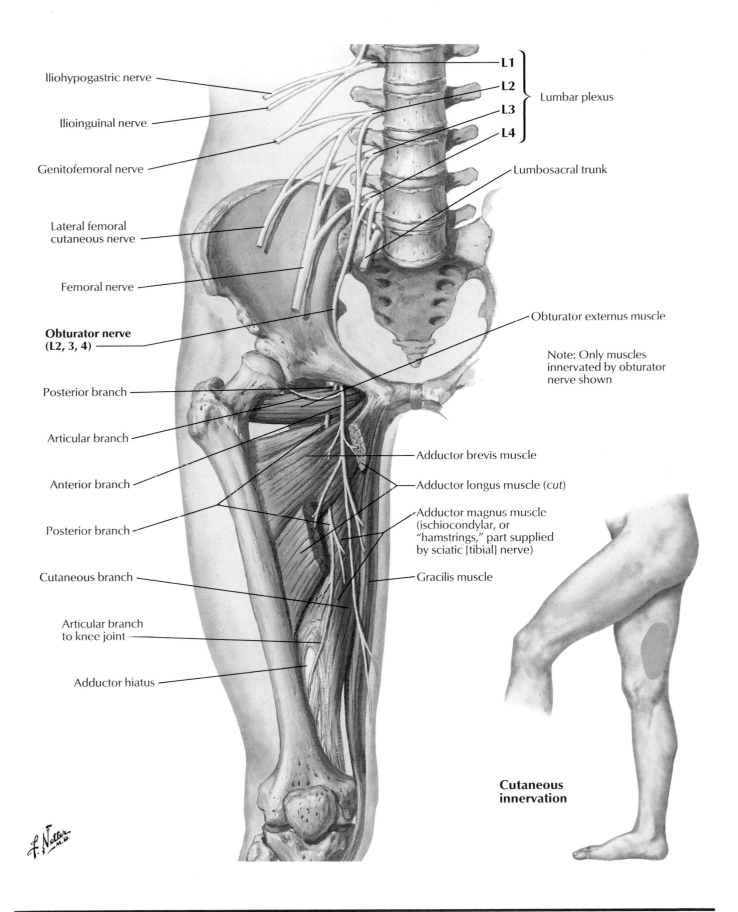

Iliohypogastric nerve

Ilioinguinal nerve

Genitofemoral nerve

Lateral femoral cutaneous nerve

Femoral nerve

Obturator nerve (L2, 3, 4)

Posterior branch

Articular branch

Anterior branch

Posterior branch

Cutaneous branch

Articular branch to knee joint

Adductor hiatus

L1
L2
L3
L4
Lumbar plexus

Lumbosacral trunk

Obturator externus muscle

Note: Only muscles innervated by obturator nerve shown

Adductor brevis muscle

Adductor longus muscle (*cut*)

Adductor magnus muscle (ischiocondylar, or "hamstrings," part supplied by sciatic [tibial] nerve)

Gracilis muscle

Cutaneous innervation

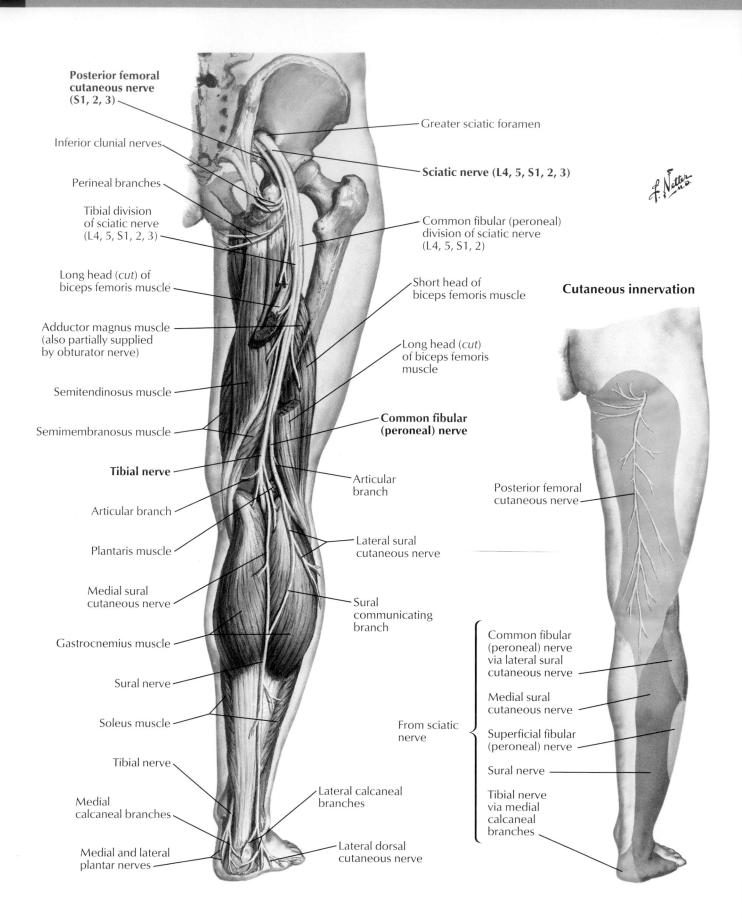

Posterior femoral cutaneous nerve (S1, 2, 3)

Inferior clunial nerves

Perineal branches

Tibial division of sciatic nerve (L4, 5, S1, 2, 3)

Long head (*cut*) of biceps femoris muscle

Adductor magnus muscle (also partially supplied by obturator nerve)

Semitendinosus muscle

Semimembranosus muscle

Tibial nerve

Articular branch

Plantaris muscle

Medial sural cutaneous nerve

Gastrocnemius muscle

Sural nerve

Soleus muscle

Tibial nerve

Medial calcaneal branches

Medial and lateral plantar nerves

Greater sciatic foramen

Sciatic nerve (L4, 5, S1, 2, 3)

Common fibular (peroneal) division of sciatic nerve (L4, 5, S1, 2)

Short head of biceps femoris muscle

Long head (*cut*) of biceps femoris muscle

Common fibular (peroneal) nerve

Articular branch

Lateral sural cutaneous nerve

Sural communicating branch

Lateral calcaneal branches

Lateral dorsal cutaneous nerve

Cutaneous innervation

Posterior femoral cutaneous nerve

Common fibular (peroneal) nerve via lateral sural cutaneous nerve

Medial sural cutaneous nerve

Superficial fibular (peroneal) nerve

Sural nerve

Tibial nerve via medial calcaneal branches

From sciatic nerve

Plate 528   **Neurovasculature**

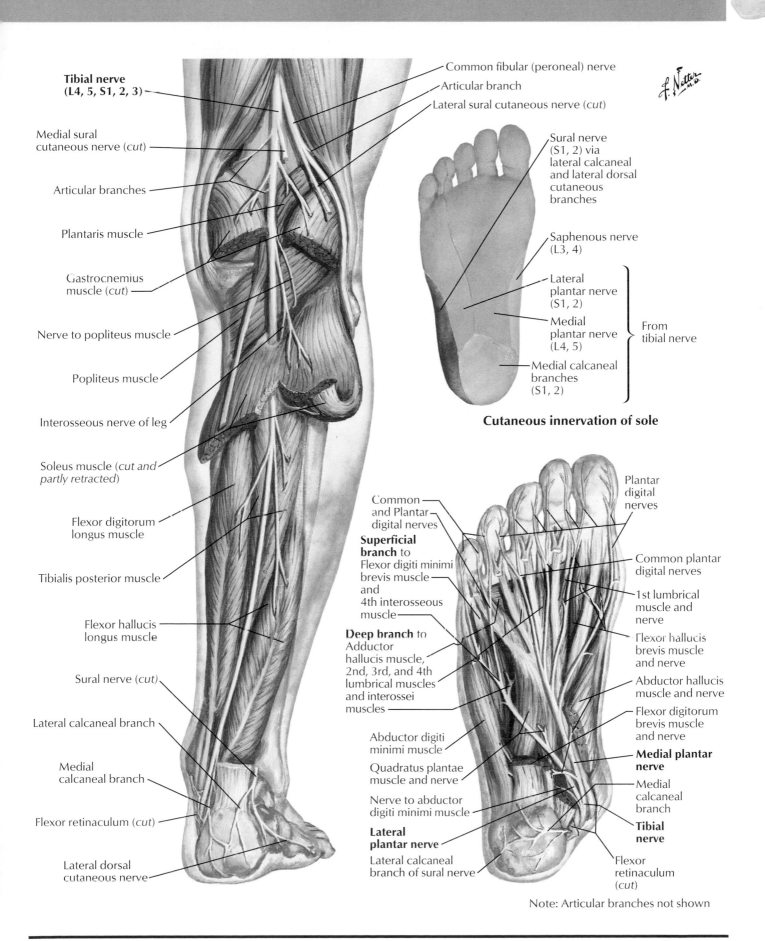

Tibial nerve
(L4, 5, S1, 2, 3)

Medial sural
cutaneous nerve (*cut*)

Articular branches

Plantaris muscle

Gastrocnemius
muscle (*cut*)

Nerve to popliteus muscle

Popliteus muscle

Interosseous nerve of leg

Soleus muscle (*cut and
partly retracted*)

Flexor digitorum
longus muscle

Tibialis posterior muscle

Flexor hallucis
longus muscle

Sural nerve (*cut*)

Lateral calcaneal branch

Medial
calcaneal branch

Flexor retinaculum (*cut*)

Lateral dorsal
cutaneous nerve

Common fibular (peroneal) nerve

Articular branch

Lateral sural cutaneous nerve (*cut*)

Sural nerve
(S1, 2) via
lateral calcaneal
and lateral dorsal
cutaneous
branches

Saphenous nerve
(L3, 4)

Lateral
plantar nerve
(S1, 2)

Medial
plantar nerve
(L4, 5)

From
tibial nerve

Medial calcaneal
branches
(S1, 2)

Cutaneous innervation of sole

Plantar
digital
nerves

Common
and Plantar
digital nerves

**Superficial
branch** to
Flexor digiti minimi
brevis muscle
and
4th interosseous
muscle

Deep branch to
Adductor
hallucis muscle,
2nd, 3rd, and 4th
lumbrical muscles
and interossei
muscles

Abductor digiti
minimi muscle

Quadratus plantae
muscle and nerve

Nerve to abductor
digiti minimi muscle

**Lateral
plantar nerve**

Lateral calcaneal
branch of sural nerve

Common plantar
digital nerves

1st lumbrical
muscle and
nerve

Flexor hallucis
brevis muscle
and nerve

Abductor hallucis
muscle and nerve

Flexor digitorum
brevis muscle
and nerve

**Medial plantar
nerve**

Medial
calcaneal
branch

**Tibial
nerve**

Flexor
retinaculum
(*cut*)

Note: Articular branches not shown

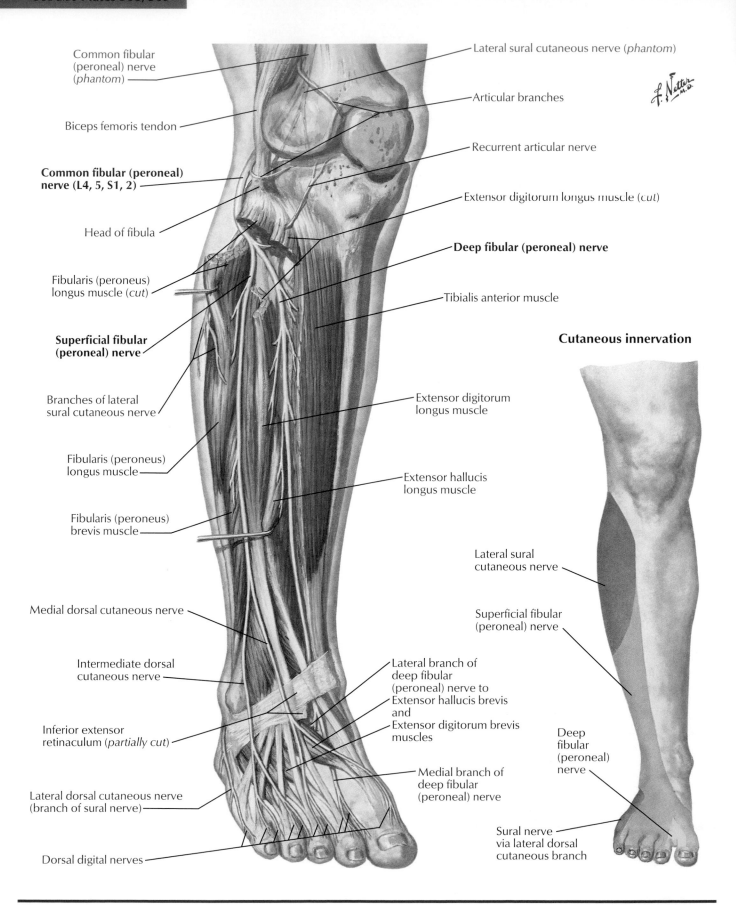

Common fibular (peroneal) nerve (*phantom*)

Biceps femoris tendon

Common fibular (peroneal) nerve (L4, 5, S1, 2)

Head of fibula

Fibularis (peroneus) longus muscle (*cut*)

Superficial fibular (peroneal) nerve

Branches of lateral sural cutaneous nerve

Fibularis (peroneus) longus muscle

Fibularis (peroneus) brevis muscle

Medial dorsal cutaneous nerve

Intermediate dorsal cutaneous nerve

Inferior extensor retinaculum (*partially cut*)

Lateral dorsal cutaneous nerve (branch of sural nerve)

Dorsal digital nerves

Lateral sural cutaneous nerve (*phantom*)

Articular branches

Recurrent articular nerve

Extensor digitorum longus muscle (*cut*)

Deep fibular (peroneal) nerve

Tibialis anterior muscle

Extensor digitorum longus muscle

Extensor hallucis longus muscle

Lateral branch of deep fibular (peroneal) nerve to Extensor hallucis brevis and Extensor digitorum brevis muscles

Medial branch of deep fibular (peroneal) nerve

Cutaneous innervation

Lateral sural cutaneous nerve

Superficial fibular (peroneal) nerve

Deep fibular (peroneal) nerve

Sural nerve via lateral dorsal cutaneous branch

Plate 530

Neurovasculature

Radiograph

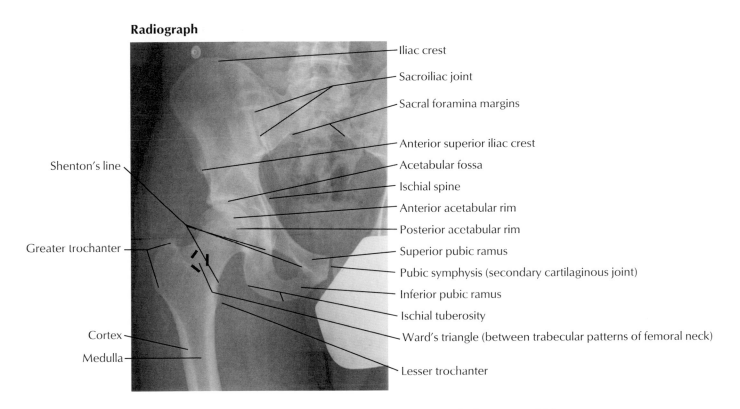

- Iliac crest
- Sacroiliac joint
- Sacral foramina margins
- Anterior superior iliac crest
- Acetabular fossa
- Ischial spine
- Anterior acetabular rim
- Posterior acetabular rim
- Superior pubic ramus
- Pubic symphysis (secondary cartilaginous joint)
- Inferior pubic ramus
- Ischial tuberosity
- Ward's triangle (between trabecular patterns of femoral neck)
- Lesser trochanter

- Shenton's line
- Greater trochanter
- Cortex
- Medulla

Arthrogram of hip

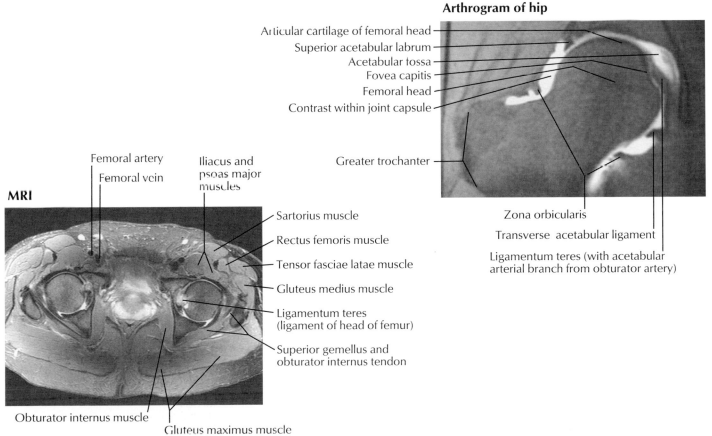

- Articular cartilage of femoral head
- Superior acetabular labrum
- Acetabular fossa
- Fovea capitis
- Femoral head
- Contrast within joint capsule
- Greater trochanter

- Zona orbicularis
- Transverse acetabular ligament
- Ligamentum teres (with acetabular arterial branch from obturator artery)

MRI

- Femoral artery
- Femoral vein
- Iliacus and psoas major muscles
- Sartorius muscle
- Rectus femoris muscle
- Tensor fasciae latae muscle
- Gluteus medius muscle
- Ligamentum teres (ligament of head of femur)
- Superior gemellus and obturator internus tendon
- Obturator internus muscle
- Gluteus maximus muscle

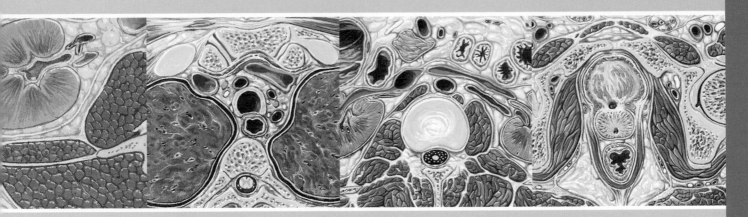

Section 8 CROSS-SECTIONAL ANATOMY

Plate No.

236
237
238

239

325

327
328
329

398

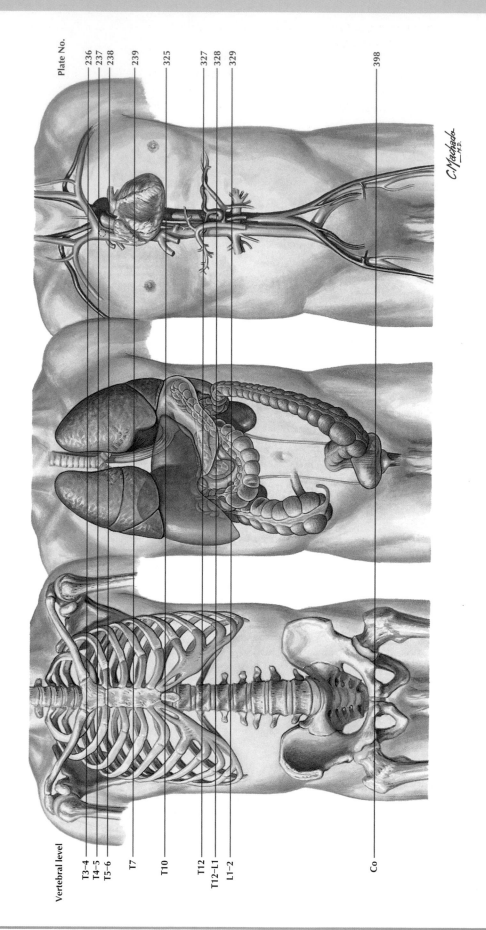

C. Machado
—M.D.

Vertebral level

T3–4
T4–5
T5–6

T7

T10

T12
T12–L1
L1–2

Co

Plate 532

Cross-sectional Anatomy

References

Plates 8, 36-38, 48-50
Lang J. Clinical Anatomy of the Nose, Nasal Cavity and Paranasal Sinuses. New York, Thieme Medical Publishers, Inc., 1989.

Plate 23
Tubbs RS, Kelly DR, Humphrey ER, Chua GD, et al. The tectorial membrane: anatomical, biomechanical, and histological analysis. Clin Anat 2007; 20(4):382-386.

Plates 25-28, 53-55, 67-68
Noden DM, Francis-West P. The differentiation and morphogenesis of craniofacial muscles. Dev Dyn 2006; 235(5):1194-1218.

Plates 31, 33, 124-130
Tubbs RS, Salter EG, Oakes WJ. Anatomic landmarks for nerves of the neck: a vade mecum for neurosurgeons. Neurosurgery 2005; 56 (2 Suppl):256-260; discussion 256-260.

Plates 65, 93, 94
Kierner AC, Mayer R, v Kirschhofer K. Do the tensor tympani and tensor veli palatini muscles of man form a functional unit? A histochemical investigation of their putative connections. Hear Res 2002; 165(1-2):48-52.

Plates 78-80
Ludlow CL. Central nervous system control of the laryngeal muscles in humans. Respir Physiol Neurobiol 2005; 147(2-3):205-222.

Plates 100-114
Rhoton AL. Cranial Anatomy and Surgical Approaches. Schaumburg, Ill, The Congress of Neurological Surgeons, 2003.

Plates 103, 138
Tubbs RS, Hansasuta A, Loukas M, et al. Branches of the petrous and cavernous segments of the internal carotid artery. Clin Anat 2007; 20(6):596-601.

Plates 115-117, 123
Schrott-Fischer A, Kammen-Jolly K, Scholtz AW, et al. Patterns of GABA like immunoreactivity in efferent fibers of the human cochlea. Hear Res 2002; 174(1-2):75 85.

Plate 157, 172
Tubbs RS, Loukas M, Slappy JB, et al. Clinical anatomy of the CI doral root, ganglion, and ramus: a review and anatomical study. Clin Anat 2007; 20:624-627.

Plate 159
Lee MWL, McPhee RW, Stringer MD. An evidence-based approach to human dermatomes. Clin Anat 2008; 21:363-373.

Plates 159, 401, 513, 470
Forester O. The dermatomes in man. Brain 1933; 56:1.

Garrett FD. The segmental distribution of the cutaneous nerves in the limbs of man. Anat Rec 1948; 102:409.

Keegan JJ. Dermatome hypalgesia with posterolateral herniation of lower cervical intervertebral disc. J Neurosurg 1947; 4:115.

Plate 165
Turnball IM. Bloody supply of the spinal cord. In Vinken PJ, Bruyn GW (eds). Handbook of Clinical Neurology, XII. Amsterdam, North-Holland, 1972, pp 478–491.

Plates 194, 195
Jackson CL, Huber JF. Correlated applied anatomy of the bronchial tree and lungs with a system of nomenclature. Dis Chest 1943; 9:319.

Plate 197
Ikeda S, Ono Y, Miyazawa S, et al. Flexible broncho-fiberscope. Otolaryngology (Tokyo) 1970; 42:855.

Plate 211
Angelini P, Velasco JA, Flamm S. Coronary anomalies: incidence, pathophysiology and clinical relevance. Circulation 2002; 105:2449-2454.

Plate 219
James TN. The internodal pathways of the human heart. Prog Cardiovas Dis 2001; 43:495.

Plate 234
Ang H-J, Gill Y-C, Lee W-J, et al. Anatomy of thoracic splanchnic nerves for surgical resection. Clin Anat 2008; 21:171-177.

Plate 279
Elias H. Morphology of the Liver. New York, Academic Press, 1969.

Robinson PJ. MRI of the Liver: A Practical Guide. New York, Taylor & Francis, 2006.

MacSween RNM, Anthony PP, Scheuer PJ, et al (eds). Pathology of the Liver. London, Churchill Livingstone, 2002.

Plates 283, 284
Odze RD. Surgical Pathology of the GI Tract, Liver, Biliary Tract, and Pancreas. Philadelphia, Saunders, 2004.

Plate 305
Thomas MD. In The Ciba Collection of Medical Illustrations, Vol 3, Part II. Summit NJ, CIBA, p 78.

Plates 323, 346, 364, 376, 394
Stormont TJ, Cahill DR, King BF, Myers RP. Fascias of the male external genitalia and perineum. Clin Anat 1994; 7:115.

Plates 337, 342, 348, 352, 357, 358
Oelrich TM. The striated urogenital sphincter muscle in the female. Anat Rec 1983; 205:223.

References

Plates 341, 346

Myers RP, Goellner JR, Cahill DR. Prostate shape, external striated urethral sphincter and radical prostatectomy: the apical dissection. J Urol 1987; 138:543.

Plates 341, 346, 363, 364

Oelrich TM. The urethral sphincter muscle in the male. Am J Anat 1980; 158:229.

Plate 383

Flocks RH, Kerr HD, Elkins HB, et al. Treatment of carcinoma of the prostate by interstitial radiation with radio-active gold (Au 198): a preliminary report. J Urol 1952; 68(2):510.

Plate 401

Keegan JJ, Garrett FD. The segmental distribution of the cutaneous nerves in the limbs of man. Anat Rec 1948; 102:409.

Plate 470

Keegan JJ. Neurological interpretation of dermatome hypalgesia with herniation of the lumbar intervertebral disc. J Bone Joint Surg 1944; 26:238.

Last RJ. Innervation of the limbs. J Bone Joint Surg (Br) 1949; 31:452.

Index

Cochlea, 46, 95, 97
  helicotrema of, 92, 96
  modiolus of, 96
  osseous, 96
  scala tympani of, 92
  scala vestibuli of, 92
  turn of, section through, 96
Cochlear aqueduct, 96
Cochlear capsule, 95
Cochlear duct, 92, 96, 97
  basal turn of, 95
Cochlear ganglion, 123
Cochlear nerve, 92, 95, 96, 97, 123
Cochlear nucleus
  anterior, 116, 123
  posterior, 116, 123
Cochlear recess, 95
Cochlear (round) window, 92
  fossa of, 93, 94
Colic artery
  ascending branch of, 288
  descending branch of, 288
  left, 257, 288, 297, 302, 378
    ascending branch of, 378
    descending branch of, 378
  middle, 281, 284, 287, 288, 301, 302, 323
  right, 287, 288, 301, 302, 315
Colic (hepatic) flexure
  left, 261, 262, 263, 264, 267, 270, 276, 278, 281, 322
  right, 261, 263, 264, 267, 270, 276, 278, 281, 317, 328
    transverse section of, 326
Colic impression, 282
Colic lymph node
  left, 296
  middle, 296
  right, 296
Colic plexus
  left, 297, 302
  middle, 301, 302
  right, 301, 302
Colic vein
  left, 292
  middle, 281, 290, 291, 292
  right, 290, 291, 292
Collar of Helvetius, 230
Collateral artery
  middle, 420, 422, 423
  radial, 420, 422, 423
  ulnar, 421
    inferior, 421, 422, 433
    superior, 422, 432, 433
Collateral eminence, 110
Collateral ligament, 446, 452, 497, 516
  accessory, 446
  fibular, 495, 497, 505, 509
    inferior subtendinous bursa of, 499
  radial, 426, 442, 446
    posterior (dorsal) view of, 443
  tibial, 495, 497, 499, 505, 507
    superficial and deep fibers of, 496
  ulnar, 426, 446
    posterior (dorsal) view of, 443
Collateral sulcus, 105, 106
Collateral trigone, 110
Collecting duct, 314
Collecting tubule, 314
  schema of, 313
Collecting vessels
  apical, 73
  basal, 73
  central, 73
  marginal, 73
Colles' (perineal) fascia, 359
Colliculus
  facial, 114
  inferior, 105, 110, 113, 114
    brachium of, 110, 113
  left
    inferior, 142
    superior, 142

Colliculus (Continued)
  seminal, 350, 364
  superior, 105, 110, 113, 114, 115, 131, 141
    brachium of, 110, 113
    of corporal quadrigemina, 106
Colli muscle, nerves to, 132
Colon
  air in, radiograph of, 333
  area for, 308
  ascending, 125, 261, 263, 266, 270, 276, 309, 328,
    329, 330, 343, 347
    axial CT image of, 324
  circular muscle of, 274
  descending, 161, 263, 270, 276, 317, 328, 329, 330, 343
    area for, 308
    innervation of, 160
    site of, 266
    transverse section of, 326
  right colic flexure of
    transverse section of, 326
  sigmoid, 161, 261, 263, 276, 343, 344, 347, 371, 372,
    373, 374, 392
    innervation of, 160
    reflected, 263
  transverse, 261, 262, 263, 265, 270, 276, 280, 281,
    282, 290, 328, 329, 330
    axial CT image of, 324
    transverse section of, 326
  tributary from, 291
Commissure
  anterior, 105, 114, 139, 144, 145, 356
  habenular, 105, 110, 114
  of labia majora, 356
  posterior, 105, 110, 114, 139, 356, 368
  of semilunar valve cusps, 217
Common tendinous ring (of Zinn), 84, 86, 120
Communicating artery
  anterior, 135, 136, 137, 138, 139, 140
    computed tomography of, 147
  posterior, 103, 135, 136, 137, 138, 140, 141
Communicating vein, 30, 167
Compressor urethrae muscle, 349, 359
Computed tomography (CT)
  abdominal, 324
  of chest, 235
  of shoulder, 468
Concha
  of auricle, 93
  inferior, 16
  nasal. See Nasal concha
Condylar canal, 13
Condylar process, 17
Condyle
  lateral, 424
    radiograph of, 498
  medial, 424, 501
    radiograph of, 498
  occipital, 10, 16
Cone of light, 93
Cones, retinal, 119
Conjoined longitudinal muscle, 372, 374
Conjoined tendon, 244, 245, 247, 253, 254
Conjunctiva, 81, 91
  bulbar, 81, 83
  palpebral, 83
    inferior, 81
    superior, 81
Conjunctival artery, posterior, 91
Conjunctival fornix
  inferior, 81
  superior, 81
Conjunctival vein, posterior, 91
Conjunctival vessels, 90
Connective tissue
  of liver, 279
  of skull, 101
  subserous, 306
Connective tissue sheath, 196
Conoid ligament, 410, 413
  attachment of, 406

Conoid tubercle, of clavicle, 406
Conus arteriosus, 206, 214, 215, 216
Conus elasticus, 78, 80
Conus medullaris, 157, 158, 329
Convoluted tubule
  distal, 313
  proximal, 313
Cooper's ligament, 88, 176, 244, 245, 247, 253, 255,
  256
Corabrachialis muscle, 407, 412, 414
Corabrachialis tendon, 414
Coracoacromial ligament, 410, 413, 414, 419
Coracobrachialis muscle, 237, 238, 417, 419, 421,
  423, 461, 462
  fascia over, 416
Coracoclavicular ligament, 410, 413
  attachment of, 406
Coracohumeral ligament, 410
Coracoid process, 179, 182, 183, 407, 410, 412, 413,
  414, 415, 416, 417, 419, 421
  radiograph of, 409
Cornea, 81, 83, 87, 88, 90, 91
Corneal limbus, 81
Corneoscleral junction, 81
Corniculate tubercle, 66
Cornuate tubercle, 67
Coronal sulcus, 368
Coronal suture, 4, 7, 8, 9, 14
Coronary artery
  left, 211, 213
    anterior interventricular branch of, 206, 211,
      213
    arteriographic view of, 213
    circumflex branch of, 211, 213, 216
    left anterior oblique view of, 213
    left (obtuse) marginal branch of, 213
    (perforating) interventricular septal branches of,
      213
    posterolateral branches of, 213
    right anterior oblique view of, 213
  opening of, 217, 218
  right, 206, 211, 212, 216
    arteriographic view of, 213
    atrial branch of, 211
    atrioventricular nodal branch of, 212,
      216
    conus (arteriosus) branch of, 212
    diaphragmatic surface of, 211
    interventricular septal branches of, 211
    left anterior oblique view of, 212
    left marginal branch of, 211
    opening of, 217
    posterior interventricular branch of, 208, 211,
      212, 216
    posterior left ventricular branch of, 211
    posterior ventricular branch of, 212
    right (acute) marginal branch of, 211, 212
    right anterior oblique view of, 212
    right posterolateral branches of, 212
  sinuatrial nodal branch of, 211, 212
  sternocostal surface of, 211
Coronary ligament, 277
  enclosing bare area of liver, 323
  hepatorenal portion of, 277
  of liver, 266
Coronary sinus, 208, 209, 211, 215, 239
  opening of, 214, 217
  valve (thebesian) of, 214
Coronary sulcus, 206
Coronary vein
  diaphragmatic surface of, 211
  sternocostal surface of, 211
Coronoid fossa, 424
Coronoid process, 7, 17, 424, 431
  radiograph of, 207, 425
Corpora cavernosa, 362
Corpora quadrigemina, superior colliculus of,
  106
Corpus albicans, 355

D

Darwin, auricular tubercle of, 93
Declive, 112, 142
Deep (Buck's) fascia, 243, 244, 245, 323, 346, 360, 362, 363, 375, 376, 381, 383
  intercavernous septum of, 362
Deep facial vein, 3
Deltoid ligament, medial, 515
Deltoid muscle, 26, 27, 149, 160, 171, 236, 238, 240, 400, 407, 410, 411, 412, 414, 416, 417, 420, 421, 423, 461, 465
  computed tomography of, 468
  magnetic resonance imaging of, 468
  origin of, 406
  reflected, 419
Deltoid tuberosity, 407
Deltopectoral groove, 400
Deltopectoral lymph node, 405
Deltopectoral triangle, 240, 411
Denonvillier's fascia, 323, 341, 346, 371, 376
Dens, 19, 21, 167
  apical ligament of, 23, 63, 65
  articular cartilage on, 21
  of axis, 7
Dental plexus
  inferior, 121
  superior, 44
Dental pulp, 57
Dentate gyrus, 105, 107, 110, 111, 118
Dentate line, 373
Dentate nucleus, 114
Denticulate ligament, 162, 163
Dentinal tubule, 57
Dentine, 57
Depressor anguli oris muscle, 25, 54, 122
Depressor labii inferioris muscle, 25
Depressor septi nasi muscle, 25, 35, 122
Dermatomes
  levels of, 159
  of lower limb, 470
  schematic demarcation of, 159
  of upper limb, anterior and posterior views of, 401
Descemet's membrane, 88
Descending pathway, 131
Diaphragm, 184, 192, 200, 203, 205, 226, 227, 230, 231, 232, 247, 256, 258, 264, 267, 277, 282, 306, 308, 309, 317, 327, 390, 486
  abdominal surface of, 189
  area for, 309
  central tendon of, 189, 256, 323
  costal part of, 189
  covered by parietal pleura, 224, 225
  cross section of, 265
  crus of, 173, 317
    left, 189, 226, 256, 262, 325, 326, 328, 329
    right, 189, 226, 256, 262, 325, 326, 327, 328, 329
  dome of
    left, 190, 191
    radiograph of, 207
    right, 190, 191
  lumbar part of, 189
  pelvic, 342
    fascia of, 344, 348, 357, 358, 362, 372, 374, 376, 385
    female, 337, 338, 339
    male, 340, 341
Diaphragmatic constriction, 227
Diaphragmatic ligament, 366, 369
Digastric fossa, 17
Digastric muscle
  anterior belly of, 26, 27, 28, 30, 33, 45, 48, 53, 61, 68, 117
  intermediate tendon of, 59
  mastoid notch of, 10
  phantom, 33
  posterior belly of, 26, 28, 33, 39, 45, 53, 59, 60, 61, 67, 68, 73, 117, 122
    nerve to, 24

Digastric tendon, intermediate, 60
  fibrous loop for, 27, 28, 53, 59
Digital artery
  dorsal, 518, 524
  palmar, 447, 448, 454
    common, 448, 450, 453, 454
  plantar, 459, 520, 521, 524
    common, 524
    dorsal branches of, 518
    to neighboring digit, 459
Digital fibrous sheath, 446
Digital nerve
  dorsal, 404, 456, 466, 471, 528, 530
  of fourth and fifth digits, 447
  palmar, 404, 447, 448, 454
    branches to phalanges, 454
    common, 450
    dorsal branches of, 456
    to fourth and fifth fingers, 448
    from superficial branch of ulnar nerve, 447
    of thumb, 448
  plantar, 520
    dorsal branches of, 518
Digital vein
  dorsal, 404, 456, 471
  palmar, 404
Dilator pupillae muscle, 88, 120, 131
Diploë, 9
Diploic vein, 99, 101
  occipital, 99
  temporal
    anterior, 99
    posterior, 99
Direct vein, lateral, 143, 144
Distal interphalangeal (DIP) joint
  in extension: medial view of, 446
  site of, 400
Distal medial striate artery (recurrent artery of Heubner), 137, 138, 139, 140
Distributing vein, 279
Dorsalis pedis artery, 518, 524
Dorsal ramus, spinal, 252, 418
Dorsal root ganglion, 131, 174, 252, 300, 303, 304, 306, 307, 320
Dorsal tubercle of radius (Lister's), 427
  posterior (dorsal) view of, 440
Dorsal venous network, 404
Dorsiflexion, of lower limb, 470
Dorsum sellae, 11
Douglas, retrouterine pouch of, 342, 344
Ductus arteriosus
  obliterated, 223
  prenatal, 223
Ductus choledochus. *See* Bile duct. common
Ductus (vas) deferens, 247, 253, 254, 255, 257, 346, 350, 364, 366, 367, 370, 371, 383, 389, 390, 396, 473
  ampulla of, 364
  artery to, 249, 257, 367, 378, 381, 383
  covered by peritoneum, 254
  in peritoneal fold, 347
Ductus plexus, 389, 390, 396
Ductus reuniens, 96
Ductus venosus
  obliterated, 223
  prenatal, 223
Duodenal cap, 268
Duodenal flexure
  inferior, 271
  superior, 271
Duodenal fold
  circular, 271
  inferior, 262, 270
  superior, 262
Duodenal fossa
  inferior, 262, 270
  superior, 262
Duodenal glands, 271
Duodenal impression, 277

Duodenal papillae
  major, 271
  minor (inconstant), 271
Duodenal wall, layers of, 271
Duodenojejunal flexure, 262, 270, 281, 317, 322
Duodenojejunal junction, 173
Duodenum, 125, 265, 266, 267, 277, 278, 280, 281, 315, 317, 322
  arteries of, 284, 286
  ascending (4th) part of, 262, 270, 271
  autonomic innervation of, 298, 299
    schema of, 300
  circular folds of, 280
  circular muscle layer of, 269, 271
  descending (2nd) part of, 262, 270, 271, 328
    cross section of, 173
    minor papilla of, 280
  inferior (horizontal or 3rd) part of, 270, 271, 323
  in situ, 270
  junction of second and third parts of, 329
  longitudinal fold of, 280
  longitudinal muscle layer of, 269, 271
  minor papilla of, 280
  mucosa of, 271
  muscles of, 271, 280
  posterior view of, 286
  reflected to left, 286
  superior (1st) part of, 268, 270, 280
    transverse section of, 326
  suspensory muscle of, 262
  veins of, 289
Dural sac
  MR sagittal images of, 377
  termination of, 157, 158
Dural venous sinuses
  coronal section through, 103
  sagittal section of, 102
Dura mater, 38, 93, 96, 100, 101, 108, 118
  lumbar, 163
  meningeal layer of, 99
  periosteal layer of, 99
  spinal, 157, 162
  thoracic, 163
  of vertebral column, 167
Dura-skull interface, 99, 101

E

Ear
  bony and membranous labyrinths of, 95
  external
    coronal oblique section of, 93
    lateral view of, 93
  middle, coronal oblique section of, 93
  tympanic cavity of, 94
Edinger-Westphal nucleus, 115, 116, 120, 131
Efferent ductule, 369, 370
Efferent fibers, 120
  of brainstem, 116
Ejaculatory duct, 398
  beginning of, 364
  opening of, 364, 369
Elastic fibers, of airway, 198
Elbow
  anastomosis around, 422
  bones of, 424
  in extension
    lateral view of, 424
    medial view of, 424
  fat pads of, 426
  joint capsule of, 426
  ligaments of, 426
  in 90° flexion, 424, 426
  opened
    anterior view of, 426
    posterior view of, 426
  radiographs of, 425
    anteroposterior, 425
    lateral, 425

Extraperitoneal (supralevator) space, 372
Extrinsic eye muscle, 90
Eye, 161
    anterior and posterior chambers of, 87, 88
    extrinsic muscles of, 84
        innervation of, 84
    innervation of, 160
    intrinsic arteries and veins of, 90
    muscles of, 117
    vascular supply of, 91
Eyeball, 87, 89
    fasciae of, 83
    fascial sheath (Tenon's capsule) of, 83, 87
    horizontal section of, 87
    transverse section of, 48
Eyelash (cilia), 81
Eyelid, 81
    arteries and veins of, 85
    tarsus of, 83

F

Face
    arterial supply sources of, 3
    muscles of, 117, 122
    sensory nerves of, 117
    superficial arteries and veins of, 3
    superficial view of, 24
Facet (zygapophyseal) joint, 239
Facets, 239
    articular
        inferior, 156
        of rib head, 181
        of sacrum, 152
        superior, 151
        thoracic, superior, 151
        of vertebral body, 180
    cervical, 20, 21
    costal
        inferior, 181
        superior, 181
Facial artery, 3, 30, 33, 35, 39, 47, 60, 61, 69, 70, 71,
        75, 85, 130, 132, 135, 136
    lateral nasal alar branch of, 40
    superior labial branch of, 40
    tonsillar branch of, 64
    transverse, 3, 33, 35, 61, 69, 85
Facial canal, 123
    prominence of, 93, 94
Facial colliculus, 114
Facial expression muscles, 25, 60
    lateral view of, 25
Facial lymph node, 72
Facial nerve (VII), 13, 33, 39, 43, 45, 46, 47, 60, 62, 92,
        94, 97, 103, 113, 115, 116, 121, 130, 132, 133, 134
    branches of, 24, 61, 161
    buccal branches of, 24
    cervical branch of, 24
    chorda tympani of, 12
    common, 70
    communication with glossopharyngeal nerve, 124
    deep, 70
    distribution of, 117
    emerging from stylomastoid foramen, 24
    geniculum (geniculate ganglion) of, 43, 45, 94, 97,
        123, 124, 130
    internal genu of, 116
    marginal mandibular branch of, 24, 30
    motor nucleus of, 122
    motor root of, 123
    schema of, 122
    in stylomastoid foramen, 12, 94
    temporal branches of, 24
    trunk of, 24
    zygomatic branches of, 24
Facial nucleus, 115, 116
Facial plexus, 130
Facial vein, 3, 30, 31, 45, 47, 59, 60, 61, 70, 85, 113
    common, 3, 31, 59, 61
    common trunk for, 59, 61

Facial vein (Continued)
    deep, 3
    transverse, 3, 70
Falciform ligament, 246, 247, 261, 266, 267, 277,
        292, 327
    nerve to, 249
Fallopian tube. See Uterine tube
False pelvis, 336
Falx cerebelli, 102
Falx cerebri, 38, 48, 101, 102, 103, 139, 142
Fascia
    alar, 34
    antebrachial, 437
        deep, thickening of, 442, 447
    axillary, 416
    brachial, 416, 423
    buccopharyngeal, 34, 60, 63
    Camper's, 243, 323, 357, 360
    cervical, 34
        investing (deep) layer of, 25, 27, 34, 63, 182, 411
        pretracheal layer of, 27
    clavicopectoral, 416
        investing layer of, 182
    cremasteric, 244, 245, 254, 367, 370
    cribriform, 250
        within saphenous opening, 473
    crural, 471, 473, 510
    dartos, 243, 346, 367, 370, 375
    deep, 455
        of leg, 510
    deep antebrachial, thickening of, 442, 447
    deep (Buck's), 243, 244, 245, 323, 360, 362, 363,
        375, 376, 381, 383
        intercavernous septum of, 362
    Denonvillier's, 323, 341, 346, 371, 376
    diaphragmatic, 230, 317
    endopelvic paravesical, 350
    extraperitoneal, 173, 245, 246, 254, 255, 392
    geniohyoid, 34
    of hand, 450
    iliac, 255, 345, 372
    infradiaphragmatic, 230
    infrahyoid, 27, 34
    infraspinatus, 168, 171
    interosseous
        dorsal, 450
        palmar, 450
    intraspinous, 248
    investing omohyoid muscle, 416
    investing subclavius muscle, 416
    of leg/lower limb, 473
        deep, 471, 473
    masseteric, 25
    medial plantar, 520
    obturator, 338, 340, 344, 345, 348, 352, 358, 372,
        382, 391
    of orbit and eyeball, 83
    over adductor pollicis muscle, 448
    paravesical endopelvic, 350
    parotid, 25
    pectineal, 245, 255
    pectoral, 176, 416
    of pectoralis major muscle, 416
    of pectoralis minor muscle, 416
    pelvic, 371
        of pelvic diaphragm, 348, 358, 372, 374, 385
        tendinous arch of, 345, 350
    penile, 243, 244, 245, 381
        deep (Buck's), 243, 244, 245, 346, 362, 363, 376,
            381, 383
    perianal, deep (investing or Gallaudet's), 346, 350,
        357, 362, 363, 371, 376, 385
    perineal
        of deep perineal muscles, 338
        deep transverse, 364
        superficial (Colles'), 346, 350, 357, 358, 360, 362,
            363, 367, 371, 375, 376, 384, 385, 391
    pharyngobasilar, 59, 65, 67, 68, 73
    plantar, 521
        lateral, 520

Fascia (Continued)
    posterior antebrachial, thickening of, 456
    presacral, 345, 376
    pretracheal, 34, 63, 196
    prevertebral, 63, 65
    psoas, 173, 317
    pubocervical
        distal (vertical) portion of, 353
        horizontal portion of, 353
    of quadratus lumborum muscle, 173
    rectal, 344, 345, 357, 364, 371, 372, 373, 374, 376
    renal, 329
        anterior layer of, 173, 317
        Gerota's, 317
        posterior layer of, 173, 317
        transverse section of, 317
    retrovesical or rectoprostatic (Denonvillier's), 323,
        341, 346, 371, 376
    scrotal, 243, 244
        superficial (dartos), 346, 370, 375, 385
    serratus anterior, 416
    Sibson's, 225
    slips of costal origin of, 184
    spermatic, 254
        external, 243, 244, 245, 253, 346, 360, 367, 370, 385
            investing spermatic cord, 251, 362
        internal, 245, 255, 367, 370
            origin of, 254
    subclavius, 416
    supradiaphragmatic, 230
    temporal, 25, 45, 54
        deep layer of, 54
        superficial layer of, 54
    thoracolumbar, 168, 171, 248
        anterior layer of, 173
        combined layer of, 330
        middle layer of, 173, 330
        posterior layer of, 169, 170, 173, 309, 330
    transversalis, 173, 230, 245, 246, 247, 253, 254, 255,
        257, 317, 323, 327, 343, 346, 347, 348, 357
        continuation of, 317
        deep inguinal ring in, 253
    transverse section of, 325
    ulna, 437
    umbilical prevesical, 247, 254, 345, 346, 348
    uterine, 345, 353
    uterovaginal, 344, 357
    vaginorectal, 345
    vesical, 344, 345, 346, 350, 357, 371, 376
Fascia lata, 243, 244, 352, 357, 387, 471, 473, 488,
        493
Fascial compartments, of leg, 510
Fascial sheath
    of eyeball (Tenon's capsule), 83, 87
    of lumbrical muscles, 450, 451
Fasciculus
    cuneate, 114
    gracile, 114
    longitudinal
        dorsal, 114
        medial, 112, 145
    mammillothalamic, 105
    transverse, 520
Fat
    in acetabular fossa, 475
    epidural, 163, 167
    of mammary gland, 176
    orbital, 48
    pararenal, 317
    perirenal, 173, 317, 329
        interlobar artery and vein in, 314
    in posterior cervical triangle, 34
    in renal sinus, 311
    retrobulbar, 83
    in retropubic space, 245, 341
    transverse section of, 399
Fat body
    of ischioanal fossa, 357, 360, 372, 398
    orbital, 83
    suprapatellar, 499

Flexor carpi radialis muscle, 419, 421, 430, 434, 437, 461, 463
  innervation of, 464
  insertion of, 438
  origin of, 438
Flexor carpi radialis tendon, 400, 435, 436, 442, 448, 449, 461
Flexor carpi ulnaris muscle, 400, 420, 430, 432, 433, 434, 435, 461, 464
  humeral origin of, 438
  innervation of, 464
  origin of, 438
    humeral origin, 439
    ulnar origin, 439
Flexor carpi ulnaris tendon, 400, 442, 448, 449, 453
Flexor digiti minimi brevis muscle, 449, 453, 464, 521, 522, 523, 524, 529
Flexor digitorum brevis muscle, 521, 522, 523, 529
Flexor digitorum brevis nerve, 529
Flexor digitorum brevis tendon, 521, 523
Flexor digitorum longus muscle, 503, 506, 529
  insertion of, 503
  origin of, 503
Flexor digitorum longus tendon, 504, 505, 506, 521, 522, 523
  groove for insertion of, 501
Flexor digitorum longus tendon sheath, 517
Flexor digitorum profundus muscle, 436, 461, 463
  innervation of, 464
  insertion of, 438
  origin of, 438
Flexor digitorum profundus tendon, 442, 446, 449, 450, 451, 452
  insertion of, 448
Flexor digitorum superficialis muscle, 431, 434, 435, 437, 463
  humeroulnar head of, 435, 461
    origin of, 438
  insertion of, 438
  origin of, 439
  radial head of, 435, 436, 461
    insertion of, 438
Flexor digitorum superficialis tendon, 400, 431, 434, 442, 446, 449, 450, 451, 461
  insertion of, 448
Flexor hallucis brevis muscle, 529
  lateral head of, 521, 522, 523, 524
  medial head of, 521, 522, 523
  medial origin of, 524
Flexor hallucis brevis nerve, 529
Flexor hallucis brevis tendon
  lateral origin of, 524
Flexor hallucis longus muscle, 506, 522, 529
  insertion of, 503
  origin of, 503
Flexor hallucis longus tendon, 504, 505, 506, 521, 522, 523
  groove for, 511
Flexor hallucis longus tendon sheath, 517
Flexor muscles
  of digits, 431
  superficial, 434
  of wrist, 430
Flexor pollicis brevis muscle, 437, 453
  innervation of, 464
  superficial head of, 463
Flexor pollicis longus muscle, 431, 435, 436, 449, 454, 461, 463
  insertion of, 438
  origin of, 438
  tendinous sheath of, 448, 449, 450, 451
Flexor pollicis longus tendon, 436, 442, 449
  in tendon sheath, 449
Flexor retinaculum, 435, 442, 449, 450, 453, 461, 504, 505, 506, 522, 523, 529
Flexor sheath, common, 448, 449, 450, 451
Flexor tendons
  common, 430, 431, 434
    origin of, 438
  fibrous sheaths of, 454, 521

Flexor tendons *(Continued)*
  in fingers, 452
  profundus, 448
  profundus and superficialis, 450
  superficialis, 448
  synovial sheaths of, 454
  at wrist, 449
Flocculus, 112
Foliate papillae, 58, 134
Folium, 112, 142
Follicles, graafian, 355
Fontana, iridocorneal angle of, 88
Fontanelle
  anterior, 14
  mastoid, 14
  posterior, 14
  sphenoidal, 14
Foot
  arteries of, 524
  bones of, 511, 512
    lateral view of, 512
    medial view of, 512
  dorsal view of, 511, 524, 525
  dorsum of
    deep dissection of, 519
    muscles of: superficial dissection of, 518
  eversion of, 470
  innervation of, 530
  interosseous muscles of, 524, 525
  inversion of, 470
  ligaments of, plantar view of, 516
  plantar surface of, 469
  plantar view of, 511, 524, 525
  right
    lateral view of, 513, 515
    medial view of, 513, 515
    superior view of, 513
  sole of
    cutaneous innervation of, 529
    muscles of, 521, 522, 523
    superficial dissection of, 520
  tendons of, plantar view of, 516
Foramen
  apical, of the teeth, 57
  of the cranial base, 12
  interventricular (of Monro), 143
  nasolacrimal, 50
Foramen cecum, 11, 13, 58, 63
Foramen lacerum, 10, 12, 13, 98
Foramen magnum, 8, 10, 12, 13, 16, 98, 126
Foramen of Luschka, 107, 108
Foramen of Magendie, 108, 114, 116
Foramen ovale, 6, 12, 13, 16, 44, 45, 55, 98
  obliterated, 223
  prenatal, 223
  valve of, 215
Foramen rotundum, 13, 44
  maxillary nerve entering, 43
Foramen spinosum, 13, 16, 45, 98
Foramen transversarium, 20, 21
  bony spicule dividing, 20
  septated, 20
Forearm
  anterior view of, 404
  bones of, 427
  cross section of, 437
  cutaneous nerves of, 404
  most distal portion of, cross section of, 458
  muscles of, 428, 429, 430, 431
    attachments of: anterior view of, 438
    attachments of: posterior view of, 439
    deep layer: anterior view of, 436
    deep layer: posterior view of, 433
    intermediate layer: anterior view of, 435
    superficial layer: anterior view of, 434
    superficial layer of, 432
  posterior view of, 404, 466
  pronated position of, 428
  radial nerve in, 466

Forearm *(Continued)*
  right
    anterior view of, 428, 430, 431
    posterior view of, 429
  serial cross sections of, 437
  superficial veins of, 404
  supinated position of, 428
Fornix, 105
  body of, 105, 107, 111, 114
  columns of, 105, 107, 109, 111, 143
  commissure of, 111
  crura of, 109, 111, 141
  crus of, 105
  imaging of, 148
  schema of, 111
  vaginal, 355
    posterior, 342
Fossa ovalis, 214, 223, 471
  limbus of, 214
Fovea
  inferior, 114
  superior, 114
Fovea capitis, 531
  arthrogram of, 531
Fovea centralis, 87, 90
Free taenia, 263, 273, 274, 371, 374
Frenulum, 274, 362
  of clitoris, 356
  of labia minora, 356
  of tongue, 51, 61
  of upper lip, 51
Frontal artery, 3
  polar, 140
Frontal bone, 1, 4, 8, 9, 10, 35, 82
  foramen cecum of, 11
  frontal crest of, 11
  glabella of, 4, 6
  groove for anterior meningeal vessels of, 11
  groove for superior sagittal sinus of, 11
  lateral view of, 14
  nasal spine of, 37, 38
  of newborn, 14
  orbital surface of, 4
  sinus of, 37, 38
  squamous part of, 14, 37, 38
  superior surface of superior part of, 11
  superior view of, 14
  supraorbital notch of, 4, 6, 14
Frontal crest, 9, 11
Frontal gyrus
  inferior
    opercular part of, 104
    orbital part of, 104
    triangular part of, 104
  medial, 105
  middle, 104
  superior, 104
Frontalis muscle, 35
Frontal lobe, 104
Frontal nerve, 44, 83, 86, 120, 121, 130
Frontal operculum, 104
Frontal pole, 104
Frontal sinus, 5, 7, 8, 36, 37, 38, 48, 49, 63
  growth throughout life, 50
Frontal suture, 14
Frontobasal artery
  lateral, 137, 139, 140
  medial, 137, 139, 140
Frontonasal canal, 37
Frontonasal duct, opening of, 49
Fundiform ligament, 243, 253
Fundus, vagal branch to, 234
Fungiform papillae, 58, 134
Funiculus, lateral, 114

G

Galea aponeurosis, 3, 101
Galen
  ansa of, 80

Gluteus medius muscle, 149, 469, 480, 484, 488, 489, 490, 491, 531
  gluteal aponeurosis over, 248, 309, 482, 483
  MRI of, 531
  origin of, 479
  transverse section of, 399
Gluteus minimus muscle, 483, 491, 498
  origin of, 479
Gonads, 369
  male, 366
Graafian follicle, 355
Gracile fasciculus, 113, 114
Gracile tubercle, 114
Gracilis muscle, 480, 481, 483, 488, 489, 490, 493, 494, 504, 527
  insertion of, 503
  origin of, 478
Gracilis tendon, 469, 480, 481, 494, 495
Granular foveola, 9, 99, 101
Granule cells, 118
Gray matter
  imaging of, 148
  intermediolateral nucleus of, 132
    preganglionic sympathetic cell bodies in, 131
    presynaptic sympathetic cell bodies in, 43
  lateral horn of, 133, 163, 321
  spinal, 162
Great auricular nerve, 2
Greater occipital nerve, 2
Greater vestibular (Bartholin's) gland
  opening of, 356, 384
Great toe
  distal phalanx of, 525
  medial side of, vein of, 471
  proximal phalanx of, 525
Groin
  left, 242
  right, 242
Gubernaculum, 366, 369
Gut
  enteric plexus of, 304
  prenatal, 223

H

Habenula, 109
Habenular commissure, 105
Habenular trigone, 110, 114
Hair cells
  inner, 96
  outer, 96
Hamate, 449
  anterior (palmar) view of, 440, 441, 444
  coronal section: dorsal view of, 443
  hook of, 430, 436, 442, 446, 454
    anterior (palmar) view of, 440, 444, 446
    radiograph of, 445
  posterior (dorsal) view of, 440, 443
  radiograph of, 445
Hand. *See also* Finger(s)
  in anatomical position, 441
  anterior (palmar) view of, 447, 453, 460
  arteries of, palmar view of, 454
  bones of, 444
  bursae of, 450
  cutaneous innervation of, 460
  deep dorsal dissection of, 457
  deep palmar dissection of, 448
  dorsal fascia of, 450
  dorsal venous network of, 456
  dorsum of, 441
    lymph vessels passing to, 405
  in extension, 441
  in flexion, 441
  lateral (radial) view of, 455
  lymphatic drainage pathways of, 456
  muscles of, 453
  nerves of, 454
  posterior (dorsal) view of, 453, 456, 457, 460
  radiograph of, 445

Hand *(Continued)*
  right
    anterior (palmar) view of, 444
    posterior (dorsal) view of, 444
  spaces of, 450
  superficial dorsal dissection of, 456
  superficial palmar dissection of, 447
  superficial radial dissection of, 455
  tendon sheaths of, 450
  veins of, 454
Hartmann's pouch (infundulum), 280
Hasner's valve, 82
Haustra, 273, 276
Head. *See also* Brain; Skull; *specific parts of head*
  autonomic nerves in, 130
  bones and ligaments of, 15
  cutaneous nerves of, 1
  lymph vessels and nodes of, 72
  surface anatomy of, 1
Heart, 125, 161
  anterior exposure of, 206
  apex of, 206, 208, 239
    radiograph of, 207
  base of
    posterior view of, 208
    posteroinferior view of, 208
  conducting system of, 219
  diaphragmatic surface of, 208
  in diastole, 216
  drawn out of pericardial sac, 209
  fibrous skeleton of, 216, 217
  inferior border (acute margin) of, 206
  in situ, 205
  left border of, 190, 206
  left bundle of, 219
  left side of, 219
  nerves of, 220
    schema of, 160
  in pericardium, 227
  right border of, 190
  right side of, 219
  in systole, 216
  valves of, 216, 217
Heiss, loops of, 349
Helicotrema, 92, 95
Helix, 1, 93
  crux of, 93
Helvetius, collar of, 230
Hematoma
  epidural, 99, 101
  subdural, 101
Hemiazygos vein, 186, 188, 210, 232
  accessory, 186, 201, 225, 232, 238
    junction with azygos vein, 232
Hemispheric vein, cerebellar inferior, 142
Henle's loop, 313
Hepatic artery
  branch of, 279
  common, 257, 264, 271, 280, 281, 286, 287, 297, 300, 306, 327
    arteriogram of, 285
    in peritoneal fold, 264
  fine branch of, 306
  intermediate, 284
  left, 280, 283, 284
  portal vein branch of, 278
  proper, 265, 266, 270, 271, 277, 278, 280, 281, 283, 284, 286, 300, 326
    arteriogram of, 285
    bifurcation, 327
    in right margin of lesser omentum, 323
  right, 280, 283, 284
Hepatic duct
  common, 277, 278, 280, 284, 327
  left, 280
  right, 280
Hepatic flexure, right. *See* Colic (hepatic) flexure, right
Hepatic lymph nodes, 294

Hepatic plexus, 125, 298, 299, 301
  anterior, 306
  branches to cardia, 299
  common, 297
  posterior, 306
  pyloric branch of, 125
  vagal branch of, 234, 298
Hepatic portal vein, 232, 265, 271, 277, 278, 279, 280, 281, 283, 284, 289, 290, 291, 292, 294, 323, 327
  prenatal, 223
  in right margin of lesser omentum, 323
  tributaries of, 292
Hepatic vein, 226, 232, 258, 266, 277, 278
  prenatal, 223
Hepatoduodenal ligament, 264, 265, 267, 270, 278
  transverse section of, 326
Hepatogastric ligament, 265, 267
Hepatopancreatic ampulla (of Vater), 280
  sphincter of, 280, 306
Hepatorenal recess, 327
Hering, carotid branch of, 33, 124, 129, 130
Hering-Breuer reflex, 204
Hesselbach's inguinal triangle, 247
Heubner, recurrent artery of, 137, 138, 139, 140
Hilar (bronchopulmonary) lymph nodes, 224
Hilum, of kidney, 311
Hip
  arthrogram of, 531
  bony attachments of, 479
    anterior view of, 478
    posterior view of, 479
  extension and flexion of, 470
  lateral view of, 474
  medial view of, 474
  MRI of, 531
  muscles of
    lateral view of, 482
    posterior view of, 483
  nerves of, 491
  radiograph of, 531
Hip bone
  auricular surface of, 474
  lateral view of, 474
  medial view of, 474
Hip joint, 475
  anterior view of, 475
  anteroposterior radiograph of, 476
  lateral view of, 475
  ligaments of, 480
  nerve to, 491
Hippocampal fimbria, 118
Hippocampal sulcus, 111
Hippocampus, 107, 109, 110
  alveus of, 111
  fimbria of, 105, 107, 109, 110, 111
  superior dissection of, 111
His, bundle of, 219
Horizontal cells, retinal, 119
Houston, valves of, 373
Humeral artery
  ascending branch of, 415
  circumflex
    anterior, 414, 417, 419, 420, 421, 422
    posterior, 415, 417, 420, 421, 422
  descending branch of, 415
  posterior circumflex, 414
Humeral ligament
  lesser, 410
  transverse, 410
Humeral vein, circumflex, 403
Humerus, 423, 424, 426
  anatomical neck of, 407
    radiograph of, 409
  anterior view of, 407
  capitulum of, 407
  condyles of
    lateral, 407
    medial, 407
  coronal fossa of, 407

Humerus *(Continued)*
  deltoid tuberosity of, 407
  epicondyles of
    lateral, 419, 420, 433
    medial, 407, 419, 420, 421, 433, 434
  greater tubercle of, 407, 410, 414, 419
    radiograph of, 409
  head of, 407
    articular cartilage of, arthrogram of, 468
    articular cartilage of, MRI of, 468
    computed tomography of, 468
  intertubercular sulcus of, 407
  lateral supracondylar ridge of, 407
  left, shaft of, 236
  lesser tubercle of, 407, 410, 419
    radiograph of, 409
  medial supracondylar ridge of, 407
  muscle origins and attachments on, 408
  olecranon fossa of, 424
    radiograph of, 425
  olecranon of, 400, 429, 432, 465
    radiograph of, 425
  posterior view of, 408
  radial fossa of, 407, 424
  radiograph of, 409
  right, surgical neck of, 236
  shaft of, 237, 238
  surgical neck of, 407
    radiograph of, 409
  trochlea of, 407
    radiograph of, 425
Hyaloid canal, 87
Hydatid of Morgagni, 355
Hymenal caruncle, 352, 356
Hyoepiglottic ligament, 77
Hyoepiglottic muscle, 63
Hyoglossus muscle, 26, 28, 33, 53, 59, 64, 127
Hyoid bone, 15, 26, 27, 28, 30, 33, 59, 60, 61, 63, 65, 67, 74, 76, 77, 80
  body of, 15, 53
  greater horn of, 15, 53, 68, 75
    prominence caused by, 66
  lesser horn of, 15, 53
Hypochondrium (hypochondriac) region
  left, 242
  right, 242
Hypogastric nerve, 303, 320, 389, 390, 394, 395, 396, 397
  left, 297, 302, 392
  right, 297, 302, 392
Hypogastric plexus, 160, 319, 389, 390, 392, 396
  inferior, 160, 161, 303, 319, 389, 390, 392, 394, 395, 396
    nerves to, 297, 487
    nerve to sigmoid and descending colon, 302, 390
    right, 302
  superior, 297, 302, 303, 319, 320, 343, 389, 390, 392, 394, 395, 396, 397
Hypogastric (neurovascular) sheath, 345
Hypoglossal canal, 10, 12, 13
  hypoglossal nerve in, 12
Hypoglossal fossa, 11, 50
Hypoglossal nerve, 13, 32, 33, 45, 46, 47, 59, 69, 71, 73, 103, 113, 128
  distribution of, 117
  in hypoglossal canal, 12, 127
  meningeal branch of, 127
  schema of, 127
  vena comitans of, 70
Hypoglossal nucleus, 115, 116, 127
Hypoglossal sinus, 8
Hypoglossal trigone, 114
Hypoglossus muscle, 60, 65, 68
  dorsal lingual vein coursing medial to, 70
Hypophyseal artery
  inferior, 138, 146
  superior, 138, 146
Hypophyseal fossa, 7

Hypophyseal portal system
  primary plexus of, 146
  secondary plexus of, 146
Hypophyseal portal vein
  long, 138, 146
  short, 146
Hypophyseal vein, efferent, 138, 146
Hypophysis, 103, 106, 145. *See also* Pituitary gland
  arteries and veins of, 146
  in sella turcica, 36
Hypothalamic area, lateral, 134
Hypothalamic artery, 138
Hypothalamic sulcus, 105, 114, 145
Hypothalamic vessels, 146
Hypothalamohypophyseal tract, 145
Hypothalamus, 107
  arteries and veins of, 146
  nuclei of, 145
    arcuate (infundibular), 145
    dorsomedial, 145
    mammillary body, 145
    paraventricular, 145
    posterior, 145
    supraoptic, 145
    ventromedial, 145
  parasympathtetic part of, 303
  sympathetic part of, 303
Hypothenar eminence, 400
Hypothenar muscles, 447, 448, 450, 464
  nerve to, 454
Hysterosalpingogram, of uterus, 354

I

Ileal artery, 287, 288
Ileal orifice, 276
  muscle fibers of, 274
  papillary, 274
Ileal vein, 290, 291
Ileal vessels, 290
Ileocecal fold, 273
Ileocecal junction, fibers around, 274
Ileocecal lips, 274
Ileocecal recess
  inferior, 273
  superior, 273
Ileocecal region, 273, 274
Ileocolic artery, 273, 287, 301, 302, 315
  colic branch of, 273, 288
  ileal branch of, 273, 288
Ileocolic lymph nodes, 296
Ileocolic plexus, 301, 302
Ileocolic vein, 290, 291, 292
Ileum, 261, 276, 324, 329
  circular muscle of, 274
  fibers to, 274
  longitudinal muscle of, 274
  mucosa of, 272
  musculature of, 272
  terminal part of, 263, 273, 274, 343, 347
Iliac artery
  circumflex
    ascending branch of, 249, 257
    deep, 249, 257, 489, 500
    superficial, 245, 257, 500
  common, 257, 266, 315, 316, 378, 380, 381, 392
    left, 297, 382
    right, 308, 324, 382
    ureteric branch from, 316
  external, 257, 266, 297, 315, 378, 380, 381, 382, 392, 489, 500
    right, 308
  internal, 257, 288, 297, 315, 316, 352, 378, 380, 381, 382
    anterior division of, 380, 382
    posterior division of, 382
    right, 308
Iliac crest, 149, 155, 168, 169, 170, 171, 240, 241, 248, 308, 309, 317, 332, 335, 469, 482, 483, 484, 490, 491

Iliac crest *(Continued)*
  anterior superior, 531
    radiograph of, 531
  iliac tubercle of, 335
  inner lip of, 241, 332, 335, 336, 474
  intermediate zone of, 241, 332, 335, 336, 474
  outer lip of, 241, 332, 335, 336, 474
  radiograph of, 531
  tuberculum of, 241, 332, 474
Iliac fossa, 335, 336, 343, 474
Iliac lymph nodes
  common, 259, 296, 318, 386, 388
  external, 259, 296, 318, 388, 473
    lymphatic pathways to, 388
    medial (inferior), 386
  internal, 259, 296, 318, 388
    lymphatic pathways to, 388
  lateral (superior) external, 386
Iliac plexus, 392
  external, 297
  internal, 297
Iliac spine
  anterior inferior, 241, 256, 332, 336, 340, 474, 475, 480, 481
  anterior superior, 240, 241, 243, 244, 253, 254, 256, 331, 332, 335, 336, 357, 360, 469, 474, 475, 480, 481, 482, 484, 488
  posterior inferior, 155, 474
  posterior superior, 149, 155, 335, 336, 474
Iliac tubercle, 335, 336
Iliac tuberosity, 241, 332, 474
Iliacus muscle, 256, 308, 345, 372, 398, 480, 484, 486, 487, 526, 531
  fascia of, 372
  insertion of, 484
  MRI of, 531
  muscular branch of, 486
  origin of, 478
Iliac vein
  circumflex
    deep, 250, 258
    superficial, 240, 250, 258, 331, 471
    tributaries to, 250
  common, 258, 379
  external, 258, 379, 489
  internal, 258, 291, 352
Iliac vessels
  circumflex
    deep, 247, 255, 345, 383
    superficial, 383, 488
  common, 263, 381, 383, 392
  external, 247, 253, 255, 273, 291, 342, 343, 344, 345, 346, 347, 354, 372, 381, 383
    covered by peritoneum, 254
  internal, 381, 383, 435
Iliococcygeus muscle, 337, 338, 339, 340
Iliocostalis cervicis muscle, 169
Iliocostalis lumborum muscle, 169
Iliocostalis muscle, 169, 327
Iliocostalis thoracis muscle, 169
Iliofemoral ligament, 475, 492
  of hip joint, 484
Ilioinguinal nerve, 254
  anterior scroal branch of, 251
Iliohypogastric nerve, 157, 171, 260, 308, 330, 389, 394, 484, 485, 486, 527
  anterior branch of, 485
  anterior cutaneous branch of, 251, 260, 389
  lateral branch of, 485
  lateral cutaneous branch of, 248, 472
Ilioinguinal nerve, 157, 260, 308, 309, 330, 389, 394, 484, 486, 487
  anterior labial branches of, 260
  scrotal branch of, 471
Iliolumbar artery, 257, 316, 382, 383
Iliolumbar ligament, 155, 309, 335
Iliolumbar vein, 258
Iliopectineal bursa, 475, 484

Interosseous muscles (Continued)
plantar, 524
superficial tibial nerve to, 529
Interosseous nerve
anterior, 436, 463
posterior, 433, 466
Interosseous palmar fascia, 450
Interosseous tendon slip, to lateral band, 452
Interpectoral lymph nodes, 178
Interpeduncular cistern, 108
Interphalangeal joint, 516
capsule and ligaments of, 446
distal
in extension: medial view of, 446
site of, 400
in extension: medial view of, 446
in flexion: medial view of, 446
proximal
in extension: medial view of, 446
site of, 400
Interphalangeal ligament, 446
Intersigmoid recess, 263, 315
Intersphincteric groove, 372, 373, 374
Interspinalis cervicis muscle, 170
Interspinalis lumborum muscles, 170
Interspinous ligament, 155, 156
Interspinous plane, 242
Intertendinous connections, 458
Interthalamic adhesion, 107, 109, 110, 114, 144, 145
Intertragic notch, 93
Intertransversarius muscle, 170
Intertransverse ligament, 181
Intertrochanteric crest, 475, 477, 491
radiograph of, 476
Intertrochanteric line, 475
Intertubercular plane, 242
Intertubercular tendon sheath, 410, 414, 419
Interureteric crest, 350
Interventricular artery, anterior, 211
Interventricular foramen (of Monro), 105, 107, 108, 110, 114, 144
left, 107
Interventricular septum, 218
membranous part of, 214
muscular part of, 210, 214, 215, 218, 219
Interventricular sulcus
anterior, 206, 239
posterior, 208, 209
Intervertebral disc, 156
cervical, 21, 22
lumbar, 152, 155, 329, 330, 429
lumbosacral, 336
thoracic, 188
cross-section of, 237, 238
transverse section of, 328
Intervertebral foramen, 174
for C3 spinal nerve, 21
lower margin of, 151
lumbar, 152, 155, 156
radiograph of, 153
sacral, 154
Intervertebral vein, 166, 167, 210
Intestinal artery, 287, 288
Intestinal gland, 305
Intestinal trunk, 259
Intestinal vein, 290, 291
Intestine, 161. See also Large intestine; Small intestine
innervation of, 160
intrinsic autonomic plexus of, 305
mesenteric relations of, 262, 263
Intraarticular sternocostal ligament, 180
Intraculminate vein, 142
Intralaminar nuclei, 110
Intramuscular plexus
circular, 305
longitudinal, 305
Intraparietal sulcus, 104

Intrapulmonary airway, schema of, 198
Intrapulmonary blood circulation, schema of, 199
Intrapulmonary lymph nodes, 202
Intrarenal artery, 312
Intratrochlear nerve, 2
Intrinsic autonomic plexus, of intestines, 305
Iridocorneal angle, 87, 88, 90
trabecular meshwork and spaces of, 88
Iris, 81, 87, 89, 90
arteries and veins of, 91
folds of, 88
major arterial circle of, 88, 90, 91
minor arterial circle of, 88, 90, 91
Irritant receptors, 204
Ischial spine, 241, 332, 334, 336, 338, 339, 340, 378, 391, 474, 475, 491
radiograph of, 531
Ischial tuberosity, 155, 334, 335, 336, 341, 357, 358, 360, 362, 363, 372, 375, 474, 475, 483, 490, 491
radiograph of, 333, 476, 531
Ischioanal fossa, 358, 372
anterior recess of, 247, 376
fat body of, 357, 360, 372, 398
posterior recess of, 376
preanal communication between right and left, 376
pus in, 376
roof of, 362
root of, 385
transverse fibrous septum of, 372, 374, 375
Ischiocavernous muscle, 342, 350, 352, 357, 358, 359, 361, 362, 363, 371, 375, 384, 385, 391
fascia of, 363
Ischiococcygeus muscle, 256, 341, 378, 382, 390, 392, 487
nerve to, 487
Ischiocondylar muscle, 527
Ischiofemoral ligament, 475
Ischiopubic ramus, 335, 336, 341, 346, 357, 358, 360, 362, 363, 364, 375, 475
Ischium, 474
body of, 474
radiograph of, 333, 476
ramus of, 474
spine of, 155
transverse section of, 399
Island of Reil. See Insula

J

Jejunal artery, 287, 288
anastomotic loop of, 272
Jejunal vein, 290, 291
anastomotic loop of, 290
Jejunal vessels, 290
Jejunum, 261, 262, 263, 270, 271, 272, 281, 328, 329, 330
mucosa of, 272
musculature of, 272
transverse section of, 326
Joint capsule, 492, 507, 516
attachment of, 499
Jugular foramen, 8, 13, 103, 124, 125, 126
Jugular fossa, 12, 94
jugular foramen in, 10
Jugular lymphatic trunk, 202
Jugular lymph nodes
anterior, 72
external, 72
Jugular nerve, 129
Jugular notch, 1, 27, 175, 179, 190
Jugular trunk, 72
left, 295
right, 295
Jugular vein
anterior, 30
communication to, 70
termination of, 70
external, 3, 30, 31, 70, 74, 192, 200, 232
internal, 3, 27, 28, 29, 30, 32, 33, 34, 46, 47, 59, 60, 61, 70, 73, 74, 75, 76, 92, 97, 127, 183, 184, 192, 202, 205, 226, 232

Jugular vein, internal (Continued)
computed tomography of, 147
inferior bulb of, 75
in jugular fossa, 12
left, 206
right, 167, 200
right, superior bulb of, 167
Jugulodigastric lymph node, 72, 73
Juguloomohyoid lymph nodes, 72, 73
Jugum, 11
Juxtamedullary glomerulus, 314
Juxtamedullary renal corpuscle, 313

K

Kerckring, valves of, 271, 272
Kidney, 161, 270, 380
anterior relations of, 308
anterior surface of, 311
arteries and veins of, 314
base pyramid of, 311
blood vessels of, 311
cortex of, 311, 313, 314, 328
cross section of, 173
fibrous capsule of, 317
gross structure of, 311
hilum of, 311
inferior pole of, 311
in situ
anterior view of, 308
posterior view of, 309
innervation of, 160, 319, 320
schema of, 320
lateral border of, 311
left, 191, 281, 282, 308, 315, 317, 322, 327, 329
anterior surface of, 312
anterior view of, 312
axial CT image of, 324
cross section of, 265
frontal section of, 312
posterior surface of, 312
renal cortex of, 328
superior pole of, 326
lobulated, of infant, 311
lymph vessels and nodes of, 318
major calyces of, 311
medial border of, 311
medulla (pyramids) of, 311
minor calyces of, 311
parenchyma of, blood vessels in, 314
posterior relations of, 309
prenatal, 223
renal capsule of, 311
renal columns of, 311
renal sinus of, 311
retroperitoneal, 264, 267, 278, 281
right, 191, 266, 267, 277, 281, 308, 309, 315, 317, 322, 329
axial CT image of, 324
cross section of, 265
sagittal section through, 317
sectioned in several planes, 311
superior pole of, 328
superior pole of, 264, 311, 328
surface anatomy of, 311
Knee
anterior aspect of, 496
anterior view of, 495, 497
arteries of, schema of, 500
bursa of, 496
collateral ligaments of, 497
cruciate ligaments of, 497
extension and flexion of, 470
interior of, 496
joint capsule of, 494, 496
lateral view of, 494
medial view of, 494
posterior view of, 497, 499
radiograph of, 498

Knee (Continued)
  right
    in extension, 495, 497
    in flexion, 497
    posterior view of, 499
    sagittal view of, 499
    slightly in flexion, 495
    superior view of, 496
Kohn, alveolar pores of, 198

L

Labbé, inferior anastomotic vein of, 101
Labial artery
  inferior, 35
  posterior, 359, 384
  superior, 35, 69
Labial nerve
  anterior, 393
  posterior, 393, 394
Labial vein
  inferior, 70
  superior, 70
Labia majora
  anterior commissure of, 356
  groove or space between, 356
  posterior commissure of, 356
Labia minora, 342, 359
  frenulum of, 356
Labioscrotal swelling, 368
Labium majus, 342, 348, 352, 356, 368
Labium minus, 342, 348, 352, 356, 368
Labyrinth
  bony, 95
    right, 95
    right, superior projection of, 97
    schema of, 96
  membranous, 95
    posterolateral view of, 95
    right, lateral projection of, 97
    schema of, 96
  orientation of, within skull, 97
Labyrinthine artery, 13, 135, 137, 138, 139, 141
  left, 135
Lacrimal apparatus, 82
Lacrimal artery, 85, 136
  recurrent meningeal branch of, 100
Lacrimal bone, 4, 37, 50
  of newborn, 14
  orbital plate of, 6
Lacrimal canaliculi, 82
Lacrimal caruncle, 82
Lacrimal gland, 44, 86, 117, 132, 160
  excretory ducts of, 82
  orbital part of, 82
  palpebral part of, 82
  schema of, 161
Lacrimal lake, 82
Lacrimal nerve, 44, 83, 85, 86, 120, 121, 130
  communicating branch of, 44
  cutaneous branch of, 44
  meningeal branch of, 86
  palpebral branch of, 2
Lacrimal papilla
  inferior, 82
  superior, 81, 82
Lacrimal punctum
  inferior, 82
  superior, 82
Lacrimal sac, 81
  fossa for, 4, 6
Lacrimal unctum, 81
Lactiferous duct, 176
Lactiferous sinus, 176
Lacuna
  lateral (venous) of Trolard, 99, 100
  magna, 365
Lacunar (Gimbernat's) ligament, 244, 245, 247, 253, 255, 256
Lambda, 9

Lambdoid suture, 7, 8, 9, 14
Lamina
  cervical, 20
  internal medullary, 110
  lumbar, 152, 153, 155, 156
  posterior limiting, 88
  spiral
    hamulus of, 95
    osseous, 95
  of thyroid cartilage, 67, 77
Lamina affixa, 110
Lamina cribrosa, 87
Lamina propria, gingival, 57
Lamina terminalis, 105, 106, 114, 145
Large intestine
  arteries of, 288
  autonomic innervation of, 302, 303
    schema of, 303
  lymph vessels and lymph nodes of, 296
  mucosa and musculature of, 276
  veins of, 291
Laryngeal artery, superior, 33, 75, 76, 135, 229
Laryngeal inlet, 62, 66, 229
Laryngeal nerve (X)
  inferior, 80
    anterior branch of, 80
    posterior branch of, 80
  recurrent, 32, 34, 71, 80, 125, 129, 234
    left, 74, 76, 187, 200, 203, 204, 205, 206, 220, 225, 226, 234, 236, 237
    right, 74, 75, 76, 80, 125, 206, 220, 229, 234
  superior, 69, 74, 75, 80, 125, 129, 130, 134, 204, 234
    external branch of, 71, 75, 76, 80, 125
    internal branch of, 65, 66, 67, 71, 75, 76, 78, 80, 215, 229
Laryngeal prominence, 77
Laryngeal vein
  recurrent, 226
    left, 75
  superior, 70, 229
Laryngeal vessels, 78
Laryngopharynx, 63
  opened posterior view of, 66
Larynx, 134, 161, 204
  anterior view of, 77
  anterosuperior view of, 77
  cartilage of, 77
  innervation of, 160
  intrinsic muscles of, 78
    action of, 79
  medial view of, 77
  nerves of, 80
  normal: inspiration, 78
  posterior view of, 77, 78
  right lateral view of, 77, 78
  sensory branches to, 80
  superior view of, 78
Lateral aperture, 108
Lateral band, 452
Lateral direct vein, 143
Lateral dorsal cutaneous nerve, 471, 472, 530
Lateral ligament, 18, 515
Lateral recess, 114
Lateral sulcus, 104, 106
Latissimus dorsi muscle, 168, 171, 173, 174, 175, 182, 236, 239, 243, 244, 248, 252, 309, 327, 330, 407, 411, 412, 414, 416, 417, 419, 421, 423
  costal origin of, digitations of, 248
  MRI of, 468
  nerve to, 414
  transverse section of, 325
Latissimus dorsi tendon, 237, 238, 421
Left bundle, of heart, 219
Left lateral aperture, 107
Left lateral recess, 107
Leg
  anterior view of, 503
  cross section of, 510
  cutaneous innervation of, 530
  fascial compartments of, 510

Leg (Continued)
  interosseous nerve of, 529
  muscles of
    attachments of, 503
    deep dissection of, 506
    deep dissection of: anterior view of, 508
    intermediate dissection of: posterior view of, 505
    lateral view of, 509
    posterior view of, 506
    superficial dissection of: anterior view of, 507
    superficial dissection of: posterior view of, 504
  posterior view of, 503
  right, bones of, 501
Lens, 81, 83, 88, 90
  axis of, 89
  capsule of, 87, 88, 89
  cortex of, 89
  equator of, 89
  nucleus of, 88, 89
  supporting structures of, 89
  suspensory ligament of, 87
Lenticular process, 93
Lenticulostriate artery, 137, 138, 139, 141
  anterolateral, 139
  lateral, 137
Lentiform nucleus, 109, 139
  globus pallidus of, 107, 109
  putamen of, 107, 109
Leptomeninges, 163
Lesser occipital nerve, 2
Levator anguli oris muscle, 54, 122
Levator ani muscle, 247, 256, 276, 292, 303, 323, 339, 342, 349, 350, 357, 358, 362, 363, 371, 372, 373, 374, 376, 378, 382, 384, 390, 398, 487
  fibers to anal canal, longitudinal muscle from, 340, 341
  fibromuscular extension of, 341
  iliococcygeus part of, 338, 340, 341, 375
  levator plate of, 338
  medial border of, 341
  medial edge of, thickened, 323
  median raphe of, 339
  nerves to, 485, 487
  pubococcygeus part of, 338, 340, 341, 375
  puborectalis part of, 340, 341, 371, 375
  tendinous arch of, 256, 337, 338, 339, 341, 345, 348, 350, 352, 358, 372
  transverse section of, 399
Levator costarum muscle, 170
Levator labii superioris alaeque nasi muscle, 54
Levator labii superioris muscle, 25, 54, 122
Levator palpebrae superioris muscle, 81, 83, 84, 86, 120
  insertion of, 81
Levator plate, 338
Levator scapulae muscle, 26, 31, 34, 168, 171, 411, 414, 415, 465
  communication with cervical plexus, 32
  nerves to, 128
Levator veli palatini muscle, 47, 52, 64, 65, 67, 68, 94, 125
  fold caused by, 66
  interdigitating fibers of, 52
Lienorenal ligament, 264, 266, 282
Ligamenta flava, 22
Ligament of ovary, 343
Ligament of Treitz, 262
Ligaments. *See also specific ligaments*
  of ankle, 515
  of elbow, 426
  of foot, 516
  lumbosacral, 155
  of pelvis, 335, 336, 354
  of wrist, 442, 443
Ligamentum arteriosum, 200, 206, 215, 225
  aortic arch lymph node of, 202
  prenatal, 223
Ligamentum flavum, 155, 156, 330

Nasal nerve
external, 35
lateral
inferior, 130
posterior, 130
superior, 130
posterior, 132
Nasal retinal arteriole, 90
Nasal retinal venule, 90
Nasal septum, 16, 38, 40, 42, 63, 66
bony, 8
coronal section of, 48
growth of, 50
schematic hinge of, 40
Nasal slit, 13
Nasal spine
anterior, 4, 8, 38
posterior, 38
Nasal vein
dorsal, 3
external, 70
Nasal vestibule, 36, 38, 47
Nasal wall, lateral, 8
Nasion, 4
Nasociliary nerve (V₁), 44, 83, 86, 120, 121, 130, 131
Nasofrontal vein, 3, 70, 85
Nasolabial sulcus, 1
Nasolacrimal canal, opening of, 37
Nasolacrimal duct, 82
in nasooptic furrow, 50
opening of, 36, 50, 82
Nasolacrimal foramen, 50
Nasooptic furrow, nasolacrimal duct in, 50
Nasopalatine nerve (V₂), 12, 41, 43
communication with greater palatine nerve, 41
groove for, 38
passing to septum, 42
Nasopalatine vessels, groove for, 38
Nasopharynx, 66, 92, 103
median section of, 63
opened posterior view of, 66
Navicular bone, 511, 515, 524, 525
lateral view of, 514
radiograph of, 514
tuberosity of, 511, 516, 524
Navicular fossa, 346
Neck
autonomic nerves of, 129
bones and ligaments of, 15
fascial layers of, 34
lymph vessels and nodes of, 72
muscles of
anterior view of, 27
infrahyoid and suprahyoid, 28
lateral view of, 26
scalene and prevertebral, 29
nerves and vessels of, 31, 32
posterior triangle of, 168, 172
right anterior dissection of, 32
superficial veins and cutaneous nerves of, 1, 30
surface anatomy of, 1
Nephron
Henle's loop of, 313, 314
schema of, 313
Nerve IX, 60
Nerves. *See also specific nerves*
of abdomen, 297
of abdominal wall, 251, 260
of back, 171
of buttocks, 491
of cranial base, 46
of cranial fossa, 142
of esophagus, 234
of external genitalia
female, 393
male, 389
of extrinsic eye muscles, 84
of female reproductive organs, 395
of fingers, 459

Nerves *(Continued)*
of hand, 454
of heart, 220
of hip, 491
of larynx, 80
of lower limb, 471, 472
of male reproductive organs, 396
of nasal cavity, 42
of neck, 31, 32
of oral cavity, 62
of oral region, 71
of orbit, 86
of pelvic viscera
female, 392
male, 390
of perineum
female, 393
male, 391
of pharyngeal region, 71
of pharynx, 62
of shoulder, 465
of upper limb, 461
of ureters, 397
of urinary bladder, 397
at wrist, 449
Nerve X, 60
Nerve XII, 60
Neurohypophysis, 138, 145, 146
Neuropathways, in parturition, 394
Neurovascular compartment, 423
Newborn, skull of, 14
Nipple, 175, 176, 331
Nose, 35. *See also* Nasal cavity
ala of, 1
anterolateral view of, 35
inferior view of, 35
mucous glands of, 161
transverse section of, 47
Nostril, 1
Nuchal line
inferior, 10, 16
superior, 10, 16, 168, 169, 170
Nucleus ambiguus, 115, 116, 124, 125, 126
Nucleus pulposus, 21, 152
Nutrient artery, 492
Nutrient foramen, 501

O

Obex, 114
Oblique aponeurosis
external, 330
internal, 330
Oblique capitis superior muscle, 172
Oblique fissure, 192
of left lung, 237
Oblique line, 17, 77, 501
Oblique muscle
external, 168, 169, 171, 173, 175, 176, 182, 185, 240, 244, 245, 246, 247, 248, 249, 251, 252, 253, 254, 256, 309, 327, 328, 330, 331, 343, 411, 412, 482
aponeurotic part of, 243, 244, 245, 246, 253, 255, 357, 361
costal origin of, digitations of, 248
fascia over, 360
muscular part of, 243
inferior, 84, 120, 182
internal, 168, 169, 173, 183, 244, 245, 246, 247, 248, 249, 253, 254, 256, 309, 330, 343
aponeurosis of, 246
fascial sheath of, 83
in lumbar triangle (of Petit), 168
tendon of origin of, 173
superior, 83, 84, 86, 117, 120
Oblique pericardial sinus, 209, 239
Oblique popliteal ligament, 499
Oblique popliteal membrane, 496
Oblique vein, of left atrium (of Marshall), 208, 209, 211, 215

Obliquus capitis inferior muscle, 169, 170, 172
Obliquus capitis superior muscle, 169, 170
Obturator artery, 257, 315, 316, 344, 345, 378, 380, 382, 383, 390, 398, 475, 500
accessory, 378, 382
acetabular branch of, 475, 492, 531
anterior branch of, 475
posterior branch of, 475
Obturator canal, 336, 338, 340, 344, 345, 348, 382, 489
Obturator crest, 336, 474
Obturator externus muscle, 479, 481, 489, 527
origin of, 478
transverse section of, 399
Obturator foramen, 241, 332, 335, 474
radiograph of, 333, 476
Obturator groove, 474
Obturator internus muscle, 247, 256, 337, 338, 339, 341, 350, 363, 372, 378, 382, 483, 487, 490, 491
fascia of, 338, 348, 372, 382, 391
MRI of, 531
nerve to, 485, 487, 491
origin of, 478, 479
transverse section of, 399
Obturator internus tendon, 341
MRI of, 531
Obturator lymph nodes, 386
Obturator membrane, 336, 352, 475
Obturator nerve, 247, 260, 315, 380, 390, 398, 484, 485, 486, 487, 526, 527
accessory, 260, 485, 486
anterior branch of, 489, 493
articular branch of, 527
cutaneous branches of, 471, 489, 527
muscles innervated by, 527
posterior branch of, 489, 527
Obturator vein, 258, 291, 379, 398
Obturator vessels, 247, 253
accessory, 253, 255
right, 383
Occipital artery, 3, 33, 69, 70, 100, 135, 136, 172
descending branch of, 33, 172
mastoid branch of, 100, 135
medial, 140
meningeal branch of, 3
occasional branch of, 13
occipital groove for, 10
sternocleidomastoid branch of, 33, 69
Occipital bone, 6, 8, 9, 14, 22
basilar part of, 8, 10, 11, 22, 29, 36, 37, 38, 52, 65, 67
clivus of, 11
condylar canal and fossa of, 10
condyle of, 11
external occipital crest of, 10
external occipital extuberance of, 10
external occipital protuberance of, 8, 10
foramen magnum of, 8, 10
groove for inferior petrosal sinus, 11
groove for posterior meningeal vessels of, 11
groove for superior sagittal sinus of, 11
groove for transverse sinus of, 11
hypoglossal canal of, 8, 10
inferior nuchal line of, 10
inferior petrosal sinus groove of, 8
internal occipital crest of, 11
internal occipital protuberance of, 11
jugular foramen of, 8
jugular process of, 29
occipital condyle of, 8, 10
pharyngeal tubercle of, 10, 63
superior nuchal line of, 10
superior view of, 14
transverse sinus groove of, 8
Occipital condyle, 8, 10, 16, 29, 98, 127
lateral mass for, 19
superior articular surface for, 19
Occipital crest
external, 10, 16
internal, 11

Occipital emissary vein, 99
Occipital groove, 10
Occipital horn, 108
Occipitalis muscle, 117, 172
Occipital lobe, 104
  left, projection on, 119
  right, projection on, 119
Occipital lymph nodes, 72
Occipital nerve
  greater, 171, 172
  lesser, 2, 31, 32, 128, 131, 171
  third, 2, 172
Occipital pole, 104
Occipital protuberance
  external (inion), 8, 10, 16, 149
  internal, 11
Occipital sinus, 102, 142
  groove for, 11
Occipital sulcus, transverse, 104
Occipital vein, 3, 70
  internal, 144
Occipitofrontalis muscle
  frontal belly of, 122
  occipital belly of, 122, 172
Occlpltomastoid suture, 16
Occipitotemporal gyrus
  lateral, 105, 106
  medial, 105, 106
Occipitotemporal sulcus
  lateral, 106
  medial, 105
Oculomotor nerve (III), 13, 46, 84, 86, 103, 113, 115, 116, 120, 130, 142
  branch of, 161
  distribution of, 117
  inferior branch of, 83, 86, 120
  schema of, 120
  superior branch of, 83, 86, 120
Oculomotor nucleus, 115, 116, 120
  accessory, 115, 116, 120
Olecranon, 400, 429, 432, 465
  radiograph of, 425
Olecranon bursa, 426
Olecranon fossa, 424
  radiograph of, 425
Olfactory bulb, 42, 48, 106
  afferent fibers from, 118
  contralateral, fibers of, 118
  efferent fibers to, 118
Olfactory cells, 118
  schema of, 118
Olfactory mucosa, 42, 118
Olfactory nerve fibers, 118
Olfactory nerve (I), 13, 41, 118
  distribution of, 117
  schema of, 118
Olfactory nucleus, anterior, 118
Olfactory stria
  lateral, 118
  medial, 118
Olfactory sulcus, 106
Olfactory tract, 42, 105, 106, 113, 119
Olfactory tract nucleus, lateral, 119
Olfactory trigone, 119
Olfactory tubercle, 119
Olivary complex, inferior, 116
Olive, 113
Omental appendices, 263, 276, 330
Omental bursa, 323
  cross section of, 265
  lesser sac, 327
  lesser sac of, 265, 266
  posterior wall of, parietal peritoneum on, 327
  with stomach reflected, 264
  superior recess of, 266, 277
    probe in, 264
  superior recess of (lesser sac) of, 323
Omental foramen (of Winslow), 264, 265, 267, 278, 323, 327

Omental ligament, 278
  lesser, 278
    right free margin of, 271
Omental taenia, 273, 276
Omental vein, 232
Omentum
  greater, 261, 265, 267, 276, 278, 323, 329, 330
    elevated, 263
    overlying transverse colon and small intestine, 261
  lesser, 265, 267, 323, 327
    anterior layer of, 280, 298
    attachment of, 266
    hepatic branch of anterior vagal trunk in, 125
    posterior layer of, 298
    right free margin of, 270, 281
    right margin of, 264
Omohyoid bone, phantom, 33
Omohyoid muscle, 28, 30, 34, 53, 192, 407, 411, 416, 417
  inferior belly of, 1, 26, 27, 28, 31, 127, 128, 415
    communication with cervical plexus, 32
    nerve to, 71
  invested by cervical fascia, 182
  invested by fascia of infrahyoid muscle, 416
  superior belly of, 26, 27, 28, 127, 128
    communication with cervical plexus, 32
    nerve to, 71
Operculum
  frontal, 104
  orbital, 104
  parietal, 104
Ophthalmic artery, 3, 13, 39, 46, 85, 131, 135, 136, 138, 141
  continuation of, 85
  in optic canal, 83
  supraorbital branch from, 69
  supratrochlear branch from, 69
Ophthalmic nerve (V₁), 2, 44, 45, 46, 86, 102, 120, 130, 131, 132, 133, 134
  frontal branch of, 13
  lacrimal branch of, 13
  meningeal branch of, 86
  nasociliary branch of, 13
  schema of, 121
  tentorial branch of, 44, 86, 121
Ophthalmic vein
  inferior, 85
  superior, 13, 83, 85, 91, 103
Opponens digiti minimi muscle, 449, 453, 464
Opponens pollicis muscle, 449, 453, 454, 463
Optic canal, 8, 13, 83
Optic chiasm, 48, 103, 105, 106, 113, 119, 138, 139, 143, 144, 145
Optic disc, 90
Optic nerve (II), 13, 46, 48, 83, 86, 87, 90, 103, 106, 131, 141, 142
  distribution of, 117
  internal sheath of, vessels of, 91
  meningeal sheath of, 83, 84, 87, 91
  in optic canal, 13, 83
  schema of, 119
  in visual pathway, 119
Optic radiation, 119
Optic tract, 106, 107, 111, 113, 137, 142
Oral cavity, 38, 48, 63. See also Lip; Oral region; Teeth; specific parts of oral cavity
  afferent innervation of, 62
  floor of, 53
  inspection of, 51
  roof of, 52
Oral region
  arteries of, 69
  nerves of, 71
  veins of, 70
Ora serrata, 87, 89, 90
Orbicularis oculi muscle, 122
  orbital part of, 25
  palpebral part of, 25, 81
Orbicularis oris muscle, 25, 35, 54, 60, 122
Orbiculus ciliaris, 89

Orbit, 90
  arteries and veins of, 85
  fasciae of, 83
  fat in, 48, 83
  left, growth of, 50
  medial wall of, 48
  muscle attachments and nerves and vessels entering, 83
  muscles of, 48
  nerves of, 83, 86
  right, frontal and slightly lateral view of, 4
  superior view of, 86
  surface view of, 4
Orbital fat body, 83
Orbital fissure
  inferior, 4, 6, 16, 83
  superior, 4, 13, 83
Orbital gyri, 106
Orbital operculum, 104
Orbital plate, 14
Orbital septum, 81
Orbital sulci, 106
Orbitofrontal artery
  lateral, 137, 139, 140
  medial, 137, 139
Orbitofrontobasal artery, medial, 137, 139, 140
Oropharynx, 227
  medial view of, 64
  median section of, 63
  opened posterior view of, 66
Osseous cochlea, 96
Osseous spiral lamina, 95, 96
Ossicles, articulated, 93
Osteomeatal unit, 49
Otic capsule, 95, 96
Otic ganglion, 18, 45, 55, 121, 122, 124, 130, 132, 134, 161
  schema of, 133
Oval (vestibular) window, 14, 95
  base of stapes in, 92, 96
Ovarian artery, 316, 380, 392, 395
Ovarian plexus, 392, 395
Ovarian vein, 380
Ovarian vessels, 315, 343, 384
  tubal branches of, 384
Ovary, 315, 342, 343, 352, 369, 380, 392
  ligament of, 342, 343, 344, 352, 353, 355
  posterior view of, 355
  right, 354
  suspensory ligament of, 342, 343, 344, 354, 355, 369, 380
    ovarian vessels n, 345

P

Pain, referred, common area of, 306, 307
Palate
  growth of, 50
  hard, 48, 63, 64
  mucous glands of, 161
  soft, 38, 51, 63, 64, 66
    muscles of, 65
Palatine aponeurosis, 52, 65
Palatine artery
  ascending, 39, 64, 69
    tonsillar branches of, 39, 64
  greater (descending), 39, 40, 46, 52, 69
    left and right, 39
  lesser, 40, 46, 52, 64
    left and right, 39
    tonsillar branch of, 64
Palatine bone, 8, 50
  greater palatine foramen of, 10, 38
  horizontal plate of, 8, 10, 16, 36, 37, 38, 52, 56, 98
  lesser palatine foramen of, 38
  lesser palatine process of, 10
  nasal crest of, 38
  orbital process of, 4, 37
  perpendicular plate of, 8, 37, 38
  posterior nasal spine of, 10, 37, 38

Palatine bone (Continued)
  pyramidal process of, 10, 14, 16
  sphenoidal process of, 37
Palatine fold, transverse, 52
Palatine foramen
  greater, 12, 37, 38, 40
  lesser, 12, 37, 38, 40, 52
Palatine glands, 52, 63, 64
Palatine nerve
  descending, 132
  greater, 12, 41, 43, 44, 46, 52, 71, 121, 130, 132
    communication with nasopalatine nerve, 41, 62
    posterior inferior lateral nasal branch of, 41, 42
  lesser, 12, 41, 43, 44, 46, 52, 62, 71, 121, 130, 132
Palatine process, 7, 8, 56, 98
Palatine raphe, 52
Palatine vein, 70
  external, 70
Palatine vessels, 12
Palatoglossal arch, 51, 58, 60
Palatoglossus muscle, 52, 58, 59, 60, 64, 125
Palatomaxillary suture, 10
Palatopharyngeal arch, 51, 58, 64, 66
Palatopharyngeal muscle, 58, 125
Palatopharyngeal sphincter (Passavant's ridge), 65
Palatopharyngeus muscle, 52, 59, 64, 67, 229
Palbebral conjunctiva, 83
  inferior, 81
  superior, 81
Palm, 441
Palmar aponeurosis, 430, 434, 442, 447, 448, 450
  septa from, 448
Palmar arterial arch
  carpal, 453
  deep, 453, 454
  superficial, 448, 449, 454, 461
    distal limit of, 454
Palmar carpal arterial arch, 453
Palmar carpal ligament, 448, 449
  continuous with extensor retinaculum, 404, 434, 435, 447
Palmar carpometacarpal ligament, 442
Palmar crease, proximal, 400
Palmar digital artery, 447, 448, 454
  common, 448, 450, 453, 454
  to neighboring digit, 459
Palmar digital nerve, 404, 447, 448, 463, 464
  branches to phalanges, 454
  common, 450, 463, 464
  dorsal branches of, 456
  to fourth and fifth fingers, 448
  from superficial branch of ulnar nerve, 447
  of thumb, 448
Palmar digital vein, 404
Palmar interosseous muscle, 450
Palmaris brevis muscle, 447, 464
Palmaris longus muscle, 430, 434, 463
  origin of, 438
Palmaris longus tendon, 400, 434, 435, 437, 442, 447, 448, 449
Palmar ligament, 452
  plates of, 446
Palmar metacarpal artery, 453, 454
Palmar metacarpal ligament, 442, 446
Palmar radioulnar ligament, 442
  radiocapitate part of, 442
  radioscapholunate part of, 442
Palmar ulnocarpal ligament
  ulnolunate part of, 442
  ulnotriquetral part of, 442
Palmar venous arch, superficial, 448
Palmate folds, 355
Palpebral arterial arch
  inferior, 85
  superior, 85
Palpebral artery
  lateral, 85
  medial, 85

Palpebral artery (Continued)
  superior lateral, 85
  superior medial, 85
Palpebral ligament
  lateral, 81
  medial, 81, 83
Pampiniform venous plexus, 250, 367, 381, 383
Pancreas, 125, 266, 322, 323
  acini of, 198
  anterior view of, 294
  arteries of, 284
  autonomic innervation of, 307
  body of, 264
  cross section of, 173, 265
  head of, 280, 281, 328
    arteries of, 286
    posterior view of, 286
    reflected to left, 286
    retroperitoneal, 264
  in situ, 281
  innervation of, 160
  lymph vessels and nodes of, 294
  posterior view of, 294
  tail of, 282, 308
    artery to, 284
    intraperitoneal, 264
  transverse section of, 326
  uncinate process of, 281, 329
  veins of, 289
Pancreatic artery
  dorsal, 283, 284, 286, 287
  greater, 284, 286
  inferior, 284, 286, 287
Pancreatic duct
  accessory (of Santorini), 271, 281
  extrahepatic, 280
  of Wirsung, 271, 281
Pancreatic lymph nodes, superior, 294
  left, 293
  right, 293
Pancreatic lymph vessels, 294
Pancreatic notch, 281
Pancreaticoduodenal artery
  anastomotic branch of, 286
  anterior inferior, 284, 286, 287, 288, 291, 300
    plexus on, 298, 299
  anterior superior, 283, 284, 286, 287, 291, 300
    plexus on, 298, 299
    retroperitoneal, 264
  inferior, 284, 286, 288, 301
    common portion of, 287, 288
  posterior inferior, 284, 286, 287, 288, 291, 300
    plexus on, 301
  posterior superior, 283, 284, 286, 287, 300
    plexus on, 301
Pancreaticoduodenal lymph nodes, 294
Pancreaticoduodenal plexus, 301
Pancreaticoduodenal vein
  anterior inferior, 289, 292
  anterior superior, 289, 292
  posterior inferior, 289, 292
  posterior superior, 289, 292
Pancreatic pain, common areas of, 307
Pancreatic vein
  dorsal or superior, 291
  great, 289
Papilla
  duodenal
    major (of Vater), 271, 280
    minor, 271, 280
  fibers to, 274
  filiform, 58
  foliate, 58, 134
  fungiform, 58, 134
  keratinized tip of, 58
  parotid, 51
  renal, cribriform area of, 313
  vallate, 58, 134
Papillary duct, openings of, 313

Papillary muscle, 210, 239
  anterior, 214, 215, 217, 219
    left, 218
    right, 218
  posterior, 214, 215, 217, 219
    left, 218
    right, 218
  septal, 214, 217, 218
Paraaortic plexus, 260
Paracentral artery, 139, 140
  medial frontal branches of, 139
Paracentral sulcus, 105
Paracolic gutter
  left, 263, 330, 343, 347
  right, 263, 273, 330, 343
Paracolic lymph nodes, 296
Paradidymus, 369
Paraduodenal fossa, 262
Parahippocampal gyrus, 106, 107, 118, 150
Paramedian artery, 138
Paramesonephric duct, 369
Paranasal sinus
  age-related changes in, 50
  bones of, at birth, 50
  coronal section of, 48
  horizontal section of, 48
  lateral dissection of, 49
  mucous glands of, 161
  sagittal section of, 49
Pararectal fossa, 343, 344, 347
Pararenal fat, 317
Parasternal lymph nodes, 178
Parasympathetic fibers, 120
  of autonomic reflex pathways, 304
  of stomach and duodenum, 300
  of submandibular gland, 132
  of tracheobronchial tree, 204
Parasympathetic nervous system, schema of, 161
Parathyroid gland
  inferior, 76
  posterior view of, 76
  right lateral view of, 76
  superior, 76
Paratracheal lymph nodes, 223, 233
  left, 202
  right, 202
Paraumbilical portocaval anastomosis, 292
Paraumbilical vein, 247, 292
  in median umbilical fold, 247
  tributaries of, 250
Paraurethral glands
  openings of, 356
  primordium of, 369
Paravertebral anastomosis, 165
Paravesical fossa, 344
Paravesical pouch, floor of, 352
Parenchyma, renal, 311
  blood vessels entering, 311, 314
Parietal artery, 3
  anterior, 139, 140
  branch to angular gyrus, 139, 140
  posterior, 139, 140
  temporal branches of, 139
Parietal bone, 4, 9, 10
  groove for middle meningeal vessels of, 11
  lateral view of, 14
  mastoid angle of, 11
  of newborn, 14
  squamous suture of, 14
  superior view of, 14
  tuber (eminence) of, 14
Parietal emissary vein, 3
Parietal foramen, 9
Parietal limb, 214
Parietal lobe, 104
Parietal lobule
  inferior, 104
  superior, 104

Radial nerve *(Continued)*
posterior antebrachial branch of, 460
posterior cutaneous, 403, 404
posterior view of, 460
superficial branch of, 402, 404, 435, 437, 455, 456,
457, 460, 461, 466
Radial notch, of ulna, 424
Radial recurrent artery, 421, 422, 435
Radial styloid process
anterior (palmar) view of, 440
posterior (dorsal) view of, 440
Radial tubercle, distal, 400
Radial tuberosity, 419, 424, 427
radiograph of, 425
Radiate artery
cortical, 312, 314
cortical lymph vessels along, 318
perforating, 312
Radiate ligament, 181
Radiate vein, cortical, 314
Radicular artery
anterior, 165
posterior, 165
Radicular vein, segmental, 166
anterior, 166
posterior, 166
Radiocarpal joint. *See* Wrist
Radiocarpal ligament, 443
Radiograph
of ankle, 514
of chest, 207
of elbow, 425
of hand, 445
of hip, 531
of hip joint, 476
of knee, 498
of lumbar vertebrae, 153
pelvic
female, 333
male, 333
of shoulder, 409
of wrist, 445
Radioulnar joint, 443
Radioulnar ligament
dorsal, posterior (dorsal) view of, 443
palmar, 442
radiocapitate part of, 442
radioscapholunate part of, 442
Radius, 424, 428, 429, 430, 431, 433, 436, 437,
453
annular ligament of, 426
anterior border of, 427
anterior (palmar) view of, 441
anterior surface of, 427
articular surface of, radiograph of, 445
articulation with lunate bone, 427
articulation with scaphoid bone, 427
carpal articular surface of, 427
coronal section of, 427
dorsal view of, 443
distal end of, radiograph of, 445
dorsal tubercle (Lister's) of, 440
in flexion, 441
groove for extensor digitorum muscle, 427
groove for extensor indicis muscle, 427
groove for extensor pollicis longus muscle, 427
head of, 419, 424, 427
radiograph of, 425
interosseous border of, 427
interosseous membrane of, 427
muscle attachment and insertion sites on, 439
neck of, 424, 427
radiograph of, 425
radiograph of, 425
right
in pronation: anterior view, 427
in supination: anterior view, 427
rotator muscles of, 428
sagittal section through, 441
sites of muscle origins and insertions on, 438

Radius *(Continued)*
styloid process of, 427
radiograph of, 445
tuberosity of, 419, 424, 427
radiograph of, 425
ulnar notch of, 427
Rami communicantes, 394
gray, 129, 131, 132, 133, 160, 162, 163, 174, 185,
203, 224, 225, 234, 252, 260, 297, 300, 303,
319, 320, 390, 392, 395, 396, 397, 486,
487
white, 129, 131, 132, 133, 160, 162, 163, 174, 185,
203, 224, 225, 234, 252, 260, 297, 300, 303,
304, 320, 390, 392, 395, 396, 397, 486
Rathke's pouch, vestigial remnant of, 50
Rectal artery
inferior, 378, 382, 384, 385
middle, 257, 288, 302, 315, 345, 378, 380, 382, 383
superior, 257, 288, 297, 302, 303, 315, 345, 380,
390
bifurcation, 378
branch of, 288
Rectal lymph nodes
middle, 296
superior, 296
Rectal nerve, 359, 390, 391, 393, 394
inferior, 303, 390, 391, 393, 394, 485
superior, 303
Rectal plexus, 258, 302, 303, 319, 390, 392
external, 291, 373, 379
internal, 373, 379
middle, 302
perimuscular, 291, 379
superior, 297, 302
Rectal portocaval anastomosis, 292
Rectal vein
inferior, 292
left middle, 291
left superior, 291, 292
middle, 258, 292, 379
right inferior, to internal pudendal vein, 291
right middle, 291
right superior, 292
superior, 379
tributaries of left and right superior veins, 291
Rectal vessels, superior, 266
Rectocervical space, 344
Rectococcygeus muscle, 256
Rectosigmoid artery, 378
Rectosigmoid junction, 276, 371, 373, 374
Rectourethralis superior muscle, 341
Rectouterine fold, 344
Rectouterine ligament, 344
Rectouterine pouch (of Douglas), 342, 355, 371
Rectovaginal space, 344, 345
Rectovesical pouch, 323, 346, 371
Rectovesical space
prerectal, 376
retroprostatic, 376
retrovesical, 376
Rectropubic space, 323
areolar tissue in, 346
vesical venous plexus in, 346
Rectum, 161, 256, 263, 276, 308, 323, 338, 342, 343,
345, 348, 364, 373, 380
ampulla of, 348
anterior view of, 379
arteries of, 378
circular muscle layer of, 373, 374
in situ
female, 371
male, 371
longitudinal muscle layer of, 373, 374
lymphatic pathway along, 388
MR sagittal images of, 377
muscularis mucosae of, 373, 374
nerves of, 160
posterior view of, 378
retracted, 392
termination of, 398

Rectum *(Continued)*
transverse folds of
inferior, 373
middle, 373
superior, 373
transverse section of, 399
veins of, 379
female, 379
male, 379
Rectus abdominis muscle, 175, 182, 183, 185, 240,
244, 245, 246, 247, 251, 252, 253, 254, 323, 327,
330, 331, 343, 345, 346, 347, 357
axial CT image of, 324
MR sagittal images of, 377
transverse section of, 325
Rectus capitis anterior muscle, 73
communication with cervical plexus, 32
nerves to, 128
Rectus capitis lateralis muscle, 29
communication with cervical plexus, 32
nerves to, 128
Rectus capitis major muscle, posterior, 170, 172
Rectus capitis minor muscle, posterior, 169, 170, 172
Rectus femoris muscle, 469, 480, 482, 488, 489, 493, 526
insertion of, 478
MRI of, 531
origin of, 478, 479, 480
transverse section of, 399
Rectus femoris tendon, 469, 480, 493, 495, 507
Rectus muscle
inferior, 83, 84
lateral, 83, 84, 86, 117, 120
fascial sheath of, 83
tendon of, 87
medial, 83, 84, 86, 120
cheek ligament of, 82
fascial sheath of, 83
tendon of, 87
superior, 83, 84, 86, 120
fascial sheath of, 83
tendon of, 91
Rectus plane, right lateral, 242
Rectus sheath, 183, 243, 244, 253, 330, 357
anterior layer of, 182, 244, 245, 246, 251, 346, 357
cross section of, 246
posterior layer of, 245, 246, 249
Recurrent artery
of Heubner, 137, 138, 139, 140
interosseous, 422
radial, 421, 422, 436
tibial
anterior, 500
posterior, 500
ulnar
anterior, 422, 436
posterior, 422
Recurrent laryngeal nerve, 32, 34
Recurrent process, 118
Red nucleus, 106, 115, 116
imaging of, 148
Reissner's membrane, 96
Renal artery, 311, 312, 316, 380
anterior branch of, 312
in situ, 130
left, 257, 302, 308, 310, 317, 329, 390
ureteric branch of, 310, 312
pelvic branch of, 312
posterior branch of, 312
right, 257, 297, 300, 308, 310
ureteric branch of, 313
ureteric branch of, 312, 316
Renal capsule, 311, 313, 314
Renal column (of Bertin), 311, 314
Renal corpuscle, 313
cortical, 313
juxtamedullary, 313
Renal cortex, 313, 314, 328
Renal ganglion, 319, 396
left, 321
right, 321

Renal impression, 277, 282
Renal medulla, 313, 314, 328
 efferent glomerular arteriole descending into, 314
Renal pelvis, 311, 329
Renal plexus, 302, 319, 390
 left, 321
 right, 297, 321
Renal segments
 arteries of, 312
 vascular, 312
Renal sinus, 311
 fat in, 311
 interlobar artery and vein in, 314
Renal vein, 311, 316, 380
 in situ, 310
 left, 232, 258, 308, 310, 317, 322, 329
 right, 232, 308, 310, 329
Renal vessels, 323, 381
Reproductive organs. See also specific reproductive
 organs
 female, innervation of, 395
 male, innervation of, 396
Rete testis, 370
Reticular nucleus, of thalamus, 110
Retina, 90
 ciliary part of, 87, 88, 89
 iridial part of, 88
 nonpigmented and pigmented regions of, 91
 optic part of, 87, 89
 projection on, 119
 structure of, 119
Retinacular artery, 492
 anterior, 482
 inferior, 492
 superior, 492
Retinacular foramen, 477
Retinaculum, inferior extensor, 528
Retinal arteriole
 inferior nasal, 90
 inferior temporal, 90
 superior nasal, 90
Retinal artery, 90
 central, 85, 87, 90, 91
Retinal vein, 90
 central, 87, 90, 91
Retinal venule
 inferior nasal, 90
 inferior temporal, 90
 superior nasal, 90
Retinal vessels, right, 90
Retrobulbar fat, 83
Retrocecal recess, 263, 273
Retromandibular vein, 3, 30, 31, 47, 59, 60, 61, 85
 anterior branch of, 31, 61, 70
 common trunk for, 59, 70
 posterior branch of, 31, 61, 70
Retroperitoneal artery, 266
 common, 266
 external, 266
Retroperitoneal portocaval anastomosis,
 292
Retropharyngeal space, 34, 60, 63, 65
Retroprostatic space, 376
Retropubic space, 245, 345, 348, 376
 fat in, 245, 341
Retropubic venous plexus, 383
Retropyloric lymph nodes, 293
Retrotonsillar fissure, 112
Retrotonsillar vein
 inferior, 142
 superior, 142
Retrouterine pouch (of Douglas), 342, 344
Retrovesical space, 376
Retzius, cave of, 323
Retzius, retropubic space of, 245, 345, 348, 376
 fat in, 245, 341
Rhinal sulcus, 105, 106
Rhomboid fossa, 113
Rhomboid major muscle, 168, 171, 174, 185, 236,
 238, 248, 411, 465

Rhomboid minor muscle, 168, 171, 411, 465
Rhomboid muscle, 237
Ribs, 180
 angle of, 179, 180
 axial CT image of, 235, 324
 body of, 179
 costal cartilage of, 236
 cross section of, 236, 237, 238, 265
 eighth, 179
 eleventh, 179
 projection of, 309
 false, 179
 fifth, 179
 first, 15, 21, 74, 157, 179, 186, 190, 191, 205, 224,
 225, 226, 406, 417, 418
 computed tomography of, 468
 groove for, 193
 left, superior view of, 80
 synchondrosis of, 406
 floating, 179
 fourth, 179
 head of, 179, 180
 articular facet of, 181
 articulation of, 180
 interarticular ligament of, 181
 radiate ligament of, 181
 middle, posterior view of, 180
 muscle origin and insertion sites on, 180
 neck of, 179, 180
 ninth, 179, 282
 second, 176, 179, 406
 computed tomography of, 468
 seventh, 151
 head of, 239
 neck of, 239
 sixth, 176, 179
 tenth, 179
 third, 179
 true, 179
 tubercle of, 179, 180
 twelfth, 157, 168, 179, 189, 241, 317
 projection of, 309
Ring finger, 400
 distal phalanx of, radiograph of, 445
Risorius muscle, 25, 122
Rod cells, 96
Rods, retinal, 119
Rolandic artery, 139, 140
Rolando, central sulcus of, 104
Root canal, 57
Rosenthal, basal vein of, 142
Rotator cuff
 anterior view of, 413
 muscles of, 413
 posterior view of, 413
 superior view of, 413
Rotatores cervicis muscle
 brevis, 170
 longus, 170
Rotatores thoracis muscle
 brevis, 170
 longus, 170
Round (cochlear) window, 14, 92, 95
 closed by secondary tympanic membrane, 96
 fossa of, 93, 94
Round ligament
 of liver, 223, 267, 277, 330
 paraumbilical veins n, 250
 of uterus, 315, 343, 352, 354, 369, 380, 384

S

Saccule, 92, 95, 96, 123
Sacral artery
 lateral, 164, 257, 316, 378, 382, 383
 median, 164, 257, 288, 316, 345, 378, 382
Sacral canal, 154, 340
Sacral cornu, 154
Sacral crest
 intermediate, 154

Sacral crest (Continued)
 lateral, 154
 median, 154, 337
Sacral curvature, 150
Sacral foramen, 153
 anterior, 154
 fourth posterior, 337
 margins of, radiograph of, 531
 posterior, 154, 335
 radiograph of, 333
Sacral ganglion, 160, 297
Sacral hiatus, 154
Sacral lymph nodes
 lateral, 259, 386, 388
 middle, 259, 388
Sacral nerve, 485, 487
Sacral plexus, 157, 390, 395, 396, 485, 487
 right, 302
Sacral promontory, 334, 336, 338, 342, 344
Sacral spinal cord, schema of, 303, 397
Sacral spinal nerves
 dorsal and ventral roots of, 163
 S1, 157, 390
 dorsal ramus of, 171
 relation to lumbar vertebrae, 158
 ventral ramus of, 394
 S2
 dorsal ramus of, 171
 relation to lumbar vertebrae, 158
 S3
 dorsal ramus of, 171
 relation to lumbar vertebrae, 158
 S4, relation to lumbar vertebrae, 158
 S5, 157
 S6, relation to lumbar vertebrae, 158
 S1-L5, schema of, 160
Sacral tuberosity, 154
Sacral vein
 lateral, 258
 median, 291, 374
Sacral vertebrae, radiographs of, 153
Sacral vessels, median, 344, 380, 383
Sacrococcygeal ligament
 anterior, 335, 338, 345
 lateral, 155, 335
 posterior, 155, 335
 deep, 335
 superficial, 335
Sacrogenital fold, 266, 347, 372
Sacroiliac joint, 334, 340
 radiograph of, 333, 531
Sacroiliac ligament
 anterior, 335
 posterior, 155, 335, 336
Sacrospinous ligament, 335, 336, 337, 339, 341, 390,
 483, 491
Sacrotuberous ligament, 155, 335, 336, 337, 339,
 341, 358, 376, 382, 390, 391, 393, 483, 490, 491
Sacrum, 149, 155, 157, 158, 332, 340
 ala of, 154
 radiograph of, 333
 anterior inferior view of, 154
 apex of, 154
 articular facet of, 152, 154
 articular process of, 154
 articular surface of, 155
 base of, 154
 dorsal surface of, 154
 lumbosacral articular surface of, 154
 median sacral crest of, 154
 median sagittal section of, 154
 MR sagittal images of, 377
 pelvic surface of, 154
 posterior superior view of, 154
 promontory of, 154
 radiograph of, 333
 S1-5
 anterior view of, 150
 left lateral view of, 150
 posterior view of, 150

Tendons. *See also specific tendons*
  of ankle, 515
  of foot, plantar view of, 516
Tendon sheaths, 449
  of ankle, 517
Tenon's capsule, 87
Tensor fasciae latae muscle, 398, 469, 480, 482, 488, 490, 491, 493, 531
  MRI of, 531
  origin of, 479, 480
  transverse section of, 399
Tensor tympani muscle, 45, 93, 94, 117
  tendon of, 93
Tensor tympani nerve, 45, 121
Tensor veli palatini muscle, 45, 64, 65, 68, 93, 117, 121
  nerve to, 71
  palatine aponeurosis from, 52
  tendon of, 52, 65
Tensor veli palatini nerve, 45
Tentorial artery, 103
Tentorium cerebelli, 86, 102, 103, 142, 143
Teres major muscle, 149, 168, 171, 174, 236, 237, 238, 407, 411, 412, 414, 415, 416, 417, 419, 420, 421, 423, 465
  lower margin of, 422
  MRI of, 468
  nerve to, 414
Teres major tendon, 420
Teres minor muscle, 168, 171, 236, 237, 411, 412, 413, 414, 415, 416, 420, 465
Teres minor tendon, 410, 413, 420
Testicular artery, 249, 257, 367, 383, 389, 396
  left (ovarian), 308, 310
  right (ovarian), 297, 310
Testicular plexus, 389, 396
  right, 297
Testicular vein, 258
  left, 308, 310
  right, 310
Testicular vessels, 247, 253, 255, 266, 315, 330, 347, 381
  covered by peritoneum, 254
  left (ovarian), 291
  lymphatic pathways along, 388
  in peritoneal fold, 347
  right (ovarian), 291
  in spermatic cord, 381
Testis, 323, 370, 396
  appendix of, 367, 369
  arteries and veins of, 381
  descent of, 366
  frontal section of, 370
  lobules of, 370
  mediastinum, rete testis in, 370
  MR sagittal images of, 377
  pathways from, 388
  schema of, 370
  spermatic fascia over, 385
  tunica albuginea of, 370
  tunica vaginalis of, 323, 367
Thalamic veins, posterior, 144
Thalamogeniculate artery, 141
Thalamoperforating artery, 138, 141
Thalamostriate vein
  inferior, 142, 144
  posterior, 144
  superior, 99, 110, 143, 144
Thalamotuberal artery, 138
Thalami, 111
Thalamus, 105, 107, 109, 110, 111, 145, 303
  left, 142
  nuclei of, 110
  posterolateral view of, 113
  pulvinar of, 106, 113, 114, 137, 143
  schema of, 110
  stria medullaris of, 105
  in third ventricle, 114
  ventral posteromedial nucleus of, 134
Thenar eminence, 400
Thenar muscle, 447, 448

Thenar muscle *(Continued)*
  abductor pollicis brevis, 463
  innervation of, 464
  nerves to, 448, 453
  opponens pollicis, 463
  superficial head of flexor pollicis brevis, 463
Thenar space, 450, 451
  septal separation of, 448
  septum between, 450
Thigh
  arteries of
    anterior view of, 488, 489
    posterior view of, 490
    schema of, 500
  bony attachments of
    anterior view of, 478
    posterior view of, 479
  cutaneous innervation of, 527, 528
  deep dissection of, 489, 490
  fascia lata of, 357
  intermuscular septa of, 493
  muscles of
    anterior view of, 480, 481
    lateral view of, 482
    posterior view of, 483
  nerves of, 526
    posterior, 528
  serial cross section of, 493
  veins of
    anterior view of, 488, 489
    posterior view of, 490
Thoracic aortic plexus, 203
Thoracic artery
  internal, 75, 136, 177, 183, 184, 185, 192, 200, 205, 206, 210, 226, 231, 239, 249, 415
    anterior intercostal branches of, 183
    cross-section of, 237, 238
    left, 187, 225
    medial mammary branches of, 177
    perforating branches of, 177, 182, 184, 185
    perforating branch of, 414
    right, 187, 224
  lateral, 177, 182, 183, 414, 415, 417, 422
  left, 75, 188
  superior, 183, 414, 415, 417
Thoracic cardiac nerve, 187
Thoracic constriction, 227
Thoracic duct, 72, 183, 188, 192, 200, 202, 203, 205, 210, 225, 226, 232, 233, 236, 237, 238, 239, 259, 295, 297, 327
  lumbar lymph nodes to, 318
  transverse section of, 325
Thoracic ganglion
  first, 160
  sixth, right, 300
Thoracic muscle
  transverse, 210
  transversus, 174
Thoracic nerve
  dorsal ramus of
    lateral branch of, 185
    medial branch of, 185
  long, 182, 184, 251, 414, 417, 418
Thoracic spinal cord
  anteroposterior view of, 165
  schema of, 132, 204
Thoracic spinal nerves, 133, 160
  dorsal root of, 132, 133, 163
  origin of, 163
  relation to thoracic vertebrae, 158
  roots of, filaments of, 157
  T1, 131, 132, 133, 157
    relation to thoracic vertebrae, 158
  T2, 132, 133
    relation to thoracic vertebrae, 158
  T3, relation to thoracic vertebrae, 158
  T4, relation to thoracic vertebrae, 158
  T5, relation to thoracic vertebrae, 158
  T6, relation to thoracic vertebrae, 158

Thoracic spinal nerves *(Continued)*
  T7
    dorsal rami of, 171
      lateral cutaneous branch of, 248
      medial cutaneous branch of, 248
    relation to thoracic vertebrae, 158
    ventral rami of, 394
  T8
    dorsal rami of, 171
    relation to thoracic vertebrae, 158
  T9
    dorsal rami of, 171
    relation to thoracic vertebrae, 158
  T10
    dorsal rami of, 171
    relation to thoracic vertebrae, 158
    ventral rami of, 390
  T11
    dorsal rami of, 171
    relation to thoracic vertebrae, 158
    ventral rami of, 394
  T12, 157
    dorsal rami of, 171
    relation to thoracic vertebrae, 158
    ventral rami of, 248
  T1-T12, schema of, 160
  typical, 174
  ventral rami of, 185
  ventral root of, 132, 133, 163
Thoracic sympathetic cardiac nerves, 129
Thoracic sympathetic ganglion
  fourth, 220
  third, 220
Thoracic vein
  internal, 183, 184, 186, 206, 210, 239, 250
    cross-section of, 237, 238
    perforating branches of, 184
    perforating tributaries to, 250
  lateral, 250
  left, 75, 188
  right internal, 188
Thoracic vertebrae, 151
  cross action through, 163
  posterior view of, 150
  radiographs of, 153
  T1, 15, 22, 157
    spinous process of, 191
  T2, body of, 468
  T3
    body of, 236
    lower levels, transverse section of, 236
    transverse cross-section of, 236, 237
  T6
    lateral view of, 151
    superior view of, 151
  T7
    body of, 239
    posterior view of, 151
    spinous process of, 151
  T8, 210
    posterior view of, 151
  T9, posterior view of, 151
  T10, body of, 325
  T12, 157
    anterior view of, 150
    body of, 327
    lateral view of, 151, 153
    left lateral view of, 150
    posterior view of, 150
    radiograph of, 153
    spinous process of, 149, 168, 169, 171, 411
Thoracic vertebral body, fourth, 224
Thoracic wall
  anterior, 182, 183
    internal view of, 184
  internal, veins of, 186
Thoracis muscle, transverse, 183, 184, 185
Thoracoabdominal nerve, 252
  cutaneous branches of, 182

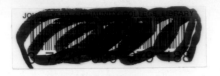